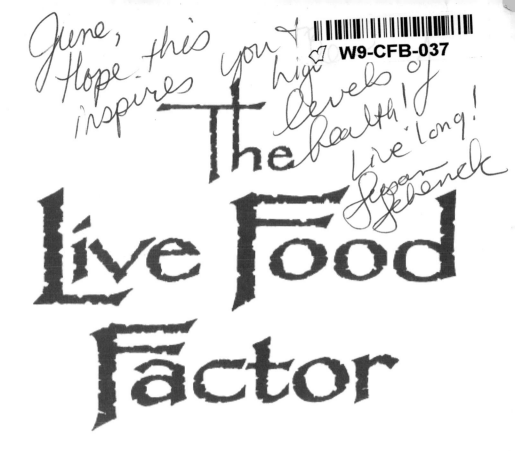

# The Live Food Factor

## THE COMPREHENSIVE GUIDE TO THE ULTIMATE DIET FOR BODY, MIND, SPIRIT & PLANET

### EXPANDED, REVISED & UPDATED

**SUSAN SCHENCK, LAc, MTOM**

**WITH VICTORIA BIDWELL, PhD, EdD**

*Forewords by*
*Dr. V. Vetrano, DC, hMD, PhD, DSci, and Victoria Boutenko*

*June, Hope this inspires you to high levels of health! Live long! Susan Schenck*

**Disclaimer**

The purpose of this book is to dispense information. It is sold for informational purposes only. The publisher, author and all others associated with the production and distribution of this book cannot be responsible for your health or how you apply the information herein to your personal life. As this book teaches, only you can be responsible for your health. This book is not intended for use as medical diagnosis or treatment.

Because there is always some risk involved when the body eliminates toxins when switching to a more healthful lifestyle and diet, the publisher, author and others associated with the production and distribution of this book are not responsible for any consequences resulting from the use of any recipes provided, suggestions given or procedures described herein.

Printed in the USA

Second Edition, 2008
First Edition, 2006

Independent Publisher award winner for Most Progressive Health Book of 2007

Published by:
Awakenings Publications
P. O. Box 712423
San Diego, CA 92171-2423

Back cover photographer: Joseph Peiri (j-pieri@sbcglobal.net)
Cover design: Bob Avery (bobavery@umich.edu)
    with logo by Gabriel Spatuzzi (gabecross84@gmail.com)

Chief Editor and Production Manager: Bob Avery
Assistant Editors: Victoria BidWell and Jacqueline Nash
Chief Editors for Natural Hygiene science:
    Victoria BidWell and Dr. Vivian V. Vetrano
Raw Diet Consultant: Bob Avery

ISBN 978-0-9776795-1-5

Nutrition/Diet        Health        Weight Loss        Beauty

*To Dad,*
*whose love of healing*
*inspired me...*
*You always said*
*I'd make a great lawyer;*
*I rest my case with this book.*

# Table of Contents

Foreword by Dr. Vivian V. Vetrano..........................................................xxiii
Foreword by Victoria Boutenko...............................................................xxix
Acknowledgments .....................................................................................xxxi
    A Special Acknowledgment for Our Chief Editor...........................xxxii
    A Special Acknowledgment for Victoria BidWell .......................xxxiii
Preface ..................................................................................................... xxxv
    Why does this book have two forewords? ...............................xxxvii
    Victoria BidWell's Preface .........................................................xxxviii
Introduction .................................................................................................xli

## Section One — Raw Power: Reasons to Go Raw

## 1 Ten Reasons to Stop Cooking .......................... 3

  1. Super Health .....................................................................................5
  2. Mental Ability and Mental Health .................................................7
  3. Optimal Weight and Beauty ..........................................................9
  4. Emotional Balance and Happiness.............................................12
  5. Spiritual Growth .............................................................................13
  6. Economy .........................................................................................17
  7. Pleasure ...........................................................................................18
  8. Ecology............................................................................................18
  9. Free Time .........................................................................................20
 10. Longevity.........................................................................................20

## 2 Rah, Rah, Raw! Raw Diet Testimonials...................... 23

"Raquel": No More Cancer, Diabetes, Asthma, Infertility, Eczema
  and Obesity! ........................................................................................23
Jessica: Her Baby Made Her Eat Raw! .................................................24
Marie Tadič: "I've Got Energy for Sale!" ...............................................25
Jenny Smith: Recovered from Twenty Years of Sleepwalking and
  Obesity ................................................................................................27
Al: Live Food for Bodybuilding and Higher Consciousness....................32

Dana Pettaway: Increased Awareness and Freedom from Vices ........ 34
Tim Tye, "The Raw Food Guy": An Awakening of the Mind and
    Creativity ................................................................................................ 37
Annette Larkins: Super Health at 63 .......................................................... 40
Mike McCright: Raw for Life ......................................................................... 43
Amy Schrift: Total Life Makeover ............................................................... 46
Sandra Schrift: Young at 68 .......................................................................... 48
Jackie Nash: Lost 45 Pounds and Became Active at 69 ...................... 50
Paula Wood: Thyroid Removal No Longer Needed ............................... 53
Samara Christy: Lost Weight, yet No Surgery Needed for Loose Skin .... 56
Angela Stokes: From Morbid Obesity to a New Life with Raw Foods .... 59
The Boutenkos: Raw Family ........................................................................ 62
Dr. David Klein, PhD: Healing Ulcerative Colitis .................................... 66
Ric Lambart: 32 Years Raw ........................................................................... 69
Dr. Vetrano, hMD, DC, PhD, DSci, and Natural Hygiene .................... 74
More Testimony… ........................................................................................... 78

# 3 Radically Raw: My Story .. 81

# Section Two — Raw Proof: The Science

# 4 A Paradigm Shift in How We View Disease and Health ........................ 97

The Two Paradigms: Conventional and Alternative .............................. 100
The Medical Model's Four Schools of Thought ...................................... 101
    Disease as a Mystery ............................................................................. 101
    Disease as Wear and Tear .................................................................... 102
    Disease as Genetic/Congenital .......................................................... 102
    Disease as Germ Inspired ..................................................................... 103
The Health by Healthful Living Model ..................................................... 104
    Crucial Alternative Terms ...................................................................... 105
The Ten Energy Enhancers: The Conditions for Health ....................... 107
The Ten Energy Robbers: The Secondary Causes of Disease ............. 108
    The Ten Energy Robbers Are the Addictors ...................................... 108
Endogenous Toxins: Bodily Generated Sources of Toxemia .............. 109
Exogenous Toxins: External Sources of Toxemia ................................. 109
Live Food — It's All about Energy! ............................................................ 110

## Table of Contents

Live Food: Our Biggest Energy Conserver................................110
Acute versus Chronic Disease ............................................111
How Acute Disease Evolves into Chronic Disease ............111
Six Ways Acute and Chronic Disease Differ.....................111
Health by Healthful Living Gets the Best Results!...................113
Your Highest Health Potential .........................................113
The Health by Healthful Living Model: One Disease, One Healing
Process ....................................................................114
Even Deficiency Diseases Can Stem from Toxemia ................115
The Politics of Poisoning People...........................................116
When Certain Cooked Foods May Be Absolutely Necessary.....119
In Deference to the Good Doctors and Their Personnel...........120
Coming Up… ...................................................................121

# 5 Bacteria and Viruses: Not Guilty as Charged!... 123

# 6 Do Drugs Work? ............. 129

Taking Drugs: It's a Black-or-White Thing................................130
The Palliation Effect of Drugs — Exposed!.............................131
The Mimicking Effect of Drugs — Exposed!...........................133
Drugs Don't Work! ............................................................134

# 7 The Simplicity of Disease Origin and Health Care... 137

So, with This Good News, Why Do Most of Us Cling So Defensively
to the Medical Model? ....................................................140
Let Food Be Thy Medicine —Hippocrates, Founder of Modern
Medicine, 400 BC ............................................................144

# 8 Cooked vs. Raw Diet Experiments and Research ........................ 147

1. Dr. Otto Louis Moritz Abramowski and His Hospital Patients...........149
2. Dr. Werner Kollath's Study Animals Thrived on a Raw Diet............149
3. Athletic Performance Improved on Raw Diet................................150
4. Dr. Edmond Szekely's 33-Year Study .....................................150

# Table of Contents

5. Dr. Francis Pottenger's Cat Study: Dietary Factors in Degenerative Disease ........................................................... 151
6. Dr. Edward Howell's Enzyme Research............................... 153
7. Calves Die on Pasteurized Milk! ........................................ 154
8. The Prisoner of War Diet Is Better Raw............................. 154
9. Lewis Cook's and Junko Yasui's Rats ................................. 154
10. Stamina, Blood Pressure and Balance Improved on Fruitarian Diet ................................................................... 155
11. Lipid Profiles and Glucose Tolerances Improved on Fruitarian Diet ................................................................... 156
12. Dr. Max Gerson: Cancer Reversals during Thirty Years of Raw Diet Clinical Practice............................................ 156
13. Mice More Peaceful on Their Natural Diet ....................... 156
14. Dr. John Douglass: Alcohol and Nicotine Addiction Reduced on Raw Diet................................................... 157
15. Sir Robert McCarrison's Monkeys: Cooked Diet Results in Colitis and Ulcers ........................................................ 157
16. Guinea Pigs Developed Several Disease Conditions on Cooked Diet................................................................ 157
17. Dr. John Douglass: Hypertension and Obesity Reduced on Raw Diet................................................................. 158
18. Energy and Endurance Increased in Mice on Raw Diet .............. 158
19. Body's Defenses Boosted on Raw Diet ............................ 158
20. Colon Cancer Risk Lowered on Raw Diet .......................... 158
21. Nutrient Status and Weight Control in Rheumatoid Arthritis Improved on Raw Diet ................................................ 159
22. Lung Cancer Risk Reduced on Raw Food ......................... 159
23. Raw Diet Is Best Vegetarian Diet for Mice........................ 160
24. Dr. Robinson's Live Food Cancer Therapy ........................ 160
25. Fibromyalgia Symptoms Reduced on Raw Diet ................ 161
26. Cancer Risk Reduced on Raw Vegetables ........................ 162
27. Blood Lipid Improvement Found on Mostly Vegetarian Diet........ 162
28. Rheumatoid Arthritis Symptoms Reduced on Raw Diet........... 162
29. Favorable Weight Loss and Amenorrhea Effects Noted on Raw Diet................................................................. 163
30. Antioxidant Status Improved on Raw Diet ........................ 163
31. Raw Diet Benefits Shown in Just One Week...................... 164
32. Pain and Joint Stiffness Decreased on Raw Vegan Diet .............. 164
33. Fibromyalgia Sufferers at Hallelujah Acres Improved on Mostly Raw Diet ........................................................ 164
34. A Largely Vegetarian Diet and Reduced Risk of Colon and Heart Diseases ...................................................... 165
35. Mostly Raw Diet and Improved Quality of Life ................. 165
36. Raw Diet Fuels Intelligence Increase ............................... 165
37. Dr. Jean Seignalet's Hospital Study: Raw Diet Yields High Patient Success Rate .................................................. 165

38.   Preadolescent Children Thrive on Live Food Diets ........................166
39.   Cancer Risk Reduced More with Raw than Cooked
      Vegetables ..................................................................................167
40.   The Roseburg Study: Sex Life, Stomach Acid and More
      Improved on Raw Diet ................................................................167
41.   Gastric Cancer Risk Reduced on Raw Diet ..............................167
42.   LDL Cholesterol and Triglyceride Levels Found Favorable
      on Long-Term Raw Diet .............................................................167
43.   Cancer Risk Reduced on Raw Cabbage ...................................168
44.   Bone Mass in Long-Term Raw Fooders .....................................168
45.   Dr. Cousens: Diabetics Improve on Raw Diet ...........................169
46.   Cancer Markers Improved on Raw Diet .....................................170
47.   Cholesterol and High Blood Pressure Reduced on Raw Diet ........170
Additional Studies in Appendix D .......................................................171
An Ongoing European Study of Cooked Foods ................................171
Numerous Individual Case Studies .....................................................171
The Most Important and Convincing Experiment of All........................172

# 9 Man's Fatal Chemistry Lab: The Great Cooked Food Experiment ...................... 173

Is Cooked Food Toxic? .......................................................................174
What Happens to the Macronutrients in Cooked Food? ......................177
      What Macronutrients Are .........................................................177
      What Cooking Does to the Macronutrients .............................179
Toxic Cookware ................................................................................183
Is Cooked Food Addictive? ...............................................................183

# 10 The Raw Ingredients ....... 187

Vitamins and Minerals ........................................................................187
Enzymes ............................................................................................188
Phytochemicals..................................................................................191
Biophotons: Light Energy from the Sun ..............................................192
Electrons ...........................................................................................192
Bioelectricity .....................................................................................193
Hormones ..........................................................................................195
Water ................................................................................................195
Essential Fatty Acids...........................................................................195
Friendly Bacteria ...............................................................................196
Oxygen .............................................................................................196
Life Force Energy ...............................................................................197
Suggested Reading............................................................................197

Coming Up… ............................................................................ 197

# Section Three — Raw Pioneers: History and Leaders

# 11 A Brief History of Raw Foodism .......................... 201

# 12 Modern-Day Leaders of Raw Foodism ............. 211

Elizabeth Baker: Active and Consulting in Her 90s ................................. 211
The Boutenko Family: Healed of Four "Incurable" Diseases................. 211
Brian Clement and the Hippocrates Health Institute .......................... 213
Lou Corona .................................................................................. 213
Dr. Gabriel Cousens, MD: Seeking the Optimal Diet for Spiritual
   Growth .................................................................................. 213
Roe Gallo: Allergic to the 20th Century ...................................... 214
Dr. Douglas Graham and Training Athletes ................................. 215
David Jubb, PhD: Living on Little Food ...................................... 216
David Klein, PhD, and Vibrance Magazine .................................. 217
Rev. George Malkmus: Why Christians Get Sick............................ 218
David Wolfe, Stephen Arlin and Fouad Dini: Nature's First Law........... 219
Paul Nison: Healing Crohn's Disease ............................................ 220
Dr. David J. Scott, DC, and Natural Hygiene................................. 220
Dr. Vivian Virginia Vetrano and Natural Hygiene ......................... 221
Many Others................................................................................ 222
Let's Go!...................................................................................... 223

# Section Four — Raw Passage: Your Journey to Raw Life

# 13 Getting Started ................. 227

The Decision ............................................................................ 227

Methods of Transitioning ..................................................................228
   Transitioning One Meal at a Time ...........................................228
   Food Elimination Transition .....................................................229
   Reduced Temperature and Heating Time Transition................229
   Instantaneous (Cold Turkey) Transition....................................230
   Fasting Followed by Instantaneous Transition .........................230
   Green Smoothie Transition .....................................................230
   Just Get Started! ....................................................................231
Invest Time in Food Preparation during the First Months...............231
(Un)Cookbooks ..........................................................................232
Educate Yourself .........................................................................234
Always Focus on the Positive! ......................................................235
Kitchen Gadgets..........................................................................235
Meal and Snack Planning ...........................................................238
Stand Firm in Your Commitment!..................................................239
Foods to Stockpile.......................................................................240
Techniques for Getting Off Cooked Foods and in Touch with
   Genuine Hunger....................................................................244

# 14 Detoxification and Healing............ 247

The Fatigue Factor.......................................................................250
Possible Detoxification Symptoms ................................................251
Are Enemas and Colonics Useful? ...............................................259
Eating Less and Enjoying More ....................................................264
The Detoxified and Purified Body, Mind and Spirit .......................265
Detoxifying Your Environment ......................................................266
Overcoming Cravings for Cooked Foods......................................266

# 15 The Fasting Factor......... 271

Fasting on Water Only versus Juice Dieting....................................272
Fasting and Freedom from Addictions...........................................274
Spiritual Benefits of Fasting ..........................................................275
Fasting and Mental Health ...........................................................277
The Natural Hygiene Fast..............................................................277
   *Fasting* and *Starvation* — Defined...........................................279
   What the Natural Hygiene Fast Is and Is Not............................280
   The Five Kinds of Rest Taken on the Natural Hygiene Fast............281
   The Natural Hygiene Fast versus the Juice Diet ........................282
   How to Break the Natural Hygiene Fast ..................................284
   Questionable Candidates for the Natural Hygiene Fast............285
Natural Hygiene Fasting Case Studies...........................................286
   Kidney Stones Passed............................................................287

Cataracts Gone ..................................................................... 287
Woman Finally Carried a Fetus to Full Term ....................... 287
Insanity Reversed ................................................................ 288
Parkinson's Tremor Gone after Several Fasts ...................... 288
Deafness, Impotence, Enlarged Prostate and Sinus Congestion
   Gone ................................................................................ 288
Ankylosing Spondylitis Healed ........................................... 289
Baby Healed from Whooping Cough ................................ 289
Extreme Emaciation Resolved via Fasting! ......................... 290
Further Fasting Cautions ......................................................... 290
The Details of Drug Withdrawal ........................................ 290
Fasting for a Heart Attack — A True Story ............................... 291
Our Final Fasting Farewells ..................................................... 294

# 16 How to Stay Raw in a Cooked World ............... 295

Staying Raw in Social Situations .............................................. 295
Eating Out ............................................................................. 297
Traveling ................................................................................ 298
How to Avoid Backsliding ...................................................... 299
Enhanced Sensitivity to Cooked Foods ................................. 301
The Glorious World beyond Temptation! ................................ 302
Paradise Health ..................................................................... 303

# 17 Nutritional Controversies ................... 307

Vegetarianism vs. Meat Eating ............................................... 307
Design/Nature Considerations ............................................ 307
Health Considerations ......................................................... 308
Spiritual Considerations ...................................................... 309
Ecological Considerations .................................................. 310
Vegans and the Vitamin $B_{12}$ Issue ..................................... 311
Restrict Your Calories for Longer Life ...................................... 315
Food Combining .................................................................... 317
Nuts and Seeds: Hard to Digest? .......................................... 318
Organic Food: Is It Really Necessary? .................................... 319
Nutritional Value ................................................................. 319
Toxins in Commercial Produce .......................................... 320
Genetically Modified Organisms (GMOs) .......................... 322
Organic Foods Even Taste Better ...................................... 324
In a Pinch... ......................................................................... 324
And a Final Warning... ......................................................... 325

Nuking Our Food by Irradiation .....................................................325
High vs. Low Glycemic Index Food.............................................327
Hybrid vs. Wild Produce ..............................................................328
The Acid/Alkaline Balance ...........................................................331
Drinking Water...............................................................................332
Controversial Foods and Seasonings.........................................336
Eating Foods in Season ................................................................337
Supplements and Super Foods....................................................338
Fiber: How Much Is Necessary? ................................................340
The Proper Dietary Proportions of Carbohydrates, Fats and Proteins ..342
  Dr. Graham's 80/10/10 Diet ......................................................343
Dr. Vetrano's "Genuine Fruitarianism — Eat Your Veggies, Nuts and
  Seeds, Too!"................................................................................346
  A Case History of Protein Deficiency.....................................350
  The Protein Needs of the Body ..............................................352
  The Digestion of Nuts and Seeds...........................................352
It's Up to You to Decide!..............................................................354

# 18 Common Pitfalls to Avoid.............................. 355

Assuming a Food Is Raw When It Isn't — Although It May Be
  Labeled "Raw" ..........................................................................355
Judging the Diet before You Give It a Chance.........................357
Overeating Fruit or Not Brushing after Acid or Dehydrated Fruit ..........359
Overeating Nuts, Seeds and Dehydrated Fruits........................361
Not Getting Sufficient Protein ....................................................362
Eating Too Much Fat.....................................................................362
Overeating and Undersleeping....................................................363
Succumbing to Social Pressure...................................................364
Trying to Gain Weight with Raw Foods Only and No Weight
  Training Whatsoever .................................................................364
  The GetWell Weight-Gain System ..........................................364
Buying and/or Preparing Too Much Food ................................366
Not Eating Enough Greens...........................................................366
Failing to Study the Raw Food Diet ..........................................366
Failing to Plan Ahead...................................................................366
Neglecting Other Areas of Health .............................................367

# 19 Frequently Asked Questions ...... 369

Isn't a raw food diet boring? ...... 369

If we've been eating cooked food throughout history, what's the big deal? ...... 370

Can't I just eat cooked foods with vitamin, mineral and enzyme supplements? ...... 373

What if I lose too much weight or muscle strength? ...... 375

I've been on the diet awhile, but still haven't lost as much weight as I would like. What can I do? ...... 375

Can't I just go on a diet of 50-95% raw food? ...... 378

How do you get enough protein? ...... 381

Won't I miss my comfort foods? ...... 383

What about my family? How can I ever get my family to eat my raw food dishes? ...... 384

Does my pet need to eat raw? If so, how can I get my pet to eat raw food? ...... 386

Aren't you hungry all the time? ...... 387

If this diet is so great and healing, why doesn't my doctor know about it? Why isn't it all over the news? ...... 388

Don't you miss eating something warm? ...... 391

Shouldn't I wait until the summer, or at least spring, to begin eating raw? Won't I be too cold eating raw in the winter? ...... 391

Why does cooked food seem to taste better? ...... 394

Doesn't cooking result in better digestion and allow for better absorption of certain nutrients? ...... 395

I have bowel problems. Can I do this diet? ...... 397

What if I just *have to* eat some cooked foods? Which ones are the least bad? ...... 397

If raw food isn't available, isn't it better to eat cooked food than to eat no food? ...... 398

Isn't there a danger of bacteria in raw food? ...... 398

Does this diet cost more money? ...... 399

Can I drink alcohol? ...... 400

Can I drink tea or coffee? ...... 400

Can I eat frozen foods? ...... 402

What do *you* eat? ...... 402

Why should I go on a raw diet if I am young and healthy? ...... 404

# 20 Raising Live Food Children ....................... 405

Can I start this diet while pregnant? .......................................405
Is it advisable for a lactating mother to go raw? ...................407
Is this diet healthful for my kid? ...........................................407
The ABCDs of Feeding Mothers, Infants and Children Hygienically .....408
    A: Feeding Mothers, Infants and Children Hygienically ...................409
    B: How to Make the Live Food Diet Fun for Kids! .............413
    C: How to Make the Other Nine Energy Enhancers Fun for Kids! ....415
    D: How to De-brand and De-drug Your Kids! ......................417

# 21 Raw Pleasure ................... 419

Victoria BidWell's Secret Touches for Perfectly Prepared, Hygienic,
    All-Raw Recipes! .............................................................421
Soups...................................................................................423
    Everybody's Favorite Celery-Cilantro Soup........................423
    Creamy Carrot Soup .......................................................424
    Cream of Tomato Soup ....................................................424
    Cream of Celery Soup .....................................................424
    Vegetable Chowder.........................................................425
    Cream of Spinach Soup ...................................................425
    Corn Chowder ................................................................425
    Creamy Cauliflower Soup ................................................426
    Lorenzo's Tomato-Avocado Soup ....................................426
Entrées .................................................................................427
    Spaghetti........................................................................427
    Nori Rolls ........................................................................427
    Chinese Stir "Fry"............................................................428
    Tomato Raviolis ..............................................................428
    Buddy and Cherrie's Barbecue "Chicken" Nuggets.........429
    Burritos ..........................................................................429
    Beet Burgers...................................................................430
    Raw Pizza .......................................................................430
Desserts................................................................................431
    Raw Cake .......................................................................431
    Raw Candy.....................................................................431
    Carob Cream..................................................................432
    Peanut Butter & Carob Cups...........................................432
    Ice Cream.......................................................................432
    Frozen Fruit Ice Cream ....................................................433
    "Pumpkin Pie" Pudding ..................................................433
    Carrot Almond Cookies ..................................................433

# Table of Contents

Peppermint Patties ....................................................................... 433
Buddy and Cherrie's Carob Nut Taffy ....................................... 434
Sandy's Apple Pie in Ten Minutes ............................................ 434
Buddy and Cherrie's Cashew Ice Cream .................................. 435
Frozen Persimmon Pudding ....................................................... 435
Beverages ...................................................................................... 436
Seed Milk ...................................................................................... 436
Nut Milk ....................................................................................... 436
Banana Milk Shake ..................................................................... 436
Smoothie ...................................................................................... 436
Carob Mint Soda ......................................................................... 437
Super Smoothie ........................................................................... 437
Pineapple Spinach Drink ............................................................ 437
Strawberry Shake ........................................................................ 437
Green Drink .................................................................................. 438
Beverages from *The Health Seekers' BeverageBook* Manuscript
(Upcoming Book) ........................................................................ 438
The Waldorf Classic ..................................................................... 438
The Sweet Waldorf Classic ......................................................... 438
The Barely Sweet Waldorf Classic ............................................. 439
The Pear Waldorf ......................................................................... 439
The Nutty Waldorf Variations ..................................................... 439
The Pineapple Slushy .................................................................. 439
The Sweetest Tomato Beverage ................................................ 439
The Mellowed-Out Grape — Choice 1 ...................................... 439
The Mellowed-Out Grape — Choice 2 ...................................... 439
The Mellowed-Out Grape — Choice 3 ...................................... 440
Dr. Scott's Refreshment .............................................................. 440
The Hygienic Retreat Traditional Trio ....................................... 440
Mango, Go! Go! Go! .................................................................... 440
Nutty Mango, Go! Go! Go! ......................................................... 440
Ginger Mango, Go! Go! Go! ....................................................... 440
Ginger Nutty Mango, Go! Go! Go! ............................................ 441
Chunky Mexican Salsa — In a Glass! ........................................ 441
Mexican Salsa In a Glass — Variation 1 .................................... 441
Mexican Salsa In a Glass — Variation 2 .................................... 441
Mexican Salsa In a Glass — Variation 3 .................................... 441
Banana Cream Pie In a Glass ..................................................... 441
Veggie Smoothie ......................................................................... 442
Plumb Yummy Smoothie ............................................................ 442
The Ginger-Mint Pear Smoothie ................................................ 442
Golden Delicious Smoothie ........................................................ 442
Banana Nutnog ........................................................................... 443
Sauces, Dressings, Condiments ................................................ 443
Tahini Sauce ................................................................................ 443
"Thousand Island" Salad Dressing ............................................ 443

Honey Mustard Dressing ............................................444
Oil and Vinegar.......................................................444
Curry Spinach Dressing ............................................444
Raw Mustard ..........................................................444
Tomato Sauce.........................................................445
Parmesan Cheese ...................................................445
Natural Hygiene Salad Dressings, Sauces and Dips ........445
Cashew Tang .........................................................446
Tart Cashew Crème .................................................446
Cashew V-4 Crème .................................................446
Apple-Sweet Cashew Crème ....................................446
Almond Tang..........................................................446
Almond V-2 ...........................................................446
GetWell's Waldorf Special Sauce ..............................446
Tomato-Pecan Dip ..................................................446
Sunny Tomato Topping ............................................446
Piña-Tahini ............................................................446
Taste of Brazil ........................................................447
Hawaiian Dream.....................................................447
Tomacado .............................................................447
Applecado .............................................................447
Avocado Special.....................................................447
Avobutter...............................................................447
GetWell Guacamole ...............................................447
Dieter's Delight Sauce .............................................447
Fig Ambrosia..........................................................447
Fruit Fixin's Sauce ...................................................448
Old-fashioned Apple Sauce ......................................448
Mexican Salsa ........................................................448
GetWell's Fruit Jam Formula .....................................448
Victoria BidWell's Nut and Seed Butter Secrets ............448
Victoria BidWell's Favorite Recipe: Traditional Cranberry Relish ......449
Appetizers and Dips.....................................................449
Raw Hummus..........................................................449
Nori Rolls ...............................................................449
Creamy Spinach Dip................................................449
Deluxe Macadamia Nut Cheese................................450
Pecan Pesto ...........................................................450
Pumpkin Seed and Macadamia Nut Cheese ...............450
Guacamole ............................................................451
Sunflower Seed Pâté ...............................................451
Salads and Salad Trimmings..........................................451
Arabian Salad ........................................................451
Cheesy Spinach Salad.............................................452
Waldorf Salad.........................................................452
Coleslaw ...............................................................452

Holiday Salad ........................................................ 453
T. C. Fry's Super Salad .......................................... 453
Marinated Kale .................................................... 453
Arame Salad......................................................... 454
Dill Coleslaw........................................................ 454
Greek Salad ......................................................... 455
Pecan Croutons .................................................... 455
Salad Sprinkles .................................................... 455
Buddy and Cherrie's Mock Potato Salad ................ 455
Snacks ...................................................................... 456
Cauliflower Pâté ("Mashed Potatoes").................. 456
Garlic Cilantro Flax Crackers................................. 457
Barbecue Flax Chips............................................. 457
Breakfast Dishes ....................................................... 458
Al's Cereal........................................................... 458
Trail Mix .............................................................. 458
Sample Menus for One Week ..................................... 459
Day 1 .................................................................. 459
Day 2 .................................................................. 460
Day 3 .................................................................. 460
Day 4 .................................................................. 460
Day 5 .................................................................. 461
Day 6 .................................................................. 461
Day 7 .................................................................. 461
Sample Seasonal Hygienic Menus .............................. 462
Veggie Volt! Tomato Bolt! Ginger Jolt! Instead Of Coffee!.............. 464

# Appendix A: Killer "Foods" to Avoid ............ 465

The Four White Evils: Wheat, Dairy, Sugar and Salt ................................. 468
Grains, but Especially Wheat! ............................................................. 468
Dairy ................................................................................................ 471
Table Salt.......................................................................................... 474
Refined Sugar ................................................................................... 476
Excitotoxins........................................................................................... 477
Soy ........................................................................................................ 479
The Corruption of Our Food Supply through Processing,
Refining and Preserving................................................................... 480

# Appendix B: The Drug Story ................ 485

# Appendix C: Radical Branches of the Raw Food Movement ............... 503

The Green Smoothie Diet ........................................................503
Nonvegan Branches ...............................................................505
    Beyond Raw Food: Guy-Claude Burger and Instinctive Eating .......506
    Aajonus Vonderplanitz and the Raw Animal Food Diet ...................511
Issues with Raw Meat, Dairy and Eggs.....................................514
Meat: To Eat or Not to Eat .....................................................518

# Appendix D: Studies from Scientific Journals.......... 523

If You Want More Studies… ....................................................528

# Appendix E: End Cooked Food Habits via Behavior Modification ..................... 529

The Addiction Syndrome at Its Very Worst ...............................529
Self-Correction Strategies for Cooked Food Eating or Overeating ......531
Mind/Body Connection Exercises for Ending Food Addictions ............535

# Appendix F: Natural Hygiene and the Nondietary Health Factors................. 541

The Medical Mentality at Its Very Worst ...................................542
Natural Hygiene at Its Very Best .............................................543
*Nerve Energy* — A Formal Definition........................................544
    How to Restore Your Nerve Energy!......................................545
    Nerve Energy Is Not Plain, Old "Energy"! ...............................545
Dr. Vetrano with Victoria on the Priceless Benefits of Adequate
    Rest and Sleep .................................................................545
    The Two Primary Needs of Sleep ........................................546
    Miseries of Sleep Deprivation..............................................546

The Lifesaving Benefits of Sleep .............................................. 546
Recuperation and Recovery Come from Rest and Sleep!............. 547
Dr. J. H. Tilden: The Seven Stages of Disease ........................... 547
The Seven Stages of Disease.............................................. 548
The Natural, Physiological Laws of Life .................................... 549
T. C. Fry's Twenty-Two Health Essentials ................................. 553
Overcome Ailments and Achieve Health: Establishing the
Essentials of Health.............................................. 553
The Food Combining Rules — Summarized ............................... 555
Classification of Foods for Food Combining Rules....................... 556

# Appendix G: How to Get Strict with the Ten Energy Enhancers ....................... 559

# Bibliography ........................ 563

General Bibliography................................................................ 563
Recipe Book Bibliography........................................................ 575

# Resource Guide.................... 579

Related Web Sites ................................................................. 579
Raw Food Chat Groups ......................................................... 586
Resources for Food and Kitchen Supplies ............................... 587
Resources for Healing and Fasting Supervision ....................... 592
Raw Food Events ................................................................. 598
Raw Restaurants................................................................... 599
United States....................................................................... 599
Alaska ........................................................................... 599
Arizona .......................................................................... 599
California........................................................................ 600
Colorado........................................................................ 605
Connecticut .................................................................... 605
District of Columbia .......................................................... 605
Florida ........................................................................... 605
Georgia ......................................................................... 606
Hawaii ........................................................................... 607
Idaho ............................................................................ 607
Illinois ........................................................................... 607
Maine............................................................................. 608
Maryland........................................................................ 608

Massachusetts ...............................................608
Michigan.........................................................609
Minnesota ......................................................609
Nevada...........................................................609
New Jersey .....................................................609
New Mexico ...................................................610
New York.........................................................610
Ohio ................................................................612
Oregon............................................................612
Pennsylvania ..................................................612
Texas................................................................613
Utah.................................................................613
Washington .....................................................614
Canada .................................................................614
British Columbia ............................................614
Ontario ...........................................................615
Québec ...........................................................615
United Kingdom ...................................................615
England...........................................................615
Raw Chains and Franchises ...............................616

# Glossary ................................. 617

# Index ...................................... 623

# Final Farewells ...................... 655
The Hygiene HighJoy Hotline: 360-855-7232 ...............................655
Victoria BidWell's Vita-Mix Code: 06-000271 ...........................655
Our Hygiene Homestead in The Woods ......................................656
Final Encouragements from Victoria BidWell ...........................658
It's Detox Time! ......................................................................659
Susan and I Answer, "Where Do We Go from Here?" ..............659
Author Contact Information ........................................................660

# Foreword by Dr. Vetrano

*The Live Food Factor* comes like a giant locomotive, roaring down the tracks of two parallel, historic events. First is the growth of the Natural Hygiene movement, the grassroots of which were formally planted in American soils in 1832. And second is the blossoming of the raw food movement, which was planted, as some believe, before Adam and Eve in The Garden, or as some speculate, by our earliest, common, humanoid ancestors. The genius of the second edition of *The Live Food Factor* is that our newest raw food author Susan Schenck with our pioneering Natural Hygiene teacher Victoria BidWell have brought these two movements together, railroad tied with similarities, rather than driving their rails apart by differences. In so doing, these two women have created *the raw food and Natural Hygiene masterpiece of all time* in the form of a take-it-home, learn-it-yourself, do-it-yourself owner's manual on alternative health care.

My daughter Tosca and her husband Gregory and I read first in awe and then further studied *The Live Food Factor* manuscript over a two-week period. We put our heads together to collaborate on this foreword. But Greg alone shares one insight that sums up the value of this masterpiece simply and with a salesman's insight: "The cliché today is that if you attend just one seminar or buy just one book that inspires you to put into practice just one new idea that improves the quality of your life in just one way, the cost involved will be well worth it. Well, this new, little book — and I use the word 'little' as a term of endearment, considering the book has reached biblical proportions of more than 700 pages — has so many practical ideas! When put into practice, each one will improve the quality of a health seeker's life enormously. *The Live Food Factor* can only be considered a *treasure chest*! It is filled with well-organized, magnificently indexed jewels, with strings of wisdom pearls, and with how-to-do-it precious coins that will bring high health and high joy to anyone willing to put in the time and energy to do the Natural Hygiene right and eat the foods live. Truly, the book is worth more than its weight in gold when weighed on the scales of life at its best!"

When I started first by looking at the Table of Contents, it was full of everything from "Hygienic soup" to nuts. The book's subtitle promises "The Comprehensive Guide": this is a huge understatement. The book's completeness is astounding — both in content and authors, doctors, scientists, facts, recipes, and how-to-do-it instructions.

I must say that *The Live Food Factor* is *the very best book on alternative health care ever done*. It contains more 1900s research and more 2000s research on the benefits of raw foods as well as on the flip side of the coin — the health dangers of cooked foods — ever amassed in one place: certainly more than one may discover even if putting in a month's worth of Internet searching!

Since the 1980s, Victoria and I have been writing and editing our work together. And Victoria only entered Susan's picture with this second edition, which I am now *thrilled and honored* to endorse and help promote. Susan's exhaustive research and Victoria's expertise in keeping Natural Hygiene physiologically correct, combined with all their how-to-do-it tips, cheerleading, and you-can-do-it motivators, *make this book the best book on the market now in the field of alternative health care*. It will probably remain so for the next 100 years as long as each edition is updated with new research. Someone will have to go to an enormous amount of work to outdo *The Live Food Factor*.

I totally enjoyed each chapter and thought to myself, "This book these two women put together is really going to be a big seller. First, because raw foodism is very popular right now. And second, because the raw fooders need *all healthful living practices*, since raw foods *alone* do not insure health." I predict this book will be passed around to reach best-seller proportions, supplying not only the truth as do others, but also the proof as none others do. Its science and long lists of how-to tips will be reproduced and repeated, part and parcel, across America and around the world — including in personal conversations, in magazines and newspapers, and on radio and television shows and web sites.

Victoria is presently editing five of my books in which we plan to feature some of the Natural Hygiene teachings and raw food practical tips from *The Live Food Factor*, as well as promote the book. Victoria, Susan and I plan to carry on a global, joyful campaign to get the word out on live food and health by healthful living habits. I can hardly wait! I just turned 80 years of age, and now I can see that the best is yet to come!

Until now, Dr. Shelton was the most researched and prolific writer in the field of Natural Hygiene. He excelled at explaining the principles of Natural Hygiene in the now archaic, oratory prose, sometimes lofty and elegant in presentation and filled with poetic language that some of us absolutely love, but which is definitely not the wave of the future in literary style. Out of 40 book volumes, many of which were several hundred pages, and 40 years of monthly *Hygienic Review* periodicals, Dr. Shelton did offer the people a great deal of inspirational essays and encouragements to live hygienically. His volumes were filled with theory, teachings, admonitions, research, and debates. But he never did put together a single manual filled with both theory and day-to-day tips on putting that theory into practice. In short, *The Live Food Factor* does one thing that all of Dr. Shelton's books combined do not. It makes Natural Hygiene exceedingly simple to understand and inspirationally easy to do. Susan and Victoria, however, do share Dr. Shelton's and my rhetoric: we all tell the reader how very wonderful life can be when lived from the clear vantage point of high energy and high health. These two women have promised high fun to all who jump on for the train ride!

To point out that Dr. Shelton based his writing on extensive personal research is an understatement. To make this same observation about Susan's work in *The Live Food Factor* would be a *gross understatement*. Susan Schenck has done her research *like none other*! Susan and Victoria together have created a blessing very special that will help all who read the book and/or otherwise learn from their compilation of information as the nuggets of knowledge ripple out, person-to-person, media-to-person. These two have compiled the best of all of

Natural Hygiene into one compact book, easy to read and understand, plus much, much more. The marvelous, detailed index prepared by Bob Avery makes traveling through this train of great thought a great pleasure.

I am told that one critic of the second edition complained that passages in *The Live Food Factor* were too happy, that when he read them, he wondered what the authors had been smoking. I have known Victoria with sisterhood intimacy since 1976. Recently, I spent one very long phone call with Susan getting to know her. Granted, both women have their ups and downs. But they are both undoubtedly of the same ilk: joyful, positive, confident, very fun, full of love, and wanting to help others be all they can be. This should be the natural human condition. I think it is genius to promote being healthy as a natural high! I hope people who are basically depressed will give up their old drugs of fear and pessimism, coffee, smokes, prescription medicines, and recreational substances and give Natural Hygiene and live foods a try. If they can get used to being healthy and happy, they might like it!

The precise explanation in *The Live Food Factor* of how acute disease develops and then evolves into chronic disease finally shows the health seeker that the body builds disease into its cellular structure and bodily fluids as energy-robbing habits are practiced — and that health is just as surely so built with our energy-enhancing habits. This is done in no uncertain, incorrect, or confusing terms whatsoever; and I have edited these explanations three separate times in their preparation. So many other books on alternative health care and with teachings prefatory to recipe collections are riddled with these very errors, and that makes it totally impossible for me to endorse them.

Dr. Shelton's greatest call was "Health for the Millions! Not Just for the Few!" Today, I call farther and wider: "Health for the *Billions*! Health for *All*!" With globalizing technology enabling all humanity to share all knowledge virtually instantly, we can literally give health information to the billions. We are approaching seven billion on earth. And every single one of us, not withstanding racial and genetic individuality, operates according to the natural, physiological laws of life. Now, *nowhere is there a better owner's operating manual for the body and mind* than *The Live Food Factor* to show us how to make it through to the ends of our lives with "health and happiness" written into our eulogies.

The cliché "A picture is worth a thousand words!" comes alive in the Chapter 2 testimonials. Here are "before pictures" of sickness and sadness. And "after pictures" of health and happiness. Here are pictured many pleased people who played what Victoria calls the "superlative health lottery" and won, who took a gamble and persevered with a lifestyle on the right track that paid off to the tune of new and healthy bodies, dispositions, and new hopes being fulfilled with fresh, live foods for their fuel of choice.

The case histories are the best I have ever seen anywhere! Yes, critics may say, "They are just anecdotal. They don't prove a thing." But these are *real* people who have experienced *real*, life-disabling diseases that in many cases, even under conventional medical care, could have succumbed to the worst of outcomes. Yet these people chose the alternative with the best of outcomes. They built health while escaping the negative future consequences that so often result when turning to conventional medications, surgeries, and treatments.

But there's more. If you open to Chapter 2 right now, you will see wonderful, healthy practitioners who not only talk the talk, but walk the walk. You will see happy families and smiling children who have learned that mangoes, bananas, and dates are much sweeter and more healthful than any candy bar or sugary cereal. You will see people who have been deprogrammed and who do not live in constant fear of that "mysterious" virus, contaminant, or bacterium that is lurking around the next corner and crouching in the seat next to you on the plane, bus, or train. You will see and cheer — "Rah, Rah, Raw!"

I was especially impressed with Victoria's teachings on the Natural Hygiene fast. With the tragedy of Dr. Shelton's *Fasting Can Save Your Life* having gone out of print, *The Live Food Factor*'s Chapter 15: The Fasting Factor is now the best the health seeker can find as an overview. The explanation of the Natural Hygiene fast is so well organized, so physiologically correct, so perfectly worded, that even a reader who had never heard of fasting could understand what the Natural Hygiene fast *is* and *is not* and the benefits to be derived from both this type of fasting and juice dieting. In fact in my upcoming book on fasting, which Victoria is editing, we will write all this great information into the opening chapter as an overview statement on the Natural Hygiene fast. Why would I want to rewrite something that is already perfect?

I raised Tosca on strict Natural Hygiene. In turn, Tosca raised four healthy, happy children on the same. Tosca shares, "Mom and I are both especially pleased and excited to endorse the hygienically correct new chapter in this second edition of *The Live Food Factor*. I will be forever grateful that Susan was wise enough to see the necessity of this addition. The book could only have been correctly called 'comprehensive' if it had included our most dearly beloved babies and little ones! After all, we all enter the world as infants who all need the best start possible. Since Dr. Shelton's *The Hygienic Care of Children* is now out-of-print, virtually no new health seekers can take advantage of his instructions. I am especially grateful to have shared my successes with my four little ones in this new Chapter 20: Raising Live Food Children. In four simple lists — 'The ABCDs of Feeding Mothers, Infants and Children Hygienically' — mom and Victoria and I have laid out the scientific and psychologically correct basics for mothers and other adults who feed kids, while Susan has answered three urgent questions parents frequently ask."

As I began my quest for conventional accreditation to teach Natural Hygiene, it was gratifying to see, learn, and understand how its basis was laid out in the beginning according to our genetic code. But it also became ever discouraging to discover how the mis-truths, mis-directions, and out-and-out lies were also laid out so solidly to look like the concrete truths and yet were built on shifting sands, constantly moving and rearranging themselves to keep the lies from ever being exposed. Tell the people a lie long enough, over and over again, and soon it will appear true. And that's what conventional medicine is all about.

We hear about "health care" practically every day. How our governmental agencies will provide more and more at a lower cost. But what they are talking about is "disease care." My family and I are exceedingly healthy, as are my clients who follow healthful living habits strictly. We will never have to worry about finding the right doctors or nurses to take care of our diseases because we know what causes and what eliminates disease. Now you, too, can all have the sharpest cutting edge advantage in print by owning this book!

In summary, *The Live Food Factor* is a book for *all* people. Prospects for the raw food diet fall into three camps: those newcomers who are open-minded to trying raw foods, the backsliders who fall off the raw food diet, and the skeptics who don't believe the raw diet holds benefit. *No other book speaks to all three groups* as fully and intimately as does *The Live Food Factor*. It addresses all three camps with *truth and proof* and so much practical help and inspiration: the uninformed health seeker as well as the addicted, eating disordered struggler and the skeptic who demands to know, "Where is the proof?"

Even though the best ever yet, *The Live Food Factor* should not be used alone. It is best used as a companion to Victoria's *The Health Seekers' YearBook with The Best of Common Health Sense*. This statement can be made for several reasons. But the most important is that Victoria's book contains a chapter, "The Year in Live-Food Menus," as well as hundreds of other recipes and recipe formulas to make an unlimited number of dishes and drinks. This is what every new raw fooder and hygienist wants: menu and recipe ideas while transitioning to the ideal of whole, raw food meals. Susan and Victoria serve up raw menus and recipes that can be trusted to move health seekers forward into high energy and health and not backwards into acute and chronic disease! Just be sure to hygienize the raw food recipes Susan serves, and let genuine hunger be your spice of life.

I consider Victoria BidWell to be the best writer/editor/teacher in the Natural Hygiene movement today. So begin with *The Live Food Factor* and follow up with *The Health Seekers' YearBook with The Best of Common Health Sense*. You can't imagine what these two women, both scholars — yet both so childlike and joyful in their sense of life — have waiting for you! I am so pleased to be part of Susan's Paradise Health and Victoria's Hygiene Joy revolution! *I am happy to add to our roaring train campaign, my own term complementing theirs: a state of mind, body, and spirit I have always called "Hygiene Euphoria" — a natural high better than any drugs can induce and lasting as long as we follow the natural, physiological laws of life.*

**DR. VIVIAN VIRGINIA VETRANO, DC, HMD, PHD, DSCI**
(Endorsed by **DRS. TOSCA** and **GREGORY HAAG**)

*Dr. Vetrano is a published author and clinician with over 50 years of experience in helping sick patients regain wellness through natural means. You can read more about her life beginning at pages 75 and 221.*

# Foreword by Victoria Boutenko

*The Live Food Factor* is destined to become a classic. This book represents the most comprehensive study of the raw food diet and the raw food movement ever put on paper. When I received the manuscript, I simply couldn't put it down and read the book in two days.

In this book, Susan Schenck does what has never been done before. She brilliantly combines the concepts of raw food eating and Natural Hygiene. Both viewpoints are masterfully explained. I especially appreciated the additional information contributed by prominent Natural Hygiene experts Victoria BidWell and Dr. Vivian V. Vetrano. As a result, we have a unique source of valuable information that is useful for all readers: novices and experienced health seekers alike.

In my classes, people have asked me over the years, "Where is the scientific research backing up the raw food diet?" I'm thrilled that now we have *The Live Food Factor*, which contains data that is thoroughly backed up with a list of over 60 scientific studies.

The author has put a huge amount of work into her research. I am impressed with the multitude of sources of information that Susan was able to pull together and study meticulously. I am a raw food teacher, writer and researcher myself. I have taught hundreds of workshops about this subject for many years, and I have learned a great deal from Susan Schenck's book. I placed a whole pack of Post-It notes inside the book for future reading and reference.

I appreciate the author's scientific approach, where she not only praises raw vegan doctrine, but also discusses the wide spectrum of variations of a raw food lifestyle. Schenck listed even the most radical trends in the raw food movement, provided authentic experts' opinions and added her own personal reasoning.

I highly recommend this book to all readers interested in improving their health.

VICTORIA BOUTENKO

*Victoria Boutenko is the author of the books* 12 Steps to Raw Foods, Raw Family, *and* Green for Life. *Her testimonial and photo appear beginning on page 62.*

# Acknowledgments

I would like to acknowledge the following people for the parts they played in making this book possible:

First of all, I wish to acknowledge Bob Avery for assuming the roles of chief editor and production manager, as well as his vetting of factual information. Please take the time to read the special acknowledgement for him that follows.

I am very grateful for Victoria BidWell and her love and enthusiasm that have propelled my book to a new level. Please read the following special acknowledgement I wrote for her.

I also want to thank Dr. Vivian Vetrano for her efforts in writing a foreword and for taking time from her busy schedule to edit all of Victoria BidWell's writings on Natural Hygiene throughout the book for scientific accuracy.

I am grateful for Victoria Boutenko, one of my great raw food teachers, for all her books and her efforts in contributing a foreword to this book, her study on cooked food addiction and especially her testimonial contribution to this edition of the book.

My heartfelt thanks go out to all of you who contributed testimonials, notably Jacqueline Nash, who also provided much-needed professional editorial input.

Additional editorial assistance, proofreading and textual suggestions were contributed by Joan Kurland, Sara Pess, Lynn Pollock and Barbara Vensko, for which I am very grateful.

I am also very grateful to Joe Alexander for his wonderful calligraphy for the front cover and his enthusiasm for the project.

I further must thank Gabriel Spatuzzi for his work on the cover design and his hard work on my web site.

For donated recipes, I am indebted to my friends Buddy and Cherrie, as well as to Lorenzo and Marycie Haggarty, who also contributed their inspiration and advice for improving this book.

I must also express my deep appreciation to every raw food author or teacher quoted or profiled in this book: Dr. Gabriel Cousens for his research into the scientific aspects of the diet, David Wolfe for his zeal to inform the world, and especially Dr. David Klein for contributing a testimonial for this second edition.

I am pleased to thank Joan Kurland, Dana Pettaway and other raw friends for hosting raw, alternative, social activities locally and Helene Idels for promoting them.

I am thankful to Cilantro Live, Rancho's, Life Restaurant and Couleur Alive Café for making live food available in San Diego restaurants.

And *most of all*, I wish to thank *Al, my husband*, for following me on this raw journey and for being the biggest fan of my writings. Thank you for all the encouragement and emotional support that made this happen!

# A Special Acknowledgment for Our Chief Editor

Bob Avery found the raw food diet after years of searching to heal himself of minor ailments. He has been practicing it for over 15 years now. Upon discovering it, he immersed himself in information until people began to consult with him, though he never charged for it. A semi-retired computer geek, he went on to become the man in charge of a well-regarded but now defunct health-oriented newsletter known as *The Natural Health Many-To-Many*, or the M2M for short. Old copies continue to circulate as collector's items. For more information on his former project, check out the web page www.rawtimes.com/m2m.

Since the Internet boom, Bob has facilitated the spreading of knowledge about health and the raw diet to many people over the years, much of it on a one-to-one basis via e-mails and chat rooms. Working tirelessly at nights, and sometimes going with only four or five hours of sleep, he has helped numerous newcomers to the diet by answering their questions and assuring them that what they are going through is normal.

Most of all, I thank Bob for the herculean feat of coaching me off cooked foods and onto live foods! I first met Bob in an environmental chat group and was intrigued with what he had to say about the raw diet, although I felt it would be very deficient in protein and hopelessly boring.

I prided myself on having studied nutrition for years, both as a part of my professional education and as a layperson, so I had a lot to say about this raw diet. He had a comeback for virtually every argument I came up with, and it is rare that someone can out-argue me on a topic I have researched. I finally realized I could not argue about something I hadn't actually experienced, so I decided to give it a try. I was totally convinced after just one week!

I am deeply grateful not only for Bob's assistance in educating me on health issues, but also for editing this book for factual information, grammar, style, typography and layout. I recall a scene in the movie *One True Thing* in which William Hurt plays a writer who criticizes his writer daughter and says something to the effect of, "You have to deliberate over *every single word*!" I thought, "That *can't* be! Why would one have to be so picky about every single word?" Well, after working with Bob, *I have learned to belabor every word.*

I am likewise appreciative for how he put his heart and soul into the project. I could never have done it without him. Whenever I felt that the book was done, he would push me on to greater levels, saying, "No, we need an index!" or "No, we need cartoons!"

Then when *he* felt that the book was done, I would notice that some new raw food book had just been released, and I would say, "No, I have to read this new book and integrate its message into ours!" To his chagrin, I even postponed publication of the first edition for six months waiting for *Green for Life*. I am thankful for how Bob hung in there patiently while I kept making changes over the six years of perfecting this project.

In addition to spreading the word about how to be healthy, Bob loves gardening, bridge, chess and dancing.

# A Special Acknowledgment for Victoria BidWell, PhD, EdD

Victoria BidWell is the author of many books, courses, periodicals, pamphlets and other teaching materials on the alternative health system known as *Natural Hygiene*. Her most well known works include *The Health Seekers' YearBook*, *Common Health Sense* and *The Salt Conspiracy*. She is currently working on *The Health Seekers' BeverageBook*.

In 1976 at age 29, Victoria was drawn to Natural Hygiene in her efforts to heal herself of an eating disorder. Her dysfunctional relationship with food began at age 16 with the trauma of her mother's illness and death by cancer three years later. From 1967 to 1977, Victoria taught English to high school students. She left teaching students to tell the world exactly how the body heals itself.

It took seven years to get focused and start her own company, now in its 23$^{rd}$ year. She worked closely with her mentor, T. C. Fry, from 1983 until his death in 1996. During those years, she wrote extensively for T. C. Fry's Life Science publications and lectured in seminars. She served as master teacher while correcting the tests for the Life Science Health System the last two of those years. Victoria describes herself as a "passionate woman with a mission to share, share, share — how to get well and stay well!"

I am very grateful to Victoria for her editing efforts in making this book accurate according to the science of Natural Hygiene, for her contributions throughout the book, and especially for the new materials prepared just for this book. I am also especially grateful for the use and reprinting of many essential teaching materials she and Dr. Vetrano wrote and edited together. Many of these teaching tools have been taken directly from *The Health Seekers' YearBook — A Revolutionist's HandBook for Getting Well & Staying Well — with The Best of Common Health Sense.*

Just as with Bob, Victoria's concern for every word reminded me of the movie *One True Thing*. Her intensive training in both linguistics and semantics has turned her into a precision wordsmith!

It has not always been easy working with Victoria. When we finally met in person, I joked that she reminded me of a character in the Stephen King movie *Misery* — a deranged woman (played by Kathy Bates) who locked up her favorite writer and forced him via tortuous tactics to rewrite *his* novel to *her* liking! But I have no regrets and have learned a lot about writing in the process.

Most of all, I am thankful for the enthusiastic energy and love that Victoria has put into this book's updates. Her upbeat cheerleading efforts have motivated me to continue on with this second edition and inspired me with a vision of this book's fullest potential. Upon studying my first edition, she saw the potential for this second edition to become the colorful yarn that knits the Natural Hygiene and raw food worlds together into one magnificent tapestry. She has worked tirelessly while collaborating with Dr. Vetrano and me to actualize this potential — even seeing it reach out and speak to the billions worldwide!

Victoria is a practicing Christian. She lives on a half-acre piece of property in the spectacular Cascade Mountains of Washington State. The HighJoy Homestead, as she has named it, has been donated by Ken and Sandra Chin, a Christian husband and wife team. Victoria also runs a second half-acre setting three miles down the Skagit River, Our Hygiene Homestead in The Woods, a schoolhouse and guesthouse for health seekers.

Victoria gets her high-voltage charge in life by playing with and riding her gorgeous and outrageously wild equine companion, a white Arabian appropriately named Captain HighJoy America! He is a 100% raw fooder. In fact I watched him absolutely tremble with raw food excitement when I fed him a big pan full of carrots and apples, one bite at a time throughout the better part of one evening while we all watched *Misery* together. Victoria offers many raw edibles through her company, and she never sells a raw treat that doesn't meet with High's approval!

During the 24 months and 2,400 hours that Victoria worked on my book, she spent a huge amount of her nerve energy (see page 544) on our project, putting other projects on hold. She sacrificed summer swims, HighJoy rides and even her cooked food indulgences!

She has struggled for years with cooked food addiction, but she credits our book with her trimming away 40 excess pounds and her determination to go all-raw one more time — for the last time!

Victoria has taken two degrees symbolized by the credential acronyms after her name. The PhD was granted by T. C. Fry in 1986 from his College of Life Science in Austin, Texas. The EdD was granted by Dr. Henry Anderson in 2008 from his City University Los Angeles. But you will never see Doctor or Dr. in front of Victoria's name. She makes this clear statement here as to why:

> Although I clearly understand that the etymology of the word *doctor* comes from the Latin verb meaning 'to teach' or 'to learn', I will always correct you if you call me "doctor." For in deference to all the Natural Hygiene doctors who took all those 7 years of sciences or more and who received *real doctor degrees* and did their internships in Natural Hygiene, I am a mere health educator. They are the *real doctors* of our Natural Hygiene movement today.

Dedicated to helping others learn about the superlative, alternative health care system of Natural Hygiene, Victoria invites anyone to call or contact her if she may be of any service whatsoever. You may contact her via addresses and phone numbers below.

GetWell♥StayWell, America!
Box 558, Concrete, Washington 98237
GetWell♥StayWell, America! and Our Hygiene Homestead in The
    Woods Phone Inquiries: 360-853-7048
The Hygiene HighJoy Hotline for *Live Food Factor* Inquiries:
    360-855-7232
Web site: www.getwellstaywellamerica.com
E-mail: victoriabidwell@aol.com

# Preface

I _had_ to write this book because the raw food diet is _the best kept secret_ on the planet. The results of my years of research into the raw diet via reading, talking to people, attending lectures and workshops, experimenting on my own and coaching others are summarized in this book.

I debated, however, about how to present the material. Some people advised me to avoid a lot of science because it makes for dull reading; on the other hand, facts backed by science are what convince most people. Without research backing it up, many will reject theory based on case studies as "mere anecdotal evidence." If hard science turns you off, _simply skip Section Two_, but please at least read Chapter 4, which is the most important science chapter.

This book will also arouse some disagreement among my friends and colleagues. Acupuncturists I know will think I am a heretic since Chinese medicine advocates a macrobiotic diet, a diet of whole foods, most of which are cooked, especially when a patient has what is known in Chinese medicine as a "cold" condition (not to be confused with the common cold).

A number of my friends and family in the medical profession may be put off by some of the facts I point out about the pharmaceutical companies. I don't mean to offend _any_ of you; I am just sharing the facts. While the body does respond to the ingestion of many drugs with symptom relief, there is a much better, more healthful way that identifies, addresses and eradicates the root causes of illness and disease.

One thing I can say with nearly 100% certainty: my mother would still be alive if I had known about this diet seven years ago because she wanted to live and would have been willing to change her diet. I wrote this book in the hope that perhaps the information might spare somebody else's mother or loved one from _senseless and needless death by cancer or from some other dread disease._

Even my raw food friends and fellow authors who are strict vegans (see the Glossary) may think I am a heretic to present a small bit of favorable evidence for eating raw animal foods, at least for certain people with certain conditions. This was the most difficult chapter for me to write, as I was trying not to offend any of my vegan colleagues and friends, since vegans make up the vast majority of raw fooders.

I pondered about whether or not to omit certain chapters. I decided that certain things, however, just had to be said. I am really a "truth warrioress" at heart, with a voracious appetite for seeking and teaching the truth.

I have always been a pioneer, although — I believe Stuart Wilde was the one who said this — a pioneer is often someone with an arrow in her back! But I can also be a bit of a wimp at times when it comes to having an arrow in my back. I therefore put the truly, majorly controversial — _and therefore juiciest!_ — things in the appendices. That way they won't detract from the main message, which is pure and simple: let (raw) food be your medicine!

Oh, and by the way, I have always been annoyed by footnotes. I don't like having to flip to the back of the book looking for the reference to something so totally unbelievable that I just have to know the source. So, for your convenience, I have included the references in parentheses within the main body of the text.

After the first edition of this book came out, I received many e-mails that made all of my work on it worthwhile. A man who is blind hired a college student to read the book to him. Before they were finished, the student announced she too was changing to a raw diet! Others have thanked me that finally their loved ones were convinced to change their diets because of the science section. One friend told me her 92-year-old father felt it was not too late to improve his health: he went raw and lost 55 pounds!

Perhaps my favorite one was from a woman who said that every morning she raced her husband to the book, as both of them were eager to read it. I got a lot of "I couldn't put this book down!" feedback, which made me glad because one of my missions with this book has been to pack it so full of astonishing information that the reader will simply delight in every page.

I have even had a man who has studied raw food diets and theories for decades tell me that he highlighted new things on nearly every page. I hope this book will prove to be an equally rewarding adventure in learning for you too!

I forwarded all these comments to my editor, Bob Avery, since this feedback was a great compliment to all his hard work and talent.

## Note to Reader

This book is intended to be read from cover to cover, as many of the facts, concepts and ideas presented are built upon from chapter to chapter. So the first time it is read, it is best read chronologically. But if you find a topic you're not interested in and end up skipping parts, that's certainly better than putting the book aside and not finishing it at all.

My editors and I have taken pains to back up all of our statements so that only truth is presented throughout. However, if you come across something that you find hard to believe or you believe is not true, please do not let this keep you from learning what the book has to offer. Rarely is there a book that is totally free of error or opinion. Indeed, many of the greatest historical and supposedly factual books contain errors, half-truths or slants of the authors and/or publishers.

While newspaper publishers may employ "fact combers," the truth is that they, more than anyone, are guilty of "sins of omission" by disallowing information that offends the corporations that pay for their advertisements. For instance, we cannot read in newspapers about the effects of all the harmful food additives mentioned in Appendix A or about research on the ill effects of cell phones on the brain because that could offend the food and mobile phone advertisers. As Mark Twain once said, "If you don't read the newspaper, you are uninformed; if you do read the newspaper, you are misinformed."

If any statement or claim in this book seems to contradict your religious beliefs or any other cherished opinions, I invite you to move beyond that and see the bigger picture. Take advantage of this great health education opportunity by passing over your disagreements. I urge you to withhold judgment just for the moment and continue reading. It is not our intention to offend anybody.

I therefore invite you to read this book with an open mind so that you may be able to receive whatever assistance or helpful insights it may provide.

## Why does this book have two forewords?

When I sent the first edition of this book to Victoria BidWell, a noted author on Natural Hygiene (an alternative health system which includes raw food as one of its basic tenets — see the Glossary), I was hoping she would sell it on her site. She called me up and said she would like to be part of the next edition by editing out parts in which I claimed that the raw food diet heals people. She called this the "biggie," a major error in conception.

She explained to me that *the body* always does the healing, and the raw diet simply doesn't drain the body of energy like cooked food does, therefore enabling the body to have more energy for healing. (See Chapter 4.) The raw diet also provides superior nutrition for assisting the body in healing itself. Although I had pointed this out in Chapter 1, my semantics throughout the book were still, "This diet heals," instead of, "This diet provides what the body needs to heal itself." She corrected these mistakes.

While working on the book, Victoria became more and more excited about its potential. She kept offering things from her books to add to make it *even more complete and comprehensive.* She has included so many teachings from so many of her publications that it would have been distracting to reference page numbers. Thus excerpts from her work don't cite page numbers while most excerpts quoted from other authors do. After 20 months of collaboration, her contributions led to the book's being a "with."

Victoria became so thrilled with the book that she asked Dr. V. V. Vetrano, the world's foremost female expert on Natural Hygiene, to write a foreword. Then she felt that the book wouldn't be complete without a foreword from the other Victoria B. who is "galloping throughout the book," Victoria Boutenko, the world's top female promoter of raw diet.

I was overjoyed when both these women agreed to write forewords! I now have these three V's — Victoria, Victoria and Vivian — heavily quoted throughout my book, each of them having contributed to the book, two having offered their testimonials in Chapter 2.

*One of the things many people loved about my first edition is that I didn't take a strong stance on many controversial issues.* The book was an overview of most of the branches of raw foodism. I don't have all the answers, having been a student of raw food for only six years. I think of myself as a kind of Lois Lane of the raw food movement, an objective reporter who also likes to do a bit of muckraking on the food and drug corporations.

My stance on everything in life is to be eclectic, researching in depth and selecting the best from everything. I don't have a dogmatic bone in my body. Besides, what is right for one person (such as eating raw eggs or a nearly all-fruit diet) may not work for another. We each have to experiment to see what works with our own physiology, according to its unique biochemical individuality, genetic predisposition and present state of health and specific needs.

*One of the things many people <u>criticized</u> me for in my first edition is that I didn't take a firm stance on many issues.* This is where Victoria BidWell and Dr. Vetrano's contributions come into play, since they adamantly advocate that the late Dr. Herbert M. Shelton's teachings on Natural Hygiene are the best, as long as they are updated as science uncovers new information. For those of you who need strong opinions for guidance, their advice is a great place to start — and possibly end.

A concern I had was that with Victoria's items and co-writing of Chapters 4, 14 and 15, the book would be too Natural Hygiene oriented and therefore lose some of the strength of the first version's more objective overview. But I feel that Victoria BidWell's writing offers a lot. Most of it is general enough that it is accepted in *all corners of the raw food movement.*

Besides, as raw food branches go, Natural Hygiene is a very good one for people who prefer not to be eclectic. It offers so much more than just the diet for health, as you will see in reading Appendix F. Thanks to my condensing of BidWell's tendency to wordiness, the chapters read much more like Victoria Boutenko's great style: easy to read, easy to understand and full of love.

Victoria BidWell, as a lifelong horse lover, uses equine allusions from time to time in her writings. She gave me a lively metaphor for the additional influence of the three V's in this book: "We are four horsewomen of the raw food movement, the good girls, galloping throughout the chapters, helping health seekers with the forces of freedom, joy, gratitude and health on our side as we stand up against the misinformation, hopelessness and greed of the bad guys."

I am thankful for the huge roles of these three women and Bob Avery as backup teachers for me and for all of you. The accumulated experience of us five is at least 125 years of studying and teaching the power of eating a live food diet. We four have gone where no man has dared to go before: joining together strict Natural Hygiene and eclectic raw foodism — all to the great advantage of the bodies, minds, spirits and planet of our readers!

## Preface by Victoria BidWell, PhD, EdD

I <u>had</u> to help Susan with this book because, to me, <u>*Natural Hygiene is the best kept secret*</u> on the planet! Today, with Dr. Vetrano's editing, we have lifted *The Live Food Factor* up to the very top of the raw food and Natural Hygiene bookshelves for all health seekers to use in our troubled times.

The food supply in today's supermarkets has never been more contaminated and less nutritious, more addicting and less wholesome, more disease promoting and less user friendly. We must wake up, get informed and take action to insure that healthy foods are our choices and that these healthy foods are always healthfully prepared. *The Live Food Factor* is the single best wake-up book in the marketplace today. It is deliberately designed to inspire us to insure our physical and mental health and to improve life on the planet.

In the 60s, we the youth chanted *Make a Difference!* and *Make the World a Better Place!* Today, we can go further. My slogan for *The Live Food Factor* is *Choose Life! Do Right! Eat Live! And Get High!* The *getting high* refers to the natural, feel-good pleasures of being healthy. The *getting high* also refers to rising high above all the misinformation that contributes to sickness. The *getting high* further refers to being so well in body, mind and spirit that our values are so high on the humanitarian tone scale that we take grand stands for peace, love, joy, safety, reaching out to help those in need and being good stewards of the animals and plants and God-given resources of our planet Earth.

*The Live Food Factor* comes as an inspired gift from God and bright beacon of hope for all. It is <u>revolutionary</u>. It calls for a return to natural foods and living in tune with Nature in a time gone sick with unnatural foods and living in tune with consumerism. The book provides that which no one else has taken the time and energy to do: expose not just the truth about, but also the proof of, the enormous and joyous benefits of the raw food diet contrasted against the long list of health hazards resulting from eating cooked food. This book will educate and motivate health seekers around our globe — and hopefully you in each of your homes — to avoid the pain and suffering inherent in food choices designed for profits rather than grown for health.

It is now common knowledge that we all should be eating more foods raw — primarily fruits, veggies, nuts, seeds and sprouts — and that cooking foods destroys nutrients. But that common knowledge so casually referred to in most of the several hundreds of books out there has not been backed up by a serious amount of scientific documentation on formal studies and reports and from informal experiments and anecdotal case histories. Susan's centering of our 600+ pages around nearly 70 studies, consequently, is what puts *The Live Food Factor* in a category all by itself and at the top of the alternative health care, take-home-manual, must-read bookshelf. It was this research and the ambitious and broad scope of her project that caught my attention. We worked together over 20 months, sometimes with hilarious agony, always with great hopes.

What were the comedies? This is Susan's book presented in Susan's writing style. We have made many compromises in our two very different styles, even bargaining for some of them that were optional in both of our English textbooks. I am from the old school of Standard English. The one- and two-sentence paragraphs and new punctuation rules of her *Chicago Manual of Style* open English resulted in lively debates and made me moan. Susan's having to throw the protoplasmic poisons of table salt and raw chocolate out of her recipes resulted in further debates and made her groan. I gave up and mastered the open English. But she let me go on record to say that I would be happier to see three times more punctuation and three times fewer paragraphs in our book. Still, I hope that those of us from the old school of Standard English will come to appreciate this new way of writing. It is the wave of the future.

Some one person was destined to get the raw food word out with all the studies. But who on earth would have bet odds on a new author, working away for five years — while teaching in public school full time four of those years — to be the prime mover to get out the truth and proof on how to get well and stay well with raw foods and healthful habits? Someone hardly even imagining the potentially explosive impact of her message of truth and proof, taken to heart and practiced by health seekers in the billions? Someone simply doing all this work because she just wanted to convince her 83-year-old medical doctor father, her loved ones and her doctors, all of whom, more or less, rejected her enthusiasm of the raw food diet with skeptical variations of one question: "Where's the documentation?"

Dr. David J. Scott once encouraged me, "If you can get just one person to change just one habit in the direction of health, you have been a successful health educator." Surely, we can all become successes by this standard! Our *Live Food Factor*, put to such use by us health seekers and leaders in both the raw food and alternative health care movements, will provide the catalyst for the paradigm shift for so many others in need of help. Their shift to alternative health care will bring merciful benefits: these blessings will come <u>with</u> *raw foods and healthful living habits* and <u>without</u> *nearly so many surgeries, medical treatments and drug prescriptions.*

Susan and her editor are amazing. They got the first edition into a format that caught my attention. What a lot of work that must have been! But it was Susan alone who had the gumption to do the research and write the first edition. Susan was the prime mover. It was merely I who made corrections and precisions and contributions as backup editor, co-writer and prime Natural Hygiene teacher. I am so grateful to Susan Schenck for allowing me to be part of this paradigm shift for the billions — to the superlative, alternative health care system of Natural Hygiene via *The Live Food Factor.*

Dear health seekers, do indulge yourselves in *The Live Food Factor.* But let these joyful indulgences be just the beginning of the ride of your life! Please pass the platter around to your circle of doctors, associates, friends and loved ones so that they can also benefit from our urgent and all-important message. Simply put, the now clear fact is that raw foods provide the body with the very best fuel for the creation of the very highest levels of health and happiness known to man, woman and child. I pray that each of you prospers accordingly in body, mind and soul as you enjoy live foods and add healthful living habits to your day and night routines — one habit at a time, one success at a time.

# Introduction

There is one custom dating back 500-1,000 generations prevalent in virtually every culture on earth — cooking. What if you could attain immeasurably stronger defense mechanisms against all illnesses, a clearer mind, a happier emotional state and even a more highly developed spiritual level merely by omitting this custom?

The raw food diet has been portrayed by the media as the latest diet craze. Out of ignorance, some "experts" will even recommend that this diet could be "unsafe" for children. Hmmm... I wonder how all those children survived for eons before cooking was invented.

Yet this diet is here to stay. People discovering its benefits develop such a zeal that they want to tell the world. It is so much more than a weight-loss diet. It is truly the diet that unveils our latent capacity to live in peace and harmony with mental and spiritual clarity.

I will always recall my first introduction to the world of living food. In 1989, I had a housemate who ate 80% "live" food, as she called it. Why wasn't I convinced after a year of living with her?

Hmmm, live food? Well, that's fine, I thought, but I would just as soon eat what I love and spend money on supplements (enzymes and vitamins) for the things lost in the fire of cooked food. Besides, her diet was *so boring*! Just fresh juice, salad and "health-food" chips for the 20% of allowed cooked food.

Little did I know that supplements could never compensate for ingredients in live food that are impossible to put into a tablet or liquid supplement, and little did I know at that time how to make raw food more appealing than cooked food. I had no idea of the variety of tastes that I was missing out on!

As I explain in Chapter 3, I was searching for the elusive "fountain of youth," the "silver bullet" that would give me more energy and halt or reverse aging. I thought it would be something that would probably cost a lot of money.

When I discovered the living food diet, and experienced it firsthand, I realized that this was *it*! I quickly read everything I could find on the topic, frequently "google-ing" the words "raw food" into the Internet search engine, as well as at the Internet bookstore Amazon.com. I read about 70 books related to nutrition, including everything on raw food that I could find, within a year and another 30 the next two years. I attended numerous workshops and lectures by long-term raw fooders.

Usually when we think of a diet, we think of weight loss. This book will show you that the power of what you eat — and refuse to eat — goes far beyond weight control. When properly nurtured, the body can heal itself of cancer, infertility, thyroid problems, asthma, diabetes and even sleepwalking, in addition to obesity. Surgery can almost always be avoided. You will read testimonials like these, and more, in Chapter 2.

Even if you have already begun your journey into living foods, you will have with this book a compilation of nearly all the scientific studies that have been done to date illustrating the superiority of the raw diet (Chapter 8), as well as many that implicate cooking in causing disease (Appendix D).

In this book, I have answered the most frequently asked questions about the living foods diet. Is cooked food *really* toxic? And more importantly, could it be that relieving the body of the toxicity of cooked food (explained in detail in Chapter 9) would give your body a big enough boost to *heal itself of disease*? What personal testimonials and experiments support this claim? (See Chapters 2 and 12.) Could it really be that a raw food diet can boost your mental ability, as well? (See Chapters 1, 2 and 8.)

Won't a raw food diet make me feel cold and be impossible to do in winter? How can I get my family to go raw? Does my pet also need this diet? And perhaps the most frequently asked question: *How do you get enough protein?* (See Chapter 19.)

In this book you will find answers to all those questions and many more. You will learn how the raw food diet is a huge benefit for the environment and future generations. (See Chapter 1.) You will discover various ways to transition, choosing the way that is most comfortable for you. (See Chapter 13.) You will learn how to make the diet work for you in practical terms, such as while traveling and in social situations. (See Chapter 16.) There is even a chapter with over 100 delicious raw recipes to get you started. (See Chapter 21.)

What, you say? You've already tried this diet, but failed? In Chapter 18, you will learn of the many snares that trip people up when starting a living foods diet and how to avoid them. You will learn about the addictive nature of cooked food, as I have experienced myself, and how to break the addiction.

But wait — if this diet is so great, why isn't it making the news? One would think that such a dietary change that can enable the body to heal itself of diseases thought to be incurable (such as cancer and even AIDS) would be all over the front pages of newspapers and on the six o'clock news. Why do mainstream media publications portray the raw diet as just another Hollywood diet fad?

You will discover, as I have, that there are powerful financial interests behind the cover-up and why this movement does not have big money to support its research. (See Appendices A and B.) You will learn why it may never be more than a grassroots movement — at least for a long time to come.

In this book, you will learn how to empower yourself, taking back control of your health from the giant food processors and drug corporations.

In Chapter 4 and Appendix F, you will learn the secret long known by the natural hygienists: the body is the only true healer. Your body can cleanse itself and heal itself of all disease if you practice the *ten energy enhancers* strictly enough and soon enough: cleanliness, pure air, pure water, adequate rest and sleep, a nontoxic raw diet, right temperatures, regular sunlight, regular exercise, emotional balance and nurturing relationships.

Additional appendices will enlighten you on some of the radical branches of the raw food movement, scientific studies condemning cooked food, behavior modification techniques to break free from the cooked food habit and *strict living* strategies especially recommended for the immune impaired and those seeking their highest health potentials.

When Victoria BidWell entered the picture with our second edition, she told me she *had to help with my message in whatever ways she could* to get the raw food word out within a correct Natural Hygiene context. Now our work is done. We hope you will run with our message, that you will share it with others in need and that you will contact us if we can be of any help whatsoever — with your raw journey!

As I mentioned earlier in the Preface, my mom would still be alive if she'd had this information. It is worthy of repetition to restate that I simply *had to write this book.* I have never been fully convinced of the idea of predestination, but I can state with firm conviction that this book was born of forces beyond my control. I couldn't sleep at night knowing that I was not sharing with others the *best kept, best secret you may ever learn in your lifetime*!

# Section One

# Raw Power:

## Reasons to Go Raw

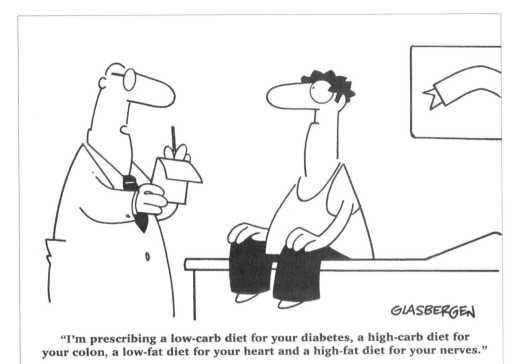

"I'm prescribing a low-carb diet for your diabetes, a high-carb diet for your colon, a low-fat diet for your heart and a high-fat diet for your nerves."

# 1
# Ten Reasons to Stop Cooking

*If cooking becomes an art form rather than a means of
providing a reasonable diet, then something is clearly wrong.*
—Tom Jaine, British editor of *The Good Food Guide*

Imagine you have discovered the most exciting secret formula that has completely transformed you. You are now at your ideal weight. Your hair is thick, your skin soft and smooth. You have recovered the vitality and energy levels of your youth, and you don't recall feeling such mental clarity and bliss *since preadolescence.* Your body heals itself of all disease, even minor ailments such as athlete's foot, acne, premenstrual syndrome (PMS), constipation and allergies. *You feel alive, in the zone, in the flow.* You have discovered the exhilaration formula, the fountain of youth.

Well, such a formula does exist. Only it is not a pill, potion, drug or lotion. It is simply a return to mankind's original diet: raw, natural, basic food — the lost art of noncooking, just eating food in its natural state.

Many who have tried the raw food diet feel such a mental, physical, emotional and spiritual shift, indeed, such a *radical transformation*, that they find it easy to believe that the "fall from grace" referred to in the mythology of numerous cultures arose from the cooking of food.

There was a time, eons ago, which most ancient storytellers spoke of, when people lived in harmony with nature and in tune with many of our untapped mental abilities, living in peace with all other creatures. Could the end of these times have resulted from the invention of widespread food cooking, thus damaging the fuel we depend on for our optimal health and well-being?

In some traditions, heavenly images include a garden of paradise, abundant with luscious fruit. By contrast, the image of hell is one of fire and brimstone.

Perhaps we don't have to wait until the afterlife to experience these states. Could it be that those archetypes were generated from earthly observations? Eat a diet of fruit and other botanical abundance from the garden, and you'll have "heaven on earth." Eat foods prepared over fire, and you'll manifest hell on earth!

When God threw Adam and Eve out of the Garden of Eden, he said to Eve, "I will greatly multiply your pain and your conception; in pain you shall bring forth children" (Genesis 3:16).

Interestingly, women on raw food diets do not experience nearly as much pain in childbirth, and often their menstrual bleeding is scanty to nonexistent and painless.

Could it be that Adam's and Eve's legendary fall from the Garden of Eden was not from *eating* the apple, but rather from *cooking* it? Whatever the case, cooking represents a foolish attempt to improve on the perfection of God's (or nature's) creation. It's doomed to failure, as we shall show.

We are told that *Homo erectus*, who may have been the first to tend fires on a regular basis, first appeared on earth about 1,800,000 years ago. For those of you who think we should have adapted to cooked foods by now, author Severen L. Schaeffer presents an excellent analogy:

"If we were to imagine the course of evolution as a road 25 miles long, men would be coming into existence only 70 yards from the end, the discovery of cooking 25 feet from the end and the development of agriculture about five inches before our time. Coca-Cola would appear roughly $1/200^{th}$ of an inch into the past" (*Instinctive Nutrition*, Severen Schaeffer, p. 9).

Truly, the vast majority of our evolution as humans has been spent eating food in its pure, natural, whole state — unheated, unprocessed, unsprayed with chemicals. You still may think, "Well, couldn't we have adapted by now?"

If we have only been cooking for 10,000-20,000 years, it would be impossible to have genetically adapted so quickly to these chemical changes in the food. This will be discussed in more detail in Section Two. Widespread genetic changes of significance need a million or several million years to occur.

Archaeological findings tell us that the use of fire for cooking may have begun roughly 400,000 years ago. Agriculture and cattle ranching, with the consequent consumption of grains and dairy, began only about 10,000-20,000 years ago. The widespread use of cooking began about the same time, but it has only been within the past century that such a large percentage of cooked food has been consumed — for some, 95-100% of the diet.

The belief that early paleolithic man routinely cooked his food is incorrect. Anthropologist Dr. Vaughn Bryant studied the fossilized excrement of early paleolithic people and concluded that they were primarily raw food eaters and, from studying the skeletons, that they were in excellent health. Thus it appears that cooking became customary only after the Stone Ages.

Why did man start to cook? There are many theories. Some anthropologists suggest that as man migrated to colder climates, the only way he could eat the frozen food he found was to thaw it out with fire. Since then cooking has become an art form and is now thought to be a near necessity.

Culinary arts have been a part of virtually every historical culture, dating back thousands of years. Every country's inhabitants have generated recipes that swell their pride, just as they are proud of creativity in the literary or musical arts.

Now I am going to suggest something *very radical*. Maybe cooking is not only unnecessary, but also deadly. Could this be one case in which creativity is not progress and in fact is sending people to premature deaths? You may think, "Well, my grandfather ate cooked food and lived to be 100." What if our natural lifespan is much greater than 100? And what if we have the potential to be very, very healthy even as we get closer to the ends of our lives?

A diet of raw, living food is not just another weight-loss diet. This is about energy transferred from the sun to the food to your body. This is about the life force and the enzymes in the food nourishing your body — hence the terms "living food" and "live food," often used to describe uncooked food in its pure, original state. If merely giving up the heating of food could transform your health and well-being, extend your life and youth, and raise you to a level of health you never even envisioned, wouldn't you gladly throw out the pots and pans?

Let us now take a closer look at some of the main benefits that a live food diet can bring you. In fact let's look at *ten reasons to stop cooking.*

# 1. Super Health

The Greek doctor Hippocrates, considered to be the founder of modern medicine, uttered the famous words, "Let food be thy medicine."

How far we have fallen from his wisdom! First, let it be made clear that nothing, no outside object, "cures" or "heals" the body. *The body always heals itself,* and it alone has the wisdom and capability to do so. As French philosopher François Voltaire (1694–1778) once observed, "The art of medicine consists in amusing the patient while nature cures the disease."

But in order for nature to do the healing, it must be aided by the right nutrients, or building blocks. Thousands of modern-day people have enabled their bodies to heal themselves from all kinds of degenerative diseases using raw food diets in combination with other healthful living practices.

As we shall see in Chapter 12, many have written books (or have been written about) describing their journeys to health and full recovery from cancer, diabetes, heart disease and many other ailments.

A number of doctors have recognized the therapeutic value of raw diets in treating a host of conditions, including the following: diabetes, ulcer, cancer, jaundice, Grave's disease, arthritis, fibromyalgia, asthma, ulcerative colitis, menstrual difficulties (including PMS), hormone disturbances, diverticulosis, anemia, circulatory diseases, weak defense mechanisms against infection, hypertension, neuralgic conditions, gastrointestinal disorders, renal diseases, gout, obesity, myasthenia gravis and various skin diseases. Many of these ailments are not normally associated with nutrition. Section Two will present the science behind these seemingly outrageous claims.

It is very common to heal from supposedly "incurable" ailments and no longer need medications on a 90-100% raw diet, especially when the diet is adopted as part of a total healthful living package.

I personally have met several people who had to take the drug Valtrex every day for many years for herpes. After going raw, they threw the drugs out and never had a breakout again. I have met people who no longer need medications for diabetes. I have also read of, and heard reports of, people with full-blown AIDS who became disease free, sometimes the virus even disappearing from their blood and not showing up on blood tests. A number of the authors of raw food books cited in this book were healed of cancer or other serious diseases using raw diet alone.

Bodily defense mechanisms are vastly enhanced on a living food diet. A clinic in Germany (*Klinik in der Stanggass*, Berchtesgaden) documented the influence of a raw diet on the body's defenses against infection. Their researchers found raw diet effects that yielded antibiotic, antiallergenic, tumor-inhibiting, immunomodulatory and anti-inflammatory results. These scientists recommend uncooked food as an adjunct to drugs in the treatment of allergic, rheumatic and infectious diseases.

Eskimos traditionally ate nothing cooked until very recent times. They are the only Native American culture that has no history of belief in a "medicine man" because they were extremely healthy until introduced to cooking.

Most people think of health as the absence of observable pathology or dysfunction. Dr. Herbert M. Shelton was a renowned leader of the Natural Hygiene movement, a health reform movement that became prominent in the 1800s. He was quick to query, "Why must we accept as 'normal' what we find in a race of sick and weakened beings?"

At his death, Shelton was writing a book to be called *Normal Man*, his vision of what *true* normal really is for our species. Perhaps we have yet to realize the full scope of our health potential.

Some people are motivated to get on the raw food bandwagon even though they were relatively healthy already. Some do it to prevent degenerative diseases. Much to their surprise, they soon encounter what can only be termed "ultra health" or "super health."

Gone is the need to sleep eight hours a day. Some even jump out of bed fully awake after three to six hours of sleep, with no desire for coffee or other stimulants. Excess fat melts off without any feeling of deprivation. The desire to overeat is diminished, as natural appetite control reestablishes itself.

Women find complete freedom from PMS. For most, even their periods, which are simply a form of detoxification, dwindle down to one day. Birthing labor is sometimes painless and very brief. Women who have been eating raw diets for several years prior to the onset of menopause report having neither signs nor symptoms that indicate they are passing through menopause. The only way they discover that they have gone through the passage is via blood tests for hormone levels.

Temperature extremes are suddenly tolerated more easily. Body odors vanish or greatly diminish after a year or two of eating mostly or 100% raw. Skin becomes soft and smooth. Hair grows thick and wild. Bad breath becomes a thing of the past. Air travel does not entail jet lag.

Various other complaints, like athlete's foot, acne, allergies, colds, flus, dandruff, herpes or cold sores simply vanish.

The physical senses sharpen. The person's psychic ability and feeling of being "in sync," or "in the flow of synchronicity," flourish. The person finds himself or herself more dynamic, radiant, charismatic and confident.

There is a feeling of lightness that everyone new to the raw diet comments on because far less energy is required for digestion. Digestive time is also reduced: while 48-100 hours are needed for cooked food, only 18-36 may be needed for raw food. This is a huge energy savings!

Athletes eating raw food diets have found their athletic performance enhanced. Dr. Elmer in Germany and Dr. Douglas Graham in the USA both experimented with athletes they train by having them go on purely raw food diets. The athletes improved remarkably in strength, energy and stamina.

Victoria Boutenko, raw food teacher and author, tells how her husband was able to do 1,000 pushups after going raw. She feels certain that once Olympic athletes discover the raw diet, many world records might be impressively broken.

Jan Dries tells of a cancer patient on his raw diet regimen who was actually skiing better than before she fell ill (*The Dries Cancer Diet*, p. 67). Comedian Dick Gregory became a remarkable athlete on a diet of raw foods and juices with occasional fasting. He ran 900 miles on fruit juice alone in 1974.

Since the vast majority of your body's cells die and get replaced within days to many months, a whole new "you" will exist after one to two years of a raw food diet. Only this will be the first time your body will be composed primarily of the best possible construction materials: nutrient-rich, living food.

A common thing people say when confronting dietary reform is, "Well, I have to die of something!" This feeling of resignation relieves them of all responsibility to watch their diets. Dr. Robert Young, a nationally known microbiologist and nutritionist, responded to this "common cultural myth. . . . I disagree with this because I feel that it's NATURAL TO DIE HEALTHY!" (*Sick and Tired? Reclaim Your Inner Terrain*, p. 83).

If you have no interest in achieving abundant health, consider that some illnesses show virtually no symptoms until the eleventh hour. For example, most people don't know they have cancer until it is in very advanced stages, and the doctor gives them about a year and a half to live, despite the tumor's having been there for up to a decade or so already. For about 40% of the people who have heart disease, the first symptom they experience is death by heart attack! (Sorry, the living food diet cannot bring you back from the grave.)

Although living foods can help your body heal itself even in advanced stages of disease, it is not wise to wait until you are ill. In the Chinese medical classic, the *Nei Jing,* it is said, "To administer medicine after an illness begins is . . . like digging a well after becoming thirsty or casting weapons after a battle has been engaged." Therefore, even if you are currently content with your state of health, consider this diet as a powerful way to help *prevent future disease.*

# 2. Mental Ability and Mental Health

The concept "you are what you eat" applies not only to physical health, but also to mental health. Diet affects ideas, perceptions and even dreams.

Eating a raw food diet definitely provides the nutrients the brain needs to get rid of brain fog, make the mind sharper and give one a "competitive edge" at work. One's short-term memory sharpens. Concentration and mental stamina improve. A raw fooder is also more alert, as excessive energy expenditure needed for digestion of cooked food is spared. The raw fooder doesn't fall asleep after eating dinner.

Raw food activist Viktoras Kulvinskas warns us, "When one eats a heavy meal, his energy goes from his head to his stomach." Digestion of cooked foods or unnatural foods consumes a great deal of energy. The clean body of a raw fooder thus contributes to a pure mind.

Dr. Edward Howell, who studied the role played by food enzymes for over 50 years, found a connection between enzyme deficiency, typical of cooked food diets, and a decrease in brain size and weight. He also found that the brain becomes smaller under the influence of obesity. Obesity generally vanishes with a raw food diet.

As you increase the fresh, raw food in your diet, you will notice an increase in positive thinking. This is partly because your body is being nourished properly, and the energy previously expended in digesting cooked food is now being used to cleanse your body of toxins. Especially if you do not overdo the phosphorus-rich acidic foods (meat, nuts, seeds, grains, beans) and eat plenty of fresh green leafy vegetables, your body will alkalinize, automatically creating the conditions for more powerful, positive thinking.

Visualization exercises, imagination and meditation will all happen much more easily. In time, your inherent psychic abilities may even blossom. Your natural intuition and instincts will sharpen. Decisions can be made with more clarity. Synchronicity will bring things into your life with ease and flow.

In his classic book *Mucusless Diet Healing System*, Professor Arnold Ehret wrote, "If your blood stock is formed from eating the foods I teach, your brain will function in a manner that will surprise you. Your former life will take on the appearance of a dream, and for the first time in your existence, your consciousness awakens to a real self-consciousness. ... Your mind, your thinking, your ideals, your aspirations and your philosophy change fundamentally."

Prominent raw food author and publicist David Wolfe says, "Raw food nutrition returns to you lost powers and abilities. I like to say that it bestows superhuman abilities — especially in physical endurance, clarity of thought and sixth sense perception." He sometimes works with corporate leaders to teach employees about this. He knew a man who was a raw food enthusiast for 37 years and became the number one insurance salesman for his company out of a field of 13,000 people. Nobody could compete with him.

Creativity may also increase. Raw food teacher Joe Alexander paints this intriguing, poetic picture of life on raw foods, "As an artist, when I ate cooked foods, I painted bleak, grotesque surrealist-type pictures with drab and dull, muddy colors . . . but when I became a raw food eater, all of a sudden I began to paint instead vibrantly alive pictures with lush abundance of healthy shapes and brilliantly beautiful colors" (*Blatant Raw Foodist Propaganda!* p. 75).

Valya Boutenko was in third grade and unable to concentrate on reading for longer than fifteen minutes at a time when her parents made her switch to a raw diet. Once her body became fully nourished with live food, she could read five hours at a time. "The biggest change I noticed from going on raw food is that I gained much mental clarity. I was amazed to discover that I can understand every subject. I'm sixteen and in college now. It's easy for me to write essays now for my writing class" (*Eating without Heating*, Sergei and Valya Boutenko, p. 13).

Leslie Kenton, health and beauty editor of the British periodical *Harpers & Queen*, and her daughter Susannah found that on a high-raw diet, they could write and research efficiently for seven or eight hours rather than just three or four as before (*Raw Energy*, p. 81).

Being a raw fooder somehow also makes people more open-minded. This is undoubtedly because the brain is clearer. However, I think it is also because taking such a radical leap makes a person begin to wonder if there are not other mental leaps to be taken and adventures to experience.

Joe Alexander declares that raw food eaters live in a more real world. "Their attitudes and opinions become transformed, energized by the reality of the Life-Force, whereas in most cooked food eaters, their attitudes and desires and opinions are programmed into their minds by parents, school, friends, clubs, organizations et al. and thus come from a very limited and superficial reality indeed, not from the deeper wisdom and reality of Nature at all" (*Blatant Raw Foodist Propaganda!* p. 59).

Mental health is tremendously enhanced. Many raw fooders find that they become freed from former addictions. For many, the desire to smoke cigarettes, drink alcohol or do drugs (prescription as well as recreational) falls away as the body becomes healthier: one experiences a natural high. Furthermore, those who work with juvenile delinquents and former prisoners have found that abnormal nutrition alone can contribute tremendously to the creation of a criminal mind. Children behave much better in school when on raw diets. Hyperactivity ceases, and brains fed with raw foods rich in omega-3 fatty acids (such as present in flaxseed) are able to focus better.

Part of the reason a raw food diet helps a person so much mentally is not only because live foods feed the brain, but also because unnatural foods are *eliminated* from the diet. (See Appendix A.) Working for several decades at the Hippocrates Health Institute, Brian Clement has seen mental problems like paranoia, depression, manic depression and schizophrenia disappear on raw foods combined with psychological therapy. Over the years, he found out that mental illness is exacerbated by hormonal imbalances from eating meat pumped with hormones, pesticide poisoning from commercial produce and a high level of body acidity from eating animal and processed foods. Eating a raw, organic diet is directly linked to the amelioration or elimination of these problems.

# 3. Optimal Weight and Beauty

The raw diet promotes beauty. To begin with, one reaches his or her ideal weight more readily and maintains it with much less effort than on a cooked diet. Many people lose 15 pounds in a month or two with no feeling of deprivation whatsoever. Obese people lose much more than that while eating raw fats, including raw "ice cream," avocados, nuts and olives. Raw fats (from avocados, olives, nuts, seeds, coconut butter et al.) are actually needed by the body to maintain youthful skin, hair and glands. They are rich in the essential fatty acids linolenic acid and linoleic acid, both of which are denatured by heat.

Raw food pioneer Dr. Ann Wigmore pointed out, "The effectiveness of live foods and fresh juices, especially wheatgrass juice, has bankrupted many complex theories about why we become fat and how to reduce quickly. . . . Among our guests at the [Hippocrates Health] Institute, the average weight loss per week is between four and fifteen pounds" (*The Wheatgrass Book*, p. 59).

Studies have shown that raw food is less fattening than the same food cooked. According to Dr. Edward Howell, raw fats are not fattening and seem to belong in "a special pigeonhole in nutritional speculations" (*Enzyme Nutrition*, p.109). While cooked fats accumulate in the body and become very detrimental to our health, raw fats contain lipase (deficient in many obese people), the enzyme involved in metabolizing fat properly.

The word *Eskimo* means 'raw eater', as the Eskimos traditionally ate nothing cooked, subsisting chiefly on raw meat and blubber. Dr. V. E. Levine examined 3,000 primitive Eskimos during three trips to the Arctic and found only one person who was overweight.

Cooked starches are also very fattening. Farmers have even learned that it is necessary to feed their animals cooked food to fatten them up for maximal profit. Hogs do not get fat on raw potatoes, but cooked potatoes make them gain weight.

In addition to reaching your body's ideal weight, many other beauty factors blossom on a raw diet. Cellulite, which is thought to result from eating heated fats, gradually disappears with the consumption of freshly squeezed grapefruit juice and raw fruits and vegetables. On a raw diet, improved elimination of cellular waste and increased lymphatic drainage help remove cellulite.

As your body's old cells are replaced with new, healthier cells through superior nutrition that only a raw diet provides, your hair may grow in thicker and at times wilder. It may even regain color after having been gray, as did Ann Wigmore's. Your skin may become as soft and smooth as it was in your youth. Your nails become strong, clear and shiny. Facial lines may fade or disappear. The face's pasty, white complexion becomes ruddy, or rosy. People may remark on how much younger you look. Your eyes will sparkle. You will smile more because you feel so good.

The Hippocrates Health Institute, one of the places where people have gone to learn about the raw food diet, was once described by *Cosmopolitan* magazine as the "well-kept secret" of beauty and rejuvenation of various famous Hollywood movie stars and celebrities. Now the news media are letting the secret out.

When Demi Moore appeared in a bikini in the Charlie's Angels movie *Full Throttle* and looked every bit as great as the women younger than her, the word went out that the secret was her raw food diet. Other celebrities who have caught the wave include Alicia Silverstone and Woody Harrelson.

Model Carol Alt shares in her book *Eating in the Raw* that the raw diet helps her stay beautiful, slim and young looking. She attributes her current youthfulness and stamina to having eaten primarily raw food for eight years. She explains that in her thirties she had to starve herself and exercise a lot to stay trim. As a raw fooder, she is able to eat anything she wants as long as it's raw. She now maintains her weight effortlessly, without ever feeling excess hunger. In addition, she claims she has better abdominal definition without exercising than she did as a cooked fooder who exercised regularly. She also has fewer wrinkles.

Health and beauty are intertwined. Dr. Herbert Shelton wrote, "The woman who maintains her health and youthfulness will retain her attractiveness. If she permits her health to slip away from her, if she values indulgences and frivolities more than she does health and impairs her health in the pursuit of false pleasure, she will lose her BEAUTY, and no art of the cosmetician and dressmaker will be able to preserve it for her."

Researcher Arnold De Vries wrote, "In the final analysis, we must regard beauty, health and youth as intimately related. To the extent that you preserve one in your physical being, you also preserve the others. The uncooked fruit and vegetable diet, pure water, sleep and rest, sunshine, strong relationships, exercise, fresh air, fasting if necessary and abstinence from drugs, vaccines, serums and other toxins are the prime requirements in your attempt to preserve your youth, health and beauty as long as you can" (*The Fountain of Youth*).

The face becomes more beautiful with a raw diet. "Skin loses its slackness and puffiness and clings to the bones better," write Susannah and Leslie Kenton (*Raw Energy*, p. 90). "The true shape of the face emerges where once it was obscured by excess water retention and poor circulation. Lines become softer. Eyes take on the clarity and brightness one usually associates with children or with super-fit athletes."

Nutritionist Natalia Rose, author of *The Raw Food Detox Diet*, profoundly praises the raw food diet as being the key to permanent weight loss. It's a lifestyle in which a woman can even attain her perfect shape without formal exercise or counting calories or grams of fat or carbohydrates and regardless of having had several children. The skin tone improves as cells become healthier and tighter. One dares to go out without make-up.

Tonya Zavasta describes her lifelong obsession with attaining beauty, which she finally discovered in her 40s through a 100% raw food diet. In her book *Your Right to Be Beautiful*, she explains how each of us can fulfill our full beauty potential, which is robbed by the energy drain placed upon the body by toxic waste accumulations from eating cooked foods, dairy, wheat, salt and drugs. "Beauty lies latent under cushions of retained fluids, deposits of fat and sick tissues. Your beauty is buried alive" (p. 134).

She goes on to explain that on a diet of uncooked foods, "The landscape of the body will change. Fat that has accumulated in pockets under the eyes and at the jaw will melt away. The lumpy potato look of one's face will give way to sleek and smooth contours. The surface of the skin will become soft and smooth but still firm and supple. Visible pores will diminish. A sallow skin with a yellow pallor will turn into a porcelain-like complexion" (p. 137).

Tonya further describes the radiance and glow produced internally when there is "an abundance of clear, pink, almost transparent cells that light up the face," which is produced by superior blood circulation. Even the most beautiful supermodel would be enhanced by a raw food diet. She notes that the modern-day version of beauty is more in harmony with health than perhaps ever before. "The quest for beauty, instead of a narcissistic preoccupation, becomes a noble pursuit."

Tonya came across many women who would not eat a raw diet for their health, preferring just to take medications. However, they would go raw for beauty, as there is no pill for it. In her book *Beautiful on Raw*, ten women contributed their own experiences of how raw diets added to their beauty.

Various observations were that hair grew out with color instead of gray, sometimes with natural waves or curls. Fingernails grew strong, long and shapely. Cellulite vanished effortlessly. Puffiness in the body and face disappeared, and the skin cleared up. These women often get complimented on the "glow" of their faces. They feel confident without make-up. Their inner beauty and confidence also radiate. They look younger than ever and have no fear whatsoever of getting old. One of the women is 64 and still gets checked out by "the young whippersnappers" when she is at the gym!

Interestingly, many of these women, before eating raw, had never been called "beautiful" by anyone, even when they were much younger. One of the women wrote about suddenly becoming aware of the benefits of being attractive, benefits which one who had always been beautiful would take for granted. People were nicer to her, cops didn't give her tickets, and salespeople waited on her first.

The authors of *Raw Food/Real World* explain, "People who eat only raw, plant-based foods have an unmistakable shine, like a pregnant woman in her second trimester or someone newly in love. They have a radiant, positive energy."

In his book *Raw Spirit*, Matthew Monarch relates that after he went raw, a woman passing him on the street offered him a modeling job! He writes, "Your appearance takes on a divine essence while on a Raw Diet. Your facial features become more defined; your skin glows, and your spiritual energy vibrates at an almost tangible rate. You become gorgeous" (p. 17).

# 4. Emotional Balance and Happiness

The word *war* spelled backwards is *raw*. On a raw diet, one loses the impulse to be at war with the world, feeling peace inside and out. The burden of digesting "dead" food, as well as all of the modern-day chemicals in food, can create mild to extreme stress on the brain as well as on the body. Dead, denatured food, with all of its toxins, pollutes the consciousness.

With the emotional balance that results from a natural diet of uncooked food, the frequency and intensity of mood swings dampen. Mind chatter calms down. You now have the capacity to deal with stress, frustration and emotional pain like never before. You will feel less overwhelmed, as well as more grounded and capable. You no longer need antidepressant or antianxiety medications.

Emotionally, the raw food diet helps put you at your peak. Your mind stops racing. You become more optimistic, even blissful, euphoric. You find joy where there used to be drudgery. You are at peace.

The Kentons explain how the raw diet affected their emotions (*Raw Energy*, pp. 119–121). "Instead of getting caught up in the emotional hassles when differences arise with other people, we can stand back and see what is happening. We no longer identify so much with what we think — we feel less threatened by someone who doesn't agree." They go on to say that life on the high-raw diet is "not the endless seesaw of minor ups and downs we once thought it."

They wonder, as I often have, if many of the negative feelings we get are not so much psychological in origin as physiological, "a sign that body chemistry is out of balance and toxins are building up." They read that Dr. Max Bircher-Benner discovered raw foods could not only help his patients recover from illness, but also help them fulfill their potentials in every area of their lives.

Nutritionist Natalia Rose explains that eating raw — and therefore cleansing, since your body has more energy for detoxification — makes you more emotionally centered, with a clearer mentality. She has observed in her clients that internal cleansing gives them the desire to clear and cleanse their living spaces and also create clear, honest communication with others. A sense of confidence develops, as well as respect for others.

She relates that her clients start to experience a "state of inner ecstasy" when they eat according to raw food energy principles. They experience "unprecedented rushes of energy and bliss" (*Raw Food Life Force Energy*, p. 2). "When your cells oscillate true vitality, you'll feel like the wealthiest person alive!" (ibid., p. 35). She claims that even when inactive she feels more euphoric, light and energized than she used to after an intense workout.

# 5. Spiritual Growth

People with low physical vitality have little energy available for spiritual focus. Therefore, a high-energy diet, i.e., an uncooked diet, can naturally enhance one's ability to commune with God, pray, meditate and perform whatever other spiritual practices one might do on one's path.

Entire books have been written about the spiritual benefits of a raw food diet. These include *Man's Higher Consciousness* by Hilton Hotema, *Why Christians Get Sick* by Baptist minister George Malkmus and *Raw Gorilla: The Principles of Regenerative Raw Diet Applied in True Spiritual Practice* by Da Free John.

Dr. Gabriel Cousens, MD, has written two books on the spiritual power of a raw diet: *Spiritual Nutrition and the Rainbow Diet* and another one published years later, *Spiritual Nutrition: Six Foundations for Spiritual Life and the Awakening of Kundalini.*

Victoria Boutenko, a famous raw food teacher, has also written a yet-to-be-published book about the spiritual power of raw food. In a lecture entitled "The Spiritual Power of Raw Foods," Victoria explained that when we rely on indulgences, we burn ourselves out. As we eat more raw foods, we rely less and less on these indulgences because we become happier without artificial stimulation.

When we rely on stimulation and momentary pleasure, we drain our vitality. It physically exhausts our hormones and neurotransmitters. Stephen Cherniske explains it like this: "Have you ever felt a 'letdown' after an exciting event — even something really good? The intense stimulation subsides and is then replaced by a creeping sense of depression or languor. This happens because your dopamine receptors, the brain cells associated with excitement, have all been fired. What follows is a metabolic rebound that you must experience until your stores of dopamine are replenished" (*Caffeine Blues*, p. 111).

Perhaps, as Victoria pointed out, that is why rich people who have funds for all kinds of gambling and other recreational highs do not derive lasting happiness from those events. With living food, we actually learn to find happiness from within.

The spiritual power of raw food is a concept that is even central to one religion. The Essenes are a religious group, dating back to the Hebrews, who are raw fooders and believe Jesus was an Essene and therefore a raw fooder.

Yogis of the Hindu tradition from India found that they could meditate better by eating only raw food. When less energy is needed for digestion, energy flows up to the body's higher chakras (energy centers) and enables one to experience higher states of consciousness. There is an ensuing "spiritual high" that makes one feel closer to the "Source," whatever version of that one may believe in.

Renowned spiritual teacher Da Free John claims, "Anyone who engages the raw diet properly will more and more naturally discover this sattvic disposition" (*Raw Gorilla*, p. 17). A sattvic disposition is one that is spiritual and peaceful.

The Mormons were probably the first group in the USA to discover the spiritual power of the raw food diet. Joseph Smith and his core group ate a primarily live food diet after discovering that it enhanced their spiritual sensitivity.

Victoria BidWell points out, "Biblical scripture teaches this same principle of spiritual growth as being a product of internal bodily purity and increased energy enhanced by a raw food diet. In the book of Genesis, God created the Edenic foods before creating Adam and Eve. Jesus' teachings instructed men and women to take care of their holy temples (bodies) and avoid defiling (poisoning) them in thought or action."

Gabriel Cousens was looking for a diet to enable him to meditate better and to enhance his communion with the Divine when he found the raw food diet. He wrote *Spiritual Nutrition and the Rainbow Diet*, in which he outlines an ideal type of raw food diet to promote spiritual growth. According to him, "Enzymes represent special high-energy vortex focal points for bringing Subtle Organizing Energy Fields into the physical plane for all general functions" (p. 101).

Cousens has claimed that in his experience working with thousands of people turning toward live foods, the vast majority responded by becoming more open and moving toward a more spiritual life, whatever their particular religious tradition. Raw food, he says, opens one up to a lot of prana, the vital force that makes you feel high naturally.

"The light is switched on with raw food. You start seeing the Divine in everything," he stated at a lecture. He claims that a live food diet turns us into superconductors of both electrical energy and cosmic energy, enhancing our sensitivity to the Divine (*Spiritual Nutrition*, p. 305).

Christians have also discovered the power of a living foods diet in a big way. Reverend George Malkmus freed himself of cancer using a 100% raw diet. He later got his Baptist congregation onto a vegetarian, primarily raw diet, citing — as do other raw diet Christian teachers — Genesis 1:29 as biblical proof that this is the divine plan for our optimal health and spiritual well-being: "Behold, I have given you every herb yielding seed which is upon the face of all the earth, and every tree which bears fruit yielding seed; to you it shall be for food."

In his book *God's Way to Ultimate Health*, Malkmus quotes Tom Suiter, a Baptist pastor, "If we practice the laws of health, then we shall start a revolution in this nation that could shake us to our spiritual foundations."

Joe Alexander, author of *Blatant Raw Foodist Propaganda!* boldly makes this comparison, "The raw fooder would enjoy a higher standard of living in a little hut than a junk food eater could in a palace. And raw foodism aids greatly in developing the spiritual maturity necessary for truly worthwhile achievements in life."

I once heard raw food activist David Wolfe say that he grew up as an atheist but that after being on raw food for some time, he *just knew* there was a spiritual realm! He experienced synchronicity and laughter for no reason. He has written in his book *The Sunfood Diet Success System* that the body decalcifies the pineal gland on a raw food diet. The pineal gland is thought to be the source of the "third eye," or psychic center of the body. Indeed, children who are raised on a 100% raw food diet have been known to be more psychic, as are animals in the wild.

Wolfe has also made the comment, "The Bible says the body is the temple of the soul. Unfortunately, I used to treat mine like an amusement park." Many of us could say the same.

Raw food has also been called "sunfood" because it contains sun energy, which is absorbed into our cells. It can be thought of as "densified sunlight." Light and its absence dramatically affect our consciousness.

Dr. Rudolf Steiner, PhD, founder of the Waldorf schools and anthroposophical medicine, taught that outer light released into our bodies stimulates the release of inner light within us. The more light we absorb and assimilate, the more conscious we become. He felt that plant nutrition connects us to unrevealed cosmic forces, enabling us to go beyond the limitations of the mundane personality.

Many people report feeling an energy current flowing through their bodies after having eaten raw for some time. Professor Ehret wrote about this, "Your soul will shout for joy and triumph over all misery of life, leaving it all behind you. For the first time you will feel a vibration of vitality through your body (like a slight electric current) that shakes you delightfully" (*Rational Fasting*, p. 89).

Matthew Monarch was catapulted into spirituality by the raw food diet. He describes what happened after six months of being 100% raw and doing a seven-day deep tissue cleanse: "Since then, I've had an orgasmic-like vibration in the center of my forehead. When it first happened, I felt like a wild tiger in the high mountains looking over a cliff into the distance; I felt clear, awake, alive" (*Raw Spirit*, p. 52). His research indicated that the pineal gland had awakened, and the vibration has only gotten stronger over the years.

Comedian-turned-raw-fooder Dick Gregory reported in *Dick Gregory's Natural Diet for Folks Who Eat*, "As my body was cleansed of years of accumulated impurities, my mind and spiritual awareness were lifted to a new level. I felt closer to Mother Nature and all her children. I felt more in tune with the universal order of existence." He also described, as a result of the cleansing his body went through, losing the "six basic fears": poverty, death, sickness, aging, being criticized and losing love.

Victoria Boutenko points out that Dr. Edward Howell's enzyme research indicates that a person typically has only 30% of his limited enzyme-generating capacity left by age 40. (See Section Two for more information on enzymes.) She says that while we can still walk, talk and think at this point, we have only 30% of our enzyme potential left. These enzymes have to give about 75% of their catalytic capacity to detoxify the body. "We become less sensitive to other people and to ourselves. We may survive physically but not spiritually" (*12 Steps to Raw Foods*, p. 5).

Raw activist Tonya Zavasta declares that her body is no longer an obstacle to meditation, prayer and self-realization. She proclaims that using her method of eating raw and only eating within an eight-hour period, which she calls "quantum" eating, "you will find enlightenment without even searching for it." She adds, "Instead of *having* a body, you will experience *being* in the body. ... You will feel weightless, you love the now so much. There is no place you would rather be but in your body. ... This creates a euphoric feeling, the ecstasy of enjoying the now" (*Quantum Eating*, p. 283).

Many spiritual leaders teach that mankind is on the brink of a major shift in consciousness. Those who radically change the way they eat, switching to 100% raw food diets, may experience such a shift. If enough people discover the best kept secret of the raw food diet, revolutionary changes in mass consciousness and the patterns of human thought habits would take place spontaneously. The hundredth monkey theory postulates that if just one in a hundred makes such a powerfully positive shift in consciousness, the other 99 will follow.

# 6. Economy

On a raw food diet, you will save money on food. You will save by eliminating processed foods. By the time you buy a processed food, it has gone through numerous steps and been passed through many hands between the farmer and you. Cost is added at every step. You will save on eating in restaurants unless you are fortunate enough to have several raw food restaurants where you live. You will save on junk food by eating simple fruit for snacks instead. You will also spend less on your grocery bill after eating raw for a year or so because, after your body rebuilds with raw materials, you will need less food. Consider that you will receive at least three times the nutrients from a raw fruit or vegetable than from a cooked one. In addition, you will save money on food immediately if you cut out meat.

Moreover, if you have been on a raw diet for a few years and have completely detoxified, you will no longer need to spend money on many personal-care products, such as perfume, mouthwash and deodorant. You will use less soap and laundry detergent because, since you will have far less toxic sweat, your clothes stay fresh longer.

Money spent on energy will also be saved. Since you may tolerate heat better, you might use the air conditioner less. You might even take up biking or walking to a lot of places you would have previously driven, thus saving on gasoline. You will save on the electric or gas bill because you will not use a stove or oven. Nonsmokers get a fire insurance discount. Since another major source of house fires is stove or oven use, raw fooders should also get a noncooking discount!

You will save money on health care, doctors' bills and nutritional supplements. You may even decide, like some people have, to save money by eliminating or scaling down health insurance. You will feel in nearly total control of your health, no longer afraid of being a helpless victim of disease. And even if you come down with an acute illness, your natural defenses will be strong enough to shake it off with a bit of fasting, followed by a tightening up of healthful living practices. After thoroughly educating yourself and becoming your own doctor, under no circumstances would you submit to toxic drug treatment, so why have costly health insurance? You might wish to purchase catastrophic insurance only, which is considerably cheaper and could be used in case of accidents.

Joe Alexander claims you will also save money on recreational drugs because the 100% raw food diet offers a better high than LSD, cocaine, speed and marijuana.

Sarma Malngailis (*Raw Food/Real World*) confirms, "Eating only raw plant foods . . . can give you so much energy; it's like a natural version of Ecstasy, and you never crash."

In addition, many raw fooders lose interest in mass entertainment and take up new, less expensive activities, such as organic gardening, hiking and camping. They also spend less on cars, being content with simpler, older models.

# 7. Pleasure

It may be hard to imagine now, but after you have been eating raw for several months, food will begin to taste much better. You will derive more and more pleasure from the simplest foods, eaten in their whole, natural states. On occasion, eating will approach ecstasy.

Cooked food loses so much of its taste that it has to be heavily spiced up with unhealthful additives such as monosodium glutamate (MSG) — a poisonous taste enhancer hidden in almost all canned and processed foods, disguised with many different misleading names. (See Appendix A.) In addition, cooked food is often "enhanced" with deadly table salt, as well as dressings and condiments. Once these are detoxified from your body, you will no longer crave them. Your tastebuds will open up to the ecstasy of whole, raw, natural foods.

When it comes to the sheer pleasure of eating raw food, perhaps no one puts it better than Juliano, the raw food chef genius, owner of a raw food restaurant in Los Angeles and author of *Raw: The Uncook Book*: "Why raw? Not because it guarantees me optimal health like the other 80 million species who eat only raw. Not because it's the last word in nutrition. Not for saving time or money. Not for the endless energy it provides me. Not because it helps the planet because, instead of discarding packaging that creates trash, I discard seeds that give life. No, not any of these reasons. So, why raw? Taste and pleasure and only taste and pleasure."

In an interview with *Newsweek* (April 12, 2005), outspoken raw fooder David Wolfe was quoted as calling his eating plan " 'sensual nutrition' rather than restrictive. 'There's such an erotic and beauty side to these foods,' he says. 'They're alive, and the colors are bright and vibrant.' "

Natalia Rose explains that she actually eats more calories on a 95% raw diet than when she weighed 30 pounds more because what she eats exits the body quickly and is not stored as waste or fat (*The Raw Food Detox Diet*, p. 88).

Pleasure from eating on a raw diet increases, but the addictive aspect is gone. While one experiences more eating pleasure, it is balanced; there is less attachment to it than with cooked food.

Sexual pleasure seems to work in the same fashion: while it may also become much more intense on a raw food diet, it is paradoxically less addictive and more balanced. The addiction, or strong compulsion, will diminish, but the enjoyment will be much greater because one is in far superior physical shape.

# 8. Ecology

On a raw food diet, there is vastly less trash produced. There is a minimal amount of packaging to throw away. In fact some raw fooders who grow their own food and compost their vegetative waste into their gardens find that they have stopped producing trash altogether!

Furthermore, much forestation has been depleted in order to produce wood for cooking in areas where people are too poor to own a stove. For those who cannot afford wood to cook with, cattle dung is often used. I remember traveling in India and having to breathe in the polluted air as people burned water buffalo dung in order to cook.

When on a raw diet, you also don't destroy any of the nutrients, so you don't need as much food. People who have been on a 100% raw food diet for years need to eat even less food than the "newly raw," as veterans absorb so much more of the nutrients since digestion has become much more efficient.

Eating raw food saves the earth. The conventional diet based on grains demands the plowing up of soil every year, which causes erosion, leading eventually to sterile deserts. The raising of cattle also creates serious erosion, with the legacy of destroyed land turning into desert. A raw food diet, on the other hand, encourages the growth of trees. Trees reach down deep into the ground and mineralize the earth's surface soil by pulling the minerals up to the stems, leaves and branches, which eventually fall to the topsoil for recycling.

The diet most Americans eat is rapidly destroying the planet for generations to come. Of prime concern is the fresh water used for cattle ranching. As Howard Lyman points out in his book *Mad Cowboy: Plain Truth from the Cattle Rancher Who Won't Eat Meat*, the water required to produce just ten pounds of steak equals the water consumption of the average household for an entire year! It took millions of years for the Ogallala Aquifer, the largest underground lake in the world, to form. This vast water supply is in America. However, the meat industry is draining it dry very rapidly. It will be nearly exhausted in half a century, as Lyman explains in his book.

John Robbins, vegetarian activist son of one of the founders of the Baskin-Robbins ice-cream franchise chain, estimates the date of depletion much sooner, at about the year 2020, in his video *Diet for a New America*. He cites a study from the University of California explaining that it takes 49 gallons of water to make a pound of apples, 24 gallons of water to create a pound of potatoes, but *5,000* gallons of water to make a pound of beef! Most people who eat meat are unaware of the true costs. When we eat meat, we are depleting one of our children's most precious natural resources.

Water is also spared because people on raw diets don't need to drink as much since the food they eat doesn't have the water cooked out of it. On a diet of cooked food, the body also needs more water to produce massive amounts of gastric juices to digest the cooked food and to dilute the pathogens in the process of eliminating them from the body.

Using our resources to produce fruits, vegetables, nuts and seeds, we could undoubtedly feed many more people. It is often reported by vegetarians that by using the same land area to grow food for people instead of cattle, a vegetarian diet feeds many more people than a diet that includes meat. Yet a raw food diet feeds even more people, using the same land space, than a conventional cooked vegetarian one does. Of course a raw food diet feeds many, many more people than the Standard American Diet (SAD) of meat and potatoes. According to Dr. Douglas Graham, "The Standard American Diet requires one hundred times the land of a raw food diet to produce the same amount of food. A [typical] vegan diet requires two and a half times as much land as does a raw food diet."

"We could feed forty people a pound of grain each, or one person a pound of beef," Graham asserts, "but nutritionists figured out long ago that we can feed 2½ times as many people from an acre of fruit than we can from an acre of grains" (*Grain Damage*, p. 35).

When asked about the issue of famine in the third world, raw fooder Guy-Claude Burger of the instinctive eating movement (see Appendix C) responded, "When you love the fruit, you love the tree as well. One plants and looks after one's orchard. Under the rule of cooked, starchy foods, fruit was demoted to the rank of snacks."

Raw food pioneer Dr. Ann Wigmore went to India and taught some beggars to sprout their grains and beans. The nutrient content of their diets increased so much from eating the food uncooked and sprouted that they were able to stop begging since they needed less food.

In addition to helping the ecology simply by being on raw diets, raw fooders report feeling closer to the earth and all of its creation. They more consciously make efforts to avoid polluting it, frequently taking up gardening, which reduces the need to consume scarce fossil fuels used in transporting foods long distances.

# 9. Free Time

No longer will you have to scrub the pots and pans of all that sticky, cooked food! You will no longer scrub endlessly at the greasy stains on the stove, oven and sink. Washing dishes and utensils used in raw food meals is simply a matter of rinsing. Sink drains will not clog up with grease.

During the six to twelve month transition stage, you may wish to experiment with many raw gourmet dishes that will take some preparation. But after a year or even less, you will become content to eat food in its most natural state. You will free up hours previously spent on food preparation and dishwashing. Eventually, you may also reduce your sleep time by a few hours a night. In a culture where time is often more precious than money, this is perhaps one of the greatest gifts a raw diet has to offer.

# 10. Longevity

Of the millions of animal species on earth, only humans habitually eat cooked food. There are the notable exceptions of farm and zoo animals, domesticated pets and wild animals foraging in our trash cans. These also develop the degenerative diseases that humans get from eating cooked food diets.

Only humans deliberately heat what they eat, and only humans tend to die at or below half their potential lifespans due to lifestyle-related illness. Typically, an animal in an unpolluted environment will live seven times past its age of maturation. Humans, who reach physical maturity in their late teens or early twenties, should be living to at least 140 years, full of health and vigor up to the last few years.

The great historian Herodotus claimed that the Pelasgians, who ate a diet of raw fruits, vegetables, nuts and seeds, lived an average of 200 years. This would make them the longest-lived people in recorded history.

On a raw food diet, you will not only have more time freed up from less sleeping time, less food preparation time and less dishwashing time, but you will also likely add many years to your life. You may be one of the modern-day pioneers in pushing the boundaries of our lifespan. You could extend your "middle years," living in full vigor and health many years past 100.

Gabriel Cousens, MD, stated in a lecture that there are two types of genes: the genotype, which you are born with and never changes, and the phenotype, which is affected by environment, such as diet and lifestyle. Eighty percent of longevity is dependent on environmental factors, especially what we eat. Only 20% comes from the genotype. What you eat feeds your genes. When you eat the phytochemicals from raw foods, you can turn on the antistress, antiaging and anti-inflammatory genes. Resveratrol, a phytochemical found in red fruits and vegetables, is especially effective in turning on the antiaging genes.

An important factor in the role raw foods play in prolonging our years is their enzymes. (See Chapter 10.) One is known as the "antiaging enzyme," superoxide dismutase (SOD), because it discourages the formation of chemicals known as *free radicals* that do serious damage to the body's cellular life.

The media tell us that we are living longer than ever before. This is misinformation. Some statistics show that the average current life expectancy is longer than the average life expectancy was, for example, 100 years ago, but these include the many babies that died. If you factor in all of the infant mortality of those years, the average life is bound to be shorter. Currently, due to better hygiene (see Glossary), fewer babies die, which adds many years when calculating average life expectancy.

Go visit a cemetery from the 1800s and early 1900s. You will marvel at all the gravestones for babies! So a big part of why the statistics tell us that we can expect to live longer is simply that fewer infants die nowadays.

According to the United States Department of Health and Human Services, the USA ranks 21st in life expectancy among all industrialized nations. People in modern America are not only *not living longer*, they are generally *getting sick much younger*. With the increased consumption of cooked foods (sometimes a food is heated three times before it is eaten!) as well as of processed and refined foods, we as a people are actually living shorter lives than our great-grandparents did, at least the ones who made it past 50.

Cancer, for example, hit only 1 in 8,000 people in 1900, according to Dr. William Donald Kelley, an expert on treating cancer. Now about 2 in 5, 40% of us, can expect to develop a cancerous condition. If such diseases as cancer were primarily caused by genetics, one would expect the rate of disease to remain somewhat stable, or even diminish (since many with the cancer gene would die before being able to reproduce).

Instead, most diseases are on the rise because they are *environmentally rooted*, our bodies not being designed to deal with the continual barrage of environmental pollutants in today's civilized societies. Our increasingly unhealthful lifestyles and polluted environments result in toxic body ecologies. The movie *Safe* graphically illustrates this by showing the effects that environmentally induced diseases have on people's lives.

Also consider that much of the talk of our alleged increased length of life is due to medications and life support devices that prolong the agony of a sick body for a few years more while vastly draining one's financial resources. Yes, we are living longer in hospitals and nursing homes. But what quality of life is this? Would it not instead be better to prolong the *healthy years*, maintaining an agile, active body, quick mind and steady emotions until the very end?

Eating a raw food diet will extend your youth and middle years, barring an early death from an unnatural cause like an accident. But even if someone eating raw gets killed in an accident before living out his or her maximal lifespan, the raw food diet still will not have been in vain. As David Wolfe says, "It's not about adding *years* to your *life*, but adding *life* to your *years*."

Now that we have explored ten reasons to eat raw, let's look at the amazing results achieved by some real-life adherents to this transformational diet.

# 2
# Rah, Rah, Raw! Raw Diet Testimonials

*Health is a state of complete physical, mental and social*
*well-being and not merely the absence of disease or infirmity.*
—Constitution of the World Health Organization

This chapter presents testimonials from people who have been consuming at least 80% of their dietary calories in the form of raw food. Some of them wrote their own stories; the rest I interviewed and then prepared summaries of their stories.

## "Raquel": No More Cancer, Diabetes, Asthma, Infertility, Eczema and Obesity!

"Raquel" (not her real name) is probably one of the most astounding cases I have personally encountered that demonstrate the power of raw food. She'd had several miscarriages when a doctor told her she could never have children due to "some hormonal thing," as she put it. She'd had cervical cancer and was told she needed another laser surgery shortly before she switched to a raw diet. She had endured asthma, eczema and Type II (adult onset) diabetes for many years before going raw. She was also overweight enough to qualify as "obese."

At the time of this writing [2005], Raquel is 26 and free from all of those maladies. She switched to a raw diet at the age of 20 under the influence of Paul Nison. (See Chapter 12.) She had been a self-proclaimed "junk food vegetarian" before that, just like many people not eating meat but living on unhealthful meat-free food. She'd had tonsillitis. She suffered eczema all over her body. She'd had asthma her whole life and diabetes since the age of seventeen, as well as cervical cancer since the age of thirteen. She'd also had frequent bladder infections, migraines and insomnia.

After reading about the raw food diet, Raquel made the commitment to eat this way *within one day*. Within five months, her allergy to animals and asthma disappeared. She went to visit her mother on the Fourth of July and was able to be around her mother's dogs with no allergic reaction. In October, she experienced a brief bout of asthma, which she rode out without an inhaler, and the symptoms soon vanished. She thought it might have been a detoxification crisis.

Without counting calories or using any deprivation diet, she also lost 85 pounds!

In fifteen months, Raquel became pregnant and was able to carry the pregnancy through to term. She ate a diet of 95% raw food during her pregnancy and gained only 30 pounds, which was unusual because everyone else in her family had gained at least 60 pounds during pregnancy.

Raquel explains that her raw diet freed her from painful menstrual cramps, and she reasoned that the diet would also free her from pain in childbirth. This belief inspired her to deliver her baby at a birthing center.

Her research indicated that the use of epidurals had several negative effects, including an increased likelihood of the baby's becoming hooked on amphetamines as an adult. She became convinced that birthing was not the "emergency" that hospitals viewed it to be and that it could in fact be a sensual, wondrous experience. She proceeded to have a *pain-free delivery* lasting six hours and gave birth to a very healthy, beautiful baby boy weighing seven pounds seven ounces.

Raquel's son, whom she fed a diet of about 80% raw food, was in perfect health his first three and a half years, never suffering from the usual childhood illnesses such as earaches, fever or even colds. Then when he spent three months with his grandmother and was fed a cooked food diet, *he came down with ten colds*! It was one continuous illness lasting the duration of his visit.

In addition to total physical healing, Raquel experienced a sharper mental awareness, as most raw fooders report. She used to have "brain fog," feeling she was "in the clouds." Now she is down-to-earth, working full-time and going to school to become a dietician while caring for her son as a single mother.

Later Raquel went from eating 95-100% raw to eating only 80% raw. While her illnesses never came back, she did gain back 30 of the 85 pounds. This motivated her to resume the 95-100% raw diet.

"I'm Cuban," she notes, "and we Latinos are more sensitive to cooked food than people of many other ethnicities."

# Jessica: Her Baby Made Her Eat Raw!

Jessica had never heard of the raw food diet. You could say that her body was her teacher — *or maybe even her unborn baby!* It was through a pregnancy plagued by morning sickness that she was forced to go raw. Her baby daughter, now three months old, was her raw food instructor. A month or two into the pregnancy, she developed a strong aversion to anything cooked. It made her nauseous. Through trial and error, she began to realize that the same food eaten in its raw, natural state did not make her sick, whereas eating it cooked provoked nausea.

Prior to this pregnancy, Jessica had been on the typical American diet. Now she had to rethink her whole way of eating. She went online and discovered that there was a whole niche of society that was eating this way! Through intense research, she grew satisfied that she could obtain the essential nutrients for her baby and herself by eating a raw diet without meat or even many eggs.

This pregnancy proceeded much more smoothly than a prior one, and she had all the "happy hormones," as she put it. When she had been pregnant with her son, she had craved pizza, ice cream and Cajun chicken. With her daughter, she craved raw broccoli, bananas and kale. While she would prepare herself a smoothie, she pictured a happy little vegan girl inside of her.

She felt happy, with almost no mood swings, thanks to the raw diet. There was one week in which she ate cooked food and became crabby, but she felt fine again after resuming the raw diet. Once in a while she craved eggs, which she ate cooked. As long as she craved them, she did not get sick. If she ate them without the cravings, the nausea would return.

When pregnant with her son, Jessica had gained three times the recommended weight for pregnant women, whereas with her primarily raw pregnancy, she stayed within the recommended weight gain limits. The delivery was by Caesarian section with her son, whereas it was by unassisted homebirth with her daughter and with everything going smoothly. She had thoroughly researched unassisted, at-home deliveries and also lived within a two-minute drive to a hospital just in case.

Jessica's daughter was born at nine pounds ten ounces. Jessica would binge once in a while on cooked meat after that. She noticed that when this happened, her breast-fed baby would get colicky. When she ceased eating the cooked meat, the colic went away, and the baby felt great. The doctor, upon examining Jessica's baby, told her to keep on doing whatever she was doing, as the child was a "textbook case" of a healthy baby.

"I feel so happy when eating raw," says Jessica. "I used to have severe depression and took antidepressants with such bad side effects that I got even more depressed. But now I am really happy. I also have more energy." Jessica additionally credits the raw diet with her loss of weight and absence of migraines and colds.

# Marie Tadič: "I've Got Energy for Sale!"

Marie Tadič is from Croatia and has a very strong character. I met her nearly four years ago [2002] when I first went raw and took colonics (see Chapter 3), as she was my colonic therapist. Like most people, she never ate a diet of primarily raw food until health challenges arose. Her major health problems began in 1984 when she had a hysterectomy during which the doctor removed part of her colon after finding a lesion there. It never healed, and for years she struggled with a chronic infection.

In 1990 she knew she had to do something drastic when she became totally constipated for ten days, followed by bloody diarrhea. She consulted an MD who gave Marie three choices: she could take medicine for her problem, get reconstructive surgery every two years, or find a diet that would correct the condition.

She did some research and came across Dr. Herbert Shelton's book *Fasting Can Save Your Life*. When she told the doctor she was choosing this route, he warned her that she would not get enough vitamins and would lose muscle, sternly suggesting that she not practice fasting. But after she spent ten days taking in nothing but water, he checked her blood and told her that everything looked great.

She then went on to consume nothing but freshly squeezed juices for six months. She learned at the Gerson Institute in Mexico how to provide the right conditions for her body to heal itself with raw juices and coffee enemas to facilitate the liver cleanse treatment.

During this time, she had more energy than ever before in her life, working fourteen hours a day. Gone were her yeast infections, constipation, diarrhea and leakage from a breast. Through consuming only raw, fresh juices, she even got rid of a stubborn frozen shoulder that acupuncture, chiropractic treatments and homeopathy had not helped. She broke her six-month juice diet on nothing but organic grapes for six weeks.

Now that it was time to resume solid foods, Marie went to a doctor who told her to eat for her metabolic type, which required the inclusion of meat and dairy. Constipation came right back, as well as arthritis. After she got off that diet and began eating about 80% raw, these ailments quickly vanished. Because of that, she got interested in colon cleansing and after taking a course and buying a colonic machine, started a colon-cleansing business.

She continued to eat about 80% raw for several years. In January of 2005, she attended a lecture by Victoria and Igor Boutenko. (See Victoria's testimonial below and Chapter 12 for more on them.) She was so impressed with Igor's strength and vigor that she committed to eating 100% raw, which she has done for some months now. She feels a huge difference between 80% raw and 100% raw. She sleeps better, and her blood pressure is better than ever. She is one "happy camper."

Having known her before, I can say *she looks younger now* eating 100% raw than she did *nearly four years ago* when I first met her (when she was eating about 80% raw), especially since she has lost inches around the waist and has more youthful skin and an even younger-looking face. She says, "I feel my body is healing the rest of the stuff that it couldn't do with a diet that was only 80% raw. I am so happy I don't have to fast and cleanse with this diet since everything I eat is good."

She also remarked that a big advantage to being 100% raw is that cooked food no longer tempts her. She doesn't salivate when smelling or seeing it; it no longer looks appealing.

Marie just turned 60, and she is working every day from 7 AM until 9 PM, both as a colonic therapist and also in two dental labs. She is fond of saying, "I have so much energy it is crazy. You want energy? I can sell it to you!" I asked her if she was like that before going raw. She replied, "No way! I was tired all the time!"

Marie also remarked on many other changes since taking the leap to 100% raw. For instance, her memory has improved. She used to be very forgetful and "in a fog." She also has more common sense and finds that when giving advice to a client, knowledge just pours out of her effortlessly. She experiences more synchronicity, earning more money because "everything just falls into place." She has also lost an allergy to metals and showed me that she was wearing a metal watch, something that formerly would have irritated her skin, making it bubble.

Spiritual changes have also occurred. "My emotions are cleansing. Emotions come up. I also get vivid dreams, and I see who needs help but doesn't ask for it, like my sister in Germany, whom I had been out of touch with. I learned she needed money, and she sent me a message in my dream. My consciousness is much higher. My consciousness is on love, sharing, service. My life is changing because I'm changing my attitude with the food I'm eating. I'm more pleasant and compassionate. I receive wisdom that was blocked before. My mind is much clearer."

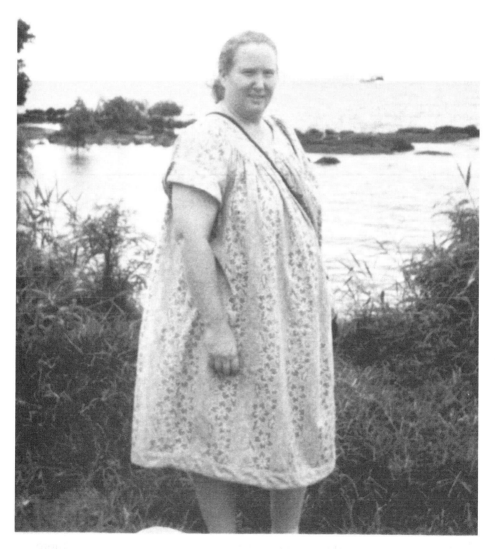

**Jenny Smith preraw in 1999 in Fiji**

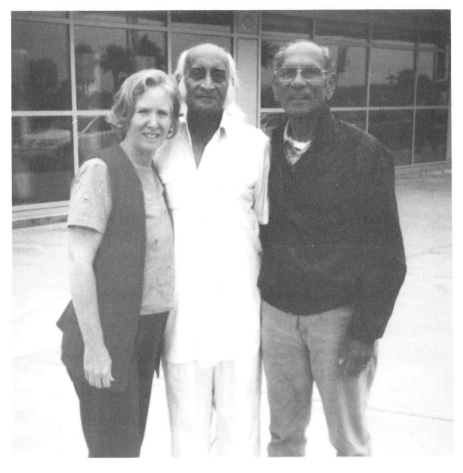

**Jenny, Indian sungazing guru Hira Ratan Manek and husband Rich Smith at the airport in July 2005**

## Jenny Smith: Recovered from Twenty Years of Sleepwalking and Obesity

Beginning in October 2000, I began a health journey, not knowing how much my life would permanently change. I was eating the typical SAD, weighing 215 pounds when I attended a health fair and learned about *fake* foods. I discovered how bad the SAD was for our bodies.

I was used to eating a diet rich in fat and refined carbohydrates and low in fiber. I learned that the answer wasn't to be found in eliminating carbs, but in dramatically reducing and/or eliminating refined, processed carbs. Thus began my journey towards health via nutrition.

In November 2000, I learned about the four deadly whites: white flour, white sugar, salt and dairy, as well as the dangers of meat. It was much too hard to give up all at once, so I started by just giving up salt. These five foods cause or contribute to over 90% of all physical problems experienced by most Americans today. I also began the popular blood type diet.

In December 2000, I eliminated white flour and used only grains acceptable for Blood Type A.

In January 2001, I eliminated sugar. In February, I switched to the Atkins diet and ate only 15-20 grams of carbs per meal, eating more eggs than chicken and fish.

In March 2001, I became a vegetarian. I also stopped eating dairy and grains, learning that these are unfit for human consumption. I had achieved a 25-pound weight loss by then.

By April 2001, with my on-going nutrition research, I became vegan, giving up all flesh and animal products. Author Erik Marcus (*Vegan: The New Ethics of Eating*) estimates that one 20-year old going vegan saves about 2,000 animals from enduring the suffering of factory farming and slaughter.

The rewards of becoming vegan included an enormous burst of self-awareness and lightness. I started drinking distilled water with added lemons. I have since discontinued this practice, as I have very little thirst eating raw foods. I soon realized that for optimal health I would need to go raw.

In May 2001, I went onto the Hallelujah Diet (85% raw/15% cooked). By this time, I had lost 42 pounds. And a most surprising thing occurred: I conceived on June 11, 2001. I was 44 with two grown children and two grandbabies! I had felt that I was infertile and had even gone two years with no prevention.

In addition, a doctor's test revealed that my HDL had risen to 48 (anything above 35 is healthy), even though it had been a mere 19 two months earlier!

By July 2001, I had lost 47 pounds. By that time, I realized I had made many choices which had led me away from the mainstream: no deodorant, tooth-paste, vaccinations, drugs, television, hydrogenated oils, white flour, sugar, soda pop or processed, packaged foods. I was proud to be following a new path and wanted to convey the importance of being different to family and friends.

In March 2002, I gave birth (gaining only 10 pounds!) to a healthy baby boy. It was an 85% raw vegan pregnancy! I gave birth at home with no problems. I called the midwife an hour and fifteen minutes before the delivery of my son, using no interventions or drugs. The cord was cut two hours and 30 minutes later, which allows ample time for the baby's blood to flow back to his own body.

In January 2003, I read *Raw Eating* by A. T. Hovannessian, which finally inspired me to commit to 100% raw. What steeled my discipline was education — I kept reading books on the topic. I hosted the Boutenkos (raw food teachers) in my home in March 2004.

I have not been 100% raw 100% of the time but usually am because I do not crave cooked foods. Family food events have no hold on me. I bring my own food, and everyone leaves me alone. It is a nonissue now. My husband and son are both on board and very adapted to eating the new standard four "food groups": raw fruits, vegetables, nuts and seeds. I follow Doug Graham's protocol of 80/10/10 — 80% carbohydrates, 10% proteins and 10% fats. It works beautifully for me.

Dr. John Baby, PhD, of Calcutta University advises that any disease can be cured if proper nourishment is given to the body. He advises a raw food diet for 41 days, whereupon almost all diseases disappear. Only pure water is to be taken; all animal proteins are prohibited, and no tea, coffee or medicines are allowed.

As of July 2005, I have continued extended breastfeeding although only at night. I have plenty of milk due to healthful eating habits. It has been documented that vegan mothers have the healthiest breast milk.

To summarize the health benefits I experienced, I started at 215 pounds (Nov 2000), eventually losing a sum total of 95 pounds, dropping to 123 pounds (Nov 2003). Then I stabilized at 140 pounds (early 2004). My cholesterol tested 155 (mid-2004). My blood pressure is 125/64, and my pulse is 63 (July 2005).

In addition, 20 years of sleepwalking ended. It ceased after I eliminated animal products from my diet. I learned it was the toxic overload that caused it.

Moreover, I have enjoyed higher levels of awareness for the first time. I do not crave junk foods now, nor am I a slave to appetite. I am free of all food addictions.

Research shows that menstrual bleeding is not normal. The cleaner you become, the less likely you are to have monthly bleeding. I have not had bleeding for three or four months but am still very fertile (white mucus discharge). I will be 48 in a few weeks.

On my journey with living foods, I experienced great opposition. I was hounded by extended family most of the time: they missed their comfort foods that I used to make; they missed the holiday foods and my homemade rolls. My husband had several severe meltdowns, thinking he was going to waste away.

When my son was 19 months old, due to an anonymous report that my son's only source of "milk" was from a coconut, Child Protective Services (CPS) visited me on two separate occasions. They closed the case after his height and weight were found to be within their government chart guidelines. It seemed CPS was more concerned about the nonvaccination issue than our food habits.

I never said the family was eating raw, only that we consumed unprocessed whole foods, fruits and vegetables. I let them assume what they wanted. It left me shell-shocked and stunned. Months later when I told a producer of the COX-TV station the story, she called and taped CPS saying they would not remove any child being fed any diet, so long as the child was growing and looked healthy. It was a load off my mind. Still, there have been several cases of children being taken from vegan parents.

My son is all-raw, and it is total freedom, as he never hollers like other children to eat candy or junk food. In fact at my grandbaby's birthday party, after a piñata was broken, the kids were diving wildly for candy. My son was picking up the foreign matter and throwing it back to them. It was such a joy to see. We explained from the get-go that there would be fake food there, which should not be eaten. He never doubted our word.

Nutritional surveys have found that one in five children eat no fruit in a week, and of those who do, the average is just two portions a day rather than the recommended five. So it makes one wonder who should be accused of having malnourished children, SAD or raw vegan parents.

My church also became a source of frustration. I was labeled a fanatic; most women stayed away from me. One woman kept telling my husband he was too skinny; another told me I was putting my son in danger by not eating meat. These days, I keep my mouth shut. I do not feel I need to justify my diet to anyone. Besides, health advice seems not to be welcomed. We have stopped going to socials centered on sugary desserts.

Most of my SAD friends left; I really cannot blame them. Most social life is centered on food. Most of my friends are on Internet chat groups or from raw support potlucks, although on occasion, I do attend raw food social gatherings.

It takes enormous power to reverse social tides. At first, I resolved to make waves, to erode ignorance. But I soon learned that it takes too much energy, and the majority do not want to leave the "herd." With more knowledge and experience, I gained confidence and pride in my lifestyle. This removed the weight from my shoulders and allowed me to act as a role model rather than a "food police cop" that family and friends grew to resent.

Those on the unconventional path are on a road less traveled. I have become quite used to it and have lately become very excited to see more and more people jump on board. I hope this information proves helpful to those coming up behind me on the path. Your health is well worth the effort.

I initially started this path when my husband asked for assistance to cure his hemorrhoids. It began many hours of nutritional study. I never resisted any part of the journey. It has been an absolute joy. I relish all that I have experienced — the good, bad and the ugly. Oh, and by the way, my husband's hemorrhoids are long gone! He joined my food regimens after his own learning curve was exhausted and only after many, many food wars. Because of my acquired knowledge, I was persistently constant, firm and unswayable — never desiring to return to the old ways.

My health journey hasn't stopped at food; I now enjoy sungazing as well, using Hira Ratan Manek's method.

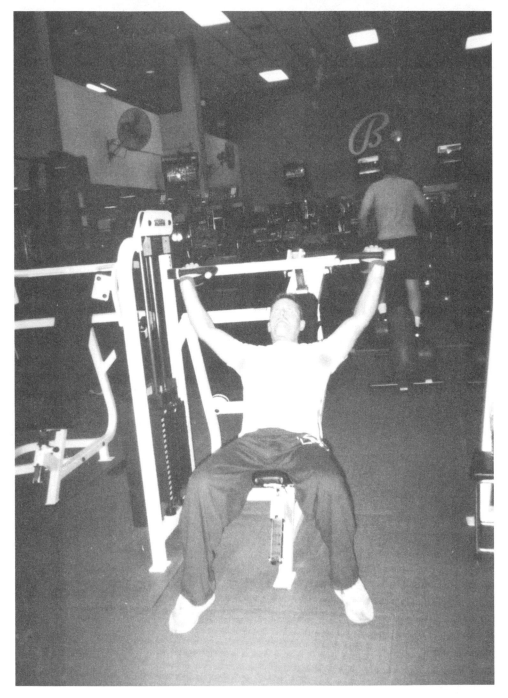

**Al at the gym in 2005 after more than three years on raw foods presses 280 pounds, something he couldn't do on a cooked food diet.**

# Al: Live Food for Bodybuilding and Higher Consciousness

Al is my husband, who was at first reluctant to eat a raw diet. He had to, by default, because I was the only one who would prepare food. Within weeks, he was absolutely astounded by the results. I didn't have to do any convincing. The experience of the raw diet spoke for itself. Although he has always taken good care of himself, he looks more youthful than ever with the "raw glow." In fact people often mistake him for late 30s or early 40s although he is 54 [2005]. Here is his story in his own words:

First of all, I have to give great credit to Susan for all of the wonderful discoveries she has brought into my life. I don't remember, but she assures me that I resisted becoming raw. It is hard for me to believe because it is so natural for me now. Before she introduced eating live, I lived on processed whey protein with little if any live salads. Now anything cooked doesn't even enter my mind as food. Because I do only eat raw, live food, I eat only a fraction of the amount of food I ate before. Susan gets full credit for the power, health and vitality that I now enjoy.

My experience is that cooked food stresses out the immune system. It takes a lot of energy that can be used for consciousness. I am interested in higher consciousness, and I've noticed that cooked food lowers my consciousness level. I've noticed that living food makes it so easy to absorb nutrients that energy can go to the higher centers of awareness so I can experience bliss. I feel blissful, especially when I am 100% raw.

I am also a bodybuilder. I've noticed that on the raw diet I'm actually stronger than when I was spending hundreds of dollars a month on strength-enhancing nutrients. Now that I'm off cooked foods, I'm actually stronger than when I spent more than a car payment a month on bodybuilding supplements.

I was initially afraid of weight loss, and with good reason, because I lost thirty pounds in just six weeks. Also, I was originally afraid that I would not get enough protein, and it was hard for me to give up my protein powders, which I drank several times a day. When I replaced them with a dehydrated, but still living, green grass powder, I was amazed that I actually got stronger and could lift heavier weights than when I ate (processed) whey protein!

After some time, I regained twenty of the thirty pounds I lost. Yet I am stronger than when I weighed more. I have heard that this is because the muscles grow back with better building blocks and though they may not be as bulky, they are superior.

Mentally, I am less forgetful. I used to have a very bad memory. It has also greatly reduced my dyslexia. It is much easier to read now.

Emotionally, I experience more peace. I think that raw food is conducive to recognizing our true, original, natural state of consciousness, which is blissful, harmonious and loving. Eating live food is simply allowing us to experience our true nature. It isn't giving us any more than who we are; it simply allows us to experience more readily who we are because there are fewer energy-draining detoxification processes involved than with cooked food. I still love the smell of cooked food, but I am rarely tempted to eat it.

The main thing about this diet is that I feel better. Even when I am going through a detox, I have more energy than I used to when eating cooked food.

I love to eat only live food. It contributes to my happiness, vitality and being more energetic, creative and youthful. This gives me the inspiration to discipline my mind to say no to dead, life-force-draining food and eat only live food.

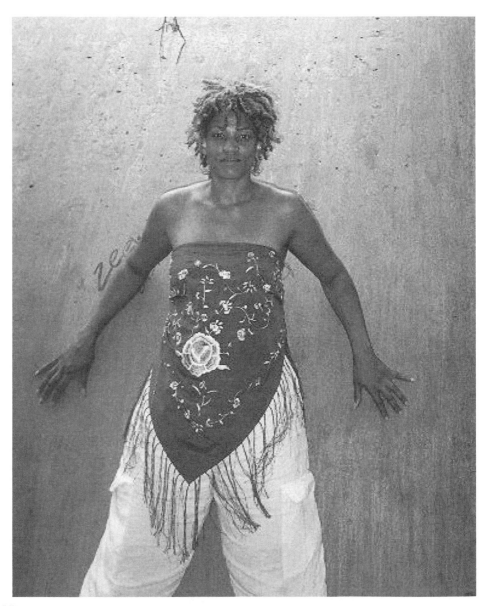

**Dana Pettaway (left) in Detroit at 160 pounds preraw in 2002 and entering the pool after 1 year raw with son Kyu, age 4, in October 2005 (below)**

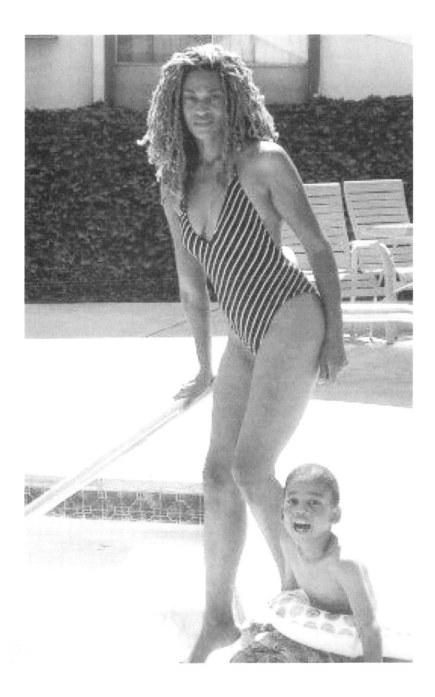

# Dana Pettaway: Increased Awareness and Freedom from Vices

Dana Pettaway just turned 36 [in 2005], yet if she had told me she was 25, I would have believed it. Before entering the world of raw food, she had been vegan for a couple of years. During the second year, she decided to cut back on her food, losing 30 pounds. She was wondering how she would keep it off when, a year ago, she saw model Carol Alt on a TV show teaching the benefits of a live food diet. Dana began her journey into raw foods at that time, the initial motive being vanity. Little did she realize that she was about to embark on a diet that would also change her very personality!

She wisely felt the need to educate herself, attending seminars and raw food preparation classes and beginning to realize there was a whole lot more to food than she had thought. As she dug deeper into the rabbit hole of nutrition and health issues, she became increasingly aware of fasting, cleansing, tinctures and food politics, such as the controversies surrounding organic and genetically modified food, the ethics of eating honey, as well as issues relating to the environment.

She realized that cleansing the inner environment wasn't enough: the outer environment also had to be clean if we are to be healthy. She began to recycle for the first time in her life. She became much more discriminating about the people she hung out with, realizing that negative people influenced her for the worse. "The more raw I've become, the more I realize I can choose to omit those negative forces from my life."

She began to hold herself accountable for violating what she now felt to be wrong, such as throwing out plastics or eating honey that had been taken away from bees that were forced to eat sugar water instead of the honey they produced.

"I changed my whole attitude and consciousness. I decided to be as pure and raw as I can be — to be *conscious, humane and not just healthy*." She started to connect with like-minded people in the local raw food community in San Diego.

Dana quickly became 100% raw and felt that anything less was not enough. Not only did she find the weight very easy to keep off, but also, to her amazement, the craving for cigarettes disappeared in a matter of weeks. She explained that while she had stopped smoking a few years prior to that, she had still craved cigarettes, especially if someone nearby was smoking. She would even have dreams that she was smoking and would wake up in sweats over the anxiety of this recurring temptation.

"Now," she says, with a look of great relief, "the idea of smoking disgusts me."

Other vices left her consciousness. She used to partake of organic wine, thinking, "Well, this is raw, after all." But even after just one glass, she woke up with puffy skin and a slight hangover. "Why am I doing this?" she thought. She quickly stopped.

Dana, like many others, found coffee harder to give up than cooked food, so she decided to at least use agave nectar (a sweetener from cactus) instead of sugar and nut milk instead of cream in her coffee. But after six months of eating raw, even this desire stopped, and she is no longer tempted by coffee. She also experienced no withdrawal symptoms!

In addition to the ease of keeping trim, Dana found a multitude of other health benefits to live food. "I felt after a month that I had found the Holy Grail."

Her long struggle with acne vanished, as did severe hemorrhoids. She acquired tons of energy, as well as the light feeling everyone who goes 100% raw gets. She also got more clarity of mind. "I became more aware of my surroundings and more clear as to my focus and life path."

She also got her son to eat raw food. "He eats a lot of the foods the other kids eat, but raw. He doesn't even know it!"

Her four-year-old is about 70% raw, eating tofu and vegan "meat" as part of his cooked food.

Her mother was a tougher sell, often calling Dana the "raw police." But Dana lovingly prepared her mom some raw dishes and fresh juice from time to time, perhaps replacing only three of her mom's meals per week with raw goodies. To her surprise, Dana's mom lost 21 pounds in one year *only because of this*!

Most amazingly, she also stopped drinking coffee. When I first met Dana's mother at a raw potluck, she announced her intention to go at least 80% raw after completing a cleansing fast she was on. When I later saw her again at the monthly potlucks, she had gone 100% raw.

Like many raw fooders, Dana wants to help spread the word about this marvelous lifestyle, although she no longer considers herself the raw police. Like others, she has learned not to be as pushy as she was initially.

"Now I think it's more about spreading awareness. If people want to own that, it's fine. Some are just not ready."

Dana is actively involved in organizing a monthly local raw food potluck. She is also writing a local raw food guide with some of the recipes and pointers she has learned, such as getting kids to eat raw food. In addition, she has started her own business selling gourmet raw food.

"I want to become a better person and surround myself with more positive people."

# Tim Tye, "The Raw Food Guy": An Awakening of the Mind and Creativity

Tim has been a 100% live food vegan for about five years [as of 2006]. Before that, he ate the SAD "to the max." As a young, single, working man, he fit the standard profile of the fast-food junkie, even a connoisseur, stopping at MacDonald's since they had the best fries and then popping over to Wendy's to get the best burgers. He claims he was in "fast-food heaven." But fast-food heaven soon turned into "health hell."

His health began a rapid decline from the stresses of PVC pipe glue exposure at work and the need to survive on canned foods during a three-month electricity outage following Hurricane Andrew in 1992. The toxic overload incurred during the hurricane experience led to chronic sinus infections, exacerbated by cheese and wheat allergies.

In 1998, at the age of only 34, he was at "death's door," suffering from chronic fatigue, listlessness, and ear, kidney and sinus infections that had grown worse and worse. He was 55 pounds overweight.

Once he had an ear infection that was so bad that his eardrums burst, oozing pus. Experiencing the worst pain of his life, he went to a hospital emergency room.

The doctors struggled to find an antibiotic that was strong enough: it took four tries and 1½ months to quell the infection. In the meantime, his liver and kidneys went into overload trying to detoxify all the debris from the infection, coupled with other toxins he had accumulated, including residues of the antibiotics themselves. His friendly gastrointestinal bacteria having been killed by the antibiotics, his chronic fatigue worsened.

Since his serum cholesterol was 285, he was put on Lipitor, a cholesterol-lowering drug. A friend who worked at the hospital said that since his liver was shot, he could die from taking this medication. Tim was so disturbed that his doctor hadn't even tested his liver before prescribing the drug that he became afraid of drug therapy. He looked everywhere for a naturopathic physician, but he had to ask around discreetly because the practice was not legal in Florida.

Finally, a friend referred Tim to her teacher at a massage therapy school. He spoke with her for just two hours, but the encounter changed his life. She empowered him with total responsibility for his own health. Under her guidance, he did a liver cleanse (see Glossary) and a two-week fast, cut out red meat and sugar, and took herbs.

He gradually got better as he looked for a health-conscious girlfriend. He got involved with a vegan woman who encouraged him to get off all animal products. But as he read *Nature's First Law: The Raw Food Diet*, he felt that they should be not only vegans, but also raw. After two weeks on the diet, they both became totally convinced.

Tim lost the last 25 pounds that he couldn't lose on the cooked diet. With a gradual, full detox, he even slimmed down to 127 pounds. People were now concerned that he was too skinny. Although he "looked like hell" for three or four months, *he felt fantastic*, better than he had ever felt before in his life! Most of the weight came back with healthy, rebuilt tissue, leveling off at a comfortable 145 pounds.

"My creativity skyrocketed," said Tim. He started writing songs about raw food. As he describes it, "I felt I wasn't even writing but was just a vessel. I was tapping into a higher source. I woke up with songs in my head." A former band member, he'd experienced creative flows before but *nothing like this*.

Tim even experimented with starting a raw food restaurant but later decided not to work so many hours after so recently regaining his health. Moreover, the community's consciousness didn't seem ready to support a raw food restaurant at the time.

Tim's mental clarity also went through the roof. Before, he hadn't read much at all. After reading a few pages, he would struggle to comprehend the material, even having to reread it. So he would put the book down and watch TV instead.

After going raw, he *couldn't stop* reading! His thirst for knowledge compelled him to devour books cover-to-cover; thus he absorbed knowledge on all manner of subjects.

He now owns a car powered by recycled restaurant vegetable oil from local restaurants as a result of information gleaned from one of his books. He has become a self-taught expert on composting after reading *The Humanure Handbook*, as well as on solar and wind power.

He also learned the importance of re-mineralizing plants and soil by reading *Sea Energy Agriculture* by Maynard Murray. He got his dying citrus trees to produce wonderful fruit once again by employing methods taught in that book.

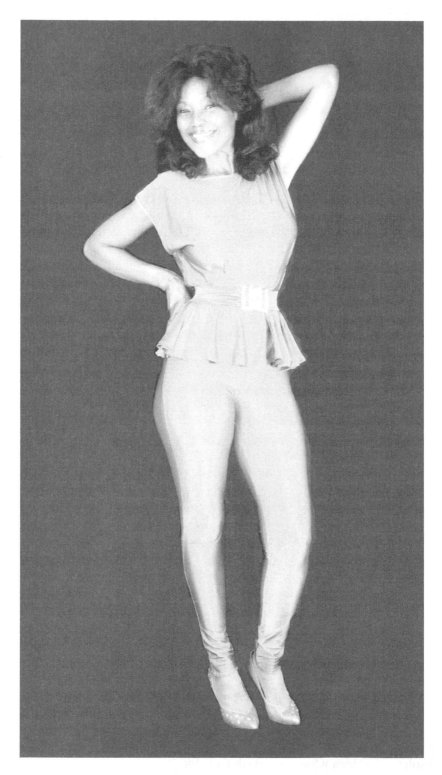

**Annette Larkins at 63**

# Annette Larkins: Super Health at 63

Just get onto the Internet and click on www.annettelarkins.com to see more photos of what being raw for decades can do for a woman! Annette's health journey, as told in her booklets *Journey to Health I & II*, began when she was 21.

Annette was born in 1942 into a family of omnivores. As an African American reared in the South, she grew up on "soul food," consisting of lots of big, greasy Sunday dinners. She was raised on chitlings, fatback, fried chicken and the like.

She very abruptly diverted from this path one day in 1963 while she was taking some pork chops out of the freezer. She intuitively felt, "If I eat these, I will throw up." At that moment, what she called a metamorphosis took place inside of her, and she never again wanted to consume animal flesh of any kind.

Later when she announced to her husband, who at that time owned a butcher shop, that she had not eaten any animal flesh in two weeks, he looked at her perplexedly and asked, "What's wrong, honey? Do you need to see a doctor?"

Her rationale for becoming vegetarian had nothing to do with health but rather inner transformation. Being unaware of the health implications, she continued fixing meat dishes for her husband and two sons while preparing vegetarian dishes for herself.

The next juncture of her journey took place as a result of being a self-described bibliophile. She has a personal library of 5,000 books in all sorts of genres! She discovered that refined sugar and flour deplete the body of micronutrients, so she gave them up. Later on, she also gave up dairy after learning that the body produces phlegm when fed dairy.

Still further on, she read books by Ann Wigmore and Viktoras Kulvinskas about raw food. It took some time for her to make the switch because she grew tired of eating salads. She said to herself, "Girl, you have got to put some *zeal* into this raw *deal*!" This led her to experiment and devise creative recipes reminiscent of the Southern soul food she'd been raised on, foods like okra, fried green tomatoes, cornbread and collard greens.

As she became 100% raw at the age of 42, Annette noticed gradual changes. Having been vegetarian for 21 years, she had commenced the raw diet with pretty good health already so her health did not change radically. But she observed that what had already been *good* became *great*. For example, her weight became balanced, with no more yo-yoing. Her small waistline got smaller. Her memory became remarkable, and her awareness heightened. Her mental focus increased, and her thoughts became clearer.

When eating cooked food, she would get painful cramps the first day of her period, so bad that she would have to stay in bed for a day. These went away on the raw diet. Five or six years after going raw, she noted that she had missed her period for three months and hoped she was not pregnant. She found instead that she was going through menopause. She had absolutely none of the typical symptoms: weight gain, emotional distress, insomnia, night sweats, memory loss. She has absolutely no idea what a hot flash feels like!

At family gatherings, her family members would make fun of her for refusing to partake of their traditional food. She never minded the teasing but stuck to what she knew was best. Sadly, she now sees who had "the last laugh," so to speak, as many of these people are quite ill with heart attacks, strokes, hypertension and diabetes. Annette, however, remains youthful and without a single health complaint! She is in super health despite inheriting what many would consider "bad genes": her mom died of breast cancer at the age of 47, and her grandmother also died of breast cancer at the age of 36.

Many people would not have liked to continue living with a spouse who remained on the omnivorous path. During her first 18 years as a strict vegetarian, Annette continued making meat dishes for her husband despite loathing the smell of cooked flesh. When he finally announced his intention to become vegetarian, she proclaimed, "Okay, but if you go back to eating meat, you must cook your own food."

He did end up going back to eating meat and took charge of his own food at that time. Three years later when Annette began eating her food raw, at least she no longer had to cook for him.

Annette compared their dietary differences to being in a marriage with political differences. "There is much more to my husband than what he eats." They will soon celebrate their 47th year of marriage. She feels very fortunate to have him as her husband, as he still treats her like a queen.

Now, however, her husband fervently wishes he had switched to her diet because his health is deteriorating, whereas hers is not. "Sadly," she said of her beloved husband, "he's *hooked on cooked*."

Annette recently was given a free blood analysis by a nutritionist who was curious to see the blood of a live fooder. The nutritionist announced to everyone at the health fair that this was the most perfect blood she had ever seen! There were no clumps whatsoever, and all cells were perfectly formed. Her blood pressure was also "like that of a child."

Annette's energy, enthusiasm and curiosity are also like those of a child! Perhaps because her health is so great, she has absolutely no fatigue, aches or pains that could slow her down. If you go to the biography section of her web site, you will be amazed at how much energy the woman has. She said to me, "If I could bottle my energy and sell it, I would be a millionaire."

She is engaged in reading, lecturing on raw food, assembling her own computers, creating her own greeting cards, sewing her own clothes, growing her own garden food and publishing her own booklets on raw eating. She published a DVD entitled "Annette's Raw Kitchen," in which she shows how she prepares her own comfort foods, including raw versions of some of the Southern soul foods she grew up on. She unpretentiously proclaims, "I'm not a chef. You won't see me throwing around any knives. If I can do this, so can you!"

She also produced a twelve-series show on a local cable TV station called *Health Alternatives with Living Foods*, which she based her DVD upon. (Her booklets and DVD are for sale on her web site.)

Annette sees herself as someone who introduces the raw diet to others. If they want to know more about the science behind it, they can read a different book. But her booklets, which include recipes, are enough to get people started.

She says the African American diet is heavily laden with fat and grease because the slaves were historically given only table scraps by their masters. Now it is time for their descendants to enter the "kingdom of living foods." Her message to the African American community is, "We no longer have shackles on wrists and ankles. Now we need to let go of the *shackles of the mind*."

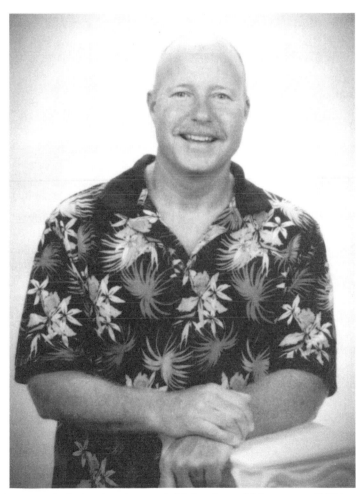

**Mike McCright in June 2004 after 2½ years 95% raw**

# Mike McCright: Raw for Life

I am Mike McCright. I am 47 [in 2005] and have been raw for about 3½ years. I remember reading an old *Organic Gardening* magazine about 25 years ago and seeing a picture of a guy in his garden; he looked about 19 — tall, lanky and healthy looking. The caption read that he ate all of his food raw. It kept him fit and young looking. He was 30 years old! That simmered in my mental file for a couple of decades.

I was having lunch at a gardening seminar in October 2001. I sat across from a vibrantly healthy man in his mid-60s. He was very energetic, more than any other man his age I had ever seen. He attributed his health to eating only raw foods. He had a girlfriend of about 60 who had gone raw soon after meeting him several months before. She had been on over a dozen prescription drugs for over three years. During the first six months of being raw, she dropped them all, as they were no longer needed. She dropped 40 pounds to boot!

I felt that it was time for change in my life. I was trying to eat more healthfully to keep my temple clean. Being reminded about that vibrant increase in health tipped the scale. I went raw after that meal.

I thought it wise to have a transition period; mine lasted two weeks. I could not then, nor now, mix cooked and raw. Cooked food is too addictive. I am currently over 95% raw, usually falling down in annual family events like Christmas and Thanksgiving.

I started out eating almost exclusively fruit. I thought, "This is great, dessert for all meals!" I noticed after about three weeks that my odors became less. I previously had bad breath almost constantly. My bad breath disappeared; my foot odor disappeared; my normal body odor largely went away; even bathroom odors were greatly diminished. I had loads of energy, no afternoon lull. I felt strong and vibrant. I ate lots of food, twice as much as before. While eating all the food I wanted, I was losing five pounds a week.

I went home to my mom's house for Christmas and found that I had little willpower around my family. I ate what everyone else was eating after the first day and got very sick. I felt awful!

I had introduced all those food toxins into my body after purifying it and let down my intestinal defenses. I also put on 15 pounds over the few days I was home. Eating cooked food causes me to put on weight extremely fast.

I came back from my mom's house, went raw again, and quickly lost the 15 pounds and a few more. My body settled on a 25-pound loss — 190 pounds after three months mainly raw. Over the next few months, I drifted down another 10 pounds. My weight has gone up and down all my life but is stable at around 180 pounds so long as I remain 100% raw.

After a couple of months of eating only fruit, I began to notice that my mouth felt different. By the third month, it was noticeably different, like my teeth were getting looser. I met other raw fooders and asked a guy who had been raw for three years about my mouth and teeth.

He explained to me that I needed greens to get the minerals I needed; fruit alone was not cutting it. I started with supplements for a boost, bought a nice juicer and started juicing greens. I also learned of the variety of wild greens in my yard and began juicing them too. Drinking a quart or more of wild green juice was like taking a power pill. I could not believe that the weeds I was composting were so good for you!

When I first began to eat greens, I didn't like them or desire them. I asked my new roommate who had been raw for five years about that. He explained that the salt I was using in my food was satisfying my need for sodium, which greens are high in. I stopped using salt and soon began to desire greens.

I have learned that my body needs plenty of greens and some fruit. If I eat too much fruit, I will have created an acidic environment in my mouth where gum disease can flourish. If I eat plenty of greens, that acidic environment will turn alkaline, and any gum disease will stop entirely.

Now when I floss, I never get any blood. The bacteria that caused my gums to bleed when flossing and slowly recede moved out and don't live there anymore! I had gum disease for almost 30 years. Now it is gone.

Salads are great, but I have plenty of nonsweet fruit in them — like tomatoes, peppers, squash and cucumber. They are fruit, not *greens*.

To get my quota of greens, I make a green drink every morning, usually of dried herbs and sometimes of wild greens as well. I also eat a salad in the afternoon and a small amount of fruit (like an apple lately) and a handful of nuts in the morning.

Early on, I ate large volumes of food to get the nutrition I needed. My body is much more efficient now, and I eat much less than the average person. If I eat more, I get fat. If I eat cooked foods more than an occasional small portion, I get sick and fat in a hurry.

I am raw for life. There is no reason to return to cooked foods. I am much healthier now than I was three years ago. Being raw was and is part of a whole new turn in my life. I am much healthier now and more outdoorsy. I get more sun and am much more active, more intuitive and much more spiritual.

I wish you well on your path. I am glad *mine* changed.

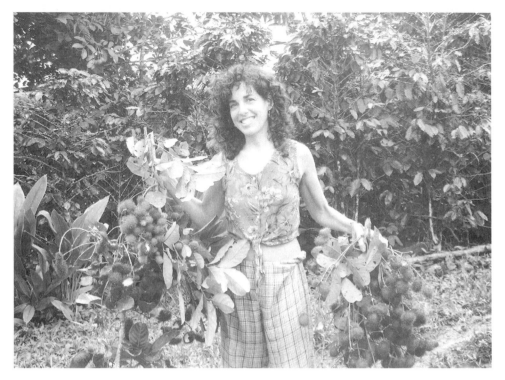

**Amy Schrift in Costa Rica in 2005**

# Amy Schrift: Total Life Makeover

Amy Schrift switched to a 100% raw diet at the age of 37 a couple of years ago [as of 2006]. Within one year, she noticed that her skin became clear and clean of blemishes, and she no longer wore any make-up. There was no longer bloating, gas and discomfort after meals. She no longer had colds, congestion or clogged nasal passages.

She stopped wearing the contact lenses that she had worn for twenty years, and her eyes have improved substantially, from -4.75 to -2.00 in less than two years. Her bowel eliminations improved to the point of effortlessness. She stopped having menstrual bleeding, which is not uncommon among serious raw fooders and is actually a sign of health in a well-nourished female. She experienced greater clarity of mind, peace, calm and feelings of joy and lightness of being. She is the only one who is pain-free of five siblings, all close in age.

Perhaps most of all, however, was the complete change of lifestyle she underwent. Eating raw brought her a sense of yearning to be closer to nature, and she simplified her life to focus on what was really meaningful and important to her.

Amy had lived in New York City, working as a musician performing a lot of gigs in restaurants that reciprocated by giving her free meals. She had begun to observe how she felt after eating various foods and stopped eating bread and pasta, noting the ill effects of wheat.

After reading a magazine article on the raw food diet, she realized this was the way to go and started attending support groups. She initially ate the raw gourmet dishes for that full, "cooked" feeling. Eventually she began to eat lighter and lighter "monomeals," consisting of eating one food at a time and then perhaps a second food later.

She now eats fruit during the day, picked fresh off trees from which she forages when possible, and eats greens and occasional seeds in the evening. "I am basically hydrating myself with my food choices and spend as much time outdoors in the sun and fresh air as possible, which may be our most important sources of nutrition.

"Being raw has made me super aware of my environment, aware of the mind-body-spirit connection. When I eat something, I try to feel the sensations it brings me on all levels."

Many changes took place after Amy switched to a raw diet. She educated herself on how to safely select wild greens, which are high in minerals, and began foraging for wild greens in New York City parks. She noticed that body odor from toxic, cooked food was gone and felt the need to shower less frequently. She started sleeping on the floor, finding it more healthful for the circulation than a mattress. She began brushing her teeth without toothpaste.

She began doing yoga, meditation and sungazing for the first three hours of every morning. Formerly an avid swimmer, she stopped swimming due to the toxic chlorine in pools. She eagerly devoured spiritual books. Despite being a musician, she stopped listening to recorded music so that she could experience deeper levels of silence and the sounds of nature to "tune in rather than tune out."

After her body cleansed, Amy realized that the New York environment was too toxic. She is currently moving to Costa Rica, where she will build her own nontoxic home on some land she bought. There she intends to live a simple life right in the midst of nature.

Amy points out, "I am healthy, not because of what I eat, but in spite of what I eat." She is convinced that eating cooked food and nonfoods is a major cause of illness and that even on a diet solely of raw foods, less is more.

She canceled her health insurance policy. "My health insurance is what I put into my mouth every day. What's yours?" she will ask others. She points out that people will even take a job they do not like just for the health insurance benefits, not realizing that they can take full responsibility for their own health!

Amy's enthusiasm for raw food is quite contagious. She persuaded several members of her extended family to switch to raw eating and has had a positive influence on her young nieces and nephews, who love to tell her how many fruits and vegetables they are eating.

"I'm definitely passionate about extolling the virtues of a healthy, living foods lifestyle. It's not just about the food; it's about rediscovering our earth connection, communing with nature, moving our bodies and getting to the essence of who we really are."

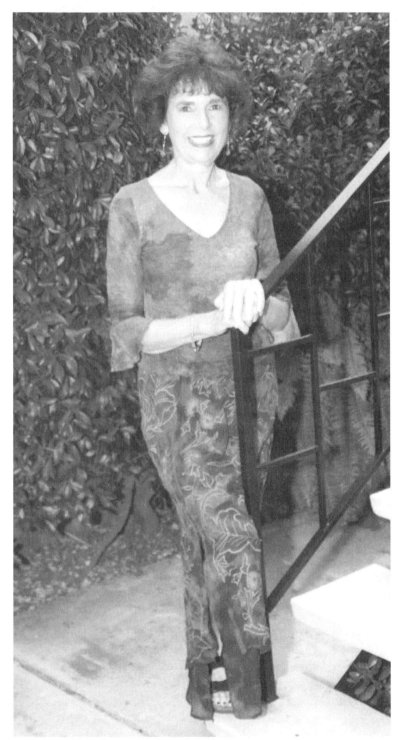

Photo by Joe Peiri

**Sandra Schrift in October 2005**

# Sandra Schrift: Young at 68

Amy's mother Sandra caught on within months. Sandra, who is 68 [in 2006], went raw about 1½ years ago. After she made the switch to 100% raw, she lost 17 pounds, and her stomach flattened. Her osteoarthritis of the knee and hip is greatly reduced. People who hadn't seen her in a while asked what she had been doing differently. Was there a new love in her life? Where did the sparkle and glow come from? She also got the courage to stop wearing make-up. She experienced more energy and a need for less sleep.

As a speaker's coach, Sandra often has to eat out. She has found a simple way to make it work. She calls the chef in advance and asks him to have a dish of uncooked salad and vegetables ready.

In her words, "I have been 95% raw since July 2004. I have more energy, need less sleep and have healthier looking skin. People say I have a glow in my face and eyes. This is a great way to diet. I lost 15 pounds and holding — no more bloat or gas. And mostly, I think I have a way of life that permeates everything I do and how I think about my environment and my community — more gentle and caring."

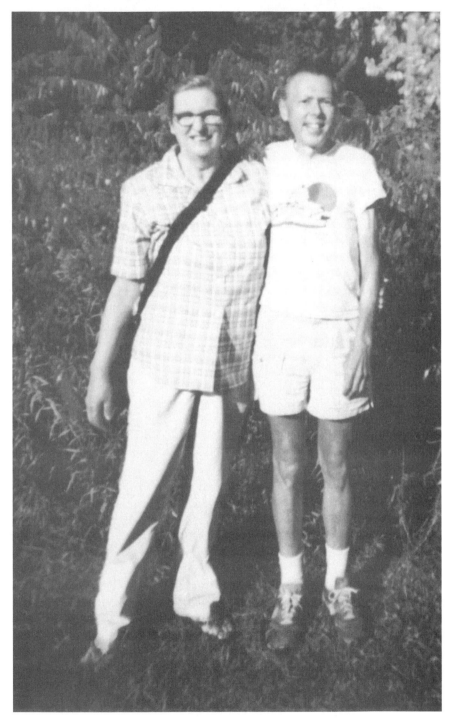

**Jackie Nash preraw in 2003 at age 68**

**with 10-years-raw Bob Avery at age 56**

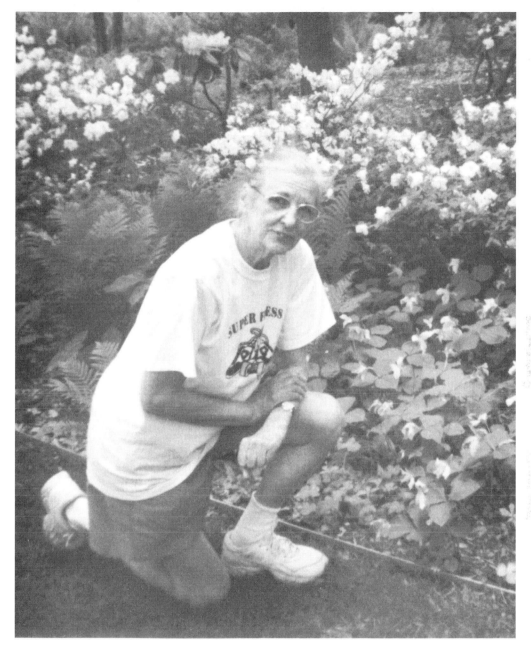

**Jackie Nash in the summer of 2005, after 1 year raw, enjoying the flowers at the Toledo Botanical Garden**

# Jackie Nash: Lost 45 Pounds and Became Active at 69

Prior to giving up cooked food, I was starting to feel my nearly 69 years: my cholesterol was high enough that I was urged to take statins; I could barely climb one flight of stairs without frequent rests, and running for a bus for more than a few yards left me red in the face and fighting for breath.

I was working approximately 30 hours a week, and after a day's work, I could not stay awake past 7 PM. My life consisted mostly of working and sleeping. The heat and humidity of Philadelphia, and then of Toledo, kept me dreading summertime when my energy would drain away in the effort to cool myself.

I started eating raw at the end of April 2004. I weighed in at that time at 165 pounds. Now a year later, eating as much as I wish, I weigh in at *a steady 120 pounds*! My dress size is a 6/8 (formerly 16/18), depending on the vendor. My cholesterol is acceptable to my demanding doctor; climbing stairs is a whole lot easier, and I am able to run for a bus for a considerable distance without any noticeable effect.

Most of the time I have plenty of energy left at the end of the day and am able to engage in whatever activities I wish, even until midnight when I make myself go to bed in preparation for an early morning start.

There have been two problem areas in this transitional period. For several months in the beginning, I was unwell for days at a time from the detoxification to which my body was subjecting me. I survived these periods without resorting to my old dietary habits because I felt so marvelous in between these bouts of misery.

The other downside is that my excess weight fell off me so quickly that my body decided I didn't need all the bone density that had been previously needed to support all the extra toxic tissue. Had I known this in advance, I would have engaged in weight-bearing exercises at the beginning of my raw food adventure.

I am currently attending a gym, under my doctor's orders, and spending an hour four times a week working on the treadmill and also building up my atrophied muscles, their true condition being visible now that there is no fat tissue to hide them, so that they will, in turn, pull on and strengthen the bones they are attached to. I go early in the morning before work and find that the combination of diet and exercise is a powerful source of increased daily energy.

Twenty-five minutes of my gym time is devoted to the treadmill. With all of its wonderful dials before me, I find I am spending most of that time at a fast walk of 4.3 miles per hour and am even starting to jog — half a mile at a time, so far — and am improving rapidly. This is remarkable to me because my bronchial tubes were severely damaged by a serious illness in my late teens, contributing in large part to my lifelong shortness of breath.

It was while pushing myself to jog, alternating in the beginning with 10 steps of jogging to 60 steps of walking, that I felt something deep in my chest give way, and all of a sudden I could take a full breath, something I had not experienced for over 50 years! Sometimes I stop whatever I am doing and inhale deeply, just for the sheer pleasure it gives me to be able to do it. This development, I assure you, would not have occurred had I not been a raw fooder for the previous nine months that led up to it.

Since I did not have any serious or life-threatening physical conditions before April 2004, it is possible that none of the above seems very dramatic. However, the quality of my life has increased immeasurably, even to such a minor effect as not being bothered nearly as much by heat and humidity. Oh, I forgot to say that my persistent minor allergies are either gone or are much improved. I feel mentally much healthier and positive.

For all the reasons above and also because my tastebuds have come back to life, I love my new raw food lifestyle.

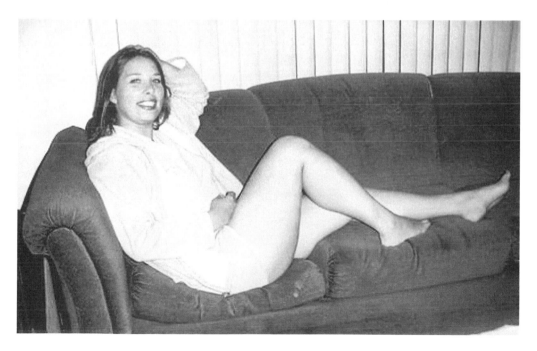

**Paula Wood preraw in June 2003**

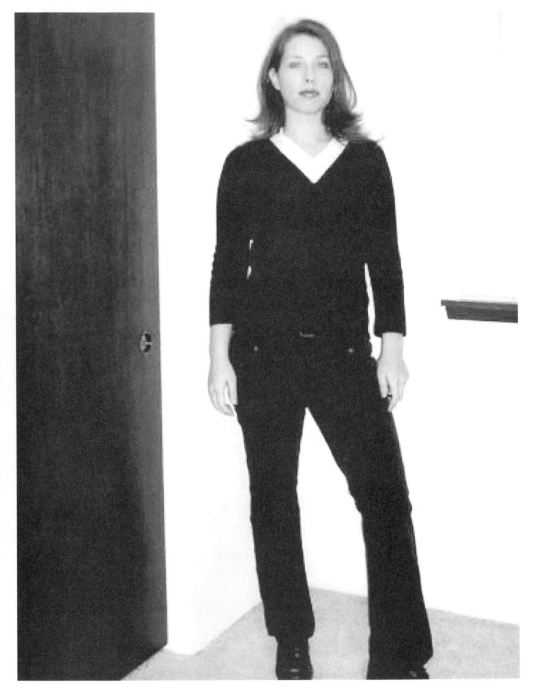

**Paula Wood raw in March 2004**

# Paula Wood: Thyroid
# Removal No Longer Needed

On September 11, 2003, I was diagnosed with cancerous tumors on my thyroid. My naturopath said I needed to have my thyroid removed immediately, possibly followed up with radioactive iodine. I had a surgery scheduled for mid-October.

Finally, about two weeks before the surgery, I told my parents and sister. You see, I didn't want to cause worry until I knew which road I was going to take, as my mother had been diagnosed with breast cancer 6 weeks before my own diagnosis.

As each day passed, and I drew closer to surgery, I became more and more distressed. After spending three days straight crying, I woke the morning of the surgery. I called at 9 AM (1½ hours before surgery, mind you) and canceled. I knew that surgery and a lifetime dependency on hormone medication was not the answer for me. At the time I was aware of no alternatives.

I ended up scheduling a second surgery, which I canceled about one week before the date. The tumor was about the size of a ping-pong ball and very visible to the human eye. I was scared to death.

Finally, I met my health coach (and now very dear friend), Arnoux Goran. Arnoux was a friend of a friend. I knew he taught about raw food. I went to a holiday/New Year's party and, after talking to him, made the decision to do my first cleanse. He agreed to coach me through it.

I began eating 100% raw food and cleansing on January 19, 2004. My first commitment was to eat raw food for the duration of the cleanse and a few weeks afterward.

I did a lot of reading, as suggested by my coach, and had many long talks about nutrients and the way my body should be working. After two weeks, I had committed to six months on raw food. I was *totally loving it*! At the end of the cleanse, I knew I could easily commit to one year of 100% raw food.

I extended the cleanse 9 days, so it was 39 days total. I lost 51 pounds, and the tumor was no longer visible to the naked eye — unless I tilted my head back; then you could see a little knob.

It was so awesome! I have an ultrasound done every three months to measure the progress. I believe that once I purge the underlying emotions that created the dis-ease within my body, the tumor will go away completely!

I am still 100% raw vegan. At this point, I am committed for the rest of my life. It's hard to fathom what I used to put into my body, and I have no desire ever to do that again!

My eleven-year-old son [in 2005] still eats the SAD. I am troubled about this and hope that one day he will see the light, so to speak, and stop being so stubborn. (He gets it from his mom!)

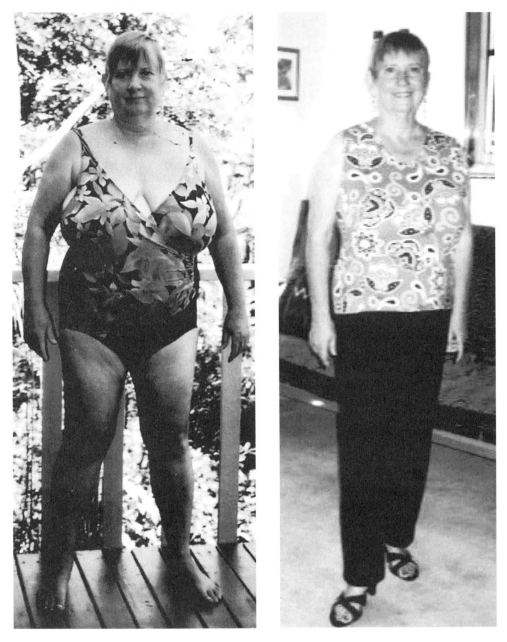

**Samara Christy before and after switching to a raw diet**

# Samara Christy: Lost Weight, yet No Surgery Needed for Loose Skin

My name is Samara Christy. I am age 57 [in 2005]. I have been, like many others, overweight for most of my life. As I got older, my inability to lose weight got increasingly worse. I would try diet after diet with my friends. They would lose 30-40 pounds, and I would lose about ten. Then in a few months, I would return to my original weight, and then over a period of about six months, I would gain an additional ten to twenty pounds.

What made matters worse was that I had been a health care practitioner for more than 25 years, and I was truly embarrassed and humiliated by my inability to lose weight. My heart would break when my clients, all meaning to be helpful, would hand me yet another diet to try. In retaliation, I threatened to wear to the healing center my super size tee shirt over my 200-lb-plus body that said, "I fought anorexia and won."

I often made jokes about my weight in an attempt to cover up my pain. When my fiancé, now husband, Ken and I were first dating, he took me on a wonderful vacation to Puerto Vallarta. We had a wonderful time as we sat on the beach and sipped margaritas and watched the sun set so magnificently, as only Puerto Vallarta is famous for. I was in love. As my fiancé and I looked dreamily into each other's eyes while we ate our sumptuous dinners, I shared my concerns that what we were eating was more than I usually ate and that I would probably gain weight on this trip. Ken looked at me incredulously and blurted out, "That's impossible!"

You see, to support me in losing weight, we would order one lunch or one dinner and ask for another plate so that we could split our meal. In fact we would split all our meals on that trip. Because I did not speak the language, and Ken spoke enough Spanish, we agreed that he would carry all the cash and pay for everything. So my fiancé knew everything that I ate because he was the only one with the money to buy anything.

When we returned from our vacation, we both weighed in on our first morning home. He had lost eight pounds, and my worst fears had been realized; I had gained five. My fiancé apologized to me, saying that he had a confession to make — that all those nights that we were dating and that we had been splitting our meals, he had just assumed that I must have been eating when I went home from our dates.

Ouch! That really hurt! Don't get me wrong. My fiancé truly loved me in spite of my weight, but unless you have lived it, you don't fully understand it.

Finally, I just gave up (see photo) and resigned myself that this was going to be my fate. I still continued to pray, "God, you have had an answer for everything else in my life, why not the weight? There just has got to be an answer — somewhere!"

Soon, a group of clients started coming to me, many of them, like me, over fifty and overweight. This group was in a ten-week program, and they all lost about 25-30 pounds in three months. Well, that really got my attention. I wanted to meet this guy who taught that class. His name is Arnoux. He may be contacted at www.thmastery.com.

He was 27 years old at the time and looked about nineteen. I began having second thoughts. What could this kid teach me? Then I remembered my wonderfully thin clients. I immediately arranged to meet with him.

Arnoux shared with me the amazing story of how he had come to embrace this program. It was hard to imagine that this handsome, articulate man/boy was born to deaf parents who were drug addicts. As a result of their drug addition, Arnoux's health was seriously compromised. Though he was never overweight, he shared with me that his doctors didn't give him long to live.

As Arnoux went from doctor to doctor, desperately looking for help, he finally discovered the raw food program and went on to heal every single one of his many ailments. Then he went on to teach what he knew to help others by creating the "How God Eats" course and making himself available as a raw food coach. His clients began to get radiantly healthy, and his hopelessly overweight and over-fifty women began to lose weight and to keep it off.

Arnoux asked me to trust him, so I decided to give his program a try. After all, what did I have to lose? — about eighty pounds to be exact. So I plunged headlong into the world of raw foods. To my shock, I too lost ten pounds the very first month.

What happened next was even more amazing. My energy level just shot through the roof! My food before, though healthy, had left me feeling tired all the time. I know that experts preach that exercise is key, but how do you exercise when you barely have enough energy to get though your day?

After a month on raw foods, I had energy to burn. I began going to Curves, where at first I could only get halfway around their circuit. Six months into raw foods, the Curves's owner offered me a job there, telling me that people were asking when I worked out because they found me supportive and inspiring, and they wanted to work out with me.

To my delight, the raw foods program worked. I lost 50 pounds in the first 5½ months, and I am still losing. I am 5'4", and I had weighed 213 pounds. I weighed 163 pounds when the after picture was taken. Not only did I lose the weight, but I am also in glowing health. To my amazement, the loose skin that many women who have lost a lot of weight have to have surgically removed didn't happen to me or to any of the other raw fooders that I met. We are all living proof that all the enzymes in raw foods completely change your skin to yummy.

Arnoux also has several techniques designed to handle the emotional reasons people can't lose weight. These techniques are contained in the complete package, "The Total Health and Weight-Loss Package."

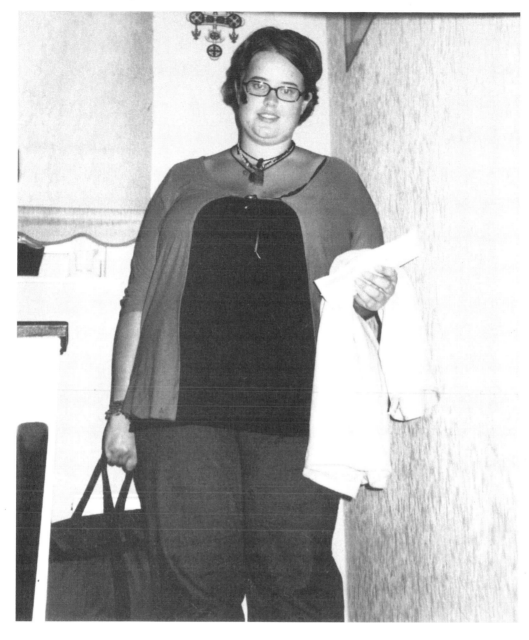

**Angela Stokes in August 2001**

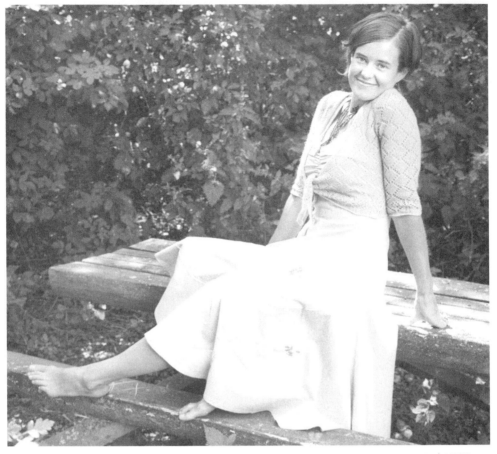

Photo by Karen Kessi-Williams

**Angela Stokes in August 2005**

# Angela Stokes: From Morbid Obesity to a New Life with Raw Foods

Just a few years ago, I weighed 294 pounds (21 stone/133 kg) and was depressed, lonely and constantly ill. These days [in 2005], after moving over to a mainly raw vegan diet since May 2002, I weigh in at a healthy and happy 135 pounds (9 stone 9 pounds, or 62 kg) for my 5'7" frame, and my life has been completely transformed.

I have lost more than half of my body weight over the last 3½ years, but my transformation has been remarkable on more than just the physical level. At the emotional and spiritual levels too, my recovery on this path has been extraordinary.

60

I frequently feel as if I am "talking about a different person" when I reflect on my life as a morbidly obese person. Things have changed in so many ways, from the little details like being able to see and feel my rib bones again to the freedom this lifestyle has brought me from isolation and living in serious denial of how much I was damaging myself.

I was not always overweight. I was a very active child and the fastest runner in my school at the age of ten. My problems began when, at the age of 11, I developed an underactive thyroid and began to gain weight. The weight gain escalated with uncontrolled overeating such that a decade later, at the age of 21, I found myself weighing in at nearly 300 pounds.

I lived in a bubble of total denial about my weight. I would not discuss the issue with anyone and showed no interest in diets or weight loss. My preraw diet consisted of enormous quantities of chocolate, fried foods, stodgy carbohydrates and greasy fats.

Everything changed the night a friend lent me a book on raw foods, and since then I have never looked back. I realized immediately that this was the answer I had always been waiting for and went 100% raw overnight. During the first year alone, I lost over 100 pounds of excess fat.

In January 2004, I set up my popular testimonial web site, www.rawreform. com, to share my message of hope with others. The response ever since has been phenomenally heart-warming, as others are inspired to lose weight naturally too and reclaim their own health on this path.

I have recently finished a book about weight loss on raw foods, which will be published soon. I also offer consultations for those who would like personal support to lose weight naturally and simply with raw foods.

Furthermore, I provide a free e-newsletter to subscribers, and my web site hosts a forum where a growing community of like-minded individuals share experiences and build networks.

I walk my talk, and my "before" and "after" photos speak for themselves. I am a living example of the healing power of raw foods and am uniquely qualified to carry this message of health to others who currently struggle with obesity and overeating.

I sum up my transformation on raw foods in the following way: I may now be half the person physically that I was before going raw, but I am so much more myself in every other way.

I am delighted to share my experience and hope with others.

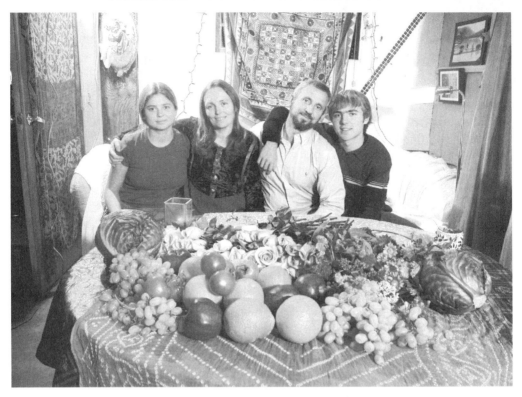

**The all-raw Boutenko family sit prepared for a feast at their home in Oregon: Valya, Victoria, Igor, and Sergei.**

# The Boutenkos: Raw Family

May I introduce you to my raw family, dear readers? Above, you see my husband Igor, our two children Valya and Sergei and me. Today, we are healthy and happy, but that was not the case not so very many years ago.

When we immigrated to the United States from Russia in 1989, I considered myself to be not very fat. I was 180 pounds, a "normal" Russian woman. The food supply in Russia had been simple, less processed, less refined, less filled with chemicals.

When I visited my very first American supermarket and saw all those multi-colored boxes and packages, I told my husband that I wanted to try them all. And I think I did! In two short years, I gained 100 pounds. We had opened a success-ful business, bought a big house and went out every night to every fancy or ex-otic restaurant in Denver and the suburbs for our eating entertainment.

From that kind of "full" life — I'd rather say *fool* life — I developed serious health problems. I was diagnosed with the same disease that took my father: arrhythmia, or an irregular heartbeat. My legs were constantly swollen from edema, and my veins were popping out. I weighed 280 pounds, and I was continuously gaining more. My left arm frequently became numb at night. Upon falling asleep at bedtime, I never knew if I would awaken to the next morning or not. I began fearing that I would die and that my children would become orphans. I remember always feeling tired and depressed.

In addition, my husband developed progressive hyperthyroidism and chronic rheumatoid arthritis. Our daughter Valya came down with asthma and allergies, and our son Sergei developed diabetes.

While the simpler Russian foods gave us a degree of good health, the American smorgasbord, in which we had all been willingly indulging, was killing us off!

My doctor told me that I absolutely had to lose weight if I wanted to reverse my situation. I signed up for a lifetime membership at a health club but never found time to go there again. I subscribed to *Weight Watchers Magazine* and had wonderful fantasies of being slim and well while reading through the issues. Then I went to the Slim·Fast workshop. Soon, I signed up for another popular weight-loss program. I got an itchy rash from eating their special food, but I didn't lose a single ounce. As a result of all the wishful thinking and these failures, I began to fall into a deep depression.

In 1993, all of a sudden, my son Sergei was diagnosed with diabetes and was told to go on insulin. This terrible event really shook me up and awakened me from my lethargy! My grandmother had just died from an insulin overdose. Being afraid to put Sergei on insulin for fear he might repeat her tragedy, I began desperately searching for an alternative solution. That was how I was inspired to discover a better way. It came in the form of a raw food lifestyle.

My husband, our two youngest children and I have been eating a raw food only diet since January 1994, more than thirteen years. We went cold turkey overnight. We emptied our kitchen of cooked foods and brought in the raw. By turning off the pilot in our stove and discontinuing all cooking, we provided the perfect environment and support system for our bodies to heal themselves of all of our so-called incurable, life-threatening diseases. During these healing miracles, we began to experience a lot more energy and began running every day.

Our health was improving so quickly that in three and a half months, all four of us ran the Bolder Boulder 10-K road race with the 40,000 other runners. In one year, I gradually lost 120 pounds, my depression vanished, and I felt happy all the time. Even Sergei's blood sugar stabilized due to his new diet and regular jogging. Since beginning to eat raw food, he has never again experienced any form of diabetic symptoms. We were greatly surprised and totally delighted not only by how quickly our health was restored to normal, but by how much healthier we were than ever before!

However, after approximately seven years of being 100% raw fooders, each one of us began to feel that we had reached a plateau at which our healing processes had stopped and from which they had even begun going backwards somewhat. More and more often, we started feeling discontent with our existing all-raw food program. I began to have a heavy feeling in my stomach after eating almost any kind of raw food, especially a vegetable salad with dressing. Because of that, I started to eat fewer greens and vegetables and more fruits and nuts. I actually began to gain weight on raw foods! My husband started to develop a lot of gray hair.

My family members felt confused about our diet and seemed often to have the question, "What should we eat?" There were odd times when we felt hungry but did not desire any foods that were "legal" for us to eat on a typical raw food diet: fruits, nuts, seeds, grains and/or dried fruit. Vegetable salads with dressings were delicious but left us tired and sleepy. We felt trapped. I remember Igor looking inside the fridge, saying over and over again, "I wish I wanted some of this stuff."

Such periods of indifference did not last. We blamed it all on overeating and were able to refresh our appetites by fasts, exercise, hikes, new recipes or by working more. In my family, we strongly believe that raw food is the only way to go. Therefore, we encouraged each other to maintain our raw diet no matter what, always coming up with new tricks.

Many of my friends told me about similar experiences, at which point they gave up being 100% raw and began to add cooked food back into their meals. In my family, we continued to stay on raw food due to our constant support of each other, but there was no doubt about it — we had plateaued.

A question in my heart burned brighter with each passing day, "Is there anything missing in our diet?"

The answer would always come back right away, "Nope. Nothing could be better than a raw food diet."

Yet however tiny, the unwanted signs of less-than-perfect health kept surfacing in minor but noticeable symptoms, such as a wart on a hand or a gray hair that brought doubts and questions about the completeness of the raw food diet in its present form. Finally, when my children complained about the increased sensitivity of their teeth, I reached a state where I couldn't think about anything besides this health puzzle. I was bewildered. I drove everybody around me crazy with my constant discussions and questioning, "What could possibly be missing?"

In my eager quest, I started collecting data about every single food that existed for humans. After many wrong guesses, I finally found the correct answer. I identified one particular food group that matched all nutritional needs for humans: *greens*. The truth was that in my family, we had not been eating enough greens. The more I read about the nutritional content of greens, the more I became convinced that greens were the most important food for humans and the missing link in our diets between good health and great health!

I began wishing I could find a way to enjoy the many kinds of greens enough to consume the optimal quantity needed to become perfectly healthy. This is when I discovered I could "chew" my greens up in the Vita-Mix. After some brainstorming, I liquefied kale leaves with a couple of bananas and water. This drink was pleasantly delicious! The sweetness of the fruit took the edge off the sometimes bitter, sometimes bland, sometimes unpleasantly strong taste of the greens of choice. I called the wonderful beverage a *green smoothie*. The solution to my greens dilemma was so unexpectedly simple! To consume greens in this way took so little time that I naturally continued experimenting with a variety of blended greens and fruits day after day.

My husband and both children have enjoyed including green smoothies in their daily menus too even though they were already experiencing what could only be called *great* health in comparison to their health at its worst. They all noticed still more benefits beyond their raw food plateaus, such as the need for less sleep, more complete eliminations, stronger nails and more mental and physical energy.

After about a month of green smoothie drinking on and off, I began to feel more energized than ever before! I noticed that many of the wrinkles on my face had gone away, and I began hearing compliments from other people about my *fresh look*! My nails grew stronger. My vision sharpened. I had a wonderful taste in my mouth, even upon waking in the morning, a pleasure I hadn't enjoyed since youth.

I now consume plenty of greens in the form of green smoothies every day. I have lost unwanted pounds, my weight has normalized again, and my tastes have changed. Plain fruits and vegetables have become much more desirable, and my cravings for the raw foods high in fats — avocados, nuts and seeds — have declined dramatically. I feel light and full of energy.

I now strongly believe that the optimal diet for humans consists of raw food with a strong emphasis on fresh greens in their many forms: as leafy greens, as edible weeds and herbs and as sprouts.

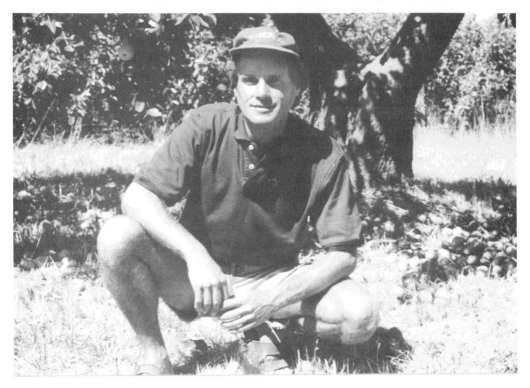

**David Klein at age 39**

# Dr. David Klein, PhD: Healing Ulcerative Colitis

Growing up in New Jersey in the 1960s, I lived a fairly typical American childhood up until 1975 when my previously robust health began to fail. A heavy eater of meat and junk food as a youth, I saw my physical and mental energies gradually deteriorate over a period of six months at age 17. Incessant diarrhea followed. A few weeks of medical treatment showed little improvement, so a colon examination was done. The diagnosis was ulcerative colitis. I spent my 18th birthday in a hospital taking prednisone and Azulfidine drug treatments. The symptoms subsided temporarily, but the drugs further ruined my health and had a devastating effect on my mental abilities.

Still feeling sickly and very weak, I experienced within a few months a recurrence of the diarrhea along with additional symptoms, including cramping and bleeding, that led to further physical deterioration. What then ensued were eight tortuous years of colitis flare-ups with off and on drug therapy. At age 26, I was reduced to a weak, sickly shadow of my former self. I was having gastric explosions every time I ate and up to ten painful bowel movements a day with mucus and blood. My nervous system became shattered by toxicity due to debilitating medications and severe demineralization.

My life became a dying hell, but I never gave in to the medical doctors' advice to just accept my illness and be patient until their impossible "miracle cure" came along. I desperately wanted my health back and doubted that the doctors knew what they were doing.

In 1984, I had the great fortune to find on Staten Island a doctor of Natural Hygiene, Laurence Galant, who introduced me to the concepts of self-healing and eating a raw, fruit-based diet. At first I thought the idea of eating mostly fruit while I was having nonstop diarrhea was crazy, yet I studied Natural Hygiene and slowly cleaned up my diet. However, I was still attached to eating chicken and other favorite cooked foods and continued to have colitis flare-ups and rely on medications.

In the fall of 1984, I had a colonoscopy exam that confirmed that I had advanced ulcerations throughout my sick colon. Surmising that I had been chronically sick, was not getting better and would eventually face cancer, the gastroenterologist recommended that I either try an experimental drug that knocks out the immune system or have my colon surgically removed. Upon hearing this, I had a heavy, decisive thought: "I have had it with this medical madness. I'll be dead soon if I don't find the answer myself!" I recognized that my life had been a gradual descent into hell that I had to climb out of right now because it was almost too late.

Over the next few days, I started focusing like never before on how to overcome my illness. I realized that I had to figure out what the MDs could not. My thinking led me to consider more closely the information on self-healing and switching to a vegan diet. The information seemed quite incredible, but I saw that it was really working for Laurence. I had also read many amazing healing testimonials.

Then one amazing night while studying T. C. Fry's Life Science/Natural Hygiene course, I beheld a healing vision. It suddenly all made sense: the picture of my new health was revealed via the Natural Hygiene healthful living system. I understood that humans are biologically fruit eaters and that fruit was the best food for my sick colon and my entire body. I was ecstatic knowing that this knowledge would set me free!

The next day, I threw away the medicines, divorced myself from all medical intervention for good, gave up all meat and dairy forever and started a three-day cleanse on fresh juices made from raw fruits and vegetables. By the second day, I was coming back to life. On the third day, I was feeling better and better. My enthusiasm and joy drove my family crazy! My gut was feeling soothed, and I was rejuvenating. I set myself free of illness, doctors and medicines for good, and my bowels were working better and better!

I adopted a fruit-based diet, which harmonized best with my mind/body/spirit. With that, my energies continually increased as I detoxified and began rebuilding. Within about six weeks, I felt that my colon was completely healed. I was able to enjoy eating and living again. With my bowels functioning better than ever, I began a new, healthful lifestyle.

Over the next few years, I diligently worked at rebuilding my depleted body, incorporating daily running and yoga, all the while studying the life sciences and all of the physical, mental, emotional and spiritual factors which determine our health. It took several years of total dedication to build robust health.

The serious health challenge I had experienced radically changed the course of my life, propelling me into the health education field that became my life's passion.

In 1993, after a year of study and training at the Institute for Educational Therapy in Cotati, California (now known as Bauman College in Penngrove, California), I became a certified Nutrition Educator and began providing nutrition and healing consultations. In 1996, I started the Living Nutrition Health Education Center, *Living Nutrition* magazine (now *Vibrance*) and the Colitis & Crohn's Health Recovery Center in Sebastopol in northern California.

In 2008, I changed the name of the magazine to *Vibrance*; it is the most widely circulated raw food lifestyle periodical in the world. My best-selling book *Self-Healing Colitis and Crohn's* has just been printed in an expanded, new edition. I have written the booklet "The Art of Rejuvenation," authored the book *Your Natural Diet: Alive Raw Foods* with Dr. T. C. Fry as a posthumous coauthor, and counseled over 1,000 clients from crippling inflammatory bowel disease to new health.

Today, at age 50, I enjoy excellent, dynamic health and vitality. I teach people that healing is easy if we understand and apply the principle that it is the body that does the healing. When we remove the unhealthful aspects of our diets and lifestyles and step out of the way, our bodies will do the healing work automatically and naturally. I happily assert that living healthfully is the easiest and most joyful way to be. I am glad to help health seekers get there and feel that for themselves.

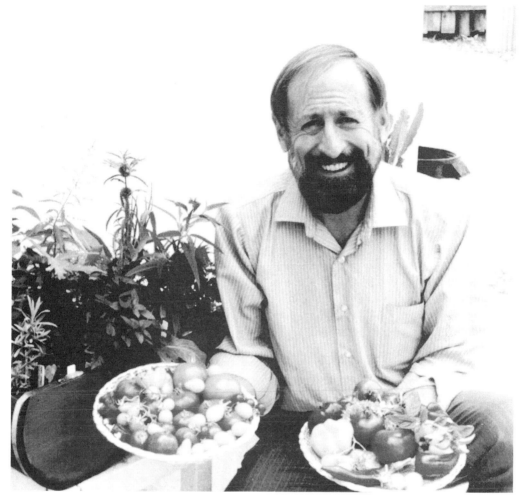

**Ric Lambart displays his hospitality at a family gathering in Leucadia, California, near San Diego in 2006.**

# Ric Lambart: 32 Years Raw

I got into raw foods via the back door. My long research into nutrition was initially undertaken not because of my own poor health, but because my first child, Patric, was not expected to live even his first year of life. Before his birth, my wife and I were worse than SAD eaters, being caught up in the epicurean practices of gourmet cooking and eating. Patric was afflicted with severe physical anomalies, including the blue baby syndrome, the variant with immediately life-threatening consequences. All of the many "experts" said that nothing could be done except to keep him isolated from any sort of germs or other contamination lest he get a cold and die, since his heart wasn't able to supply him with sufficient oxygen.

So, in search of a way outside of what medicine could do (nothing), I delved into the connection between nutrition and disease — something the medical "experts" claimed would be futile because medicine's generally rock-solid position in those days, the 1960s, was that there was simply no connection between what we ate and our health. To propose otherwise was tantamount to medical "quackery."

In short, I discovered that an extremely crucial connection did exist and that conventional nutritional information and education were almost as flawed and unscientific as was medicine itself. Its literature has been developed primarily from questionable "research," research very often conducted as the consequence of funding from the major food processing industrial giants. This fundamental conflict of interest provided very shallow and self-serving study results for anyone interested in truly finding out what real world nutrition was all about.

Further research and observations of wild animal life, which was virtually devoid of disease, brought me to the shocking and devastating conclusion that cooking food was absolutely insane — no less than a slow, "civilized" road to mass suicide. Consequently, I was able to establish that the medical authorities and "experts" were all wrong since my handicapped son remained alive and developed extraordinarily well on a strict, "healthful" (no junk foods), largely raw diet.

I also discovered that animal product consumption, particularly cooked meat, was extremely dangerous and often injurious to humans for a host of reasons. Accordingly, my family and I switched to a vegetarian lifestyle. This made me and my, by then, three children quite happy since they all loved animals and were greatly relieved to discover that it was not only not necessary to kill and eat them, but that consuming them could actually be injurious to human — and environmental — health.

Although I was soon convinced that raw foods were the only sensible foodstuffs, I wasn't quite ready to give up my cooked gourmet vegetarian fare, thereby uncovering another problem: the severely addictive nature of cooked foods. It took me almost five years to finally, totally and *permanently* stop eating dead foods. My youngest son, Eric, had started his life out right by eating only raw from day one, so he obviously never had cooked food addictions to break, as did the rest of us.

Patric was tragically killed in 1973 at only 8½, but his needs had now revealed too much truth about real health maintenance and recovery, so my daughter Catherine and I joined young Eric and went all-raw in 1976. Patric's untimely death led to a divorce in that same year, and I remarried a year later.

By the time we went all-raw, I'd concluded that supplements just weren't what we were created to be taking, so we dropped using any of them, trying instead to obtain whatever nutrients our bodies needed, including vitamins and minerals, from the food alone that we ate.

I did conclude, though, that it was essential not to mono-diet on only the few foods we liked, but to make a concerted effort to maintain a very broad spectrum of different foods in our diet. The reason behind this, since no one really knew exactly what we needed and when it was needed, was to provide a statistically sound parameter, one that would permit our biological needs to be met on a continuous basis — whatever those needs might actually be.

In short, common logic seemed to dictate the critical importance of keeping a wide range of foods on the menu. Some have called it Ric's "shotgun" approach, but that's okay since it correctly conveyed exactly what we were doing.

I would like to add, however, that while we did okay without supplementation, as have many others, not everyone seems able to do this, particularly when it comes to Vitamin $B_{12}$.

Kathy Ryan, my second wife, became Catherine and Eric's stepmother. Kathy was a fabulous woman with a diverse background: from being a UAL Flight Attendant Supervisor, to a worker in Laos and Cambodia with the Tom Dooley Foundation, to an MBA grad who became the first woman to break into the executive ranks of the Arizona Bank, to a tireless worker and financial consultant to food co-ops in Arizona, to finally a CPA.

Before I even met Kathy, she had been given only a few years to live from an *always* fatal, rare liver disease called Budd-Chiari syndrome. Once it is diagnosed, the prognosis is for 1½-3 years at the most before death. I met her almost two years after she'd been diagnosed, so she had less than a year to live. The medical experts had said in 1972 that there was nothing they could do for her. Aware of my work with nutrition, a client of mine who knew her suggested I meet her and try some nutritional approaches to her dilemma.

I worked with Kathy and first eased her into vegetarian eating in 1974. This seemed to improve her condition markedly. Next, I recommended raw foods and vegan living as well. She continued to improve. When her time to die was up, she seemed in better health than when we'd met. She went all-raw in 1976, the same year my children and I did. We married in 1977.

She continued to improve, but our place in California burned in a wild brush fire in 1982. This was horrendously stressful for her and seemed to knock down her otherwise vibrant health. Next, a visit to Arizona four years later for a bank employee reunion banquet saw her accidentally get some forbidden foods (dairy) into her system. She quickly became violently ill. We couldn't move her or even get back to California for four more days.

When we did get back home, she was still very weak and run-down, but she had a client company that was about to go bankrupt unless she could get their books in order to obtain a bank loan before their deadline. Unfortunately, she continued to work days without any sleep while still ill. She saved the company but lost her life.

Kathy collapsed and began to hemorrhage internally from the liver. She made me promise not to take her to the hospital. She died in my arms at home, but at only 44 years of age. This was some 14 years after having been told to put her life and affairs in order because she was supposed to have died by 1976 — at the latest.

While working all night at the client company in Santa Monica, California, she had stimulated herself to keep awake by munching on nuts, which she was not supposed to do. She had almost no tolerance for nuts at all. They simply destroyed her remaining good liver tissue.

In short, the dietary changes that culminated in the raw vegan diet gave her another 12 years of vibrant life. Had she been more careful and not so overdedicated and hardworking, I am sure she would have continued to live for many more years. The autopsy pathologist recognized the Budd-Chiari syndrome despite its rarity, saw the damaged and tumor-ridden liver and marveled at how amazingly healthy looking the rest of her body and organs were for her age.

Meanwhile, I have stuck to being all-raw, with benefits beyond description. Gone are my aches, pains, arthritis, gout, ulcers, cardiovascular disease, benign tumors (re-absorbed) and persistent lifelong allergies. I even seemed to grow younger, per remarks from friends, and became far more energetic than in my earlier years when I'd been an athlete in college.

Eric and Catherine grew up without the usual childhood diseases, with no need for doctors except for accidents (broken bones from falls jumping their horses) and without the typical "immunizations" experienced by their young friends, who regularly seemed to get ill despite their vaccinations.

I was able to work mostly from home and raise the children, home-schooling them in order to provide them with superior educational opportunities. That toughest, most challenging — and exciting — time of my life resulted in Catherine's entrance into college at 13 and Eric's at 9. Both graduated with honors. I genuinely believe that the exposure to such a healthy diet significantly benefited their mental evolution, not just their physical development. I'd submit that if the body's physical well-being can be substantially enhanced by way of an optimally healthy diet, then why not the brain's as well? Isn't it but another of our physical organs?

The home education also had another benefit in that it didn't immerse them in the "normal" cultural educational experience, which I felt too often tended to be mind-numbing, too easily leading to adverse peer pressure to conform rather than think independently, or "outside the box." I had attended an Ivy League college myself and felt that much of what I learned there actually tended to cripple my creativity and ability to think independently, to approach problems in new and unique ways.

I also made sure that my children were exposed to the manual arts, disciplines too often neglected in higher education, where the principal emphasis is on academics. Both Catherine and Eric were avid young equestrian competitors, so they encountered a great deal of social interaction with children of their own ages. Being so unusually young during their early college years also enhanced their ability to relate well to older people since their fellow students were of course actually adults.

Both of them first soloed an airplane (sailplane) at the minimum age of 14 and additionally became enthusiastic motorcycle and tennis buffs as well as accomplished sailors, scuba divers, and Catherine, a wind-surfer. Since they were raised in a rural setting much of the time, they didn't have the problem of prying and meddling nearby neighbors who might have otherwise objected to their being out of "normal" school and eating so strangely — without even a stove in their home.

I always caution against focusing exclusively on the goal of raw nutrition because it can too easily lead one to ignore the many other essentials of a productive life. I strongly suggest that it always be kept in mind that while sound health cannot be achieved without intelligent eating, we should always do our best to remain focused on how we can best use the resulting superior health to accomplish the most with our other gifts in life. In other words, exclusive raw food consumption merely enables us to be optimally free to realize our other unique personal gifts and potentials.

In short, I would invite you to consider that raw foodism not be the goal in one's life but rather the means by which to maximize our personal potential to make our life as meaningful and constructive as possible. After all, this is not very easily done when continuously impaired, or threatened, by illness and disease.

The famed German philosopher Hegel observed about 200 years ago, "Perfect freedom is perfect obedience to perfect law." I grasped the profoundly universal logic and truth of that observation as it pertains to the political sphere and subsequently postulated it into the health arena, to wit: since nature's laws are perfection, how can we expect to realize the freedom of optimal health unless we are willing to obey nature's sublimely perfect laws that pertain to such health?

Thus it was that my now-familiar dictum came into being:

## Raw Is Law!

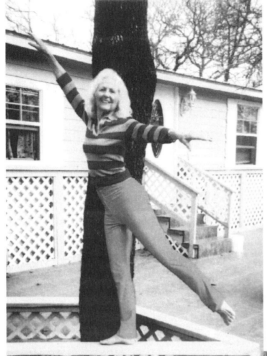

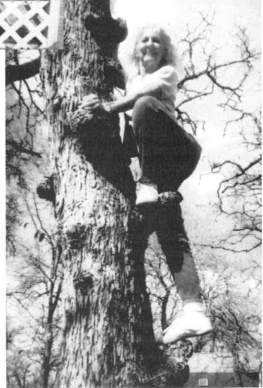

**High in the Texas hill country, Dr. Vetrano — at a playful age 80 — delights in superlative health and Hygiene euphoria.**

# Dr. Vetrano, hMD, DC, PhD, DSci, and Natural Hygiene

Naturally, I began reviewing my life story when Victoria BidWell asked me to answer the question, "What has Natural Hygiene done for you?"

Suddenly, a picture of the famous Bernarr Macfadden speaking at one of the yearly American Natural Hygiene Society conventions flashed through my mind. He was 80 years old at the time and just as handsome as he was when he was a young bodybuilder. His hair was white, fluffy and beautifully thick. I was impressed at his electrifying vitality and charisma, being that of a much younger person. It was amazing to learn that he had just parachuted out of an airplane by himself, making a beautiful, controlled landing. Macfadden was a good example of having lived hygienically. That kept him healthy and vital throughout his life.

I marveled to myself, "I want to be like that when I am 80 years old!" Then I'd look at myself in the mirror. Facing me was a chubby young woman with the shape of a pear, skinny on top and overloaded on the bottom. The question in my mind was, "How can I get rid of the fat thighs and hips?" Fruits alone were not helping, so I had to teach myself to like vegetables and vegetable salads.

I graduated from high school weighing 120 pounds at only 5'2" tall. Finally, I got down to 102 pounds. I looked and felt marvelous! I had more energy and endurance than ever: my enthusiasm for life and living was soaring! It was a natural, healthy, hygienic "high"! I still have that today at the age of 80!

At that time, I was only on the threshold of the wonderful world of Natural Hygiene. From what I had already read, I deduced that its teachings were genuine truths, so I did not hesitate one second to change my lifestyle and diet completely. I was like a sponge soaking up every detail while reading and rereading all of Dr. Shelton's books.

I did not become a hygienist because I was sick. I got sick after I was already living hygienically. Becoming a hygienic doctor did me in: the stress factor was the culprit. I was the type of person who had to make straight A's and would become angry when I missed even one question on exams. At chiropractic school, we were graded by numbers. If I did not make 100 on every test, I became terribly upset. I studied every minute of the day, even taking *Gray's Anatomy* to the circus when I took my daughter, where I watched and studied at the same time. Nevertheless, I always went to bed early, but I got up at 3 AM on test days to review the material before going to school. The eight years of college greatly enervated me. I was already uptight, stressed out and exhausted when I received my BSc degree from Trinity University. Yet I still had four more years of chiropractic college to do, and that included summer sessions.

I graduated from the Texas Chiropractic College summa cum laude in 1965, took the state board exam, and then dove right in to manage Dr. Shelton's Health School because he had to retire. I had finished my education, but now I had to learn how to manage a health school! With the added stress of taking on a new job and having to learn management, proofreading and all the other responsibilities concomitant to running an institution and keeping *Dr. Shelton's Hygienic Review* going, I began to have stomach problems.

I could eat absolutely nothing without pain in my upper abdomen. Watermelon wouldn't even stay down. I'd get nauseated and vomit. After a day's work, I'd wake up at night with extreme pain in the abdomen, also causing vomiting. Often, I had to check the guests when my stomach felt like knives were making hamburger meat out of my insides. I knew that I needed more rest. However, supervising an average of 20, and many times 50, fasters on any given day, I ended up being on call 24 hours a day and working 16 hours a day, 7 days a week.

Nevertheless, I arranged to get away every afternoon from 1:00 to 2:30 PM. I would take a short sunbath and lie down for the rest of the time. I'd go home as early as possible and be in bed before 9 PM. I finally had to take Sundays off. I would stay in bed the whole day, sometimes fasting. This lifestyle kept me going, but it delayed the recovery of my health. Then several unjust lawsuits were filed against Dr. Shelton, the health school and me. That was cataclysmic, stressing me out still more.

Later on, something else happened that worsened my condition tremendously. While riding double on a big horse with my granddaughter, a truck frightened the horse. He pitched, bucked, twisted and circled like a wild bronco. We both fell off, me first. Then she toppled onto me. I knew I had a fracture the moment I hit the ground from the pain and the crack I heard. It was an impacted fracture of my left humerus (upper arm) bone. Therefore, I did not have to wear a cast. I was able to bathe and move the arm after a week. The orthopedist said the broken arm would be shorter than the other one and that I would have limited range of motion for the rest of my life. I was determined to avoid these handicaps. So, as soon as I could, I exercised the arm and shoulder, stretching the injured arm up as far as the other could go. Now you can't tell which one was broken. They both are the same length and have the same range of motion.

Shortly after being thrown off the horse, a more serious part of the accident happened on my fifth day of a fast. After going to bed, I felt nauseated and lay there hoping it would subside. Suddenly, the nausea became a strong urge to vomit, causing me to leap out of bed and run to the bathroom barely in time before the vomitus came surging out. I vomited two or more quarts of pure red blood. Not wanting a blood transfusion, I did not go to the hospital. I fasted and rested in bed, knowing that a clot would form in the blood vessel and the bleeding would stop, which it did.

After becoming stronger and wanting to know the status of my red blood cells, I had blood tests done that showed that I was anemic. It took a year before the number of red blood cells became normal. My digestion was not good before the hemorrhage, and it was even worse after. From the symptoms and localization of the pain, I determined I had two peptic ulcers, one in the pyloric region of the stomach and one in the duodenum.

A year or two later, I went to see a hygienic doctor to rest and get blood tests. I left the place very quickly because I could not eat what was served. Pure or diluted carrot juice was about all my stomach would tolerate, and I could drink no more than about four ounces at a time. Later on, through the grapevine, I heard that this doctor had intimated that I had cancer of the stomach and that I would not be around very long. Well, I am not six feet under yet! I celebrated my 80th birthday during the 2007 Thanksgiving season! I definitely gave thanks to the awesome intelligence that created this marvelous body that heals itself no matter how damaged or sick it may become!

Natural Hygiene's teachings have always helped me keep alive, if not always thriving, in spite of all the stress and emotional upheavals in my tumultuous, demanding, exciting, rewarding life! I searched for all the possible causes of my ulcers so that I could eradicate them and get well. I had no toxic habits, and I was supplying all the needs of life except one: equanimity! Victoria BidWell calls this *emotional balance* in her ten energy enhancers, while Dr. Shelton called it *emotional poise*, and T. C. Fry called it *self-control.*

It has been a huge and very difficult challenge to eliminate my hypersensitivity and excitability. I have had to force myself to relax and to maintain an internal calmness in all situations. The cultivation of poise has taken years. I have had to retrain my mind and rid myself of poor emotional/neurological habit patterns. This has required awareness and perseverance. Nevertheless, time and time again, I have had to do what they say to do here in Texas, "Bite the bullet, grin and bear it." I have no ulcers now. I thank God and Hygiene that I don't suffer with the sharp, knife-cutting pains in my stomach anymore.

The beauty of the hygienic program is that it fulfills our every need and helps us reach old age in as healthy a condition as possible. I am not undamaged. But thanks to Hygiene, I can still function on high physical, physiological, mental and emotional levels. I may not look quite as dashing as Bernarr Macfadden did at 80. But I am slender, I still have all my wits about me, and I feel young. I can ride a bicycle, dance a jig, and kick up a heel! I hope to keep doing all of this just as long as my cells are well slept, well rested, well fed and kept emotionally calm. I feel like the unsinkable Molly Brown who shouted with such high spirit, "I ain't down yet!"

Perhaps the greatest blessing of all is that I now share the Hygiene joy with my entire family! The man my daughter chose to marry, Gregory Lynn Haag, became a hygienist as soon as he first visited the health school and talked to some guests who had fasted and had recovered their health. Tosca and Gregory went to medical school together. We all three have MD degrees, but we practice Natural Hygiene. In addition, my grandchildren also live according to the principles of Natural Hygiene. They know exactly what to do should they get sick! They fast! And we all stay on the nontoxic, properly combined, raw food diet of Natural Hygiene. Amen!

# More Testimony...

There are many great books with more testimonials by raw fooders. Paul Nison's books *The Raw Life: Becoming Natural in an Unnatural World*; *Raw Knowledge: Enhance the Powers of Your Mind, Body and Soul*, and *Raw Knowledge II: Interviews with Health Achievers* are filled with extensive interviews with raw fooders, many of them long term, and many with "before" and "after" photos.

Other books attesting to the power of live food diets include *The Living Foods Lifestyle* by Brenda Cobb and *Perfect Body* by Roe Gallo.

There are also a number of web sites sporting testimonials and before/after photos. Currently, here are some of these:

www.shazzie.com/raw/transformation

www.rawandjuicy.com/photoalbum.html

www.thegardendiet.com/testimonials.html

www.rawfamily.com/testimonials.htm

www.rawfood.com/testimonialsgen.html

# COUNTERTHINK

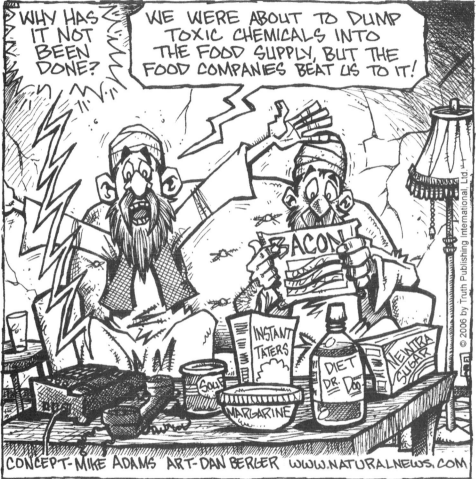

CONCEPT-MIKE ADAMS  ART-DAN BERGER  WWW.NATURALNEWS.COM

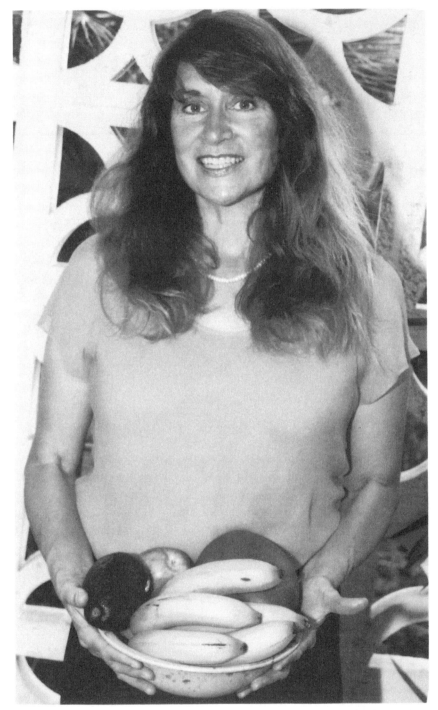

Photo by Joe Peiri

**The author at 3½ years raw just prior to her 50th birthday**

# 3
# Radically Raw:
# My Story

*The best retirement plan is to be so healthy
that you never need to retire.* —Susan Schenck (1956–)

Like most Americans, I was raised with constant reminders of the importance of food and the seemingly contradictory value of being trim. My parents were always on some diet, constantly struggling to abstain from the abundance of available food. Food was a minor obsession for my parents, and I am sure that this impacted my consciousness and influenced me to become determined to master the art and science of eating.

Growing up in the 1960s, I was always told to clean my plate because of the starving children in China. Later, as an adult, I always wanted to go to China, clasp my hands around my fat tummy, and say to the people, "See? Look at what I did for you all!"

I came from the first generation that was raised on processed food. I remember eating Campbell's soup for lunch, half the bowl filled with soaked saltine crackers. I recall that one day in particular, when I was about five years old, I tried to form a mental "time warp" into the future. I thought to myself, "On the day I get married, I will remember this moment, sitting here, eating Campbell's soup." Well, I didn't remember the incident on *any* of my wedding days, but for some reason I have often recalled that moment since.

Processed food was just becoming commonplace when I grew up in the '60s: Pop·Tarts for breakfast, Twinkies for lunch, Oreo cookies, graham crackers or ice cream after school and TV dinners for supper. When I reflect, I think I may have had an average of one fresh food item a day: an apple, a banana, a carrot or the occasional salad smothered in pasteurized, sugary dressing.

After my parents divorced when I was 14, I moved from a small town in Indiana to a larger city. Convinced that I would be more successfully popular if I lost the fat around my waist, I went on my first diet and lost ten pounds in a couple of weeks.

In spite of the fact that this did not add anything to my popularity or confidence, I was so proud of myself that I kept strict tabs on my eating. I memorized the entire calorie book and counted calories every meal, every snack, every day, diligent never to allow myself to go over 1,600 calories a day.

I slowly slipped into anorexia nervosa, the golden cage of needing a figure like that of Twiggy (a fashion model of the late '60s who made it stylish to be skinny), but at the same time being obsessed with forbidden foods. When I restricted my intake to 1,300 calories a day, I slimmed down to 96 pounds at the age of 16 at 5'4".

My diet consisted of things like sugar-free sodas, sugar-free diet gelatin, sugar-free gum, low-fat cheese, lettuce, sugar-free Kool-Aid, canned tuna, canned green beans and dry air popcorn. I thought it was a glorious time that we lived in: technology had enabled man (and best of all, me!) to defy the law of calories by eating all these delicious synthetic "foods."

My diet was so full of chemicals and so nutrient-deficient that it was no wonder I came down with asthma, allergies and hypoglycemia. My blood sugar became so unbalanced that I sometimes fainted. I spent nearly a week in the hospital for tests, as my parents were quite concerned about my sudden illness.

The asthma and allergies got so bad that sometimes I would gasp for air, unable to sleep, so the doctor had me take asthma medication. I quickly became addicted to over-the-counter asthma pills, which were a mild form of speed (amphetamines). This went on for about a decade as I battled an addiction to stimulants that kept my nervous system very hyperactive.

At that time, few doctors knew about anorexia. This was nearly a decade before pop singer Karen Carpenter's death made the public aware. Like many anorexics, I had elaborate food rituals. For example, I would spend eight hours creating gourmet Christmas cookies and then eat only one.

After I'd been anorexic for about three years, suppressing my desires to eat and dreaming every night about food, the dam suddenly burst. I became bulimic and gained 60 pounds within months. This was very depressing, as I had always had full control of myself until then. In fact my willpower had made me feel superior to everyone I knew. Losing my willpower and my figure shattered my self-image.

The full-blown bulimia, or binge/purge syndrome, lasted for seven years. It was seven years of hell that completely changed my life.

On a positive note, it made me a much more compassionate person. Within months, I transformed from the most judgmental person I have ever met to a non-judgmental person with insight into why people do the most insane things. I developed the insight to *seek to understand the reason* behind the actions or words I disagreed with, *rather than condemn the doer or speaker*.

But I hated this disease. Worst of all, perhaps, I believed that I was alone, that no one in the world was sharing my illness. When I confessed my compulsive behavior to a doctor, counselor or psychologist, no one had any idea what was going on with me. I even took eight psychology classes at the university, hoping to find some insight that would lead me to a cure. I knew that I couldn't wait for some doctor to treat me or for someone to find the cure or magic pill. *I had to heal myself as soon as possible.* I couldn't wait for medical science to figure things out.

One day I picked up a copy of the magazine *New Woman* and read an article explaining that B vitamins from brewer's yeast reduce stress. I started reading about nutrition and trying out various high energy and high mineral foods, such as bee pollen and brewer's yeast. Several months before that, I had also begun to exercise regularly.

Gradually I freed myself. I no longer felt the mood swings, stress and compulsive behavior to binge and purge. After seven years of hell, I was free! (Well, relatively free, at least.) *From that time on, I knew that nutrition played a key role in mental, emotional, spiritual and physical health.*

In retrospect, I realize another reason I was able to rid myself of eating disorders was that I was living in Mexico that year. I wasn't exposed to most of the food additives and chemicals found in American food. (See Appendix A.)

About a year later pop singer Karen Carpenter suddenly died from complications of her own eating disorder, and the topic of eating disorders suddenly sprouted in all the media. Books were written about it. Treatment centers started advertising to help women with this disease. It was interesting to me, but it didn't really matter because I had been freed. I was on to other things, like traveling around the world.

In my mid-twenties, I was still somewhat addicted to stimulants of the legal variety, such as asthma pills. To unwind at night from the stimulants, I had to drink beer. I also smoked. My vices became so habitual that I thought I had better clean myself out. For years I had longed to go to the exotic Middle East, so I went to a place where alcohol was even illegal: Saudi Arabia. After a year of teaching English in Arabia, I still indulged on occasion after returning to the USA, but the addictive compulsion was gone.

After tiring of traveling the world, I returned to the United States and got a master's degree in traditional Oriental medicine. I had an acupuncture and herbal clinic for a while but felt frustrated because I knew that these therapies alone weren't getting people well enough, fast enough. Those with chronic pain would have to spend a lot of money and come for months, even years. That was something that few could really afford.

I gave up the clinic but continued working from my home or doing house calls while searching for more of the missing pieces to the health puzzle. I realized that my calling was not so much to be a healer, but rather an educator. I've always been a teacher at heart, and I hope to empower others to heal themselves. Now I realize that healers only facilitate: it is the body alone that can heal itself.

Meanwhile, now in my mid-thirties, I was struggling to keep slim. I never reverted to the eating disorders but retained a very typical female concern for keeping my figure. My weight fluctuated within a 15-pound range, yo-yoing between 130 and 145 or so pounds. I tried low-calorie diets, low-fat diets and low-carbohydrate diets. I exercised by running, lifting weights and walking. Once a year I would take a one- or two-week juice diet. While others indulged in Oktoberfest, I experienced my annual "Octoberfast."

Whenever I went to Canada to visit relatives, I observed how much older they got, year after year. I listened as my grandmother would talk endlessly about her helplessly aging friends and relatives, mostly people I didn't even know. Their organs were falling apart, they were incontinent, they needed operations. Life as an old person was pretty miserable. My grandmother lived to be 95 but had a pacemaker, had two hips replaced, and was very fragile during the last decade or two.

As I pondered how everyone around me was aging, I vowed that this would not happen to me. Whatever it took, I would not age like this. I would grow old, but I would never lose my strength, fitness and health.

Exercise grew into a part-time job, as I incorporated yoga for flexibility, weightlifting for strength and muscles, and walking for aerobics. I was constantly reading books about health, preventive medicine and nutrition. My monthly purchase of supplements slowly grew to hundreds of dollars, often more than a new car payment. I drove my ten-year-old car around Southern California, where nearly everyone has the latest luxury auto. But I preferred to spend that money on my body, the most precious of vehicles.

Throughout my adult life, I was constantly on the lookout for the fountain of youth, as well as the elixir of ecstasy. You name the herb, drug, pill or potion, and I probably experimented with it.

Convinced that I had attention deficit disorder after reading the book *Driven to Distraction* (Hallowell and Ratey), I even took Prozac for a year. At first I thought it was splendid, but later it gave me anxiety attacks and a weight gain of 30 pounds. A key ingredient, I learned later, was fluoride, an extremely toxic substance. Read *The Fluoride Deception* by Christopher Bryson or *Fluoride the Aging Factor: How to Recognize and Avoid the Devastating Effects of Fluoride* by John Yiamouyiannis for more information on that.

Fortunately, I stopped taking Prozac before some of the other effects could manifest: thyroid damage, loss of calcium in the hipbones, brain damage and more.

A number of my closest friends also experimented with these selective serotonin reuptake inhibitor (SSRI) antidepressants that year. We all had bad results after the initial mild euphoria. Yet these drugs remain frighteningly easy to obtain from just about any doctor. Incidentally, after going raw, I discovered that my "spacey" feeling and short attention span were not due to "attention deficit disorder," but rather to wheat sensitivity.

Some people may think I was obsessed with health due to fear of death. Oddly, I have never been able to relate to that fear very much. I was born with an innate knowing that we are immortal spiritual beings here on a journey. I may have wanted to prolong my health and lifespan a bit, but death per se has never given me any angst. My spiritual life was always more important to me than my health. In fact one of the reasons for my health quest is that I found, like so many others who know about the body-mind-spirit connection, that I feel a higher spiritual vibration when I feel healthy.

Another part of the reason for my obsession with health, I confess, is that I was a total wimp when it came to pain. Even a minor ache or infection would throw me out of my comfort zone. I had completely outlawed headaches from my body. I wanted to be sure that I never, ever experienced pain and had no need for pain medications.

Another reason for my health quest, though, was that I noticed early on that how I felt had almost nothing to do with outer circumstances and almost everything to do with how my inner biochemistry was. In other words, my happiness quotient depended primarily on my level of health.

I could win the lottery but still feel miserable if I had a bad case of PMS. On the other hand, I could lose my job or go through a bad relationship breakup and feel great as long as my health was up. I was therefore determined to discover the greatest health secrets to building the highest states of well-being and felt it was my mission to teach these secrets to others.

Nutrition was always one of my passions, and I experimented with several diets throughout the years. I tried out vegetarianism for several years, as well as the trendy low-fat diet. How fortunate, I thought, to live in a time when technology can create zero-fat "butter" out of chemicals, zero-calorie spray for frying, and Olestra zero-fat chips. But to compensate for the low fat, I would eat lots of carbohydrates and fall asleep after eating zero-fat pasta.

Then I read *The Zone* by Dr. Barry Sears. This led me to a new diet, low in carbohydrates. Again, thanks to technology, I was able to eat protein powders and protein bars that fit perfectly into the 40% carbohydrates, 30% fat and 30% protein of the Zone Diet. I devoured seven of Dr. Sears's books.

Although my energy soared as a result of having low insulin levels, I noticed a dull headache and even fatigue as I ate the protein bars, which, unbeknownst to me, were loaded with excitotoxins — MSG and aspartame.

My mother discovered she had kidney cancer at the age of 73. I knew she was not going to make it to 100 with her eating habits, but it was really shocking that this would happen in her early 70s. A year and a half later she died of a stroke when the cancer metastasized to her brain. It was such an amazing thing to see her last breath.

About 50 years ahead of her time, Mom had always been a pioneer. She taught me by example not to care what others thought of me, but to follow my heart. I once gave her a card that said, "Though you raised me to be an independent thinker and my own person, I ended up being a reflection of you."

I became a free spirit and could confide in her all of my '70s, '80s and '90s experiences. She used to say, with a hint of pride in her voice, "Nothing you could do would ever surprise me!"

Mom was 30 pounds overweight, but that didn't stop her from hiking and staying very active. We traveled together in Scotland and even India.

In July 1999, I got a call from my sister Sally saying that Mom had collapsed. I flew out to visit her, and the doctors broke the devastating news that she had kidney cancer. It had already metastasized to *both* lungs. This meant surgery was out of the question. She was given six months to two years to live.

Mom took the medical doctors' advice and tried interferon. She came to San Diego for a month as a shadow of her former self. Dropping down to her ideal weight pleased her, but she had no energy for the walks on the beach that we had formerly enjoyed.

Seeing that even the interferon was not working, she went off the drugs. In about a week, her vitality came back. She was again able to walk, hike and trim the hedges. The sparkle and enthusiasm returned.

Then in September 2000, I received a hospital call informing me that Mom had suffered a stroke. The cancer had metastasized to her brain. The doctors said that no one ever recovered from this type of stroke.

My sister and I rushed to see her. We spent the next five days by her side talking to her, even though she was in a coma. I went days without sleep, holding her hand and telling her it was okay to pass on.

I thought — not even saying out loud — "Mom, you know you have to cross over. If you agree, please cough." To my astonishment, she coughed immediately! And that was the only time that I heard her cough during those five days.

Then on September 25, the nurse could tell from her breathing that the end was near. I witnessed Mom's final moments in the body. Watching her breathe ever more slowly, then stop a little, and then gasp some more was very intense. Sally and I held her hands, stroked her forehead, and reassured her that it was okay to go into the light, that we would be okay without her. Though Mom was unconscious, tears streamed down her eyes as she silently said goodbye.

Watching Mom's final breath and rebirth into a higher dimension was probably as intense as *her* watching *our* first breaths and births into this dimensional plane had been.

Sally and I felt very privileged to have witnessed this passage. We hung around awhile, as the room felt lit up with Mom's energy. I gave her body one final hug.

I later wrote, though didn't publish, a book entitled *Losing a Parent: The Ultimate Wake-Up Call*. While researching for the book, I noted that many people's lives change after a parent dies. In retrospect, I can see how Mom's death led me to want to publish this book about raw food: I want to expose the futility of drug medicine in the face of ravishing disease. I want to help someone save *her* mother, even though it may be too late for mine.

As I mentioned, I was never really afraid of dying myself. For one thing, I knew the afterlife was much better than this one. Secondly, I felt I was always two steps ahead of disease through exercising, abstaining from red meat, drinking plenty of water and taking enough supplements to feed a family of ten.

Then in my 40s, I was suddenly diagnosed with hepatitis C. During a routine exam, my liver enzymes were found to be very high. Some doctor thought I should be tested to see if I had the virus. Well, I did.

At that time, I knew zilch about hepatitis C. It scared me. I felt vulnerable for the first time in my life. I felt mortal. Even I, despite my complete focus on health, was capable of illness. It was reminiscent of the unforgettable scene in the movie *Philadelphia* when the character played by Tom Hanks realizes he has AIDS and is listening to the sad opera music.

Since I was not really afraid of death, it was bittersweet. I observed the drama of it all with a bit of detachment. If I died, okay. But if I lived, *I simply had to have good health*. Life without excellent health, I held, was not worth living.

Within a month or so, I brought the liver enzymes down to very healthy levels simply by abstaining from alcohol and consuming ample quantities of the herb milk thistle. When the medical doctor saw that my enzyme levels were to be envied by anyone, he thought maybe the test result had been faulty. So he retested me, but the test had been accurate: I still had hepatitis C.

The doctor convinced me to take interferon for six months. I felt fine, I argued. I let him frighten me when he said that as long as the virus was there, it could suddenly cause cirrhosis of the liver or even lead to liver cancer.

I finally relented. But since the drug had only a 30% chance of knocking out the virus, I decided to cover all bases and take vast quantities of herbs and liver supplements.

Along with the interferon, I took ribavirin, a viral suppressant, to increase the effect. The interferon made me so depressed that I had to take an antidepressant. A side effect of the antidepressant was insomnia, so I had to take a heavy-duty sleeping pill.

I was inundated with various drugs and their side effects. Six months later, the virus was apparently gone. But so were half my hair, my energy, my exalted life spirit and my healthy complexion. The interferon had weakened and aged me. My face was white and pasty. My hair was turning gray.

Had I known about raw foods, I never would have gone the drug route. It was so unnecessary because my liver was just fine before the drugs so long as I ate well and avoided alcohol.

Though warned I had only a one-out-of-three chance, I won the battle against the virus. Then the doctor threw me for a loop when he told me that although the drug had succeeded in combating the hepatitis, yearly checks were needed because it could come back — after everything I had been through!

How could that be? I thought the drug was supposed to *cure* me. I knew then that I had to change my lifestyle. *Something radical had to be done.*

On an Internet chat room, I met someone who told people everything about the raw food diet. I prided myself in knowing a lot about nutrition. I had read dozens of nutrition books and was convinced that a raw food diet would be too low in protein.

But this person was one of the few who knew more than I did about nutrition. It took about three months of debate before I decided to give it a try. Although I was most skeptical and a "hard sell," one week of the diet was enough to convince me. No amount of reading about the diet could equal the experience of trying it myself — for just one week.

In April 2002, I did something I hadn't done in a decade: I fasted, consuming only water and juice for two weeks. I also took a series of colonics, which are much stronger than enemas for cleaning out the colon. To my amazement, pounds of waste came out.

Then I did a liver cleanse. I merely ingested a mixture of half a cup of unheated olive oil, a cup of raw apple juice, a tablespoon of garlic, a tablespoon of raw apple cider vinegar and a tablespoon of ginger without having eaten anything all day, taken within five minutes of lying down to sleep. It doesn't work if you don't lie down on your right side afterwards. This was followed by a colonic the next day. After I did this liver cleanse, hundreds of gallstones poured out of me.

This made me realize how unnecessary gallbladder removals are, with the difficulty in digesting fats that comes as a result. (The gallbladder is a saclike organ that stores liver bile, essential for digesting fats properly.)

I felt so light and euphoric that I didn't even want to break the fast. Finally I did. I wanted to keep that light feeling. I wondered if going raw would do the trick so decided to give it a try.

Within a month of going raw, I lost about fifteen pounds. But much more than that, things I never expected I would ever be free from disappeared completely. Athlete's foot that I'd had for a decade, and nothing would rid me of, vanished, as well as the fungus on my big toenail.

My PMS was getting worse every year to the point that I was depressed three weeks out of every month. After going raw, I didn't even feel the usual depression and irritability the day before my period. Thus it was always a surprise when my period came. Before going raw, the PMS had become progressively worse the closer it got to my period. My period, a form of detox, went from three days to one.

On the raw diet, I felt lighter, more mentally clear than ever, more energetic, more alive, more joyful. My skin was as soft as when I was a teenager. Hypoglycemia was gone. Cellulite vanished. Brain fog and sluggishness became a thing of the past. My energy, previously scattered, became focused. My face, which had been whitened by the interferon, grew rosy again. I had my youthful, rosy cheeks back. Most surprisingly to me was that I regained the bounce and energy of my preadolescence.

I sensed that this was the fountain of youth I had been looking for. I gave away about eight grocery bags of dead food from my cabinets. After buying several raw food recipe books, I experimented with new food creations and invited friends over to try these delightful new taste treats. By making food that tasted so much better than cooked food, I knew I would not be tempted to go back to old eating habits.

Most exciting was that I found an ecstasy from having an alkaline body. (See Chapter 17 for more on that.) I felt joy, peace, a natural high. My energy became smooth, balanced and stable. My addictive tendencies melted effortlessly.

Although I cannot brag that I healed from cancer on the raw food diet, as can several of the people I have met since going raw, I nonetheless have my own testimony. I now have the vigor and energy of my youth. I look younger, feel younger, sleep less, and feel freer than ever. I am able to sing much better since the phlegm is gone. When I travel, I no longer get jet lag! I can also endure humid weather like never before.

A chronic upper back and neck pain is gone. When people find out that my husband is a premier massage therapist, they always exclaim, "How lucky you are! You must get massages every day!" I reply that I feel no need for massages. Thanks to a raw diet and yoga, all my muscles feel great.

Before going raw, I thought I was "regular" because I eliminated once a day. I now realize I was, like most people, chronically constipated. I now go to the bathroom two or three times a day, effortlessly and quickly.

My addictive personality is growing dimmer and dimmer. When I stick to a 100% raw diet, my weight is effortlessly stabilized. There is no longer a need to periodically go on a weight-loss diet, yet I am free to eat delicious foods such as olives, avocados and nuts that formerly would have been off limits due to their high calorie and fat content.

I no longer feel throbbing pain with minor injuries. After I'd been 95% raw for a few years, people began remarking about how shiny my eyes were. Best of all, my mood swings are gone. I feel much happier than when I ate the SAD. I am not so overwhelmed by "the things I have to get done," and most of the time I feel that life is a joy. Most amazingly, I no longer have the remotest fear of disease. I feel totally in control of my health.

As a child, I used to pray, right before going to bed, "Now I lay me down to sleep, I pray the Lord my soul to keep. If I should die before I wake, I pray the Lord my soul to take." Having experienced the death of several childhood friends, I was convinced that I too could die *any day*. I was often conscious that I had to experience life fully and also get certain things done because I could die any day from meningitis, toxic shock syndrome, a brain aneurysm or something. Like most people, I felt powerless against a number of diseases that seemed to hit randomly and destroy people with no rhyme or reason.

Another interesting phenomenon that occurred after switching to a raw diet was that in my dreams, I would find myself at a large buffet, happily selecting only the uncooked food. I couldn't help but compare this to the years of self-deprivation as an anorexic in which I would always gorge myself on doughnuts, ice cream and all sorts of other "goodies" in my dreams. Dreams give us a way to peak into our unconscious, and this confirmed to me that I was not feeling deprived even unconsciously.

People in the raw movement are prone to ask each other two questions: "How long have you been raw?" and "What percentage raw are you?" I have found that at certain times it is easier to be 100% raw. At other times, however, I allow myself the occasional "cheat" of a cooked potato once a week or so and even popcorn a few times a year, as I have found no adequate raw substitutes for these two favorite indulgences.

However, I have developed a healthy respect for the addictiveness of cooked food. Cooked food can be so addictive, especially if you are living under constant psychological stress, that I have learned it is simply easier to stay out of that addictive zone altogether and remain 100% raw. Doing so removes one more source of stress from my life.

When I am 100% raw, it is incredibly easy to decline the most elaborate of cooked smorgasbords. When I indulge in the occasional cheat, it evolves into a constant internal battle not to "treat" myself to cooked food almost daily.

I have also experimented with Boutenko's green smoothie diet. (See Appendix C.) I feel this is the next step forward and have noted dramatic improvements in my health.

One regret I have is that I did not find the raw diet sooner. Although I had come across a few people in California who told me about it — including a housemate! — it didn't register because I didn't know the science behind it. So I just assumed I could take a vitamin pill and a few enzyme pills to compensate for the nutrition lost from heating.

I never realized how much more complicated and ultimately deadly preparing and eating cooked food was. It's suicide on the installment plan. Furthermore, these raw fooders didn't hit me over the head with missionary zeal. Perhaps that is why I can often be zealous to the point of being obnoxious. And that is also why I put so much science into this book, so that the diet would make sense to the left-brained people like me.

Take heed, those of you who want to put this off until you are older or sicker: *I wish I had started sooner!* And I have never met a raw fooder who has not expressed that same wish! I am told that people who start young maintain their youth well into middle age. Furthermore, my mom would still be alive today if I had discovered this diet just a year or two prior to her death.

Another reason I didn't know about the startling benefits of raw foods is that almost all the books on the raw food diet are self-published and are therefore not found in bookstores, where I would peruse and purchase any books I wanted to read on health. All of my adult life, I used to go to bookstores every week, looking for new avenues to research to satisfy my curiosity about health, spirituality and other subjects. Yet I never encountered a raw food book.

The only way I could research this topic was by ordering books from the Internet, obscure titles that no one has ever heard of. As Victoria Boutenko points out, people are so hungry for health that they begin seeking answers, not waiting for scientific research to catch up. "We witness hundreds, if not thousands, of books on nutrition written by average people . . . sometimes without the necessary background" (*Green for Life*, p. 5).

During my first year of going raw, I bought every raw food book I could find. I read about 70 books on the raw food diet and related nutritional subjects, all of which I reference here in the Bibliography. I voraciously read the vast majority of the books you will find there. Within a year and a half, I had also read literally hundreds of health and raw food diet articles on the Internet.

Although it is not necessary to study the diet as extensively as I did, I know that educating myself about it helped tremendously with the ability to stick with it. Every week or so I would search the Net for books on the raw diet, consumed with passion to learn as much as I could because the topic was so fascinating for me.

People who enjoy life would like to live forever, or at least a long time, in order to synthesize and share all they have learned. Some people like to think they achieve immortality or regain their youth by having children. Others like to marry people young enough to be their children. Some achieve immortality by changing a law or inventing something or writing a book.

As Woody Allen said, "*I prefer to achieve immortality by not dying.*" Since that is highly unlikely, I can at least live a long, healthy life on a raw diet.

This is why I researched the raw food diet with a zeal found only in those who have discovered the secret of immortality. Many people uncovering this secret also have the same zeal, almost a missionary passion. Actor Woody Harrelson made a documentary, *Go Further*, in which one of his traveling partners got turned on to the raw diet and was shouting on the streets to people something like, "You've been lied to! No more corn dogs! You've been lied to!"

If you count my two master's degrees, as well as my continuing education, I have eleven years of university/college education. But the truth is that for many people, most of our learning occurs when we *study on our own*. What I learned in my years of college and university was *how to do research*.

As I explained in the Preface, I felt compelled to write this book. I had discovered the secret of a lifetime. I couldn't sleep at night unless I shared it with others! The results of years of my research reading, talking to people, attending lectures and workshops, experimenting on my own, and coaching others on the raw diet are summarized in this book.

As for the title of this chapter, the word *radical* is defined as 'arising from or going to a root or source', as in "a radical solution." This certainly applies to the raw food revolution we are witnessing today and how it goes to the root or source of illness, unlike orthodox treatment. *Radical* is also defined as 'departing markedly from the usual or customary; extreme', which also applies to the raw diet. A third definition is 'favoring or effecting fundamental or revolutionary changes in current practices, conditions, or institutions'. What could be more radical than changing the fundamental institutions of medicine and cooking? The final definition of *radical* is slang: 'excellent, wonderful'. Indeed, the raw diet is!

I will have to say, along with Dr. Herbert Shelton, one of the 20th century's raw food proponents, "If the views presented herein seem radical to my readers, if they seem revolutionary, I shall be happy; for I strive always to be 'radical' in the true meaning of this much abused term, to be revolutionary in a world that is reeking with decay."

The truth is not only radical, but also often too *simple* for people to accept. As Albert Einstein said, "If at first the idea is not absurd, then there is no hope for it."

So there is great hope for this diet and its power to provide the optimal nutrition needed by body, mind and soul. And there is also my favorite Einstein quote: "Condemnation without investigation is the height of ignorance."

So I invite you, dear reader, not only to *read* what I have written, but also to *investigate* for yourself to see if it is not true. Do some research on your own body. See if it does not thrive most wholeheartedly on a raw food diet, and read some of the books I quote throughout this one. But most of all, try the diet! See if your body, brain and spirit do not love you for feeding them what they truly need!

We shall deal next with the science showing how and why the live food factor is one of the most, if not *the* most, potent keys to optimal health.

If you are eager to begin implementing this diet right away, you may wish to proceed to Section IV first, which shows you how to get started, coming back to the science later. Just be sure not to skip Section II entirely, especially Chapters 9 and 10, as the science behind the raw diet is sure to leave a deep impression, reminding you why you should never revert to your old eating habits.

This is not just another fad diet, weight-loss program or disease-specific diet. This is the diet *you were genetically designed to eat* for optimal, overall well-being. Even if you are not keen on studying science, reading through the science section will explain why this is so.

# Epilogue

Shortly before we went to print with this second edition, my father died. He was diagnosed with colon cancer that had spread to the liver and bones, and in *nine days* he died! I spent the last week with him. I told him, "Dad, this wouldn't have happened if you had gone raw!" to which he replied, *"Touché!"*

At nearly 85, Dad realized his chances of surviving chemo or surgery were slim: he was an MD himself, after all. He also complained that the hospital staff woke him up every hour for blood pressure tests, and he got very little sleep as a result. I said, "Dad, you used to work in a hospital!" — to which he replied that he always allowed people to sleep. Consequently, he decided to go home to die with hospice care and his family at his side.

I will never forget the pain Dad felt those final days. "Torture! You're torturing me!" he screamed whenever anyone gently moved him. The last two days it was so bad he had to take morphine.

My father was a true Renaissance Man. He had enough talents and hobbies for several lifetimes, but he especially identified with being a WW II Royal Air Force veteran. The love of his life was flying.

The day before Dad died, I had a few minutes alone with him. I will never forget the sense of urgency in his eyes as he struggled to give me some profound words of wisdom: "Life is here, then gone tomorrow!"

As all of his family hovered around him, Dad went into a period of intense, labored breathing until he gasped his last breath. My last words to him were, *"Dad, now you don't need an airplane to fly!"*

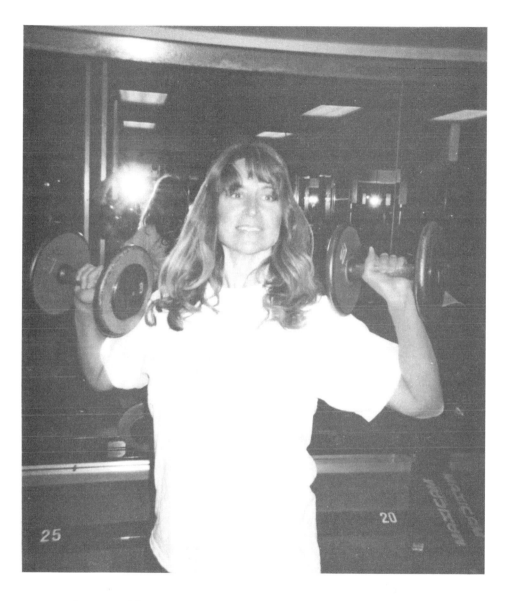

**At age 49, right after a 2-week cleanse on green juices, your author works out at the local gym.**

# CounterThink

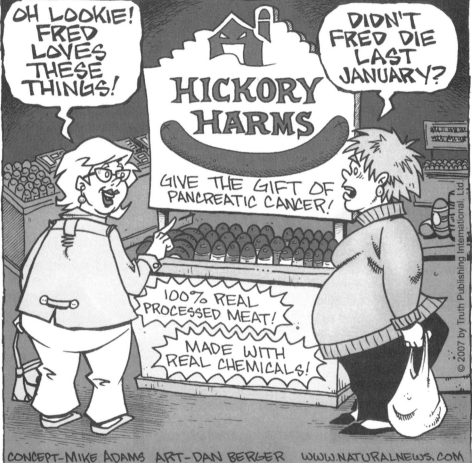

CONCEPT-MIKE ADAMS  ART-DAN BERGER  WWW.NATURALNEWS.COM

SODIUM NITRITE CAUSES CANCER.
SEE WWW.HONESTFOODGUIDE.ORG

# Section Two

# Raw Proof:

## The Science

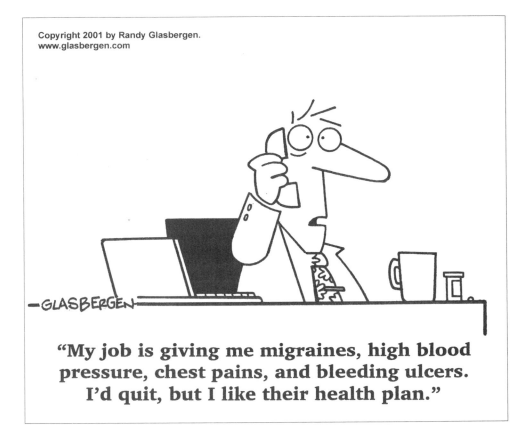

—GLASBERGEN—

"My job is giving me migraines, high blood pressure, chest pains, and bleeding ulcers. I'd quit, but I like their health plan."

# 4
# A Paradigm Shift in How We View Disease and Health

*All truth goes through three stages. Truth will first be ridiculed, then violently opposed and finally accepted as self-evident.*
*—Arthur Schopenhauer (1788–1860)*

A paradigm shift is a dramatic change in one's belief system, a fundamental change in underlying assumptions. If a scientist works from the wrong theories or from misconceptions based on wrong assumptions, he will ask the wrong questions and design and conduct irrelevant experiments resulting in erroneous conclusions that may even result in dangerous consequences. As Dr. Lorraine Day states, "Modern medicine isn't getting great results in treating disease because its scientists are looking in the wrong direction, wasting time and money on incorrect theories."

Beliefs are the hardest addictions to break. Most of us are so addicted to our convictions that we don't want anything to disrupt the cozy little belief worlds in which we feel safe. For some, preconceptions take on religious overtones. Most of us are deeply attached to our ways of thinking. Even when presented with strong evidence indicating that a painful or fear-inducing belief is untrue, that the truth is infinitely better and that the universe is far more benevolent than suspected, ignorance and insecurity lead many of us to shrug off the evidence and meld back into the comfort zone of negative but familiar beliefs.

For some of us to confess, even to ourselves, that we could greatly profit from belief or paradigm adjustments, that we have been wrong and even blinded to the truth, takes not only humility, but also courage. It takes a willingness to shift into initially frightening, although ultimately freeing, modes of seeing reality. It takes a sense of adventure!

Beliefs are so ingrained within some of us that we are willing to die, or to enlist others to die, for these cherished ideas about what is right and wrong, true and false. Dying for others may be commendable when such beliefs are deliberate sacrifices made for the greater good, but most people are too trusting of authority.

For example, some are willing to risk their lives in an unjust war rather than question the judgment of their political leaders, even though it may turn out that the war was initiated more for political imperialism and corporate interests than for "defending the nation's freedom." Suicide bombers give their lives for their causes, blindly believing they are fulfilling their destinies. Some people subject themselves to chemotherapy every day, fully trusting in the system, though the value and even safety of that treatment has now been proven highly questionable.

A paradigm shift occurs when a person begins, gradually perhaps, to see the world from a radically different viewpoint. It is not just a shift in a mere theory but in an entire perspective. Sometimes it is mind-blowing when it occurs instantaneously! Either way, once people make paradigm shifts, they often become amazed, aghast or even amused at how they could have invested their whole lives in erroneous belief systems.

Two examples of this situation are nearly always referenced when paradigm shifting is encouraged. One is the formerly popular belief that the world was flat until Christopher Columbus proved otherwise by sailing to the New World without falling off the edge in 1492.

The other is Galileo Galilei's early adoption and publicizing in 1610 of Nicolaus Copernicus's then radical theory of 1530 that the earth orbited the sun rather than being a stationary center around which the whole universe rotated. Galileo was branded a religious heretic by the Catholic Church, arrested and publicly humiliated. It was only in 1992 that the Vatican finally reversed its earlier position that the earth was the center of the universe! This belief was so impossible to let go of for some that there is even a group, the Geocentric Bible Foundation, which still believes the sun revolves around the earth!

Victoria BidWell points out the all-pervasiveness and all-importance of paradigm shifting in our times:

Human history is the story of paradigm shifts that have dramatically changed our directions, living conditions and values. We have gone from labeling members of certain groups of people *inferior* and treating them as slaves or bitter enemies to regarding and treating them as respected equals. We have gone from viewing the rich as nobility and serving as serfs under them to regarding all men and women created equal as we practice democratic ideals. We have gone from viewing women as the weaker sex: unable to own property, disallowed to vote and mandated by law to obey their husbands, to seeing and treating women as deserving esteem and opportunities equal to that enjoyed by the male gender. And we have gone from seeing earth as limitless in its natural resources and invincible in its character to understanding the delicate ecological and biochemical balance our planet must maintain to sustain us all in vibrant health.

One of the biggest paradigm shifts in all of history occurred in the 20th century when theoretical physicist Albert Einstein proposed that we live in a universe in which mass and energy are interchangeable, thus proving to the world that *it's all about energy*! He postulated that we live in a nonmaterial universe in which all matter at the most minute level is not matter at all, but energy made of differing atomic combinations vibrating at differing speeds.

Out of his and other physicists' early 20th century theories and discoveries came the quantum physics paradigm shift that resulted in television, the atomic bomb, spaceships, computers, cell phones and CAT scans.

Also deriving from this work came the pop psychology movement, backed up by psychoneuroimmunologists and molecular biologists who taught people how to deliberately change their thoughts and feelings — nonmaterial, nonmeasurable events — to bring about changes in their physical health — material, measurable events.

We are now in the midst of another radical shift — from the medical mentality to holistic health care, from the doctor as healer to the human body as healer, from lifestyle practices as unimportant to lifestyle choices as all-important, from surgeries and synthetic drugs as viable healing strategies to lifestyle changes for maximizing natural healing responses as most desirable, from diet as irrelevant in health considerations to live foods as essential for superlative health.

Yet most people arrogantly cling to erroneous theories. Imagine having dedicated the focus of your *entire life* to a theory and then having to watch some radical upstart come along and pull the rug out from under it! The closed-minded always react with a staunch, egoistic desire to protect their theories. This is true especially when a lot of money has been invested in them, as is the case with today's global trillion-dollar-a-year medical system.

Dr. Gabriel Cousens explains, "Paradigm-shifting breakthroughs often hit cul-de-sac dead ends in societal acceptance due to the vagaries of vested economic interest, political intrigue and pride of the ego" (*Rainbow Green Live-Food Cuisine*, p. xv).

Eventually though the truth emerges. Those who are heavily invested in earlier paradigms will die. Younger scientists unattached to old theories then become free to test new hypotheses without scorn from older colleagues. As anthropologist Harvey Weiss put it, "Science progresses one funeral at a time."

We have already seen the many cumulative benefits to the individual on all levels when a raw food diet is followed. Chapter 1 gave us ten reasons to go raw, but only one of those reasons is powerful enough to prompt change. *Health* is the most highly motivating reason that inspires people to sacrifice their french fries and convenience foods — and even change their social lives.

Eating raw food is not difficult, but giving up cooked food is. Let's ask some telling questions: How many will give up that mouth-watering dish of twice-baked potatoes just so their complexions will be lovelier? How many will quit making lasagna just to save the time and effort of scrubbing the melted cheese off the pan? How many will sacrifice sampling all the goodies at a potluck just to feel more spiritual? Who will give up the convenience of packaged, processed foods just to spare the landfill of paper and plastic wrappings?

On the other hand, if a person were faced with a life-threatening illness, he or she might take a closer look at the wholesome raw diet nature has provided, made from the constituents of air, soil, water and sunlight. If a person were losing his or her mental capacities, diet might become a serious consideration. If depressed, one might decide this diet worth learning about. If extra energy were desired to commune with God at a higher spiritual level, a person might see this diet as very attractive.

Let's face it. Health is one of the most important things in this life — mental, spiritual, emotional and physical health. As the subtitle of this book suggests, people want to feel good in body, mind and spirit.

If we are interested in improving any of these areas of our well-being — and they are all intertwined, each affecting the other — we may very well want to educate ourselves in healthful living practices that cooperate with the physiological laws of our being and to understand why they work. The only other choice is to go against these natural laws and sabotage ourselves in the process. Fatigue and disease penalties must be paid when we break natural health laws that change for no man or woman.

Virtually all raw fooders and other holistic health proponents no longer accept the conventional medical model of disease origin and its so-called cures via drugs, various treatments and surgery. Yet most members of conventional society still do see disease as a due to a mystery, the passage of time, genetic flaws or unfortunate encounters with malevolent microbes.

I am grateful to Victoria BidWell for her clear-cut contributions and seven lists that make up most of Chapter 4. I also thank Dr. Vetrano for taking the time from her busy schedule to edit (three times!) Chapters 4 through 7.

I came straight from the raw food studies, and my Natural Hygiene background has been much more limited. So Victoria enrolled me as her first student at The International Institute of Pure Natural Hygiene and has spent many hours giving me the Natural Hygiene Crash Course for Health Educators.

After that we collaborated in Chapters 4 through 7. Victoria helped organize and add to my ideas and get the terminology and constructs precise. Dr. Vetrano added her stamp of physiological approval. Because Victoria contributed most of the teachings in the next several sections, when the first person pronoun is used, that is Victoria sharing her experiences and work. Victoria now takes the lead:

# The Two Paradigms:
# Conventional and Alternative

First, let us consider a crucial word. *Physiology* is a general term in the sciences for 'all the processes that take place in the living body, in sickness and in health'. The adjective *physiological* means 'bodily' or 'referring to the body'.

Next, please stop to enjoy Appendices E and F. They will greatly enrich your grasp of what is to come here. *By the end of our Chapter 4, you will know more about how to get well and stay well than all MDs deeply entrenched in the medical mentality at its very worst.*

I always start helping a new health seeker by asking, "What are the only two ways to go about getting well?"

Everyone knows the answer and gives some variation of this: "Do what the medical doctors tell you or do something else."

They are all right. All the ways to try to get well other than the one conventional medical route can be lumped under the term *alternative health care,* also popularly called *holistic health care.* All alternativists reject the medical model and propose alternative treatments, cures, pills, potions and/or care. It should be noted, however: as long as the alternative health care professional is telling the patient *to do something or take something into his body that is unnatural* to get well and stay well, the alternativist mindset is just a holdover from the medical mentality.

Under the conventional medical mentality are four overriding schools of thought. Under the alternatives, if different diets to get well are included, are literally hundreds of schools of thought from Acupuncture to Zone therapy. We do not intend to cover all these alternatives. Some are just modified versions of the medical mentality and on the wrong track entirely. Some are harmless but do little good either.

One is the best of all. Every alternative program that is firmly based in correct human physiology and the health sciences — and that shows *the body is self-healing if the causes of disease are removed and the conditions for health are provided* — is on the right track. In this chapter, we lay out both paradigms: the conventional medical model and the best alternative model, best summarized as *health by healthful living.*

# The Medical Model's Four Schools of Thought

Various basic models within the medical world explain how disease in the human body gets there and how it should be handled. The most practiced within the medical model rely upon four schools of thought: (1) the mystery school, (2) the wear and tear school, (3) the genetic/congenital school and (4) the germ theory.

## Disease as a Mystery

The mystery school of disease origin and health care is based upon three assumptions. First, the body is fundamentally flawed. Second, it will break down and contract disease. Third, nobody knows why or what to do about it. In the case of disease as a mystery, how to handle it is shrouded with occult factors. We are told that the causes of some diseases and their cures are simply "baffling," "mysterious" or "unknown." These explanations are backed up by admonition and intimidation to "follow doctor's orders" and to never, ever go outside the establishment for cures.

The mystery school is turned to when the other three schools fail utterly and probably accounts for about 10%, more or less, of medical doctor and hospital case files in recent times.

## Disease as Wear and Tear

The wear and tear school of disease origin and health care also is based on three assumptions. First, the body is fundamentally flawed in design. Second, it will break down as time marches on by virtue of wear and tear. Third, disease and malfunction are inevitable. Of course this is true if the body is not cared for and is subjected to years of abuse. Dentistry, ophthalmology (eye doctoring), blood transfusions and orthopedic replacement, reconstructive and regenerative surgeries are representative of this school.

A growing minority of adherents to this school do acknowledge that lifestyle choices, primarily of wrong nutrition, underexercise and overstress, accelerate breakdown. Still, few systematic teachings for preventive medicine in the form of providing the conditions for health and removing the causes of disease have been forthcoming from MDs.

In fact most MDs and their patients have little faith in the human ability to change these lifestyle habits and even less in the human psyche to be inspired to change. Wear and tear MDs, therefore, handle diseases with a "we can fix it" approach. They administer drugs. They perform surgeries to replace worn-out parts or get rid of them completely. They prescribe hearing instruments and eyeglasses. They move tissues around in the body to inspire regeneration. And generally, they do whatever is necessary to get a few more weeks, months or years in for their patients until inevitable and final breakdown occurs.

In addition to many other diseases, such as arthritis, obesity and chronic fatigue, three of the top four killer diseases in America today (cancer being the exception) are all wear and tear situations: cardiovascular disease, adult onset diabetes and cirrhosis of the liver.

Wear and tear patients, therefore, probably account for 50%, or much more, of medical doctor and hospital case files in recent times.

## Disease as Genetic/Congenital

The genetic school of thought on disease origin and health care explains the ongoing disease processes in the body as chromosome determined, as destiny stored within DNA. No cure is offered. While it is true that some diseases are genetically determined and thus not preventable, such conditions are extremely rare.

Dr. Bruce Lipton, PhD, states, "Some diseases, like Huntington's chorea [a nervous system disorder], beta thalassemia [a red blood cell disorder] and cystic fibrosis [a disorder of multiple systems in the body], can be blamed entirely on one faulty gene. But single-gene disorders affect less than 2% of the population" (*The Biology of Belief*, p. 51). Dr. Lipton even cites a study in which the improved diet of mice resulted in their genetic diseases not being passed on (p. 71).

In the most comprehensive study on nutrition ever conducted, the health impact of genes was found to be virtually irrelevant compared to that of a wholesome natural diet (*The China Study*, T. Colin Campbell, p. 71).

Gabriel Cousens, MD, corroborates this. He points out that genes themselves don't cause disease. Rather, unhealthful lifestyle and poor diet can change gene expression in such a way as to develop disease. What we eat and the toxins to which we expose ourselves affect our genes.

Dr. Vetrano reinforces the conclusions of both men in her article "Gene Trouble," first published in *The Natural Health Many-to-Many* newsletter. Here she points out that healthful living practices greatly benefit those with sickle cell disease, hemophilia, muscular dystrophy and cystic fibrosis:

> Good nutrition is very often master of heredity. And many health seekers who have had so-called genetic diseases have recovered, employing fasting followed by an uncooked diet of fresh fruits, vegetables, nuts and seeds. Supply the body with the correct diet and with all the requisites of life, and it is possible that even genetic errors and damaged genes may be corrected fully or to some extent.
>
> Under the right conditions, reverse mutations can and do occur. The body heals its genetic structures just as it does its body structures. Furthermore, we can do something for many of those already afflicted. We do not really know just how much we can do for people with some serious genetic disease because most people seek medical care. This is understandable because the experiments which have been done, such as Pottenger's with his cats (see page 151), are not widely publicized. Hygienists have not had the opportunity to care for these cases.

Gerontologists now agree that 75% of a person's health after the age of 40 depends not on his genes, but on what that person has done to keep his genes healthy.

Various researchers have postulated that between 80% and 100% of our health status is directly determined or indirectly affected by diet, lifestyle choices and other environmental, social and psychological factors. This is why identical twins can grow up with very different results. One twin can stay very youthful and healthy well into old age by practicing healthful habits, while the other, who breaks every law in the healthful living book, inevitably experiences disease and debility early in life.

Even the Human Genome Project researchers align with this 80% determination, stating that genes are only a part of the story. The book *Genetic Nutritioneering: How You Can Modify Inherited Traits and Live a Longer, Healthier Life* by Jeffrey S. Bland, PhD, shows that scientists now have a huge amount of evidence that many diseases previously attributed to "bad genes" are now known to be caused by a bad diet that "feeds the genes," affecting them for the worse.

Genetic or congenital patients probably account for 5% or much less of medical doctor and hospital case files in recent times.

## Disease as Germ Inspired

The germ theory of disease origin and health care proposes that disease-producing microorganisms, either present in the body or by introduction, cause disease. The MDs' proposed cure is to get rid of the germs. They do this almost exclusively with drugs. The most common vehicle is the vaccination during the so-called flu season and contagion episodes. The runner-up most popular drug vehicle to ward off germs is use of antibiotic injections. Shots are mandatory and used routinely for schoolchildren and government workers. Another common vehicle for drugging against germ danger is use of prescription inhalers and pills or potions for personal use. Many over-the-counter drugs and cleaning items advertised to kill germs can also now be purchased.

This school of thought probably accounts for 30-40% or much less of medical doctor and hospital case files in recent times. The germ theory school is so pervasive in the American and global consciousness that we devote Chapter 5 to exposing the lie on which it is based.

# The Health by Healthful Living Model

Einstein laid the foundation for virtually all natural health care models when he showed the world that everything, including the human body — at its most fundamental level — is vibrating energy that follows natural laws. If we cooperate with the natural laws of our being, we will have health.

The many alternative holistic models of disease origin and health care that are on the right track are thus energy oriented. The alternative health care movement shook the world in 1986 when *Fit for Life* — the all-time best-seller in diet and nutrition in history — made *Natural Hygiene* a common household term in millions and millions of homes. Health via raw foods is the alternative movement now gaining the most momentum.

In our new millennium, the people are becoming so well informed that they are rejecting the medical route and choosing alternative care. With this system, we learn one simplicity: we get sick when we become toxic, and we become toxic because our bodies run low in energy. I simply teach that disease is an energy crisis in a toxic body! Virtually every new health seeker gets this and wants to know more!

Since 1832, Natural Hygiene has been waved under the banner Health by Healthful Living. For 24 years, I have taught Natural Hygiene under the banner of The Superlative, Alternative Health Care System! Its popularity is growing because it is systematically grounded in human physiology and the health sciences. It gets the best results for sick and suffering health seekers. For most sick people, it is the only route that gets good results at all.

When Dr. Vetrano, Susan and I speak of the "ten energy enhancers" or "health care based on natural, physiological laws of life" or "health by healthful living" from this point on, we are speaking of all alternative health care systems based on principles that are on the right track and that align with those of the systematic body of natural healing knowledge and health care known as Natural Hygiene.

# Crucial Alternative Terms

Specific terminology and definitions are used by Natural Hygiene health educators and must be grasped by Natural Hygiene health seekers. These are neither *Webster's Dictionary* nor MD textbook terms and meanings. Foundational to the health by healthful living model is the term *enervation*. Think of enervation as exhaustion so deep that the body is in trouble. Defined as follows, it is the first stage of disease: the result of the body being so low on energy that poisons created within the body and poisons taken into the body from outside sources accumulate in the fluids and cells, and finally, in the tissues and organs and systems.

*Toxemia* is almost synonymous with and often used interchangeably with two more terms: *toxicosis* and *autointoxication*. *Toxemia* refers specifically to 'the saturation of the bloodstream with toxic waste'. By contrast, *toxicosis* refers exclusively to 'the more advanced bodily condition of toxic poisoning not only of the blood, but of the tissues themselves'. And finally, *autointoxication* is a general term, simply meaning 'self-poisoning'.

Health seekers have come to me so many times, grasped these definitions and then exclaimed, "Oh, my God! I'm sick because I'm toxic!" *They get very happy and excited. Some get very angry.* Some of these people have spent *ten years* or more investing *hundreds of thousands of dollars* or more in the medical route and in alternative routes that were really just holdovers from the medical mentality — only to get decidedly worse!

Their next question is always some variation of this: "What do I do to get back the energy and end my crisis?" Great hope is on their horizons. *Within days or weeks* of doing right and eating live, they get better and better. The whole time they had been on the wrong track.

The happy answer is so simple. First are needed a few more definitions and seven lists. Being dubbed "the list lady" by Susan, I am so grateful and pleased to provide these in the following so that you too will know how to end the energy crisis in your toxic body and recover the health and high joy of your youth!

First, we use two words over and over again. *Pathology* means 'the study of disease'. The adjective *pathological* means 'diseased'. Toxin accumulation in the body ultimately leads to a downward spiral of pathological symptoms, pain and an unnatural, untimely death.

The only cure of disease in the health by healthful living model is a natural cure. It is based on providing the energy-enhancing conditions for health and removing the energy-draining leaks of disease. Only then can the body get its energy supplies up and go through its own self-initiated, self-cleansing and self-repair processes. Only then can the body raise its molecular vibration, cellular integrity and move forward into health.

Being totally natural when compared to conventional medical thinking, the health by healthful living paradigm is through the looking glass and appears so many times backwards, upside down or at least very odd. And rightly so, as the two models are opposite in so many ways. What follows, therefore, is a deprogramming from the conventional medical paradigm to the unconventional alternative. *Get ready to get turned upside down and maybe even inside out.*

Because these two models are so opposite so much of the time, the same vocabulary cannot be used for both. While many alternative health educators opt to use the terms *treatment* and *therapy*, Natural Hygiene alternativists are dead set against using these medical model terms. We want to free health seekers from the medical mentality altogether. Therefore, there are no treatments or therapies or pills or potions to take that will get you well. There is only the self-healing body receiving your natural healthful-living care to get you well. We want you to think outside the medicine bag of tricks and get into your own intelligent body as healer instead.

Likewise, many alternativists use the term *cure* freely. But we never, ever use the word *cure* except in the strictest sense that 'all cure is body initiated, body conducted and body maintained when the conditions for health are provided and the causes of disease are removed'. And the word *medicine* is never used unless the ten energy enhancers could metaphorically be considered the only "medicine" man, woman and child should ever take.

A final term must be addressed: *detoxification* and its variants *detox, detoxify* and *detoxer*. Dr. Vetrano has just issued a statement proposing that Natural Hygienists leave these terms exclusively to the medical world from which they originated in 1867. The medical model employs toxic drugs to reduce the even more toxic properties of poisons within the body system. Enervating detoxification treatments and therapies are also employed by MDs. For example, addicts are given methadone to get off heroin. Or they take sweat baths to get alcohol out of the system.

I have nevertheless asked Dr. Vetrano to allow the use of this trendy and popular term and its variants in this book, especially since the whole idea of getting pure and clean is so attractive to people who would like to have all life has to offer at its best. We want to make the use of this term perfectly clear in all our following teachings. *Detoxification* and its variants always refer to 'the natural, physiological processes of the body alone doing the cleansing, eliminating and excreting (see Glossary) of toxins as a result of discontinuing toxic substances and instituting the ten energy enhancers'. Preferred holistic synonyms for these medical-minded detox terms are *cleansing, elimination of toxins* and *excretion of wastes*.

Except for these crucial differences in the foregoing terminology and the Natural Hygiene stance behind them, all alternative health care systems correctly based in physiology and on how the body works in health and disease are on the right track.

Nearly all emergencies, far-gone cases of wear and tear, blunt force traumas and 11th hour crises absolutely require medical and/or chiropractic intervention to end suffering and save lives. Barring these extreme situations, however, the health seeker takes into the body only four energy enhancers: pure air, pure water, sunlight and wholesome raw foods in digestive-friendly combinations. The health seeker practices six other energy enhancers to inspire natural healing. For the naturalists, there is but one disease (toxemia) and but one healing process (revitalization, cleansing and repair). From this natural perspective, getting well becomes an adventure! And staying well — fun!

# The Ten Energy Enhancers: The Conditions for Health

Dr. Shelton never did consistently name or list the ten energy enhancers, although he did call them *the basic requisites of life* and *the primordial requisites of life.* T. C. Fry named and numbered an unwieldy 22. Dr. Doug Graham has issued 32. I have provided just ten that encompass all healthful living habits, if the ninth and tenth are expanded to include all that is good and wholesome to natural, normal, healthy human life. These ten lifesavers are listed in the order of psychologist Abraham Maslow's hierarchy of needs: survival needs first, aesthetic and social needs last. The ten energy enhancers, practiced consistently over time, cause the body to adapt by building health:

---

## The Ten Energy Enhancers

1. Cleanliness — inside the body and on its outside surfaces
2. Pure air
3. Pure water
4. Adequate rest and sleep
5. The ideal diet of nontoxic, properly combined, raw fruits, vegetables, nuts, seeds and sprouts, organic whenever possible
6. Right temperatures
7. Adequate sunlight
8. Regular exercise
9. Emotional balance, including freedom from addiction, high self-esteem, a purposeful life and meaningful goals
10. Nurturing relationships

---

The ten energy enhancers, practiced by us health seekers, provide our bodies with what they need to get free from addiction and to build health and achieve a natural high. All enhancers are to be instituted into our daily lifestyles if we are to get well and stay well!

# The Ten Energy Robbers:
# The Secondary Causes of Disease

The ten energy robbers (also called *the remote causes of disease* or *the secondary sources of disease*), practiced consistently over time, cause the body to adapt by building disease.

---

## The Ten Energy Robbers

1. Uncleanliness — inside the body and on its outside surfaces

2. Impure air

3. Impure water

4. Inadequate rest and sleep

5. The Standard America Diet of processed, cooked, refined, chemicalized meat, dairy, fruit, vegetables, grains and all junk foods

6. Wrong temperatures

7. Inadequate sunlight

8. Lack of regular exercise

9. Emotional unbalance, including addictions, low self-esteem, a purposeless life and meaningless goals

10. Toxic relationships

---

## The Ten Energy Robbers Are the Addictors

First, let us consider my informal and extended definition of *addiction*. It is a process over which we are powerless and that leads to self-sabotage and ultimately, when allowed to run its course, to self-destruction. Addiction works at the subconscious level. It takes the path of least resistance. It defies conscious attempts to change. It takes control. It causes the addict to think and do things that are dangerously against his or her best interests. It works against highest personal values. It leads to becoming progressively more obsessive with thoughts and feelings that lead to compulsive and destructive actions. It is characterized by fear and danger to self and others. Its sure sign is denial when confronted with a better way.

For my clinical definition of *addiction* as used in rehab centers around the world, see "The Addiction Syndrome at Its Very Worst" on page 529.

The ten energy robbers, when practiced by you or me, not only lead to addiction, but also build disease and destroy happiness. They must be removed from our daily lifestyles if we are to *get well and stay well.*

# Endogenous Toxins: Bodily Generated Sources of Toxemia

## Endogenous Toxins

▶ Metabolic waste: toxic byproducts at the cellular level

▶ Spent debris from cellular activity

▶ Dead cells

▶ Waste from emotional and/or mental stress in normal displays or in excess

▶ Waste from physical fatigue, in normal amounts or in excess

There is only one direct cause of toxemia: being critically low in energy. To be so tired is also termed *enervation*, meaning 'pathologically low on nervous system energy'. But the remote (or secondary) sources of toxemia are many. All of us autointoxicate from two sources: (1) from within the body, resulting in endogenous toxemia, and (2) from what we take into the body from the outside, resulting in exogenous toxemia.

The health seeker will learn to minimize the sources of endogenous toxemia through an energy-conservative lifestyle that is governed by the ten energy enhancers and to — as totally as possible — eliminate the sources of exogenous toxemia through an energy-wise lifestyle that excludes the ten energy robbers. Alternative health care at its best is all about energy conservation.

Endogenous (*endo-* = within + *-gen* = generated) toxins are generated within the body from the sources listed above.

# Exogenous Toxins: External Sources of Toxemia

## Exogenous Toxins

▶ Unnatural food and drink typical of the Standard American Diet

▶ Natural food deranged by processing, refining and preserving

▶ Improper food combinations resulting in endogenous toxins

▶ Medical, pharmaceutical, herbal and supplemental drugging

▶ Tobacco, alcohol and all other forms of recreational drugging

▶ Environmental, commercial and industrial pollutants

Exogenous (*exo-* = outside + *-gen* = generated) toxins are generated outside of the body and include the items listed to the left.

Over time, if a person is burning the energy candle at both ends and not getting enough rest and sleep, the endogenous and exogenous poisons accumulate far beyond the body's energy capacities to conduct a poisons-in/poisons-out balance. For the average person eating the disease-generating food supply, nearly all of which is cooked, enough energy is never available to stay clean, healthy, happy and energetic.

# Live Food — It's All about Energy!

For thousands of years, the power of the body to make good use of time set aside for fasting to bring about healing and rejuvenation has been known. And now the power of the body to make good use of the mostly or 100% live food diet in revitalizing, cleansing and healing is becoming known.

By eating live fruits, veggies, nuts, seeds and sprouts, health seekers first conserve energy. Then this conserved energy is freed up to be used by their bodies, minds and spirits to create health and happiness and wellness around the world.

Following are seven wonderfully conserving and freeing reasons I always present to show health seekers how to get *high energy* and *high joy — naturally.*

## Live Food: Our Biggest Energy Conserver

▶ Energy is conserved because the body is not required to expend energy manufacturing all digestive enzymes needed, an abundance of which are naturally present and active in raw foods. (See Chapter 10.)

▶ Energy is conserved because the body is not required to continually cleanse fluids and tissues of exogenous toxins in heated and chemically adulterated SAD foods.

▶ Energy is conserved because the body is no longer creating nor being required to eliminate the toxic byproducts (endogenous toxins) of cooked food metabolism.

▶ Energy is conserved because the body moves fiber-rich, peristalsis-stimulating, live foods through its digestive tract with a high energy efficiency when compared to the larger amount of energy required to so move cooked foods, which are fiber degraded and no longer peristalsis stimulating.

▶ Energy is conserved because live foods are nutrient rich. They thus provide the body with the best digestible, assimilable, raw building blocks and with the best raw supplies needed for energy-efficient physiological activities. (See Chapter 10.)

▶ Energy is conserved when the health seeker eats live foods in proper combination because the body does not have to detox from endogenous toxins, which are toxic byproducts of poorly combined foods.

▶ Energy is conserved when pure, live foods are eaten in modest amounts and strictly according to genuine hunger because the digestive task set before the body is moderate, easy and efficient on energy demands. In energy-draining comparison, supermarket shelf foods are addicting. SAD food consumption leads to overeating for most people. The big energy task set before the body is therefore doubled on SAD foods. The toxic food is energy demanding to digest, and a huge amount of food is hugely demanding to process.

By eating raw, you will have so much more energy, first *conserved* and then *freed up.* More energy for cleansing and healing! For rising to your calling and for living out your sweetest dreams! For giving and receiving love everywhere you turn! For making the world a better place! Raw foods = raw energy! It's so simple.

# Acute versus Chronic Disease

First, let us always understand that the word *disease* is an abstraction. There is no such concrete thing you can hold in your hand or that you can otherwise measure that can be named a *disease.* There are only abnormal, ill-health conditions of body tissues and fluids and their malfunctioning. These are always accompanied by unpleasant subjective experiences of fatigue, malaise, pain and suffering. Whenever we use the abstract word *disease,* therefore, we are always referring to these concrete realities of malfunction and misery at all levels of our wonderfully made bodies. With this clarification, the alternative model of health care separates disease into two distinct classifications in the following.

## How Acute Disease Evolves into Chronic Disease

Three points are all-important here. First, disease evolves from enervation to toxemia to acute symptoms. When these symptoms are not reversed through healthful living habits, the symptoms worsen and evolve further into chronic disease.

Second, the six ways acute and chronic disease differ are mutually exclusive. Once a person crosses the line from acute to chronic, he or she can almost never return to full and vibrant health.

Third, all people who are living the ten energy robbers will eventually develop acute and then chronic disease if accidental death does not get them first. This reality makes our live food and ten energy enhancers message of utmost urgency and a complete blessing for absolutely every person on the planet!

---

### Six Ways Acute and Chronic Disease Differ

**1.** Acute disease has been short-lived in the making, in process only a few hours, days or weeks. Due to higher energy reserves and thus a lowered adaptation to tolerate toxic saturation, natural healing takes place. Examples of short-lived acute illnesses are diarrhea, headache, indigestion, fatigue, all *-itises* in their early stages and the so-called common cold and flu.

Chronic, degenerative disease has been long-lived in the making, in process over many months or years. Due to lowered energy reserves and thus an increased adaptation to tolerating toxic saturation, natural healing does not take place without strict healthful living intervention. Examples of long-term chronic diseases include diabetes, emphysema, gangrene and all the advanced colitis, cancer and cardiovascular diseases.

---

**2.** In acute disease, the sufferer may have flare-ups, also called *healing crises*, due to a higher vitality. In virtually all cases of acute disease, complete recovery into health is reached once healthful living practices are instituted and detoxing and repair are completed.

The chronic sufferer exhibits lowered vitality and experiences progressively worsening symptoms as time marches on and does not have the vital energy to conduct any healing crises.

**3.** Acute disease may last only a few hours, days or weeks in the healing process. Even without learning about and practicing energy-enhancing habits, many people are healed of acute disease because their living habits are healthful enough and their energy reserves high enough.

But eventually and without exception, if energy-robbing habits are continued long enough, acute disease will evolve into chronic degeneration. Chronic disease will last the rest of the chronic sufferer's lifetime and be the death of him or her if strict adoption of the ten energy enhancers is not immediate.

**4.** Acute disease reflects a strong enough energy supply and reserve vitality that powerful elimination of toxic waste and repair processes are still possible.

Chronic disease reflects a long-term state of toleration of toxins. It is a state of continued elimination of enough toxins to sustain life but in compromised and lowered health. In the latter stages of chronic disease, the natural healing rate is much slower for health seekers who have weakened their defense mechanisms (also collectively and popularly called the *immune system* by conventional MDs, many holistic health educators and most of the people).

For medical model refugees deep into chronic degeneration who have so weakened themselves on fruitless medical routes, the arrest or partial recovery rates are much lower and much less dramatic. Even in chronic cases, however, the cleansing, eliminating and repair processes are still possible if the sufferer gets strict with the ten energy enhancers soon enough. (See Appendix G.)

**5.** Acute disease is designated *remedial* (or *corrective*) in nature, because the disease process itself is an orderly natural process by which the body attempts to eliminate toxins and repair itself. Acute disease results in complete reversal of the disease process — if the ten energy enhancers are strictly followed.

Chronic disease is also designated *remedial* (or *corrective*) in nature, but one cannot expect the same recovery results as in acute disease. In chronic disease, complete arrest of the disease process and possibly some reversal and even much reversal of the abnormal tissues and fluids into health can be expected.

In chronic disease, some tissue changes of a detrimental and many times irreversible nature have taken place. The tissue degenerations are sometimes reversible, sometimes not, depending on the severity and the type of tissue damage. Still, these improvements for chronic sufferers are cause for great celebration compared to the medical route paradigm where virtually all just get worse!

**6.** Acute disease uses up energy in the elimination of toxic waste and in cellular repair, such that the tissue integrity and normal organ and system functions are fully restored. The health seeker may feel enervated or exhilarated when the acute crisis passes, depending on the amount of energy expended and on the kind and amount of toxic overload expelled. This is the time to take extra rest and recuperate the energy expenditure of getting well.

Chronic disease is characterized by progressive fluid and cellular poisoning and retrograde changes such that tissues, organs and whole systems lose their full functional integrity, ending in long-term misery and/or death of the chronic sufferer.

*Obviously, our message is urgent.* Take action during the acute stages, and do not let your disease situation evolve into chronic degeneration. Once you get well, you cannot go back to your old bad habits if you intend to stay well.

# Health by Healthful Living Gets the Best Results!

Susan and I went back and forth for months about how many times we would use the term *Natural Hygiene* in our book. She did not want the book to get lopsided for Natural Hygiene when her overriding goal was to get the raw food word out. One of her arguments was so powerful and so true: *"When people get sick, they really don't care about debating models and schools of thought on disease origin and health care. They simply want to get well! They want what gets results!"* In the final analysis, the very best and speediest way to reach your highest health potential comes from practicing healthful living habits.

The healthful habit most neglected by the majority of people is eating live foods: raw fruits, veggies, nuts, seeds and sprouts. In most cases of sickness, most health seekers are greatly benefited by going on a raw juice diet or by undertaking, for a relatively short period of days or weeks, a properly conducted fast on water. (For a crash course on detoxing while on raw foods and on fasting and juice dieting, refer to Chapters 14 and 15.) The health seeker can go the faster route by fasting on water only or the slower route by drinking raw juices and/or eating raw foods. Either way, all ten energy enhancers must be followed to get the best results possible.

## Your Highest Health Potential

The extent to which you, as a health seeker, get results is determined by five factors:

## Five Factors That Determine Your Highest Health Potential

✓ Your systemic weaknesses, which are affected by your inherited predisposition and your past injuries and irreversible damage already done to your body

✓ The amount and kinds of toxins present in your body

> ✓ Your existing nerve energy reserves (see page 544)
>
> ✓ Your complete abandonment of the ten energy robbers
>
> ✓ Your strict adoption of the ten energy enhancers

At alternative centers, records show that people got marvelous results in virtually 100% of the acute cases reviewed. And most people in chronic degeneration showed arrest or partial to near-complete recoveries.

These health recoveries have been recorded in well over a million cases throughout the last three centuries. These case histories have been kept at clinics, schools and retreats run by a long list of alternativists worldwide: Dr. Harvey Kellogg, Dr. J. H. Tilden, Dr. Edmond Szekely, Dr. H. M. Shelton, T. C. Fry, Dr. William Esser, Dr. Vivian Virginia Vetrano, Drs. Tosca and Gregory Haag, Dr. David Scott, Dr. Douglas Graham, Rev. George Malkmus, Dr. David Klein, myself and many others presently practicing and referenced in the Resource Guide.

Only a very, very few health seekers who are deep, deep into chronic degeneration are too far past the pathological point of no return to recover. If they arrive at the doorsteps of alternative health care institutions in this deathbed condition and as a last resort, it is sometimes just too late for their self-healing bodies to do the work of revitalizing, regenerating, rebuilding and renewing. The body does have its limits. Still, these far-gone health seekers are very, very few in comparison to the vast majority, who are in the earlier stages of disease. Time is of the essence.

Many times, when the conditions for health are provided, results can only correctly be called *miraculous*. The real miracle, however, is simply the natural healing capabilities of the body, so wonderfully resourceful in its design.

To claim your own virtual healing miracle, see Appendix G for how to best get strict with the ten energy enhancers.

# The Health by Healthful Living Model: One Disease, One Healing Process

For the vast majority of us health seekers who do choose the alternative route, our full recoveries (acute) or arrests or partial to near-full recoveries (chronic) are doable. We are among the alternative health intelligentsia. We know that disease is as natural a process as is health. We know that in disease, the body has low energy reserves, with a too-many-toxins-in/not-enough-toxins-out imbalance established and building. We know that the body's job is to keep the blood clean and that in disease, the body has low energy reserves and resorts to putting toxins away in special areas to eliminate them when it can. We know that in health, the body has high energy reserves, with a toxins-in/toxins-out balance maintained.

We alternative paradigm shifters correctly understand it impossible to find congruent the idea that there is one cause of all disease — toxemia — with the idea that disease is caused by some mysterious force, wear and tear, bad genes or dangerous germs. We well informed correctly find it impossible to reconcile the ideas of letting the body heal itself by providing the conditions for health with drugging and cutting practices to create health. We intelligentsia are filled with truth, confidence and optimism! Many of those with the medical mentality remain in the dark, mystified by all the disease around them and very often feeling victimized, demoralized and hopeless.

Two natural healing pioneers taught the idea of one disease, one healing process. In the early 1900s, Arnold Ehret declared, "Nature alone ... heals through one thing — fasting — every disease that it is possible to heal. This, alone, is proof that nature recognizes but one disease, and that in every body the largest factors are always waste, foreign matter and mucus [phlegm]" (*The Mucusless Diet Healing System*).

At the turn of the 20th century, Florence Nightingale, mother of the nursing profession, taught, "There are no specific diseases, only specific disease conditions."

Dr. T. Colin Campbell, author of the landmark book *The China Study*, based on the largest nutritional study ever conducted, concurs with these two pioneer teachers. When asked if he could make specific dietary recommendations according to certain diseases, Campbell replied that he had come to see, through decades of research, two truths. First, diseases all have "impressive commonalities." Second, the same good nutrition benefiting the body in disease prevention can also nourish a sick body back to health.

This concludes my seven lists on Natural Hygiene as *The Superlative, Alternative Health Care System*. Now Susan takes the lead with Dr. Vetrano and me to back her up.

# Even Deficiency Diseases Can Stem from Toxemia

Concerning deficiency diseases, Dr. Shelton and Dr. Vetrano have noted that a very few situations arise not from toxic overload, but from malnutrition due to inadequacies of other basic requisites of life. Examples are scurvy (Vitamin C deficiency), beriberi (Vitamin $B_1$ deficiency) and pernicious anemia (Vitamin $B_{12}$ malabsorption).

Deficiency diseases are on the rise in the West due to increasing mineral depletion of our soils (a topic to be addressed in Chapter 17). Since some people have been known to heal even in certain cases of malnutrition during fasting, toxicity can even be at the root of certain deficiency diseases.

One possible explanation for such healings of deficiency diseases may be that the body is ridding itself of toxic interference in the small intestine. This results in improved nutrient absorption. For example, Albert Mosseri, author of *Mangez Nature Santé Nature*, reports that anemia has regressed in patients not by ingestion of iron, but rather after undertaking a fast.

Dr. Doug Graham also notes that Vitamin $B_{12}$ rises during fasts because the body is able to eliminate the $B_{12}$ analogs and other such toxins while fasting. So it appears that toxins can at times be the cause of deficiencies. (Another factor is that during fasts there is more $B_{12}$ available for recycling into the remaining cells and tissues after being liberated from autolyzed cells.)

# The Politics of Poisoning People

One hundred years ago, cancer developed in only 1 out of 2,500 (by some accounts, only 1 in 8,000). Now 2 in 5 people will develop cancer. Cancer is expected to overtake heart disease as America's number one killer disease soon, if it hasn't already. Most people will build both within their bodies. How could this be if disease were purely genetic? Some argue that the cancer rate is on the rise because we live longer. But how would this longevity factor explain why cancer is increasing at an alarming rate among young children?

These rising and alarming cancer and heart disease statistics do not stand alone. Incidences of obesity, diabetes, AIDS and other diseases are also rising. The recorded incidences of the other top killer diseases of the Westernized world, where nearly all the people overeat on the SAD foods, have all been similarly skyrocketing in the past few decades. These deadly foods are designed with one idea in mind — profits. The two primary considerations in maximizing profits are creating longer shelf lives and a deeper addiction to keep people eating, preferably all day and night. See Appendix A for how food disease industrialists lace our food with addictive toxins.

Victoria points out how we are being undone via the SAD:

A steady diet of these deadly designer SAD foods results in terrible disease, loss of quality of life, suffering and untimely fatalities.

Clearly, a systematic and lucrative poisoning of the people is at work via the unnatural food supply. If this work is not a deliberate conspiracy amongst the medical and pharmaceutical capitalists, the SAD food and advertisement industrialists and some government leaders, it may as well be for the fabulously successful results their cooperative work is getting! Consider the following:

▶ The worldwide medical/pharmaceutical industry now rivals, if not surpasses, the war machine in making more money than any other industry.

▶ The food/advertisement stockholders' profits are at an all-time high.

▶ The government bureaucrats are saving vast sums in Social Security benefits that will never have to be paid because the retired workers are killed off by their addiction to cooked and refined food laced with chemicals.

▶ Those who do live longer spend their lifetime savings on medical bills. Statistics show that 25% of all the money the average American spends on medical care is spent during the last year of life. Nice how that all works out for the powers-that-be!

There is no doubt that children and young adults are getting sicker sooner than those of the older generation. It has been predicted by gloom-and-doom statisticians that the current youth will be the first generation in history to live shorter lives than their parents. To give a political spin to what is going on, Victoria notes, "The most readily available weapons of mass destruction are in the supermarkets and convenience stores. And there is nothing hidden or secret about their locations!"

If you do the research, you will find that the rising disease statistics parallel the increasing pollution of both the food supply and our planet. We are being bombarded by toxic food, water and air. For many of us, our work environments and homes are polluted. Even our clothes, rugs and cleaning materials are made of and reek of antilife chemicals. Microwaves, computers and televisions (especially high-definition TVs) emit harmful rays. Noise offends, if not damages, our organs of hearing. Recreational and prescription drugs poison our bodies.

All these exogenous toxins, however, cannot compete in any given person with the toxins ingested when eating three "square" SAD meals a day plus junk snacks and beverages. Dr. Ralph Moss reports that according to National Institutes of Health directors Donald Frederickson and Arthur Upton, most of the toxins that contribute to the body developing cancer are from food (*The Cancer Industry: The Classic Exposé on the Cancer Establishment*, p. 231). For this reason, the need for people to make live food connections to their personal health conditions is of utmost importance.

Victoria continues with her adventures along these lines:

From 1983 to 1992, while working on endless projects to promote Natural Hygiene, I lived weeks and months at a time in the home of Marianne Fry and at the offices and retreats of the humble, half-Cherokee and half-white, eighth-grade-educated, all-American, self-made man — T. C. Fry. This was back before Thunder Cloud (T. C.) was bestowed the honorary degree that made him "Doctor T. C. Fry," a ludicrous possibility on his professional horizon. At the time, he joked about it: "The last thing I want to be called is a 'doctor' of anything!"

The Fry rhetoric was beloved by some. But it was criticized by others, especially by some of his peers, for three valid reasons. First, T. C. oversimplified and therefore misrepresented some of the teachings. Second, he pushed the dangerous all-fruit diet. And third, he made false claims, promising all the people that they all could get well from any and all diseases, all in a matter of days or weeks.

One such sensational ploy T. C. would use to wake the people up was the astounding, outrageous and then-unbelievable claim that he made to describe the frightful state of the poisoned food supply. (I say *unbelievable* because more people were in more ignorance in the 1980s.) T. C. would warn the people, "We poison ourselves 100 different ways every day!"

This particular claim, however, was true. His new followers were shocked and horrified to get this education. Now 25 years later, this book is presenting the most extensive research yet amassed to show that people on SAD foods are poisoning themselves up to several thousands of times a day, when all cooked food toxins and all other endogenous and exogenous poisons are all totaled!

Nutritionist Natalia Rose concurs that glowing health arises not only from what we put into our bodies today, but also from "the removal of waste matter built up from years of improper eating" (*The Raw Food Detox Diet*, p. 10). She explains that most diets don't work for permanent weight loss because their authors don't address the issue of removal of those toxins that cause slow metabolism and sluggish digestive and circulatory systems. As Natalia points out, "The worst offender of this system happens to be your diet" (p. 227).

She compares this toxic overload with an overloaded hospital emergency room in which, at the end of the day, only half the patients have been attended to.

Victoria provides a body-as-home metaphor rather than Rose's hospital analogy:

I compare the body's toxic overload to a dirty house wherein the cleaning lady, the plumber, the electrician, the garbage man and the carpenter did not show up to do their necessary chores, yet a house where people keep living, never picking up after themselves and never fixing anything. The house is going to get dirty, fall into disrepair and become uninhabitable. So too will become the body when overloaded with toxins.

To extend my metaphor, the body simply does not know what to do with its trash when the workers are too tired to do their jobs! So poisons pollute first the bodily fluids. Then if energy is too low to move out all the pollutants, endogenous and exogenous poisons not eliminated and left circulating in the fluids are transported to and deposited in the tissues: onto or within artery walls, in the joints, in fatty tissues, onto colon walls and other out-of-the-way places. Such deposits are determined both genetically and by the presence of weakened, damaged, unhealthy tissues. (All damaged tissues have an affinity for attracting toxins.) Note that the weakest areas of the body may be determined genetically and also have this affinity for toxins. Yet it is not genetic determination, but the presence of exogenous and endogenous toxins that actually pollutes the fluids and harms the bodily cells, tissues, organs and systems.

Cleverly and in an attempt to keep toxins out of mainstream circulation and harm's way, the body even creates its own storage containers: tumors, cysts, polyps, pustules, pimples, warts and other bulges and bumps and dropsy bags, double chins and fatty aprons. Keepers of the medical mentality have quite reasonably but entirely wrongly concluded that since there are approximately 10,000 different names for diseases, there must be approximately 10,000 different cures. All the while, the health by healthful living paradigm quite reasonably and entirely correctly theorizes one simplicity: one disease, one healing process. In the alternative health care paradigm, absolutely no ailments are mysterious. There are no multiple schools of thought about disease origin and health care.

# When Certain Cooked Foods
# May Be Absolutely Necessary

Victoria BidWell cautions us with one exception to the raw diet rule:

After a 2008 lesson with Dr. David Scott, I would like to add a huge qualification to our nearly to 100% all-raw food teachings throughout our book.

Dr. Scott and other alternative health care professionals have found that over the years, certain patients in certain advanced diseased conditions absolutely cannot tolerate a mostly raw or all-raw food diet. Violent reactions to raw food and/or a wasting away into nutrient deficiencies and/or dangerously low body weight can occur with these raw food-intolerant people.

According to Dr. Scott, these incidences of raw food intolerance are very rare. We wanted to make it perfectly clear, however, that they may be found in certain advanced diseased states. It could be that the raw fiber is too rough for their digestive systems to handle. It could be many things. Exactly why this is so is a matter of pure speculation. What is *not* a matter of any speculation whatsoever, however, is two-fold:

First, each patient has his own unique inherited predisposition and his own unique state of developed pathology. The flesh is mortal and not perfect. Breakdown inevitably occurs when the natural, physiological laws of life have been broken long enough. What the body cannot digest, absorb and metabolize — cooked or raw — will result in an inordinate energy drain, the creation of endogenous toxins and autointoxication. First, acute disease develops. Then chronic, degenerative disease evolves. But for a very few people for whatever reasons, a raw food intolerance also develops.

Second, for certain patients, this advanced diseased condition manifests not in the lungs or the joints or elsewhere in the body, but in the digestive system. Compromised digestion and/or absorption develop. Dr. Scott and others have found that in a variety of advanced pathological situations — certain cancers and colitis, for two examples — the patients can tolerate, digest and absorb certain cooked foods and absolutely cannot tolerate, digest and/or absorb certain raw foods. Speculation why is pointless. This is simply a matter of observations of thousands of patients over decades of case histories kept by many alternative health care doctors.

Dr. Scott told of patients who could not handle raw foods at all when admitted to his institute but who could thrive on them after taking one or more long fasts. The cooked foods typically given during the get well period are mild flavored and nonstimulating: steamed veggies such as zucchini, carrots, potatoes or a gruel of steamed potatoes mashed with a small amount of water.

The health seeker is given various foods to discover what will digest well. But always, in time, as his diseased state reverses into health, raw foods which are properly combined and free of all protoplasmic poisons will become the mainstay of the diet as he stays well.

# In Deference to the Good
# Doctors and Their Personnel

The following statement has been written by Victoria BidWell and endorsed by these four women: Victoria BidWell, Dr. Vetrano, Dr. Tosca Haag and Susan Schenck:

As pitifully outdated and absolutely wrong as "The Medical Mentality at Its Very Worst" (see page 542) is and the people who perpetuate it are, the collective group of individuals who have supported it and do continue certain of its practices in the traditional, allopathic paradigm have contributed much good to society.

No doubt about it, their sophisticated technological gadgetry and pharmaceutical genius enable them to prolong the lives of seriously sick and deathbed-ill people. The good doctors and their staff, with their space-age life-support systems, keep people in severe degenerative conditions alive when no hygienic intervention or guidance could so do.

Furthermore, we all know at least one person who is alive today only because of spectacular, heroic medical intervention by the good doctors and their personnel. (Had this person turned wholeheartedly to healthful living practices years earlier, however, his health would have undoubtedly improved so greatly that he would not have needed the medical intervention in the first place.)

Please do understand that this book is not discounting that *the good doctors and their personnel* do good. Of course we acknowledge enthusiastically that the medically minded collective have made invaluable contributions and instituted certain practices that can only be called *blessings*: providing insulin to diabetics, offering childbirth services, reviving a stopped heart, carrying out kidney dialysis, performing organ transplants and lifesaving emergency surgeries, prescribing narcotics in cases of excruciating pain, outfitting amputees with prosthetics, performing restorative and reconstructive surgeries, giving dental aid, offering many kinds of first aid services and follow-up support to a long list of trauma and burn victims and numerous like measures. Such services provided by the good doctors and their personnel are *absolute blessings*.

This book nevertheless asserts that *on the whole*, those with their medical mentality *in no way* offer the *superlative health care program* whereby we can learn to prevent disease in its earliest stages of enervation and toxemia and enhance health by removing the remote causes of disease and providing the conditions for health. Therefore, we speak here in deference to the good doctors and their personnel and commend them for their good works. We only wish there were more of them!

If only the medical students were to turn their studies to health while in school and away from naming diseases and what drugs to prescribe for the diseases! If only the doctors were to teach the suffering people how to enhance their health through energy-conserving lifestyle practices rather than prescribing drugs and surgeries and other enervating "therapies" and "treatments"! Then we would not have the suffering class as the largest and most miserable group of Americans among us today. What good doctors and personnel we would then have!

# Coming Up...

Next, we continue with a mind-blowing exposé on the big lie that germs are the sole causative factor in many disease conditions. The medical doctors and pharmacists have given microorganisms a bad rap!

*We will see that the ten energy robbers are the true culprits in virtually all disease and that health by healthful living is the most effective means of reversing disease and creating health.*

# 5
# Bacteria and Viruses: Not Guilty as Charged!

We must look rationally at the bacterial issue. Consider the fact that many tribes ate primarily unsalted raw meat, unsalted raw fats and/or unsalted raw dairy products from the beginning. They did not wash their hands or sterilize their food before eating. Every form of natural bacteria, including salmonella, *E. coli* and campylobacter were eaten with their food abundantly and constantly. Why were they vibrant, healthy and disease free if microbes are the culprits?            —Aajonus Vonderplanitz (1947–), *The Recipe for Living Without Disease* (p. 18)

At this point, let's focus on the medical model's fourth school of thought, the germ theory of disease. Practically a mass hysteria when it took off in the late 1800s, germ phobia swept the globe.

Presently, the germ theory promoted by the medical, pharmaceutical and advertising industries remains a hugely powerful persuasive force worldwide. Even today, the public still demands pills and vaccinations to kill or stave off germs, thus carrying on the hysteria begun more than a century ago. It is, and always has been, a hysteria based upon a complete lie. It makes a lot of people a lot of money as new diseases are identified or made up and blamed on new germ culprits suspected to be responsible for new diseases that are then put on trial and declared guilty!

In our alternative model, microorganisms are termed either *friendly* or *unfriendly*, depending on whether they serve us in health or hasten our demise in disease, respectively. Bacteria remain our friends so long as we keep ourselves internally clean. When we do so, we no longer have to fret about visiting sick friends, worrying that we too will "catch the bug" going around. Wherever we may go, we no longer have to fear people sneezing on us, passing on viruses by shaking hands with us or by breathing germs upon us.

Remember the bubonic plague, or Black Death? Reportedly, one-third of the rural European population and half of the urbanites died during the Late Middle Ages pandemic, peaking in 1348, and stretching into the 1600s. The worldwide death count ended at an estimated 75 million, 20 million of those in Europe alone. What about those who didn't die? They were mostly exposed to the very same germs. Most of those not "stricken" actually cared for the sick and even buried the dead.

Maybe it is time to study radically healthy people for clues to good health instead of the pathologically sick.

Germ phobia began in the 1860s. Louis Pasteur, after whom the process of pasteurization was named, proposed that germs played the primary role in causing disease. He popularized the notion that one unique germ causes one specific disease. To get rid of the specific disease, one must rid himself of the corresponding unique germ culprit.

At the same time, biochemist Antoine Béchamp, who remains unrenowned to this day, discovered microzymas, which are the smallest living unit in all living organisms. Béchamp found that microzymas changed their forms (pleomorphism) according to the general health of the cells they inhabited.

He declared that when the body's chemistry was healthy, the microzymas developed into benign or even helpful bacteria. When the body's chemistry was out of balance, as from malnutrition or toxicity, some of the microzymas transformed into harmful forms that contributed to furthering the disease process. He summarized his findings by boldly denouncing Pasteur, declaring, "The soil [biological terrain] is everything!"

Later German doctor Günther Enderlein, through sixty years of observing human blood, proved Béchamp's theory of pleomorphism to be correct. It states that microzymas, or protits, change form according to conditions in the blood. He concluded, "The most powerful diet for bringing a diseased biological terrain back to normal is live foods."

Dr. Robert Young, PhD, DSc, explains that a healthy or diseased body is determined by four things: (1) pH balance (acid/alkaline), (2) electromagnetic charge (positive/negative), (3) levels of toxic accumulation and (4) nutritional status (*Sick and Tired?* p. 21).

He claims that an unhealthy blood cell can morph into a bacterium, which can later change into a yeast, or fungus, which could turn into a mold in an advanced state of bad health. He states that this metamorphosis of bacteria and fungi in a drop of fresh blood is one of the most dramatic things he has seen in his career.

Thus there arose two conflicting theories about what is to blame for disease: the presence of a pathogen versus the condition of the biological terrain. Pasteur's theory stated that the germs were the enemy. Béchamp's theory stated that germs cohabit with us but do not change into harmful forms when we remain healthy by taking care of our inner terrain.

Pasteur's theory ultimately won out because establishment leaders found it easier and much more profitable to convince people that they had to wage war against germs rather than teach people that they had to take good care of themselves with healthful living practices.

Pasteur's victory led to great profits for food processors from pasteurization, the process of destroying germs by heating food, especially dairy products. Since the late 1800s, vast sums have been made creating vaccinations and other drugs to kill germs. Today, the war on germs is a multibillion-dollar-per-year industry in the United States alone. Think of all the wasted money that could have been used for humanitarian purposes since then!

If only all of these people had been taught to eat right and live right, they might not have developed toxic body ecologies that poisoned their microflora into developing into unfriendly forms that then created their own toxic byproducts. But hey, what profit would there have been in that? Happily, we still have time to change our ways and profit from true health care knowledge.

There is an oft-quoted mid-1800s comparison of germs with mosquitoes originally made by the father of pathology, German physician Dr. Rudolph Virchow: "If I could live my life over again, I would devote it to proving that germs seek their natural habitat — diseased tissue — rather than being the cause of the diseased tissue; e.g., mosquitoes seek the stagnant water but do not cause the pool to become stagnant."

In other words, microorganisms can become opportunists that metamorphose from benign forms to feed on diseased tissue, but they do not cause the tissue to become diseased. The "critter," be it a bacterium, fungus, virus or parasite, has nothing to feed on in a pure body.

Over a century later modern-day author Arthur M. Baker echoes Virchow in *Awakening Our Self-Healing Body: A Solution to the Health Care Crisis*, "Virulent bacteria find soil in dead food substances only and cannot exist on living cells. Cooked food spoils rapidly, both inside and outside our body, whereas living foods are slow to lose their vital qualities and do not as readily become soil for bacterial decay."

Ironically, even Pasteur himself eventually came to realize he had been wrong, that the filthy condition of a body's internal terrain, not the mere presence of germs, was to blame for illness. Pasteur's assistants documented his deathbed confession for posterity, but the medical germ theory propagandists had already won out by then.

Today, Dr. Young points out, "The American Medical Association, pharmaceutical companies and others wish us to plan our health care around this scientific error" (*Sick and Tired?* p. 25).

Raw food experts and virtually all biologists and physiologists go a step beyond viewing germs as merely friendly or unfriendly. These experts claim that microorganisms do us a necessary service by helping us clean up our internal and external environments. If you saw a gathering of rodents and flies eating trash, you wouldn't likely blame them for creating the garbage site. Disgusting as their activity may appear, you would more likely be grateful they are helping to get rid of the trash. The same is true with bacteria. They cannot be blamed as the cause of your toxic body; they are merely the scavengers that eat the toxic buildup.

Victoria Boutenko gives us a graphic image to contemplate when she asks us to think of all the dead animal bodies that would be strewn across the land if bacteria did not decompose them! Could it be that the true role of bacteria in your body is actually to help get rid of the pathogenic debris left over from cooked food and other toxins, rather than to cause disease?

I remember when I used to "catch a cold" or "come down with the flu," now understood to be *eliminations of toxins* via *healing crises* in the alternative paradigm. I would feel really great when it was finally over! I experienced a wonderful taste in my mouth and a feeling of bliss.

Others I talked to agreed that they also experienced these sensations, but they didn't fit our establishment paradigm of disease and getting well, so no one knew why this happened. I realize now it was largely because of the "alkaline high" from my body rebalancing its chemistry and cleaning out acidic waste. (See page 331 for more on alkalinity.)

Physicist Bruno Comby, PhD, states, "Conventional medical theory regards illness as resulting from chance or from microbes or from a genetic predisposition. This view does not square with the fact that the manifestation of illness is diminished or nonexistent in animals and humans whose lifestyle and diet are more natural" (*Maximize Immunity*, p. 103).

Part of Dr. Comby's proposed "dietary theory of immunity" is the "useful virus theory." Based on his research data, he proposes that a virus can actually offer *useful genetic information* to the cell to assist it in carrying out its beneficial job of detoxification.

After years of study, he proposes that viruses, bacteria and other microbes are not harmful in and of themselves. They present harm only if the body's internal chemistry has been greatly unbalanced, the tissues greatly retrograded and its defense mechanisms greatly compromised. The body adapts to a toxic overload due to toxic diet, drugs and/or other endogenous and exogenous stressors only when the energy robbers are consistently practiced.

Microbes, including allegedly dangerous ones such as HIV, are not inherently harmful in the "soil," or body ecology, of a person eating a 100% raw or mostly raw diet. If someone is reasonably healthy, microbes can actually be *beneficial* by taking part in eliminating internal accumulations of abnormal substances. Microbes can thus fulfill a natural and useful biological role.

In fact even macroscopic parasites are affected when one eats raw foods. On several occasions, Comby and his colleagues witnessed people on raw food diets spontaneously eliminating *tapeworms* that had resisted bodily expulsion by conventional treatments. Their soil was just too clean to attract such parasites.

When someone goes cold turkey off highly toxic and addictive drugs, like street heroin or medically prescribed painkillers, he may experience a cluster of toxic elimination and withdrawal symptoms, such as nausea, vomiting, diarrhea, chills, mental/emotional aberrations and even hallucinations. No one denies that his body is simply struggling to eliminate toxins.

Yet when the same person experiences a so-called cold, which is also a cluster of respiratory tract cleansing symptoms, usually from all the bad food eaten lately, the ill-informed says his body is being "attacked" by a "bad virus." In fact the opportunistic virus was only there taking advantage of the bad soil. The presence of bacteria can even be helpful since they assist the body in cleaning up its toxic mess.

In the next chapter, Victoria BidWell tackles the most challenging question to the medical establishment: Do drugs really work?

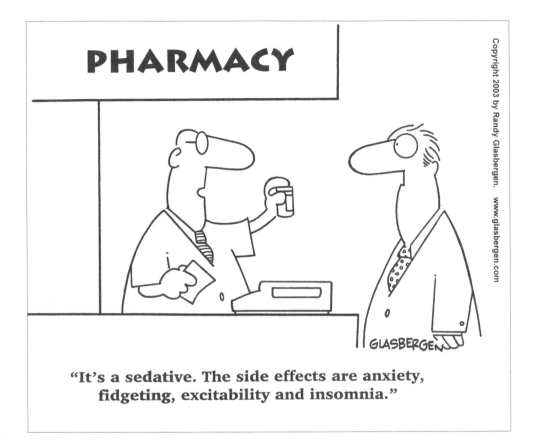

"It's a sedative. The side effects are anxiety,
fidgeting, excitability and insomnia."

# 6
# Do Drugs Work?

Researchers in Canada were curing breast cancer with linseed oil better than chemotherapy. Why wasn't this discovery front-page headline news? Women around the world should be outraged that the truth and effectiveness about linseed oil treating breast cancer is being hidden from them. Drug company executives years ago told me directly that anything that would cut into the profits of chemotherapy has to be debunked, discredited, and hidden from the public! —Kevin Trudeau (1963–), *More Natural "Cures" Revealed* (p. 23)

Victoria BidWell contributes this chapter in collaboration with Dr. Vetrano.

Let us now focus on the second greatest source of exogenous toxins for most people after cooked food: drugs of all kinds. These include the following: prescription drugs, over-the-counter drugs, nicotine, alcohol, coffee and tea, herbal drugs, synthetic supplement drugs and all illegal and recreational drugs that are swallowed, sniffed, snorted, smoked or injected.

But first, another term and its definition: *Protoplasm* is a general term for the viscous grayish translucent colloidal substance that makes up an estimated 75,000,000,000,000 (estimates range from 50-100 trillion) cells in our bodies. And all these drugs are all protoplasmic poisons — deadly to cellular life, dangerous to us!

Taking drugs to cure disease or to make it through the night is foundational to the medical model. That drugs "work," however, is the big lie of the medical model. Little concern, at least initially, is given by the doctor or patient if the drug habit leads to physiological, mental and emotional toleration and addiction. Little concern is given to the fact that when drugs have sickening ramifications, a second round of different drugs have to be taken to relieve those side effects. Through the looking glass, we call them *poisoning effects*.

Our health by healthful living model completely shatters the proposition that drugs "work" and offers the one disease, one healing process solution instead. Self-education, self-responsibility and self-care make up the backbone of this alternative health care model. The health seeker will surely need all three to get free of drug use and/or addiction and to cultivate the natural high that natural living promises.

The success rates for current drug treatment programs are pitifully low. Although most drug rehab centers do focus on some of the ten energy enhancers, few include the live food factor in their drug withdrawal and keeping clean strategies. This is so sad and so physiologically unwise because the one thing a tired, drug-ridden body needs is superlative nutrition for its worn-down mind and broken spirit.

# Taking Drugs: It's a Black-or-White Thing

*Drugs absolutely do not cure!* Drugs are all classified as toxic stimulants, in that the body responds to their poisoning presence by using precious energy needed elsewhere to reject them.

While in the body, different drugs result in different physiological and personal experiences. Some drugs clinically classified as depressants and barbiturates are called "downers" on the street because the user's physical reflexes and mental/emotional responses are impaired and are effectively narcotized into a groggy lethargy. Street drugs termed "uppers" are so called because of the excitation of brain activity into manic and/or paranoid thinking while the body moves into the fight-or-flight mode. Most drugs, however, do not alter moods and do not stimulate the user into entertaining highs or mellow lows. Most drugs just poison as they palliate (relieve symptoms) and stop any cleansing and repair process in progress.

It is erroneously stated that "drugs relieve pain" and "drugs will cure you." Certainly this is what television advertisements and medical/pharmaceutical pushers would lead us to believe. "Relieved" or "cured" may very well be seemingly correct subjective ways of describing what a person feels after taking a drug. But this relief that feels like a cure because symptoms die down is only temporary. The drug user is being poisoned with every dose unless alternative care is practiced so that his or her body can heal itself.

The health by healthful living model teaches that what we take into our bodies is either a poison or a nutrient. It's a black-or-white thing. See the Law of Utilization as defined on page 552. "The normal [health-promoting] elements and materials of life are all that the living organism is ever capable of constructively utilizing, whether it is well or sick."

All drugs are loaded with antilife chemicals, foreign to any molecules in the human body. The body cannot use them. By definition, therefore, every drug is a *poison*. By contrast, raw foods are loaded with pro-life chemicals and wholesome nutrients. And the body can use them with glorious, health-building results! In the final analysis, if the body could make use of a drug as a material with which to build healthy blood, brain and brawn, it would not be classified as a *drug* but as a *food*.

When bringing something into your body, first ask, "Does this item support life or poison life?" This distinction is what takes lifesaving insulin out of the poison-drug category and puts it into the emergency replacement-drug category unto itself. Still, the alternative model records show that thousands of insulin-dependent people with adult onset diabetes and even children with juvenile diabetes have been taken completely off all insulin to lead normal healthy lives once health by healthful living has been firmly established.

# The Palliation Effect of Drugs — Exposed!

In the health by healthful living model and through its looking glass, disease messages are best understood not as symptoms to palliate or alleviate, but as cries for correction from a tired and toxic body! During the disease process, the body has been forced to make abnormal changes in fluids and tissues. Pain, checked elimination and abnormal tissues are the pathological results of natural bodily processes. But they are abnormal and retrograde, going backwards and downwards, away from health and into disease. These processes appear backwards if yours is a medical mentality, but disease symptoms are not to be halted with drugs! Disease symptoms are the body's natural survival warnings to go no further with the energy robbers. They are cries for help *now*. They are user-friendly messages for the health seeker who wants to get well.

Disease symptoms in times of pathologically low energy (chronic disease) are paradoxically two-fold. First, they are evidence of the body's long-term and now failing ability to deal with self-poisoning. Second, they are warnings that the sick person must change his or her ways and live right immediately! If a person continues with the energy robbers, he may build up such a toxic saturation and be so low on energy that his body progresses from acute symptoms into chronic, without so much as a sniffle or cough, just with chronic weariness and the emotional doldrums.

Thus it happens that a person is suddenly "stricken" with cancer or his heart "attacks" him or he "succumbs" to a virus with no warning signs whatsoever. This leaves ill-informed, medical model thinkers confused or shocked, as they shake their heads in disbelief, muttering at the funeral, "But he was never sick a day in his life. He was healthy as a horse." We can usually spot these "drop-dead time bombs" because they are never really overtly sick. They are just so tired, lifeless, uninspired and depressed — all the time.

Alternativists explain that the body responds to a newly added drug poison by rerouting its energies to get rid of it. Efforts go from excreting other sources of toxemia and healing to eliminating the drug just taken in. MDs and ill-informed patients see it backwards and do not consider this to be a rerouting of energy to get rid of a highly undesirable drug at all. Rather, they see drug taking as a welcome palliation of symptoms and highly desirable, since it brings relief and a cure for the moment.

When elimination symptoms stop, a medicine user gets quick relief. But it is a symptom palliation illusion. All the "sniffles-and-cough-medicine-so-you-can-sleep" concoctions are classic examples of this quick relief palliation effect that poisons the body into further disease stages while symptoms are effectively masked. The medicine makers will never ever find a cure for the common cold in their chemistry labs because the only way out of disease is completed re-energizing, detoxing and repair — the very thing cold medicines are designed to stop!

Let us propose a scenario with one of these everyday people who take drugs for quick relief (palliation). As breaking the laws of life would have it, within

131

minutes or hours or days or weeks, the person wanting drug relief and/or mind-altering euphoria finds his problems have multiplied. The body now has an added drug poison within its systems, complete with poisoning effects, a building toleration to the drug habit toxins and a growing addiction. These new problems all go along with the original symptom complaint: a foggy mind and/or emotional doldrums, which inspired him to take the drug in the first place!

With lowered energy at the onset of drugging, even less energy is available for detoxing and healing. Taking drugs, therefore, may spell "r-e-l-i-e-f" in the short run, but it spells "m-i-s-e-r-y" in the long run.

Ironically, the recreational drug user who just wanted to feel good soon finds himself hooked and in hard-core addiction and *feeling horrible*. This cycle of reintoxication will simply repeat if the person gets clean in rehab but then goes back to the drugs and to living out the ten energy robbers.

The reality TV show *Intervention* gives us vicarious views of the horrors of drug addiction. Without such intervention by concerned loved ones and professionals to get clean, the chronically toxic body of the drug addict will descend into chronic, degenerative disease. Incorporating the live food factor and the ten energy enhancers into all intervention formulas would speed up drug withdrawal like nothing else in the world!

A huge and hidden price must be paid for momentary and symptomatic relief or emotional escapism. Figuratively put, drugs drive the symptoms underground. Science terms this phenomenon *palliation*. The toxins driven underground will surface and be eliminated only during long-term revitalization, cleansing and/or a healing crisis or series of crises.

Always in cases of acute disease, after the health seeker practices the ten energy enhancers strictly and refuses drugs long enough, the body will revitalize and cleanse, then repair and rejuvenate. In cases of chronic, degenerative disease, by contrast, further ingestion of drugs no longer palliates but only results in furthering the toxic saturation because the body no longer has the energy to reroute its energies or to initiate healing crises. The exogenous poisons in drugs thus go underground. Being tired and uninspired all the time is the sure-fire wake-up call that warns, "Do right or get your affairs in order."

While some drug poisons are driven underground, getting retained in already severely poisoned bodily fluids and tissues, others are eliminated only at the cost of overworking and thereby damaging the organs of excretion, especially the liver and kidneys. Proof of this is two-fold. First, the long list of side effects for prescription drugs (in print too tiny to read without a magnifying glass) announce, by the pharmaceutical industry's own admission, potential poisoning effects. Second, the shorter list of contraindications warns that taking the prescription drug will do further damage to the body if existing diseases processes are in full progress.

Furthermore, the functional integrity of the entire body's defense mechanisms (also called the *immune system*) is likewise compromised with every drug poison taken. When the army of white blood cells is pathologically low in number and weak in power, for instance, they can no longer seek out, engulf and destroy toxic or foreign matter effectively. Disease is inevitable.

Opting for quick-fix drug therapy (palliation) prescribed by MDs entrenched in the big lie that drugs "work" only gets results momentarily. Drug palliation only gets relief from annoying symptoms in acute stages, when the body still has energy for violent reaction and elimination. In chronic stages, the quick fix just quickens the arrival of the coroner.

In *Living Nutrition*, Volume 18, 2006, Dr. Vetrano explains the mystery of palliation and of how drugs seem to "work" when they are really only adding to a sick person's toxic overload:

> Antibiotics seem to "work" because the minute they enter the mouth or body, signals are sent all over the organism alerting the cells that a toxic substance is on the way, and the body cells begin preparing their defense against the invader. Your wonder body mobilizes so quickly because of the urgent importance of defending good, functioning tissues. It is a lifesaving function. . . . Symptoms disappear because the body is diverting its energies to an emergency situation. The body can no longer attend to its healing crisis — whether it be a so-called cold, the flu, or any other acute, so-called bacterial disease — and simultaneously continue the elimination of exogenous and endogenous poisons, daily or long-term accumulated. The emergency takes precedence over the acute disease.
>
> We feel energy only in its expenditure, just as some people feel rich only when they spend money extravagantly. While expending energy defending against antibiotics and other drugs, we feel stronger because additional physiological and biochemical activities are taking place. In short, the extreme defensive maneuvers of the body are inspired by the body's decision to get rid of the toxic drug stimulant. This is another one of those circumstances where the appearance is not the reality. You are expending energy eliminating the drug, so you "feel" more energy than you did previously. Your energy is being spent, and this is making you feel peppy. But, in the long run, drugs will only add to your enervation. This is why anyone staying on drugs long enough reports a crash in energy levels. For some, this crash ends in death.
>
> "Well, I sure got well by taking drugs," you may reply to my line of reasoning. "How do you know that the antibiotic did not heal me?"
>
> The answer is simply, "Drugs cannot act. They cannot do work. All healing powers reside within the living organism. I agree with you that your symptoms may disappear and that you may feel better and apparently have more energy after taking antibiotics. But don't let appearances fool you. Actually, if one gets well after taking an antibiotic, it is in spite of, rather than because of, the drug."

# The Mimicking Effect of Drugs — Exposed!

In addition to the palliation effect, drugs can have a mimicking effect. When the body takes in certain drugs, their molecular structures so closely mimic the body's corresponding natural molecules that it is fooled and uses them as though they were the real things. These mimickers have the ability to hook up to cellular receptor sites and to take part in a multitude of other metabolic pathways as if they were the real things. These facsimile drug molecules are recognized by the body to inhibit or otherwise affect physiological changes that the drug user experiences as a suppression of symptoms, as painkilling, as allergy relief and so on. The facsimiles are nevertheless foreign to the body and leave toxic byproducts to poison tissues and fluids when degraded for elimination.

Opiates, for example, copycat natural endorphins and can work at the same neuron receptor sites in a lock-and-key fashion as natural endorphins. The subjective experience is similar to that of natural endorphin molecules: the pain stops, and euphoria sets in. Both palliating and mimicking, however, are dead ends. They both drain energy and poison the body as the user attempts to get rid of what the drugs were taken for in the first place.

# Drugs Don't Work!

To view drugs as "doing work" and "acting upon you" are medical model misconceptions! The entire pharmacopoeia and all those television ads for medications pumped into the living rooms of homes around the world, all day and night — sit atop this foundational error that "drugs act upon the living organism."

Just imagine! Every person at the checkout in every pharmacy you ever happened by has bought into this lie! Every medicine cabinet screwed into every bathroom wall in every home is symbolic of this lie. Such symbols erected show the omnipresence and insidious subtlety of the great big drug lie taken for granted by the vast majority of the ill-informed people around the world. The conventional medical paradigm and its four schools of thought are all not only entrenched in the minds of the people, but sitting in their kitchen cupboards (toxic cooked food) and waiting in their bathroom cabinets (medications).

To make matters worse, there is a drug we are encouraged to take for everything. The media propaganda machinery that is in motion to brainwash the medical mentality into every person on the planet is frightening! It's bad enough that we are we told that drugs will help us deal with everyday physiological functioning, such as sniffles, restless legs, itching, headaches, poor memory, sleepless nights, inability to get an erection, ad nauseum. But on top of that, the medical powers that promote these drugs make up one new disease after another that never existed in the last century and then offer their drug solutions to the new diseases!

Furthermore, MDs reassure us, "If these drugs stop working, there are others we will try."

By taking this stock medical/pharmaceutical advice, you are making matters much worse. You are getting yourself more toxic with each dose. You are postponing recovery by not making use of effective natural healing pathways that could get you well! You are getting ever closer to the pathological point of no return so that *even if you do turn to health by healthful living*, it may be too late. *And you are unwittingly playing the guinea pig* as you take standard and/or experimental poisons! No wonder, at each and every one of the seven locations for

Dr. Shelton's Health School, waved the banner Where Health Is Built, Not Bought.

Sometimes, as with chemotherapy and radiation, the poisoning effects of the treatment kill the patient before the disease gets to. Or the drugs so greatly poison, sicken and weaken the patient that little quality of life is left to enjoy. Dr. Shelton used to say of this final solution to treating medical patients, "To cure them is to kill them!"

With genius wit and polished sarcasm, Dr. Shelton asked his most famous question and delivered his most quoted condemnation of the medical mentality at its very worst: "How is a man who is already sick to be made less so by swallowing a substance that would sicken — even kill — him if he were to take it in a state of health? The theory that disease can be removed by creating a temporary and less serious one must have been invented in a madhouse!"

Much later Dr. Bruno Comby echoed the rhetorical question in *Maximize Immunity*, "How can we hope to heal sick and weakened patients by giving them medication which engenders side effects that would make a healthy person ill?"

Two out of three Americans are presently taking some kind of medication. Most are taking multiple medications. Some are taking as many as ten different kinds and more. Since MDs seldom keep up with all the data (if it even exists) and therefore cannot caution their patients about the dangerous practice of mixing drugs, shouldn't more people be frightened to take so many kinds at once? Now we can see why Nancy Reagan's slogan Just Say No! to street drugs should have been extended to *all* drugs!

For information on how drugs became so popular and so prevalent, please read Appendix B.

Susan now takes the lead as we finish these foundational chapters that present the simple wisdom of alternative health care with the ten energy enhancers and without drugs.

# 7

# The Simplicity
# of Disease Origin
# and Health Care

Simplicity is the ultimate sophistication.
—Leonardo da Vinci (1452–1519)

Let's review. There is only *one disease*, toxic accumulation of bodily fluids and tissues, *toxemia*. And there is only one *healing process*, re-energizing the nervous system. With replenished energy, the body then proceeds to normalize its chemistry, cleanse fluids and cells and heal tissues and systems. It is that simple. English philosopher William of Occam proposed the scientific principle now known as Occam's razor. It states that the simplest theory that fits the known facts is always the best theory to use. What could be simpler than one disease, one healing process?

Most of us are dazzled by all of the gadgets, machines and knowledge that the last century has brought to medicine. As an acupuncture student in pathology class, I was in awe of all of the diseases discovered and labeled. But where has all that gotten us?

Victoria, Dr. Vetrano and I acknowledge once again all of the good that all of the good doctors are doing in emergency and trauma care, prosthetics, dentistry and other such restorative and replacement treatments. Yet these highly admirable and successful efforts account for only about 5% of people seeking medical intervention. *Where is the help for the other 95% of those who have diseases that could all have been prevented completely at their onsets with health by healthful living practices?*

After decades of fighting the war on cancer, the various cancer treatments have grown to a $120 billion per year industry! Anyone considering submitting to chemotherapy for cancer can study the recovery rates and adverse side effects of this treatment. (See Appendix B.) Better to be educated than bedazzled.

A great deal of waste is involved in the obsession with labeling diseases. Think of the hundreds of diseases and their symptom clusters that medical students have to memorize. Think of the hundreds of drugs that have to be memorized, along with their indications and contraindications. Think of all the diagnostic tests and all the expenses involved in them.

Yet many times physicians do not agree among themselves on a single diagnosis! They openly admit that approximately half of their diagnoses are incorrect. That means half of their prescriptions, treatments and prognoses are incorrect. Their patients should only be asked to pay half of their doctor, hospital and prescription bills!

The best odds are with holistic health care because disease evolves through seven stages, from enervation to chronic degeneration. (See Appendix F.) The hygienic doctor can readily assess at which stage of the *one disease* the person has arrived and can readily counsel as to the *one healing method*, which is always healthful living care tailored to the patient's specific needs.

By contrast, just think of the extreme anxiety every frightened patient goes through when medical doctors can't agree among themselves on a diagnosis! When the patient's ailment is finally labeled, all breathe sighs of relief, as if labeling the disease symptoms will somehow make everything clear.

The same holds for Oriental medicine. To pass my classes and board exams to get my license, I had to memorize all sorts of ailments — both Oriental and Western diagnoses — and hundreds of herbs with their indications and contraindications, as well as all of the acupuncture points. Yet most Oriental doctors do not agree on exact diagnoses and treatments either.

Dr. Herbert Shelton sarcastically joked about all of the *-itises* and how arbitrary the classifications were. If you have inflammation in your rectum, it is labeled *proctitis*, but when it is a quarter inch farther up the colon, it is labeled *sigmoiditis*, a completely different ailment altogether according to the medical establishment. Yet inflammation is simply one of the seven stages of the disease process. Inflammation is inflammation regardless of its location.

To summarize, the medical model of disease and health care adheres to four schools of thought: disease as mystery, as genetically flawed, as wear and tear or as the result of germ invasion.

Treatment for germ-based diseases involves "declaring war" on the common cold germ, the Asian flu bug, the AIDS virus, the SARS virus and whatever latest dastardly disease microbe is discovered. We are told we must wait for chemists to concoct specific miracle drugs that will fight each of the corresponding evil germs. We are supposed to breathlessly await the invention of new vaccines that will prevent or "cure" these diseases, even though vaccine use has been linked to high incidences of autism, encephalitis, Alzheimer's, Parkinson's and more.

The wear and tear school of medical thought teaches us that skin can be molded to look younger, hair can be moved around on the scalp to look thicker, and organs and even body parts can be removed and/or replaced just as easily as we change the oil or replace the batteries in our cars. As pointed out in our medical disclaimer at the end of Chapter 4, many of these wear and tear procedures are absolute blessings to people who have bone on bone at the hip and knee for example. Yet the vast majority of surgeries would never, and should never, be performed if doctors were simply to administer alternative health care to the sick as needed and in a timely manner.

If people were instructed in the proper care and feeding of the body, virtually all of the following surgical procedures and many more not listed could be completely avoided: gallbladder removal, colostomy, stents, tonsillectomy, appendectomy, cardiovascular surgery of virtually all kinds, regenerative surgery, tumor removal and the most common unnecessary major surgery of all, the hysterectomy.

Victoria Boutenko humorously points out that a baby's runny nose is not an indication of a "nose drop deficiency." I further ask, is a headache really an aspirin deficiency? Is a tumor a chemotherapy or radiation deficiency? Is constipation a laxative deficiency? Is indigestion an antacid deficiency? Is pain an analgesic deficiency?

All of these medications and therapies are toxic and contribute to the body's building first acute and then chronic disease. Some medications kill within weeks or months. For instance, it is estimated that chemotherapy kills great numbers of healthy cells for each cancer cell it destroys. As Aajonus Vonderplanitz remarks, administering chemo to kill cancer is akin to killing everyone on the entire planet in order to get to a few that you want dead. (See Appendix B.)

Would God or nature be so cruel as to withhold the very essentials we need for radiant health? Is our health really dependent upon alchemists experimenting in a lab, searching for the Holy Grail of medicine, that elusive combination of chemicals needed to formulate a miracle drug?

Look at animals in the wild. They are healthy, able to thrive and frolic in weather extremes and enjoy their genetically determined lifespans. In fact wild African monkeys carrying SIV (a virus related to HIV) remain perfectly healthy. Their counterparts carrying the same virus in captivity sicken and die. Wild animals do not routinely eat cooked food. We humans and our captive animals are the only species that do that. All cooked food eaters, human and animal alike, have suffered greatly for our taming and harnessing of fire.

The health by healthful living model of disease origin and health care is actually ancient knowledge, practiced and then lost repeatedly over the millennia. Now rediscovered once again, it holds that the body is genetically designed both to heal itself when necessary and to maintain health when proper conditions are provided. Once polluted or damaged, the body must first revitalize its nervous system so that it will have the energy needed to eliminate toxins and then rebuild with the correct building blocks found in live foods.

For medical doctors trained and licensed in the allopathic medical model at its very worst, natural healing and dietary approaches seem too simplistic, even naïve — if not insulting. Medical training is consistently along the lines of different pills, treatments and/or surgeries for different diseases.

They think it insignificant that "miracle pills" cannot be entirely natural in order to be patented. These drugs are toxic because anything unnatural to healthy cellular life is toxic to the body. Even some plants are toxic. Since plants cannot be patented unless genetically modified, drug manufacturers will not research and promote as medicinal any natural foods or herbs, even though they generally result in far less harm and are far less toxic than laboratory drugs. There is simply no huge profit markup in natural healing.

Yet diet is most certainly key when all of the research is examined. Dr. Campbell reached the conclusion that *"nutrition [is] far more important in controlling cancer promotion than the dose of the initiating carcinogen"* (*The China Study*, p. 66).

In other words, one's diet is far more important than how much exposure to a dangerous chemical one has had! He also reveals, "More people die because of the way they eat than by tobacco use, accidents or any other lifestyle or environmental factor" (p. 305).

In France, scientist Bruno Comby has studied the raw instinctive diet in the treatment of AIDS. He reports, "Scientifically, the dietary theory of immunity, which at first glance appears bizarre in the extreme, turns out to be unshakable, something that cannot be said for other forms of natural or holistic therapy" (*Maximize Immunity*, p. 101).

Comby has found the evidence inescapable that a 100% natural diet enhances the development of the body's natural defenses. He has witnessed full-blown AIDS patients go into 100% remission and remain so. "Observation of more than 15,000 individuals who have followed this natural diet over the past 25 years demonstrates that almost any immune disease follows a different course in people who exclusively eat foods that are natural and have not been denatured" (ibid., p. 101).

Healthful living habits, especially including the raw diet, do not bring about an instantaneous "miracle cure," but they certainly are the next best thing when the rare miraculous healing event is not forthcoming. By persisting in the ten energy enhancers patiently, one gives the body the time and the conditions it needs to revitalize so that the body's natural healing process can proceed slowly but surely, day by day.

Dr. Vetrano lightheartedly invented a new disease for the impatient patient who discovers the ten energy enhancers and cannot get well quickly enough. She named it in an article from *Dr. Shelton's Hygienic Review* entitled "The Hurry-Up Disease." She reminds those afflicted, "You did not get sick overnight, and you cannot expect to heal overnight."

Nature provides a gentle way for the body to heal itself. Nature is kind, not harsh. "Easy does it," the motto of the highly successful Anonymous rehab programs, is Nature's motto too.

## So, with This Good News, Why Do Most of Us Cling So Defensively to the Medical Model?

For many people including myself, it has taken time to switch paradigms. The reasons vary for clinging almost defensively and desperately to the medical paradigm. Different people cling for different reasons.

Many of us are so entrenched in the medical mindset that we are initially shocked and need time to digest the new ideas, try them out and verify that they are correct.

Many of us love our doctors and cannot imagine they might not know absolutely everything. We put them on pedestals and worship them as infallible gods. My father was a general medical practitioner and surgeon in a small town. I was always so proud because everyone I met knew and admired him.

Most of us, even physicians themselves, have put complete faith in the medical mentality and ask no questions. Physicians are so very sure of themselves, which engenders our faith in them. But they are only doing what they learned through so many years in medical school. Most think they are on the right track, having seen so many patients' symptoms relieved by allopathic treatments.

For people who do not take good care of themselves, wear and tear intervention is very often necessary. Some drugs, such as antibiotics and painkillers, at least appear helpful momentarily because they so successfully *palliate symptoms* and *relieve pain*, but this is only due to the masking and/or mimicking phenomena previously explained.

Most of us, including our medical doctors, totally believe in the wear and tear theory and therefore look for no better way. Physicians have been taught, as we all have, that sickness is normal and natural, especially as we age. They and their patients alike fully believe that most people are simply going to get sick sooner or later.

Most of us, including our doctors, believe that drugs can effectively weed out the root causes of illness. Few see that taking drugs to "cure" an illness is like cleaning your kitchen with dirt. Many medical doctors get frustrated at their inability to cure their patients permanently. Those few who manage to break the mold by thinking outside of the medicine bag do so at the risk of being branded "quacks," "medical heretics" or "alternative health care renegades." They fear losing their licenses or being sued for not following standard procedures.

Most of us have been completely indoctrinated into believing the medical paradigm through media brainwashing: the scientific reports, the pro-drug and doctor advertisements, the latest technological advancements and the grand wisdom behind the newest wear and tear replacement parts. In the book *Trust Us, We're Experts! How Industry Manipulates Science* by John Stauber and Sheldon Rampton, we get a behind-the-scenes view of how the powers-that-be control the masses. We are being conditioned to worship the men and women in white laboratory coats so that we will believe in medicine, automatically go to them for diagnosis and treatment, purchase pharmaceutical remedies and submit to invasive hospital procedures unquestioningly.

As David Hawkins, MD, PhD, points out, "The fact that many opinions are held by great masses of people is hypnotic. Few minds can escape the appeal of the authority of mass agreement. . . . Few can resist the propaganda of the news media" (*The Eye of the I*, p. 182).

Public relations expert Edward Bernays confessed to having been hired to promote the health benefits of bananas, bacon and even *Crisco cooking oil*. In his book *Propaganda*, he explains how people are made to depend on what medical doctors and other leaders say. "Those who manipulate this unseen mechanism of society constitute an invisible government which is the true ruling power of our country. ... Our minds are molded, our tastes formed, our ideas suggested, largely by men we have never heard of."

When you come to realize that those behind the pharmaceutical corporations and government agencies like the Food and Drug Administration (FDA) care more about money than they do about your health, *it's a bit like discovering that your mother has Munchausen by proxy syndrome*, a mental disorder in which a mother poisons her own children to seek attention. It is shocking to learn that many we have trusted to protect our health are actually poisoning us and even killing us with their drugs, surgeries and other treatments! All the while, the "health care" costs for these disease services and poison products drain all but the very rich very dry.

Another reason for clinging to the medical model is that many of us are followers. We prefer to let anyone in a position of medical authority take responsibility for our health: doctors, nurses, hospital personnel, drug peddlers. We do not want to acknowledge that we have to do a whole lot more than swallow "magic" pills and/or take treatments to get well and stay healthy. We do not want to accept responsibility.

Furthermore, many of us take the path of least resistance. In the short run, it is vastly easier to take a pill, inhale a gas, get an injection, submit to surgery or accept other invasive treatments than to change lifestyle habits — especially our diets. We do not want to learn what is poisonous. We do not want to clean up our external environments, maybe even quit our jobs if they are too stressful or if the workplace is lethal.

Choosing the path of least resistance, though limited in getting us well, requires so little effort. Taking a drug requires the very least effort and gives us quick-fix relief. Taking the path of least resistance is so much easier than making so many new decisions and so many new choices that will require so much more energy that we so do not have. To revamp our lifestyles completely — it all takes so much effort! It is so much easier to swallow a magic pill or go in for a treatment.

It is easier to have someone else do the research and reasoning concerning our bodily needs. Yet as Victoria Boutenko warns, "When we let others observe and reason for us, in a sense we consciously choose to stay blind and deaf" (*Green for Life*, p. 3).

Most people want the quick fix, even if it can't "cure" in the long run. Dr. Joel Fuhrman, author of *Fasting and Eating for Health: A Medical Doctor's Program for Conquering Disease*, prophesied that the time might come when doctors would be accused of malpractice for not prescribing the substantially more effective nutritional approach for their patients.

He is less optimistic in an interview with Shelly Keck-Borsits from her book *Dying to Get Well*, pointing out how well trodden is the path of least resistance, "The masses will continue to seek instant gratification via dangerous nutritional habits and drug seeking." Most people have just not been inspired to put much effort into building their health, due to ignorance about how to get healthy.

Another reason many of us cling so desperately to the medical model is that we have taken a victim stance in life, especially when it comes to our health. All four schools of medical thought are perfect setups for the victim mentality: We are victims of a mysterious disease. We are victims of wearing out. We are victims of our DNA. We are victims of germs. Some of us are victims of combinations or all of these mindsets. The helpless, hopeless victim falls into depression or rants and raves about how horrible it is to grow old and how his or her medicine isn't working and how bad its side effects are. "It's not my fault!" whines the victim.

Yet another reason is financial. Many people don't want to invest much out-of-pocket money in their bodies. If health insurance won't cover the alternative doctor or fasting clinic, they won't go. They spend more on car maintenance than maintaining their own bodies. They take more pride in their luxury transportation vehicles than in their souls' vehicles!

Some people are fearful of upsetting the economic structure. Alternative health care, while creating a multitude of new jobs, is also eliminating a multitude of others. Keep in mind that the SAD is part of the medical model at its very worst: until just recently, most medical doctors have claimed that diet has little or nothing to do with health. If people were to switch from SAD foods to live foods, most medical professionals, food giants, restaurant owners, pharmacists, drug salespeople, people employed by the American Cancer Society and other such organizations searching for drug cures, herbicide and pesticide producers and even many veterinarians and alternative health care professionals would all have to change or radically revamp their careers. This would upset the employee ladder from janitors to executives in every country!

Many of us resist the idea that diet is absolutely, intimately connected to vibrant health and well-being. We have been so poorly educated about health and nutrition in school and via the media that we often deny the impact of what we eat on our day-to-day and long-term experiences of health or lack of health.

When an animal becomes sick, we naturally wonder what it has been eating. When we get sick, we just self-medicate over the drugstore counter or go to an MD. Ads for pet food emphasize nutritional value. Ads for human food emphasize taste thrills, convenience and even sex appeal. Veterinarians and farmers both know that animal health depends principally on diet and that animals will adapt to unnatural, cooked and chemicalized foods by fattening up, rapidly aging and developing disease symptoms.

Pet owners, in contrast to farmers, want their animals to live long, healthy lives. Raw food diets for pets are becoming all the rage. More and more people are putting their beloved dogs and cats on raw meat instead of the more convenient canned, bagged or boxed pet food that has been heated and processed for extended shelf life. Yet few people apply this concern to their own feeding dishes or stop to even consider that just such a diet of uncooked food may also be far healthier for *them*.

Finally, and perhaps most challenging of all, some of us do not want to relinquish our favorite toxic, cooked foods and switch to health-enhancing diets. Indeed, reluctance to give up our toxic, cooked favorites in exchange for raw food health may be the biggest mental and emotional stumbling block for most potential paradigm shifters. *Too much of our identities revolve around food.*

The idea that we might have to radically change our diets to obtain health is a fate worse than living in food-related disease for some. They would sooner change their religions or even let themselves die than change their eating habits. In fact authors Roman Devivo and Antje Spors point out that our entire social structure revolves around food. It is "linked with love, sex, agreement, admiration, obedience, control, belonging, reward, indulgence and self-destruction. Our very identity of who we are contains food likes, dislikes, events, recipes and restaurants. To be outside of that paradigm can be very unsettling" (*Genefit Nutrition,* p. 181).

So why do so many cling so defensively to the medical model? Victoria BidWell answers, "They cling so because they do not yet know about the health by healthful living model and the ten energy enhancers. When they really know the alternative program, as practiced in their own thoughts, feelings and actions, they will drop the medical model like a hot potato!"

The good news about this healthful living alternative is that we no longer see ourselves as victims. No longer will we quake in trepidation every time we get sick. Some of us no longer even bother with yearly physicals or dental check-ups. Barring environmental factors beyond our influence to improve, we can be in total control of our health! The shift from cooked foods to live foods and health by healthful living habits will make us masters of paradise health.

A final and most pleasant surprise about this alternative health paradigm shift is that it doesn't cost anything! There are no costly medical bills for doctors, laboratory tests, surgery, drugs, supplements and so forth. Some may initially want to invest in new kitchen machines to make raw food preparation easy and fun and in exercise equipment or a fasting clinic visit, but the alternative health care model is free for the most part. Except for the cost of quality food and good drinking water, the other eight energy enhancers are completely free! Your body is its own healer and doesn't charge you a penny. For those of us who are used to thinking that health care and even preventive medicine should be expensive, this financial freedom comes as a huge relief and a great delight!

# Let Food Be Thy Medicine —Hippocrates, Founder of Modern Medicine, 400 BC

Eventually, a person may become disillusioned enough, sick enough and desperate enough with medical results to try an entirely different kind of "medicine" — live foods. After a few weeks of eating a 100% raw food diet, or close to it, the person is sold: natural living proves to be the best medicine. Hippocrates was right. Food can be thy medicine.

Yet it all seems so strange, so fantastical. You feel like Alice in Wonderland — everything is upside down. Suddenly, the real pharmacopoeia becomes the "farm-acopoeia"! Meryl Streep marvels, "It is bizarre that the produce manager is more important to my children's health than the pediatrician."

You start to realize that cooking food destroys its life. My parents took a photo of me on my first birthday. I was entranced by the flame of the single candle, touched it and cried. Fire can be seductive, as it exudes warmth and engenders a secure feeling. Fire dazzles as it releases aromas while the foods heat up, but don't be fooled. Fire kills food. Plant a raw seed in the ground, and watch it sprout. Watch it grow. Plant a roasted seed, and watch it rot!

Unheated food is *nature's* medicine. Our bodies heal and rid themselves of disease when properly cared for, properly nourished and not overwhelmed with toxins. Our bodies need the proper raw materials for their best building blocks, those found exclusively in natural, uncooked foods. Cooked foods are dead. Raw foods are "alive."

Look at a juicy, organic apple. *If you eat it, its life force will become yours!* That is not so with the cooked apple. Instead, the cooked apple's toxic byproducts will add to your burden! If you want more out of your years, living in pleasure and happiness, eat live food. If you want less out of life, dying in pain and misery, eat dead food. Raw food is full of nutrition the body needs and uses for rejuvenation and vigorous living: fats, proteins, carbohydrates, vitamins, minerals, enzymes, biophotons, other phytonutrients, fiber and water.

Dr. Herbert M. Shelton described the beauty of health by healthful living in *Health for the Millions*:

> When one adopts Natural Hygiene, one lives in a New World. The transition from the Old World to the new is immediate. All nature becomes more beautiful and glorious! Duties that were irksome become easy to perform. We breathe purer atmosphere. New purposes animate us. New strength, energy and power to perform are infused into us. The change in our character is equally as great! We see in every tree and shrub and in every blade of grass a beauty of which we had not before been conscious! A new spirit of love and goodwill permeates our whole lives! We develop a gentleness and kindness that are new to us. A fresh zeal enters into our relations with those around us. We have the strength to perform whatever we choose with cheerfulness and delight. Troubles, anxieties and cares dissipate, for we know that our welfare is secure and on a firm basis.

The proof is in the raw pudding. Try the live food diet yourself. Chances are, no matter how healthy and happy you are now, you will become amazed at how much more health and happiness are to be discovered and savored along your raw life journey!

Are you ready to make a paradigm shift?

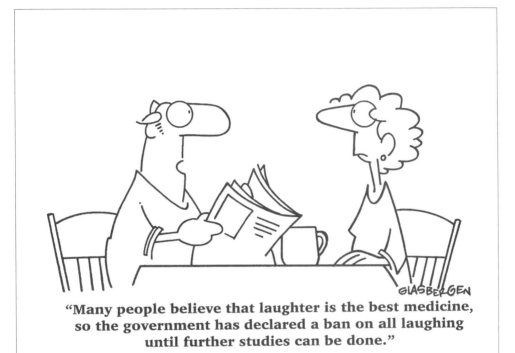

"Many people believe that laughter is the best medicine, so the government has declared a ban on all laughing until further studies can be done."

# 8

# Cooked vs. Raw Diet Experiments and Research

*The strongest arguments prove nothing so long as the conclusions are not verified by experience. Experimental science is the queen of sciences and the goal of all speculation.*
—Roger Bacon (1220–1292)

Quite a number of experiments have been done comparing the raw food diet with the cooked. I have listed numerous such studies here, many performed on people and others on animals. I wish to thank Victoria BidWell for her work in perfecting the presentation of these studies. They are now listed individually and chronologically for the most part.

This chapter presents nearly 50 scientific studies. Combined with those described in Appendix D, there are *nearly 70 studies* illustrating both the *benefits of raw food* and the *dangers of cooked food.*

Unfortunately, while selling raw produce can be somewhat profitable, the huge profits are to be had in selling artificial and processed foods. The entire pharmaceutical and processed-food industries would stand to lose vast profit-generating empires if the raw diet were to catch on. Such a pocketbook vote by the public would force the pharmaceutical industry to downsize considerably and the food industry to reduce or eliminate most of its products. Furthermore, think of all the restaurant chains that would lose profits, not to mention those making and selling cooking appliances and apparatus.

Because profitable businesses are wedded to the status quo, little funding support has been allocated for research in the area of raw diet. Those with the deep pockets simply don't want the health hazards of cooked food to be made public knowledge. As a result, most of these studies have been done by individuals so driven by curiosity and humanitarian concerns that they were motivated enough to fund their own research. Or they have been conducted in those universities where bucking the system is still possible.

If you would like to research these articles for yourself, start by going to www.ncbi.nlm.nih.gov/entrez/query.fcgi. You will see a web site called "Pub-Med," which contains the National Library of Medicine. It enables you to search for articles by ID number, subject, title and such. There you will find article abstracts and links to the journals that published them. I have included where available the PubMed ID numbers of the cited research papers for your convenience.

There is also an article "Raw Food Diets Living Food — Review of Scientific Literature Journals," which summarizes some of the findings from studies into raw food diet research located at www.living-foods.com/articles/scientific literature.html. As its author points out, the vast majority of research into the raw, or living, diet has been done in Europe. A good list of recent studies also appears at http://members.iinet.net.au/~pgraham/rawfoodstudies.htm.

I compiled for this chapter every raw food experiment I came across in all the different books I read. I thought it would be useful to have all of these experiments assembled in one book so that people could show anyone who is skeptical. I was inspired to do this by two major events.

First, when I told my doctor of my new raw diet, he scoffed, declaring that no research had been done. There was, in his tone of voice, an insinuation that I was hopelessly naïve! I have heard of numerous other raw fooders and aspiring raw fooders receiving the same treatment from their medical doctors.

Well, I handed him what little bit of research I had managed to gather at that point. But shortly after beginning my raw journey, I realized it was hopeless to work with someone so entrenched in the drug therapy paradigm and never went back to him.

Second, I had a dear friend, a medical doctor, who died of an inoperable brain tumor. When I suggested the raw diet, he had replied, "People get healed by that diet only because of their beliefs."

Certainly the power of the mind to influence healing has been proven. The scientific name for that is the "placebo effect." There is a definite body/mind connection. However, raw food diets also result in significant health improvements in animals, which clearly haven't been indoctrinated in belief systems.

Perhaps if I had already assembled this collection of experiments, I could have convinced my doctor friend. Since I hadn't yet compiled the evidence, he died, having tried only a few fruitless treatments, including chemotherapy.

Admittedly, there may be a dearth of scientific studies showing that people on raw foods can heal from advanced stages of AIDS or eleventh-hour cancer. But who has the financial incentive to fund such studies? Certainly not the pharmaceutical companies! Furthermore, what makes me laugh is that medical people not only deny the live food factor within natural foods, but also go so far as to think that eating a 100% raw food diet could be *dangerous*. How do you think man's ancestors survived for literally millions of years prior to the invention of cooking?

I admit it would be nice to have still more research performed verifying the healing power of the body when it is fed a diet of natural, living foods. Personally, I do not need it, as I am totally convinced from the experiments I have done on myself and the results observed in others. Objectively, I am thoroughly convinced by the results of the studies I'm about to show you, but maybe more research would convince the skeptics and doctors.

Perhaps, as enough of us begin to compile research on ourselves, people will eventually view with amazement how utterly naïve we were to have ever believed that drugs could heal us better than nature. Maybe then, finally, all of the skeptics and their medical doctors will wake up and smell the fruit!

# 1. Dr. Otto Louis Moritz Abramowski and His Hospital Patients

Dr. Abramowski was an Australian medical doctor who completely recovered from hardening of the arteries, loss of vigor and inability to work by means of a raw, vegetarian diet in his middle years. After turning to raw foods, he felt better than he had felt even as a young man. So enthusiastic was he that he decided to conduct an experiment at his hospital.

As told in his booklet *Fruitarian Diet and Physical Rejuvenation*, he divided over a hundred patients into two groups. The first was kept on standard hospital food and drug therapy; the second was taken off all drugs and given only fresh fruit, three pounds a day.

Several weeks into the experiment, it was abruptly terminated when the head nurse objected to the inhumanity of the experiment. She felt it would be immoral to continue giving drugs and cooked food to the first group because, she said, it was clearly killing them!

# 2. Dr. Werner Kollath's Study Animals Thrived on a Raw Diet

Just before World War II, Professor Kollath at the University of Rostock in Germany raised animals on processed food that had virtually no vitamins or minerals other than thiamine, potassium, sulfate and zinc.

Despite the depleted diet, the animals initially appeared healthy, showing no signs of deficiency. But when they reached adulthood, they displayed degenerative signs much like those of humans living in the Western world on conventional diets: osteoporosis, intestinal toxemia, dental cavities and damaged organs.

Kollath then gave these animals vitamin supplements to see if that would reverse their conditions. No improvement was noted. The chronic degeneration reversed only on a diet of fresh, living, raw food composed of many vegetables.

A control group raised on raw food all along that was never fed the processed food did not acquire the degenerative disease conditions. He labeled these differences "meso-health" and "super-health."

Researchers in Sweden and Germany later confirmed Dr. Kollath's findings. Research scientists studying raw food diets and their use in treating illness conclude that great numbers of people in industrialized societies are living in states of "meso-health" due to their highly processed and devitalized food.

# 3. Athletic Performance Improved on Raw Diet

Professor Karl Eimer, director of the Medical Clinic at the University of Vienna, had athletes eat their usual cooked diet for two weeks of highly intensive training. He monitored and evaluated their athletic performance. Next, they were put on a 100% raw food diet and continued with the same training.

Every one of the athletes improved in reflex speed, flexibility and stamina. Eimer and his colleague Professor Hans Eppinger concluded that cellular respiration and efficiency increase on a raw food diet. His article in German, "Klinik Schwenkenbecher," appeared in the July 1933 edition of *Zeitschrift für Ernährung*.

# 4. Dr. Edmond Szekely's 33-Year Study

One of the most impressive human experiments on the raw food diet was a long-term study conducted by Dr. Edmond Szekely, who guided more than 123,600 people over a 33-year period (1937–1970) on a raw diet. Though an informal observational study, its duration warrants great consideration. This study yields stunning empirical evidence of the power of the live food diet. Seventeen percent of these patients had been diagnosed "incurable." His treatment method was published in his book *The Chemistry of Youth*. He achieved amazing results in increasing people's health status in comparison to the control groups by using raw foods. Over 90% of the 123,600 patients regained their health.

Dr. Szekely was inspired to undertake this project by a trip he took to visit the Hunzas in Central Asia in the 1920s. These people lived long, productive lives (100-120 years) without the customary infirmities of aging.

Their undiminished vitality he attributed to their high consumption of sprouted seeds. "We may have learned how to extend the lifespan through the conquest of epidemics and contagious disease, but until we can achieve that level of vitality, well-being and complete freedom from degenerative disease known by the Hunzas at extremely advanced ages, we will not even have begun to penetrate the real secrets of longevity" (*The Chemistry of Youth*, p. 31).

It was at his center at Rancho La Puerta, Mexico, that Szekely claimed to have pioneered organic gardening, long before the term became popular. From his observations in what Dr. Szekely called his "Great Experiment," he classified foods into four groups. The first he called "biogenic" food, the most life-generating and cell-renewing group. These high-energy foods include all sprouts: soaked and germinated nuts, seeds, grains, legumes and grasses, such as wheatgrass.

According to Dr. Edward Howell (*Food Enzymes for Health and Longevity*), sprouting increases enzyme content by 6-20 times. Vitamin and mineral content is also greatly increased. For example, according to Ann Wigmore (*The Hippocrates Diet and Health Program*), Vitamin $B_6$ can be increased up to 500%, $B_2$ up to 1300% and folic acid by 600%. These biogenic foods contribute the most toward the healing and regenerative processes of the body, so Szekely estimated that these biogenic foods should make up 25% of a healthy person's diet, perhaps more if the person were seriously ill.

The second category he called "bioactive," which were raw fruits and vegetables, unheated and untreated. These foods contribute to health maintenance and slightly enhance an already healthy body. Dr. Szekely felt these foods should make up about half of a healthy person's diet.

The third category Dr. Szekely termed "biostatic," referring to foods that stabilize or actually slightly diminish the body's functioning and slowly age a person. These include cooked foods and even raw foods that are not fresh. Dr. Szekely allowed for these foods to be 10-25% of a healthy person's diet, not because they are needed or healthful, but because he felt most people could not stick with a diet so limited as to exclude cooked foods.

The fourth category, "bioacidic," he considered to be so life-destructive that he felt we should eliminate these altogether, even if we presently feel healthy. These are processed and/or refined foods full of additives, preservatives and/or pesticide residues. They rapidly tear down and age the body.

# 5. Dr. Francis Pottenger's Cat Study: Dietary Factors in Degenerative Disease

Probably the most well-known study on the effects of cooked versus raw food was performed by Francis Pottenger, MD, during the years 1932–1942. He was raising cats for a scientific study on adrenal glands. He ran out of the raw food he had been feeding these animals, so he gave some of them leftover cooked table scraps to economize.

He noticed health degeneration in the latter group, and so he decided to do an additional controlled experiment on the effects of raw versus cooked food. Over a ten-year period, he raised about 900 cats. Half were fed a diet of cooked meat, whereas the other half were fed raw meat. Both groups were given supplementary milk and cod liver oil.

These groups were kept in separate pens so there could be no eating from the other group's food. Pottenger was very careful to use scientifically controlled methods and even used the same male cat for breeding with both groups to minimize genetic factors. He kept such meticulous records that his study was published in the *American Journal of Orthodontics and Oral Surgery*.

The first generation of deficient cats began its cooked food diet only as adults. Their kittens were called *second-generation deficient* cats, and their "grandkittens" were called *third-generation deficient* cats.

Pottenger noticed progressive health declines with each generation. Gingivitis and gum tenderness worsened. Skulls got progressively smaller. Teeth did not grow in straight, and there was a narrowing and foreshortening of the dental arches. The calcium content of the bones worsened progressively until, by the third generation, the deficient cats had bones like sponge rubber with "spontaneous fractures on the slightest provocation."

Note: Cooked food often contributes to acidity in the body. Upon threat of death to the organism, the body reacts to acidity by drawing upon calcium and other alkaline minerals from the bones in order to neutralize this acidity.

In the second generation of deficient cats, 83% of the males were sterile, as were 53% of the females. The third generation cats were not even able to produce kittens and in fact died prematurely at about six months, the period corresponding to childhood in humans.

The deficient cats displayed these symptoms: incomplete development of the skull and bones, bowed legs, rickets, curvature of the spine, paralysis of the legs, convulsive seizure, thyroid abscesses, cyanosis of liver and kidneys, enlarged colon and degeneration of the motor nerve ganglion cells throughout the spinal cord and brain stem, with some cells affected in the cerebellum and cerebral cortex. The raw-fed cats suffered none of the above.

Behavioral differences were also documented. Cooked fooders were more irritable. A role reversal occurred, with male cats becoming submissive and females becoming more aggressive.

Furthermore, it was found that by returning kittens to the optimal diet of raw food, a gradual regeneration could occur. Yet from the second-generation deficient cats, it took *three generations* of kittens to get a litter that returned to the optimal health of the original cats! In the *second generation of cats returned to raw food*, deformities and allergies were still present due to *their parents'* having eaten cooked food! It was only *their* kittens that could achieve optimal health.

Pottenger made the following comments: "Man is rarely restricted in his dietary to a totally cooked food ration. It must be remembered that these cats do receive raw milk of market grade and that this is not sufficient to overcome the effects of cooked meat. Man seems to be more like a rat, having greater vitality than the cat, and he can apparently respond to deficient conditions in a better manner. The changes found in cats are nevertheless comparable to many of those that we see in human beings. Moreover, anthropologists today tell us that civilized man is physically steadily on the downgrade. May not the heat processing to which we are subjecting a great portion of our foods be a factor in this downward trend?"

He went on to remark that his colleague, Dr. Weston Price, dramatically documented the same downhill spiral of civilized man in his book *Nutrition and Physical Degeneration: A Comparison of Primitive and Modern Diets and Their Effects*. Although humans, rats and hogs are the most versatile mammal species on the planet, they still suffer when eating cooked food, as has been borne out by many experiments.

There was even an experiment within this experiment. At some point, various types of milk were tested: raw, pasteurized, evaporated and sweetened condensed milk. Plants that sprang up in the various pens were observed. Those that had been fertilized with the urine and feces of the cats fed raw food were vigorous and healthy. Plants fertilized with the excreta of the cats fed pasteurized milk were less healthy. The growth was very poor with evaporated milk, and almost no growth occurred with the sweetened condensed milk. The implications of using fertilizer from cooked-food animal excrement are staggering!

This criticism of Pottenger's conclusions was found in the Wikipedia online encyclopedia: "Pottenger's study was conducted in a time before the nutritional needs of cats were understood — especially the role of taurine in the diet. Since cats cannot synthesize adequate amounts of taurine, they must get taurine from food. Heat renders taurine inactive; cooked food without taurine supplements can cause health problems in cats."

While this appears rational at first glance, has anyone actually tried feeding a cat a diet of cooked food with taurine supplements? If not, how can anyone suggest that just adding taurine would compensate for *all* of the deficiencies of cooked food? The implication is simply untrue that cats need *only taurine* for optimal health and not *all the other nutrients* degraded by heat.

This presumed refutation continues, "However, this finding does not apply to humans since humans, like most other animals, synthesize their own taurine." What about all the other nutrients needed by humans that are destroyed by fire (see Chapter 9), many which have yet to be discovered?

For more complete information on this experiment, read the landmark publication *Pottenger's Cats: A Study in Nutrition.*

# 6. Dr. Edward Howell's Enzyme Research

Dr. Edward Howell spent a lifetime researching enzyme biochemistry. He pored over hundreds of published scientific studies on enzymes and reached some startling conclusions. He found that the concentration of the starch-splitting enzyme ptyalin in the saliva of young adults was 30 times stronger than that of people 69 years of age and older. In the older group, the digestive enzymes pepsin and trypsin were decreased to ¼ the strength of these same enzymes in the younger group.

He found that enzyme activity for all metabolic processes, digestive and otherwise, weakens in old age because people have been on enzyme-deficient, cooked diets throughout their lives. He concluded that the fatigue people suffer starting in their 30s and 40s is due to exhaustion of their enzyme-generating potential, which is depleted due to unnatural needs of the body for digestive juices. These unnatural needs are due to the likewise unnatural habit of cooking the enzymes to death. Destroying the enzymes in the food supply causes early aging. Howell declared that "what we now call 'old age' could become the glorious prime of life" if we take in enzyme reinforcements (raw foods).

Some of the studies reviewed by Dr. Howell also compared organ weights in humans versus animals. A cooked diet was associated with enlarged pancreases due to overwork. In addition, the brains of rats fed a cooked diet actually shrank! Their other organs became swollen and weak.

## 7. Calves Die on Pasteurized Milk!

The *British Medical Journal* published a study entitled "The effect of heat treatment on the nutritive value of milk for the young calf: the effect of ultra-high temperature treatment and of pasteurization" (Vol. 14, Issue 10, 1960).

Calves were fed their mothers' milk after it had been pasteurized. The calves died before maturity in nine out of ten cases, proving the harmful effects of cooked milk, *even for creatures designed to drink cow's milk.*

## 8. The Prisoner of War Diet Is Better Raw

Prisoners of war in Japan during WW II were fed a scanty diet of brown rice, vegetables and fruit, totaling only 729-826 calories per 154 pounds of body weight. In 1950, Dr. Masanore Kuratsune, head of the Medical Department of the University of Kyushu in Japan, thought that this diet might be a remarkable way to validate previous studies comparing raw and cooked food. He and his wife decided to be the guinea pigs. Both followed the raw version of the same diet for three periods: 120 days in winter, 32 days in summer and 81 days in spring. Mrs. Kuratsune was breastfeeding a baby during this time. Both continued to do their usual work. Remarkably, they both continued to enjoy good health. Mrs. Kuratsune even found that breastfeeding was less of a strain than before eating this raw diet.

Next, they both switched to the same prisoner diet in cooked form. They became as hungry and diseased as the prisoners of war. They quickly came down with edema, vitamin deficiencies and collapse. It became so bad that they were forced to stop the experiment.

This informal empirical study was recounted in a 1967 monograph written by Dr. Ralph Bircher-Benner of Zurich entitled *Dr. Bircher-Benner's Way to Positive Health and Vitality, 1867–1967.*

## 9. Lewis Cook's and Junko Yasui's Rats

Described in their book *Goldot*, Cook and Yasui studied three groups of rats. The first group was fed a raw diet from birth. They suffered no diseases, remained very healthy and full of energy, and were never fat. They mated with enthusiasm, producing healthy offspring. These rats were gentle, playful and affectionate, living in perfect harmony with each other.

They were killed and their bodies examined when they reached the equivalent of 80 human years. The rats were found to be in perfect health, with no sign of aging, degeneration or disease.

The second group of rats was fed from birth a diet consisting of cooked food: bread, milk, salt, junk food, soft drinks, candies, vitamins and medications — in other words, the SAD. They grew fat. They developed the same degenerative conditions that humans do on such a diet: heart disease, cancer, diabetes, arthritis, obesity, colds, bouts of the flu and so on.

Their behavior was also affected. They became nervous, mean, self-destructive and violent toward each other. They even had to be kept apart to prevent them from killing each other. Their offspring were the same. Many died prematurely.

Autopsies showed great degeneration throughout their organs. All of the organs, glands, tissues, skin, hair, blood and nervous systems were negatively affected by the diet.

The third group was fed the SAD too and also exhibited poor health. They were just as mean and vicious as the second group and had to be kept separated. But when they reached middle age, the equivalent of 40 human years, they were fasted strictly on water. Then they were given the raw, healthful diet of the first group of rats. This was alternated with periodic fasting in order to gradually detoxify the residual toxins remaining from the SAD.

They gradually became as healthy, playful and affectionate with each other as the rats in the first group. They could co-exist in harmony and displayed no illnesses.

Upon reaching the same age as the SAD-fed rats, they were put to death and autopsied. They were shown to be just as healthy as the group that was raw from birth.

*The implications of this are astounding!* First, living organisms fed a raw diet and periodically fasted experience age reversal and regeneration. Second, although we have polluted our bodies, we can reverse much of the destruction with raw food diets. Third, living organisms can experience a speeding up of the detoxification process when a period of complete physiological rest is provided while fasting on water.

The authors state, "The same principles apply to human life as there is only one truth! Thus it may be concluded that sick people may be restored to health simply by choosing the proper diet, fasting and observing the other rules of health. There is no mystery. There is no external force that will help — all healing being accomplished within the body by the body in accordance with the laws of organic life and health."

# 10. Stamina, Blood Pressure and Balance Improved on Fruitarian Diet

Inspired by a 45-year-old woman he met who was in excellent health "despite" having eaten a fruitarian diet for 12 years, Professor B. J. Meyer of the University of Pretoria in South Africa performed an experiment. He fed a control group of 50 people fruits (mostly raw, though some canned or stewed) and nuts alone for six months.

They became sickness-free, with greatly improved health and weight. Many claimed that their stamina increased, along with their ability to undertake serious physical tasks and compete in sports. The pH of their urine changed from acid to alkaline. The four subjects who were originally hypertensive had decreased blood pressures.

The February 20, 1971 issue of the *South African Medical Journal* published the results in an article called "Some physiological effects of a mainly fruit diet in man" (Vol. 45, Issue 8, pp. 191–195, PubMed ID 4928686).

# 11. Lipid Profiles and Glucose Tolerances Improved on Fruitarian Diet

In the March 6, 1971 issue of the *South African Medical Journal*, Professor B. J. Meyer published an article, "Some biochemical effects of a mainly fruit diet in man." The effect of the nut-supplemented fruit diet on glucose tolerance, secretions, plasma proteins and plasma lipids was investigated. It was found to be not merely adequate with respect to those measures, but even commendable.

# 12. Dr. Max Gerson: Cancer Reversals during Thirty Years of Raw Diet Clinical Practice

Dr. Max Gerson, MD, wrote an article entitled "The cure of advanced cancer by diet therapy: a summary of 30 years of clinical experimentation," which was published in *Physiol Chem Phys* (1978, Vol. 10, Issue 5, pp. 449–464, PubMed ID 751079). The study concluded that *even advanced stages of cancer* respond favorably to the diet of raw fruits, vegetables and raw-liver-derived active oxidizing enzymes (which facilitate rehabilitation of the liver), with no fats, oils or animal proteins. Iodine and niacin supplements were also given, along with coffee enemas.

# 13. Mice More Peaceful on Their Natural Diet

Ann Wigmore describes the following experience in her book *Be Your Own Doctor: A Positive Guide to Natural Living*. A friend of hers, John MacDonald, had a pet shop that specialized in white mice, selling them by the thousands all over the world. In the enclosure for the mice would be their "apartment complex" made of a large bale of hay. There they led happy, peaceful, playful, harmonious lives.

When John became concerned about the rising cost of grain to feed his mice, a neighbor with a boardinghouse offered to supply him with leftover table scraps. John saw this as a way to increase his profits, but when the mice began eating the same food that humans ate, quarrels broke out. Battles raged through the corridors of the baled-hay cooperative mouse house. Within a week, there were many dead mice, having been killed by other mice. Parent mice ate their young. Weaker mice were killed for no apparent reason.

Finally, John went back to feeding all of his mice grain, refusing the table scraps. Once again, peace reigned. The mice returned to sound mental health. Although this was an informal observational study, it nonetheless testifies to the link between diet and peace of mind. Maybe *peace through proper diet* is the long sought solution to war!

# 14. Dr. John Douglass: Alcohol and Nicotine Addiction Reduced on Raw Diet

Dr. John Douglass, MD, PhD, of Kaiser-Permanente Medical Center in Los Angeles, California, prescribed raw foods to his patients and noticed that common addictions, such as to alcohol and nicotine, lose their addictive power over people on raw food diets.

Experimenting with specific foods, he found that sunflower seeds in particular were especially effective at fighting the cravings of addictions. He found that when nourished on natural food in its original, raw state, the body becomes more sensitive to what is good for it and what is bad for it. (See also his other study below.)

He discussed some of his findings in an article called "Nutrition, nonthermally-prepared food, and Nature's message to man," which was published in the *Journal of the International Academy of Preventive Medicine*, Vol. VII, Issue 2, July 1982.

# 15. Sir Robert McCarrison's Monkeys: Cooked Diet Results in Colitis and Ulcers

In India, Sir Robert McCarrison fed monkeys their usual diet, but in a cooked form. The monkeys all developed colitis. Autopsies revealed that they also had gastric and intestinal ulcers. The book *Raw Energy* describes this study on page 37.

# 16. Guinea Pigs Developed Several Disease Conditions on Cooked Diet

Swiss researcher O. Stiner put some guinea pigs on their usual diet, but cooked. The animals quickly developed anemia, scurvy, goiter, dental cavities and/or degeneration of the salivary glands. When 10 cc of pasteurized milk was added to the diet, the animals developed arthritis as well. The book *Nature's First Law* refers to this study, as do several web sites. It is also reviewed in *Raw Energy*, page 37.

# 17. Dr. John Douglass: Hypertension and Obesity Reduced on Raw Diet

Dr. John Douglass, MD, PhD, of Kaiser-Permanente Medical Center in Los Angeles, California, published an article with five other researchers entitled "Effects of a raw food diet on hypertension and obesity," which was published in the *Southern Medical Journal*, July 1985, Volume 78, Issue 7, pp. 841–844, PubMed ID 4012382.

They examined responses to cooked and uncooked food in 32 people with hypertension, 28 of whom were also overweight. Patients acted as their own controls.

After a mean duration of 6.7 months, average food intake of uncooked food comprised 62% of the calories ingested. The mean weight loss was 3.8 kg (about 8.3 pounds)! Mean diastolic pressure reduction was 17.8 mm Hg, both statistically significant figures. Perhaps most interesting was that *80% of those who drank alcohol or smoked stopped spontaneously*.

# 18. Energy and Endurance Increased in Mice on Raw Diet

Dr. Israel Brekhman of the former Soviet Union performed a simple experiment with telling results. He fed mice cooked food and live, raw food at different times. When these mice ate only the raw food, they had *three times more energy and endurance* than when eating cooked food. Dr. Gabriel Cousens writes about this in *Rainbow Green Live-Food Cuisine* (p. 117).

# 19. Body's Defenses Boosted on Raw Diet

An article entitled "Raw food and immunity," published in *Fortschr Med* (June 10, 1990, Vol. 108, Issue 17, pp. 338–340, PubMed ID 2198207), summarizes research on the raw diet, "Uncooked food is an integral component of human nutrition and is a necessary precondition for an intact immune system. Its therapeutic effect is complex, and a variety of influences of raw food and its constituents on the body's defenses have been documented. Such effects include antibiotic, antiallergic, tumor-protective, immunomodulatory and anti-inflammatory actions. In view of this, uncooked food can be seen as a useful adjunct to drugs in the treatment of allergic, rheumatic and infectious diseases."

# 20. Colon Cancer Risk Lowered on Raw Diet

Quite a few controlled studies of the raw food diet's effects have been performed at the University of Kuopio in Finland. Researchers in the department of physiology published a paper called "Shifting from a conventional diet to an uncooked vegan diet reversibly alters fecal hydrolytic activities in humans" in *The Journal of Nutrition* (1992, Vol. 122, Issue 4, pp. 924–930, PubMed ID 552366).

The test group adopted a raw vegan diet for one month and then resumed a conventional diet for a second month, while the control group consumed a conventional diet throughout the study. Blood levels of the chemicals phenol and p-cresol, daily urine output and fecal enzyme activities were measured.

Within one week of commencing the raw vegan diet, fecal urease had decreased by 66%, cholylglycine hydrolase by 55%, beta-glucuronidase by 33% and beta-glucosidase by 40%. These values remained lowered throughout the diet. Within two weeks of resuming the conventional diet, however, the fecal enzyme activities returned to the higher, baseline values.

In plain English, these results suggested that the raw vegan diet resulted in a bodily adaptation: a definite decrease in bacterial enzymes and certain toxic products that have been implicated in colon cancer risk.

# 21. Nutrient Status and Weight Control in Rheumatoid Arthritis Improved on Raw Diet

The department of clinical nutrition of the University of Kuopio in Finland also wrote an article entitled "Effect of a strict vegan diet on energy and nutrient intakes by Finnish rheumatoid patients." It was published in the *European Journal of Clinical Nutrition* (October 1993, Vol. 47, Issue 10, pp. 747–749, PubMed ID 8269890).

Forty-three Finnish rheumatoid arthritis patients were divided into two groups. The experiment lasted three months. The experimental group of 21 patients ate uncooked vegan food and had tutoring by a living-food expert. The control group of 22 ate their usual diets and had no tutoring.

It was found that shifting to an uncooked vegan diet resulted in a significant increase in the intake of energy and many nutrients. The raw vegan dieters also lost 9% of their body weight.

# 22. Lung Cancer Risk Reduced on Raw Food

A study published in the *Japanese Journal of Cancer Research* (June 1993, PubMed ID 8340248) showed that the odds of incurring lung cancer among smokers and former smokers are reduced with raw vegetable and fruit consumption. The study was entitled "Protective effects of raw vegetables and fruit against lung cancer among smokers and ex-smokers: a case-control study in the Tokai area of Japan."

# 23. Raw Diet Is Best Vegetarian Diet for Mice

Dr. Stanley Bass, ND, DC, PhC, PhD, DO, DSc, DD, spent four years experimenting on hundreds of mice, feeding them every form of vegetarian diet imaginable. He published his results in 1994 in *In Search of the Ultimate Diet: Testing Nutritional Theories on Mice*. This report is available at his website, www.drbass.com.

He found that on diets completely devoid of animal products, such as fruitarian and vegan diets, the mice would become cannibalistic, particularly toward their vulnerable newborns. There was a great deficiency of B vitamins, especially $B_{12}$, Vitamin D and other factors perhaps not yet discovered. In humans, *it could take years for such deficiencies to show up* in a person's health status.

After two years of experiments, he determined that a 75-85% raw vegan diet supplemented with raw animal products was best for his mice. He found raw egg yolks to be the best supplement, as the mice on that diet had the healthiest babies. Eggs are the most complete source of protein and all other essential nutrients.

In part two of his mouse studies, *Discovery of the Ultimate Diet: Testing Nutritional Theories on Mice, Volume 2* (1996), Dr. Bass concluded that it was possible to remain in perfect health on a 100% raw diet that included a minimum of ½-1 ounce of animal food, such as one raw egg yolk, a day.

I called him to find out why he had earlier suggested that the ideal for humans might be only 75-85% raw. He said that was simply because most people cannot stay on a 100% raw diet. He admitted that a 100% raw is ideal, provided there is at least a "silver dollar-sized amount" of daily animal protein.

His advice to include small amounts of animal foods echoes recommendations of the late hygienic doctors John Tilden and Christopher Gian-Cursio. However, it should be noted here that modern science has determined that the protein requirements of rodents exceeds those of humans and other primates.

# 24. Dr. Robinson's Live Food Cancer Therapy

As President and Research Director of the Linus Pauling Institute of Science and Medicine, Dr. Arthur Robinson studied the effects of ingesting live foods, including wheatgrass, as opposed to taking synthetic Vitamin C, on cancer in laboratory mice.

He used various groups of mice, giving them skin cancer with ultraviolet radiation and then feeding them on differing diets that included supplementary Vitamin E and varying amounts of Vitamin C. The control group got "standard mouse feed" only. Some of the groups got raw foods similar to those recommended by Dr. Ann Wigmore.

It is important to point out that although Dr. Robinson was aware of a low-calorie, raw food diet's nutritional contribution toward empowering the body to *totally reverse* cancer, this experiment was designed merely to test the effects of the raw food diet in *slowing down* cancer growth.

Cancer incidence decreased by about 75% for those on living foods alone. This could be duplicated with Vitamin C supplementation only by giving doses so massive as to be nearly lethal for the mice and far beyond any reasonable range for humans to consume.

However, when high protein, high fat foods were added to the diet, even raw ones like nuts and seeds, cancer suppression stopped. Only when subjects were fed raw fruits and vegetables, which are lower in calories, was cancer reversal noted.

In other words, if these rodent results translate to humans, a diet considered healthful and ample for a healthy person could nevertheless be deadly to a person with cancer, who really needs calorie restriction in addition to a raw produce diet to starve the cancer.

"The effect is so large that, in my opinion," states Robinson, "if diet restriction were practiced by all cancer patients in the United States, the resulting life-extension might equal or surpass that resulting from the combined efforts of the entire current medical oncology effort."

Interestingly, Robinson also found that Vitamin C supplementation at less massive megadoses of from 1-5 grams daily actually resulted in *accelerated* cancer growth. Only near-lethal doses of about 100 grams could yield the same cancer-suppressing effect as the raw fruit and vegetable diet.

This discovery was so disturbing to Dr. Linus Pauling that Robinson and Pauling terminated their 16-year professional collaboration! Dr. Pauling was not willing to accept the fact that artificial Vitamin C supplementation in moderate megadoses accelerates cancer growth.

Robinson's study, "Suppression of squamous cell carcinoma in hairless mice by dietary nutrient variation," *Mechanisms of Ageing and Development*, July 1994, pp. 201–214, is described in an article entitled "Living Foods and Cancer" that can be found at www.nutritionandcancer.org.

# 25. Fibromyalgia Symptoms Reduced on Raw Diet

Researchers in the physiology department of the University of Kuopio in Finland found that a raw vegan diet had beneficial effects on fibromyalgia sufferers.

Fifteen control patients continued their omnivorous diet while 18 ate the raw diet for three months. Those eating the raw diet experienced significant improvement compared to the control group. Their pain lessened, joint stiffness diminished, sleep patterns improved, and general health improved. Serum cholesterol and urine sodium were lowered. A majority of the patients, overweight to begin with, lost weight.

Results were published in an article called "Vegan diet alleviates fibromyalgia symptoms," which appeared in the *Scandinavian Journal of Rheumatology* (2000, Vol. 29, Issue 5, pp. 308–313, PubMed ID 11093597).

# 26. Cancer Risk Reduced on Raw Vegetables

The *Journal of the American Dietetic Association,* October 1996, Issue 10, pp. 1027–1039, PubMed ID 8841165, published an article entitled "Vegetables, fruit and cancer prevention: a review." A review of 206 epidemiologic studies on humans and 22 studies on animals examined the correlation between fruit and vegetable intake and cancer risk. It found that a diet predominating in raw vegetable consumption correlated more strongly with reduced cancer incidence than conventional diets of cooked food.

# 27. Blood Lipid Improvement Found on Mostly Vegetarian Diet

A study entitled "Effect of a diet high in vegetables, fruit and nuts on serum lipids" was published in *Metabolism* (May 1997, Vol. 46, Issue 5, pp. 530–537, PubMed ID 9160820). The effects of a diet high in leafy green vegetables, fruit and nuts on serum lipid risk factors for cardiovascular disease were assessed. Ten healthy volunteers consumed their habitual diet for two weeks and then for another two weeks ate a diet largely consisting of vegetables, fruits and nuts.

After two weeks on the plant diet, the lipid risk factors for cardiovascular disease showed significant reduction in comparison with the control diet. The reduction in total serum cholesterol was 34-49% greater than would be predicted by differences in dietary fat and cholesterol.

The researchers concluded, "A diet consisting largely of low-calorie vegetables and fruit and nuts markedly reduced lipid risk factors for cardiovascular disease. Several aspects of such diets, which may have been consumed early in human evolution, have implications for cardiovascular disease prevention."

# 28. Rheumatoid Arthritis Symptoms Reduced on Raw Diet

Researchers in the department of physiology of the University of Kuopio in Finland also performed a study that found that a raw food, vegan diet benefited patients with rheumatoid arthritis. In this study, the benefits were found to be both subjective and objective. Subjectively, the patients felt better. Objectively, joint stiffness was reduced, and significant increases of antioxidants (protective chemicals) were found in the blood of the raw fooders.

This study was published in the *British Journal of Rheumatology* (March, 1998, Vol. 37, Issue 3, pp. 274–281, PubMed ID 9566667). The article is entitled "Uncooked, lactobacilli-rich, vegan food and rheumatoid arthritis."

# 29. Favorable Weight Loss and Amenorrhea Effects Noted on Raw Diet

Published in the *Annals of Nutrition and Metabolism* (1999, Vol. 43, Issue 2, pp. 69–79, PubMed ID 10436305), this study was called "Consequences of a long-term raw food diet on body weight and menstruation: results of a question-naire survey." It was performed at the Institute of Nutritional Science at Justus Liebig University of Giessen, Germany.

The study involved 216 men and 297 women who ate raw diets varying from 70-100% raw for 3.7 years. An average weight loss of 22 pounds (9.9 kg) for men and 26 pounds (12 kg) for women was observed. About 30% of the women under 45 years of age experienced partial to complete amenorrhea (cessa-tion of menstrual bleeding). Those who ate a large percentage of raw foods (over 90%) were beneficially affected more than those who ate a moderate percentage of raw food (under 90%).

The study concluded that raw diets are associated with a high loss of body weight and amenorrhea. The writers of the article stated, "Since many raw food dieters exhibited underweight and amenorrhea, a very strict raw food diet cannot be recommended on a long-term basis." This statement reflects three signifi-cantly mistaken cultural biases ingrained in our belief systems concerning health.

The first myth is that being underweight is not healthy. In fact many studies show that the lean person lives longer and in better health than the so-called nor-mal weight or overweight person.

The second myth is that menstrual bleeding is normal and healthy. In fact monthly bleeding is a sign of advanced toxemia. This fact is backed up by obser-vation of other primates. Female apes in the wild, eating their natural diets, do not bleed with menstruation. Some modern-day apes do bleed slightly, perhaps due to environmental pollution and zoo diets that are seldom nearly 100% raw.

The third myth is that monthly bleeding is a requirement for fertility. Ovula-tion generally occurs at the opposite pole of the monthly fertility cycle whether or not discharge of the resulting placental lining is accompanied by bleeding.

In humans, menstrual bleeding is thought by raw food experts to be a sign of toxicity and/or Vitamin C deficiency. It would be nonsensical to state that people should not be on a raw food diet for a long-term basis when that is how we, as all animal species, evolved over millions of years!

# 30. Antioxidant Status Improved on Raw Diet

An article called "Vegan diet in physiological health promotion" appeared in *Acta Physiologica Hungarica* (1999, Vol. 86, Issues 3–4, pp. 171–80, PubMed ID 10943644). It was again authored by members of the department of physiol-ogy at the University of Kuopio.

Subjects eating a diet of raw vegan food displayed increased levels of caro-tenoids and Vitamins C and E. The results also showed lowered cholesterol concentrations, as well as urinary phenol and p-cresol. Several fecal enzyme levels that are considered harmful were also lowered. The patients that had arthritis reported a lessening of pain, stiffness and swelling of joints. Those with fibromyalgia lost weight. Upon resuming their normal diet, the pathological conditions returned and worsened.

# 31. Raw Diet Benefits Shown in Just One Week

The ambitious Finnish group at the University of Kuopio also published a study entitled "Effects of eating an uncooked vegetable diet for 1 week" (*Appetite*, Vol. 19, pp. 243–254, PubMed ID 1482162). This study concluded that such a vegetable diet was shown to be of some benefit in the short term but that any longer-term use required further evaluation.

# 32. Pain and Joint Stiffness Decreased on Raw Vegan Diet

Yet another study conducted at the University of Kuopio in Finland entitled "Antioxidants in vegan diet and rheumatic disorders" was published in *Toxicology* (November 30, 2000, Vol. 155, Issues 1–3, pp. 45–53, PubMed ID 11154796).

A living food diet of uncooked berries, vegetables, roots, nuts, germinated seeds and sprouts was fed to one group, whereas the control group ate the typical omnivorous diet.

The raw food eaters reported decreased joint stiffness and pain, as well as improvement in their health. They also experienced improvement in objective health measures when tested.

# 33. Fibromyalgia Sufferers at Hallelujah Acres Improved on Mostly Raw Diet

A study was done at Hallelujah Acres, a center founded by Rev. George Malkmus, who advocates an 85-100% raw food diet. The study is entitled "Fibromyalgia syndrome improved using a mostly raw vegetarian diet: an observational study," published in *BMC Complementary Alternative Medicine* (2001, Vol. 1, Issue 1, p. 7, PubMed ID 11602026).

Fibromyalgia patients generally suffer from chronic pain, fatigue, poor quality sleep and depression. Thirty patients were put on a mostly raw vegan diet. After several months, 19 of the patients experienced significant improvement as measured by tests like shoulder pain at rest and after motion, abduction range of motion of shoulder, flexibility, a chair test and a six-minute walk.

# 34. A Largely Vegetarian Diet and Reduced Risk of Colon and Heart Diseases

A study entitled "Effect of a very-high-fiber vegetable, fruit, and nut diet on serum lipids and colonic function" (*Metabolism*, April 2001, 50[4]: pp. 494–503, PubMed ID 11288049) demonstrated that a very high vegetable fiber intake reduces risk of cardiovascular disease and colon cancer.

# 35. Mostly Raw Diet and Improved Quality of Life

Michael Donaldson, Director of Research at Hallelujah Acres, published the study "Food and nutrient intake of Hallelujah vegetarians" in *Nutrition and Food Science* (2001, Vol. 31, Issue 6, pp. 293–303).

For 28 months, 141 followers of the Hallelujah Diet, which is 100% vegan and at least 85% raw, kept dietary journals. Members reported significant improvement in health and quality of life after adopting the diet. Mean daily consumption of fruits and vegetables was 6.6 servings and 11.4 servings, respectively. The mean energy intake was 1,460 calories for women and 1,830 calories for men. It was found that with some modification, this diet pattern allows people to adopt a low-calorie diet sufficient in most nutrients.

Critics of this study may argue that the results are subjective. Ask the patients if they care!

# 36. Raw Diet Fuels Intelligence Increase

Renowned raw food teacher Victoria Boutenko performed a raw food study herself. A university professor conducted the experiment. The control group did not eat raw food. The experimental group ate raw food for only two days. (She wanted them to do it for a week, but none thought he could!) The subjects were given an intelligence test before eating raw and after.

Although many people still believe that IQ is something static, her amazing findings were that after eating raw for only two days, the average IQ was raised by 40%! Victoria discussed her findings at a workshop. She may be contacted through her web site at www.rawfamily.com.

# 37. Dr. Jean Seignalet's Hospital Study: Raw Diet Yields High Patient Success Rate

Dr. Jean Seignalet of the hospital St. Eloi in Montpellier, France, undertook a large-scale experiment with a diet he prescribed to hundreds of patients. The diet consisted of as much raw food as possible and excluded all dairy and wheat products. Success was defined to consist of remission with a 50% reduction in disease or ailment symptoms. He tested people with dozens of different diseases and syndromes.

Success rates for all ranged from 75-100%. Patients enjoying a 100% success rate included those with the following medical conditions: systemic lupus, scleroderma, juvenile diabetes, Crohn's disease, acne, atopic eczema, hay fever, rhinitis, allergic conjunctivitis, edema and more. Patients enjoying a 92-98% success rate included those with these conditions: fibromyalgia, ankylosing spondylitis, psoriatic arthritis, multiple sclerosis (MS), depression, spasmophilia, irritable bowel syndrome, urticaria and asthma. (See *L'Alimentation ou la Troisième Médecine* [Nutrition or the Third Medicine], Dr. Jean Seignalet, Édition François-Xavier de Guilbert, Paris.)

# 38. Preadolescent Children Thrive on Live Food Diets

Dr. Gabriel Cousens of the nonprofit Tree of Life Foundation in Patagonia, Arizona, decided that research needed to be published on the effects of live food diets on children since so many raw food parents get harassed by the authorities for "child abuse."

Preliminary results as of June 2004 showed that the heights of 74% of the children were above the lowest $25^{th}$ percentile and the weights of 68% of the children were above the lowest $25^{th}$ percentile. All children were above the $10^{th}$ percentile. The heights of 37% of the children were above the 75% percentile. Over 60% of the children were above average for both weight and height as measured by the National Center for Chronic Disease Prevention and Health Promotion.

Dr. Cousens notes that these children are also not under the influence of the stimulating effects of growth hormones to which the majority of nonvegan children are exposed since the vegans do not consume meat and dairy, which contain hormones. He also notes, "The preliminary conclusion of our data is that a live food diet has no major positive or negative effect on height and weight. None of the children in the study have a score above the top $90^{th}$ percentile or below the lowest $10^{th}$ percentile. Therefore, the children fall into the middle 80% of normal height and weight."

This study has not been published, as it is not yet finished. The preliminary results were written in a handout passed out at the 2004 Raw Food Festival in Portland, Oregon.

Note: Dr. Cousens is very aware of one risk for children on a raw vegan diet: the potential lack of Vitamin $B_{12}$. He is very careful to monitor the children for this, which all responsible parents of raw vegan children should do. (See Chapter 17.)

# 39. Cancer Risk Reduced More with Raw than Cooked Vegetables

A study entitled "Raw versus cooked vegetables and cancer risk" was published in *Cancer Epidemiology Biomarkers & Prevention* (Vol. 13, Sept 2004, p. 1422–1435). It consisted of a review of the medical literature from 1994 to 2003 that summarized the relationship between raw and cooked vegetable consumption and the risk of various cancers.

Twenty-eight studies were examined. Most showed a direct correlation between consumption of vegetables, raw or cooked, and lower cancer risk. Nine of 11 studies linked eating both raw and cooked vegetables to lowered cancer risk, but only four studies linked eating only cooked vegetables to lowered cancer risk.

# 40. The Roseburg Study: Sex Life, Stomach Acid and More Improved on Raw Diet

Victoria Boutenko and Dr. Paul Fieber, MD, conducted this study on the effects of raw green smoothies on patients who had low levels of hydrochloric acid (HCl). HCl is necessary in the gastric juices for proper protein digestion.

Twenty-seven participants drank a quart of green smoothies prepared by Victoria's husband every day for 30 days, adding it to their normal diet. Three participants dropped out; 66.7% of those 24 remaining showed vast improvement in their HCl levels. The doctor did not expect to see such dramatic results in such a short period of time.

The participants reported many other beneficial effects, such as improved sex life — one man even saying it was like being 15 years younger! — reduced cravings for bad foods, better sleep and elimination and much more. For further details on this study, read *Green for Life* by Victoria Boutenko. See Appendix C for more on her revolutionary raw green smoothie diet.

# 41. Gastric Cancer Risk Reduced on Raw Diet

A study published by the Kaunas University of Medicine in Lithuania found that higher consumption of raw vegetables, such as cabbage, carrots, garlic and broccoli, is linked to a decrease in the risk of stomach cancer. This study appeared in *Medicina* (Kaunas) 2005, 41 (9): pp. 733–740.

# 42. LDL Cholesterol and Triglyceride Levels Found Favorable on Long-Term Raw Diet

An article published in the October 2005 edition of *The Journal of Nutrition* (135, Issue 10, pp. 2372–2378, PubMed ID 16177198) is entitled "Long-term consumption of a raw food diet is associated with favorable serum LDL cholesterol and triglycerides but also with elevated plasma homocysteine and low serum HDL cholesterol in humans."

A reduction of some cardiovascular disease risk markers manifested in subjects on raw foods. However, the study emphasizes that raw fooders must make certain to take Vitamin $B_{12}$ supplements, or they may accumulate excess homocysteine, a risk factor in heart disease and a marker for $B_{12}$ deficiency. (See Chapter 17.) Additionally, some raw fooders in the experiment had lower amounts of HDL, known as the "good" cholesterol.

The study makes mention that there was a high consumption of raw fruits and vegetables, but perhaps the participants were not eating sufficient nuts. Almond consumption, for example, was found to be associated with increased HDL in a study published in *Circulation, Journal of the American Heart Association* (2002). A study published in *The Journal of Nutrition* (2003) found that macadamia nut consumption yielded the same results. Additional studies have found that pistachio and walnut consumption correlated with improved HDL to LDL ratios.

# 43. Cancer Risk Reduced on Raw Cabbage

In 2005, a study done at the University of New Mexico showed that women migrating from Poland to the USA tripled their risk of breast cancer. This resulted because they no longer consumed at least three servings a week of raw cabbage and sauerkraut. These staples of the native Polish diet were found to contain glucosinolates that correlate with lowered cancer risk. Brussels sprouts, broccoli and kale also contain glucosinolates. See www.medscape.com/view article/515835.

# 44. Bone Mass in Long-Term Raw Fooders

Dr. Luigi Fontana, MD, and associates at the Washington School of Medicine in St. Louis, Missouri, published a study entitled "Low bone mass in subjects on a long-term raw vegetarian diet," which appeared in the *Archives of Internal Medicine* (Vol. 165, Issue 6, March 28, 2005, pp. 684–689, PubMed ID 15795346).

This was a cross-sectional study of 18 volunteers aged 18-85 who had been eating a raw vegan diet for a mean of 3.6 years. They were compared with people of their own age who ate a conventional diet. Both groups were measured for body mass index, bone mass, bone mineral density, markers of bone turnover, levels of Vitamin D and inflammatory markers, such as C-reactive protein and insulinlike growth factors.

The raw vegans were found to have less inflammation, indicated by low levels of C-reactive protein, which is made by the liver in response to inflammation in the body. The presence of inflammation is a sign of disease progression and aging.

The raw vegans also had lower levels of the human hormone IGF-1, which meant lower risk of breast and prostate cancer. Their bone turnover rates were normal. They had higher levels of Vitamin D, which Fontana initially thought was going to be a problem area since vegans don't consume dairy fortified with Vitamin D. He attributed their high Vitamin D levels to their being conscientious enough to expose themselves to sufficient sunlight. Those on the raw diet also had lower body mass indices and lower body fat percentages.

Interestingly, the raw fooders also had low levels of the hormone leptin, which is associated with high bone density. They exhibited lower bone mass in significant places, such as the hips and spine, which theoretically could lead to osteoporosis and fracture risk. However, they didn't have the biochemical markers that typically accompany osteoporosis.

Fontana proposed that despite having lower bone mass, those on the raw diet actually might have good, healthy bone quality. He hypothesized that since their bone turnover markers were normal, their Vitamin D levels above normal, and their inflammation levels low, it was possible that the raw fooders didn't have increased risk of fracture. He theorized that perhaps their lower bone mass is related to the fact that they weigh less because they take in fewer calories.

# 45. Dr. Cousens: Diabetics Improve on Raw Diet

A study of the raw food diet's effect on diabetes has been documented in the film *Raw for 30 Days*. The following summary is provided on Dr. Gabriel Cousens's web site, www.treeoflife.nu/diabetes.html. It should be noted that their dietary program consisted of 100% vegan, low-glycemic food, along with some mineral supplements, the proteolytic enzyme supplement Vitalzyme, and Natural Cellular Defense, another commercial supplement.

Over the years, a significant number of people have returned to a normal, nondiabetic physiology from the diabetic physiology through our antidiabetic program at the Tree of Life. According to the research of the *New York Times*, there are 21 million diabetics and 40 million prediabetics, and diabetes is "incurable."

In order to test our clinical experience, in February 2006, we invited six people who were eating the traditional American fast and junk food diet and had been insulin-dependent diabetics for an average of five years. It represented a final test of our program. We invited an independent movie producer to film the month-long program, and we did "before and after" studies regarding the effect of a month of raw food and specific supplements.

The results were outstanding. Although one person whose blood sugar dropped from 500 to 200 in two weeks dropped out of the program because he was not willing to . . . [continue] the live food program, the others had exceptional results. Within four days, all participants except the Type I diabetic were off insulin and oral antidiabetic medications. By the end of one month, two people had blood sugars regularly averaging between 70 and 85. Two had dropped from an average blood sugar of approximately 250-450 to around 120. All their blood tests became essentially normal. In other words, by the end of 1 month, the Type II diabetics had achieved a level of health according to their blood tests and daily blood sugar readings that was considered comparable with a normal nondiabetic physiology; i. e., the physiology of a healthy person. The Type I diabetic went from an insulin intake of 70 units to 5 units. Succeeding with a group who knew virtually nothing about live foods or the live food lifestyle and who had no particular interest in it was a real test for this program.

Although no program can guarantee any results for healing diabetes in one month, we feel this program offers a reasonable, healthy, optimistic and realistic way to ameliorate diabetes.

Of course one can only stay in a nondiabetic physiology if he or she continues to follow the healthy program outlined and experienced in the 30-day program. If someone does not stay on this program, we cannot expect he or she will stay with the normal healthy physiology.

# 46. Cancer Markers Improved on Raw Diet

A study published in the December 2006 issue of The *American Journal of Clinical Nutrition* (PubMed ID 17158430) assessed blood cancer markers in three groups of 21 people each.

The first group ate a low-protein, low-calorie diet consisting of uncooked and unprocessed plant food. The second group ate a customary Western diet but ran an average of 48 miles a week. The third group consisted of sedentary people on the standard Western diet.

When the three groups were compared, the lowest levels of the very powerful cancer-promoting human growth hormone IGF-1 were found in the group of raw food eaters. Additionally, the raw eaters exhibited low levels of the inflammation marker C-reactive protein, blood insulin and cancer-promoting sex hormones.

# 47. Cholesterol and High Blood Pressure Reduced on Raw Diet

An experiment filmed for British television enlisted nine volunteers to go on what was called an "evo diet." They ate up to five kilos a day of raw fruit, vegetables, nuts and honey. The experiment lasted 12 days. For the last five days, they were given standard portions of cooked fish "as a nod to the hunter and gatherer."

The diet was based on research showing that if we ate as we evolved to eat over thousands of years, our cholesterol and blood pressure levels would be healthy. The results were published in the January 11, 2007 issue of *BBC News Magazine*:

Once they were over the withdrawal from caffeinated drinks and some foods, they enjoyed good energy levels and mood. So the moments of "unhappiness and grumpiness" that the TV crew was primed to capture failed to happen. . . . Overall, the cholesterol levels dropped 23%, an amount usually achieved only through anticholesterol drugs, statins. The group's average blood pressure fell from a level of 140/83 — almost hypertensive — to 122/76. Though it was not intended to be a weight-loss diet, they dropped 4.4kg (9.7 lbs), on average.

# Additional Studies in Appendix D

Most of the studies summarized in this chapter are about the *power of the body to thrive on wholesome raw food.* For those who need further convincing, additional experiments reported in the scientific literature are summarized briefly in Appendix D that prove the *failure of the body to thrive on toxic, cooked food.*

# An Ongoing European Study of Cooked Foods

The Europeans are taking the toxicity of cooked food so seriously that they have initiated a multination study entitled "Action 927, thermally processed foods: possible health implications." This study began in 2004 and will end in 2009.

# Numerous Individual Case Studies

There are thousands of published and over a million unpublished case histories of dramatic healing with the assistance of live food diets. Often shrugged off as "anecdotal" by medical doctors, these cases cannot be so cavalierly dismissed when the numbers are so large. Interview any of the doctors listed in the reference section of this book. The late Dr. Shelton alone had over 40,000 cases of improvement for fasters on file by 1985.

Also read some of the published accounts: *Roger's Recovery from AIDS* tells about the use of raw foods in the complete remission of full-blown AIDS. *Raw Food Treatment of Cancer* recounts medical doctor Kristine Nolfi's healing from her own cancer. *Why Christians Get Sick* includes Rev. George Malkmus' story of raw juices and his healing of colon cancer. *How I Conquered Cancer Naturally* is about Eydie Mae Hunsberger's use of raw foods in her healing from breast cancer. More such books are listed in the Bibliography.

Also check out the videos by Dr. Lorraine Day, such as *Cancer Doesn't Scare Me Anymore* (www.drday.com). When Dr. Day got breast cancer, she tried dozens of alternative treatments. None of them worked until she discovered Natural Hygiene and raw foods via the teachings of the Seventh Day Adventists.

Interestingly, the Guinness world record for sleep deprivation was recently broken by Britisher Tony Wright, who attributed his 11 days and nights without sleep to his raw food diet!

# The Most Important and Convincing Experiment of All

Finally, if not one of these experiments convinces you, it is time to try the most important experiment of all, the one on yourself! The living food diet speaks for itself.

About two weeks of a nearly or 100% raw food diet changes the most skeptical and cynical of people, who need no "scientific proof" at that point. Raw foods really do bring priceless benefits to tired and toxic bodies, minds and spirits. The direct experience of just two weeks is sufficient to satisfy virtually all who want personal proof.

The next few chapters explain the scientific theory behind the raw food diet so that you will understand how toxic it is to eat cooked and how important it is to eat raw.

But if you can't wait to get started, skip ahead to Section Four. You can come back to the rest of Section Two later for more science.

# 9
# Man's Fatal Chemistry Lab: The Great Cooked Food Experiment

We cannot escape from being entangled in the
conclusion that intractable disease is as old as cookery.
—Dr. Edward Howell (1898–1987)

Even if you are not a "science person," I encourage you to read this. Reread it if you backslide into cooked foods or are tempted to. Even if you don't understand some of the terms, you will get the gist of the message, and it will become ingrained into your mind that "cooked food is poison." You may not understand what the presence of certain chemical byproducts means. You may not even be able to pronounce the terms. But you should be aware that you do not want these chemicals in your body!

A couple of terms used in this chapter include *carcinogenic*, which means 'cancer causing', and *mutagenic*, which means 'causing mutations in the DNA sequence of a gene or chromosome'. Mutations are often precursors to cancer, and so the two are related.

As stated in *Diet, Nutrition and Cancer* (p. 277), "Initiation of the carcinogenic process may involve an alteration in the genetic material of a cell. Therefore, it is reasonable to suppose that chemicals that alter DNA (i.e., cause mutations) will have a high probability of being initiators of carcinogenesis."

People have asked me, "But why focus on the negative?"

I have concluded that both the positive aspects of a raw diet and the negative aspects of a cooked one are important to recognize. It is too easy to backslide into the world of cooked food if you do not understand the rationale behind avoiding fired foods.

I know some people who merely pop a few pills of dehydrated fruits and vegetables and think they can get away with eating whatever they like after that. They are sadly mistaken. It is not simply a matter, as the American Cancer Society would say, of eating a certain number of fruit and vegetable servings per day.

The implication here is that once you finish your quota of the good stuff, you can eat pretty much whatever you want. This is clearly not the case. What you *refuse* to eat is as much a health factor as what you *choose* to eat, especially in a world in which cooked food is everywhere.

Cooking and organic chemistry operate primarily in the temperature range between 68° F and 572° F (20° C and 300° C). When you were in chemistry lab at school, you no doubt learned that heating things changed their chemical structures. Why would heating food be immune to this chemical process?

Think of a kitchen as a chemical laboratory, producing a multitude of new chemical substances that do not normally occur in a natural setting. And think of modern man as unknowingly being immersed in the grandest chemistry experiment ever by eating cooked and denatured, chemical-laden food.

When various foods are commingled and cooked, thousands of new molecules are created that are unnatural to our bodies' biochemistry. Serious researchers have ascertained that the human body has not adapted to these numerous complex molecules that we have been ingesting for only a few thousand years.

In fact the extensive adaptations that would be required may be biologically impossible. For it is doubtful the body's design could ever adjust to the 10,000-plus novel chemicals — protoplasmic poisons — laced into the modern food supply.

# Is Cooked Food Toxic?

In Chapter 5, we explained that it is the body's internal environment, not the germ, gene or wear and tear that is most responsible for our state of health. One of the keys to maintaining a healthy biological terrain is staying free of toxic accumulations. As we shall see, cooking food renders it toxic.

*Are we playing with fire when we cook our food?* Man is the only creature on earth that cooks its food. Animals in the wild do not cook. When these creatures die of old age, they remain free of the degenerative diseases of civilization, such as cancer, diabetes, arthritis and heart disease, so long as they haven't been subjected to heavily polluted water or air.

In the 1930s, research done in Switzerland showed that people's leukocytes (white blood cells) increased after eating cooked food. This leukocytosis was otherwise known to happen only after exposure to toxic substances, trauma or infection. Because cooking is so deeply ingrained in all cultures, when "digestive leukocytosis" was first observed, it was assumed to be normal.

It occurred to no one that the ingestion of cooked food was the toxic impetus for the body to marshal huge numbers of leukocytes to disarm those toxins and restore homeostasis (see Glossary). The leukocytes are defender cells that appear in force to neutralize dangerous substances that show up in the body from either endogenous or exogenous sources.

Dr. Edward Howell found that the leukocytes were also the body's main repository and backup supply of digestive enzymes outside of the pancreas. When the body's limited supply of pancreatic digestive secretions is overtaxed by the absence of sufficient food enzymes, these auxiliary helpers are called in to assist in the digestive process, leaving them temporarily unavailable to carry out their normal defensive and restorative functions within the body.

Dr. Paul Kouchakoff discovered that eating raw food or food heated at very low temperatures, less than 118° F (48° C) provoked no digestive leukocytosis. He also found that refined, homogenized, pasteurized, preserved or otherwise denatured foods stimulate the body to greatly increase the white blood cell count.

Since then Dr. Howard Loomis has repeated Dr. Kouchakoff's results with hundreds of patients in his clinical work. He found that overstimulating the body's natural defenses three to four times a day by eating cooked food is very stressful to the human body.

Cooking and processing food destroys nutrients by changing their molecular shape, size and chemical potential. The ensuing biochemical chaos results in the accumulation of indigestible and harmful substances, residue and debris. Moreover, cooked food is prepared in utensils that emit toxic metal, plastic or paint particles.

After you cook, look at what sticks to the pots and pans: grease, sticky starches, gooey cheese! This is a reflection at the macroscopic level of what sticks to your entire gastrointestinal tract at the microscopic level. On the other hand, raw foods cling neither to the pots nor to your intestines. In addition, look at the clogged sink drains common among those who prepare cooked foods. Raw fooders' drains don't clog up with grease and don't need to be roto-rooted. Neither do their arteries clog up and need stents, angioplasties or bypass surgeries!

Cooking has been proven to produce millions of different "Maillard molecules," sugar/protein combinations. In 1916, the chemist Louis Maillard proved that brown pigments and polymers that occur in pyrolysis (i.e., chemical breakdown caused by heat alone — in a word, *cooking*) are formed after the reaction of an amino acid group of a protein with the carbonyl group of a sugar.

The substances generated are endless chains of new molecules that are variously toxic, aromatic, peroxidizing, antioxidizing, mutagenic and carcinogenic. For example, in a broiled potato alone, Maillard identified 450 novel chemicals and tested them one by one for toxicity. Every one of the first 50 he tested was proven to be carcinogenic to laboratory animals. At that point, his employer terminated that line of research and gave Maillard something else to work on before he could test the others.

This remarkable proliferation of biologically incompatible chemicals resulted just from cooking a potato all by itself. Try to imagine, if you can, what chemical mayhem occurs in most kitchens when that potato is cooked together with butter, vegetable oils, sour cream, herbs, spices, condiments and various other food items. And this represents only one small side dish of a typical cooked meal! It is believed by some that the chemical byproducts of cooking food are *so chaotic and unpredictable that our biochemistry will never, ever fully adapt to them.*

Maillard's research was swept under the rug. It would have been devastating to the food processing industry had his conclusions become widely known. But they were later published in 1982 in a French journal (*Cahiers de diététique et de nutrition*, Vol. 17, pp. 39–45). The name of the article, translated into English, was "Pyrolysis and risks of toxicity."

Marilyn Willison of the Hippocrates Health Institute writes, "We should not cook our food. During the apparently harmless process, vital enzymes are destroyed; proteins are coagulated, making them difficult to assimilate; vitamins are mostly destroyed, with the remainder changing into forms that are difficult for the body to utilize; pesticides are restructured into even more toxic compounds; valuable oxygen is lost, and free radicals are produced."

One researcher who found out how chemicalized foods are made even more toxic with heat was Dr. William Newsome of Canada's Department of Health and Welfare Food Research Division, Bureau of Chemical Safety. He discovered that cooked, fungicided tomatoes had 10-90 times more ETU, a mutagen and carcinogen, than raw tomatoes from the same garden.

Dr. Bernarr Zovluck, a holistic doctor who has been eating a raw diet for over 50 years, writes, "Cooking causes the inorganic elements to enter the blood, circulate through the system, settle in the arteries and veins, and deaden the nerves. After cooking, the body loses its flexibility; arteries lose their pliability; nerves lose their ability to conduct electrical signals properly; the spinal cord becomes hardened; the tissues throughout the body contract, and the human being becomes prematurely old. In many cases, this matter is deposited in the various joints of the body, causing joint disease. In other cases, it accumulates as concretions in one or more of the internal organs, finally accumulating around the heart valves." See his article "Why Raw?" on his web site www.healself.org.

Moreover, cooked food is bad for the teeth. Harmful bacteria thrive only on dead, cooked food, and this encourages plaque buildup, cavities and gum recession. Cooked foods are highly acidic, so the body has to draw upon calcium and other alkaline minerals from the teeth and bones to neutralize that acidity. Decreased dental exercise from the softness of the cooked food also leads to dental abnormalities, such as crooked teeth.

Cooked food promotes obesity. Because you do not get fed the full spectrum of nutrients you need on a cooked diet, your body will often remain hungry even when it is calorically overfed, causing you to overeat. Since the toxic residues of all this cooked food leave an abundance of particles in your body that are not properly metabolized, the weight piles on as toxins are stored in fat cells and tissues. As the toxins build up, so does disease potential.

Dr. Gabriel Cousens sums up the hazards of eating cooked food: "Cooking coagulates the bioactive mineral and protein complexes and therefore disrupts mineral absorption, including calcium absorption. Cooking also disrupts RNA and DNA structure, which minimizes the amount of complex protein that our bodies are able to take in. It destroys most of the nutritive fats and creates carcinogenic and mutagenic . . . structures in the fats, as well as producing free radicals" (*Rainbow Green Live-Food Cuisine*, p. 109).

I once saw a cookbook entitled *Healthy Cooking*. This is an oxymoron because no cooking is healthful! No doubt about it, cooked food is toxic.

Food destruction by pyrolysis is a function of both time and temperature. The longer something is cooked and the higher the heat applied to it, the more toxic it becomes. If meat is seared for a few seconds, it will be vastly less toxic than meat that is well-done. Also, the higher the temperature at which something is cooked, the more toxic it becomes. For example, lightly steaming vegetables would produce less toxicity than baking them.

Microwaving may be the most destructive form of cooking because of the extreme violence with which microwaves rip apart food molecules. (See page 397.)

The cause/effect relationship between eating cooked food and physical degeneration usually goes unnoticed for two reasons:

First, the time lag between eating and serious illness is great. It is a cumulative effect, with the disease process slowly progressing from acute to chronic degeneration over decades. As Bruno Comby says, when we eat cooked food, we are "committing suicide on the installment plan." Because of this gradual, cumulative, toxic effect, illness is thought to be a part of the normal aging process.

Second, there is no modern-day society free of cooked food that we can hold up as a comparison. The cooking habit is deeply ingrained within the human psyche. Maybe our minds have adapted to it, but our bodies certainly have not.

# What Happens to the Macronutrients in Cooked Food?

Biologists agree that nourishment for the living human organism includes air, water, sunlight and food.

Food is a complex chemical package comprising (a) a number of micronutrients: enzymes, minerals, vitamins and various known and unknown phytonutrients; (b) three basic macronutrients: proteins, carbohydrates and fats; (c) indigestible nonnutritive matter: fiber, and (d) other indigestible nonnutritive and/or antinutritive matter.

Victoria BidWell offers us the following crash course in macronutrient definitions, adapted from *The Health Seekers' Yearbook* (edited by Dr. Vetrano):

## What Macronutrients Are

All natural foods contain a mix of all three macronutrients. Since different foods have different proportions of each, specific food items are usually thought of as chiefly proteins, carbohydrates or fats. Let's take a closer look at the composition of these macronutrients.

### Proteins

*Proteins* are the cells' vital construction materials. Proteins comprise about 75% of bodily tissue solids. They are continually required for cellular growth and repair, especially of muscle tissues, and for the production of hormones and enzymes. Proteins catalyze chemical reactions, regulate numerous metabolic functions and defend us against a multitude of potentially destructive agents.

*Amino acids* are the building blocks of proteins. Proteins are huge conglomerations of amino acids, called *macromolecules*, which come in various shapes and sizes. Proteins are not normally used as a fuel source but can be enlisted as such in times of dire need if neither of the body's preferred sources, carbohydrates and fats, is available.

The liver can synthesize 14 of the 22 amino acids needed by the body, but eight of them are deemed *essential* because they must come directly from food sources. All eight of these essential amino acids can be found in a variety of plant foods and all animal foods.

The body has the ability to store amino acids in its *amino acid pool*. It can also decompose and recycle some of the protein waste from dead and dying cells. As much as 90% of our daily protein needs are met by this recycling process.

Barring accidental injury, most of the major construction work has already been completed in adult bodies. Therefore daily dietary needs are not large. Most people need an average of 25-40 grams of protein daily, depending on body size, physical activity and stress levels. Meat and dairy promoters would have you believe that you need to consume 70-100 grams of protein each and every day because their expensive food products are very protein rich.

It should be noted, however, that raw protein is about 50% more assimilable than cooked protein. Excessive protein consumption, especially cooked protein, can lead to decades of chronic, degenerative diseases as excess acidity from eating these foods builds up in the body.

The raw fooder may thrive on a plant-based diet by eating moderately of those plant foods most abundant in protein: raw nuts, seeds, avocado and durian. Leafy greens and broccoli contain more modest amounts by weight, though often sufficient, followed by lesser amounts in other vegetables, with smaller amounts even being present in all fruits as structural components of their cells.

## Carbohydrates

*Carbohydrates* manifest in two types: simple and complex. The simple carbohydrates are termed *sugars*. The complex carbohydrates include *starches*, glycogen and fiber. The simple sugar *glucose* is the body's greatest need because this is the fuel that continuously provides each of its trillions of cells with energy for all metabolic activities. Most sugars and carbohydrates may be readily converted into glucose as needed through enzymatic activity. Sugars are the easiest, most energy-efficient macronutrients for the body to utilize as fuel.

*Sucrose*, or table sugar, is but one variety of simple carbohydrate. The sugars are sweet to the taste and abundant in all fruit, chiefly occurring in the forms *fructose*, *glucose* and *sucrose*. There are also a number of other sugars that occur in some foods.

The simplest of the sugars, called *monosaccharides*, need no chemical breakdown to be absorbed directly through the small intestines into the bloodstream. Fructose and glucose are the most common monosaccharides in food. Fructose still needs to be converted into glucose in the liver in order for the body to use it in its energy production cycle.

More complex sugars may be *disaccharides, oligosaccharides* or *polysaccharides*. Sucrose, being a combination of both glucose and fructose, is the most common disaccharide in food. These are digested by salivary enzymes in the mouth and upper, or cardiac, portion of the stomach in a process called *predigestion*.

*Starches* are complex carbohydrates, or polysaccharides (many sugars). They are initially nonsweet to the tastebuds, occurring abundantly in all grains and many vegetables, particularly root vegetables, corn and winter squashes.

Because of their polysaccharide structure, they are slower and more energy expensive to digest than simple sugars. Starches must be broken into monosaccharides and ultimately glucose before they can provide metabolic energy. They begin to predigest and sweeten to the taste in the mouth as the salivary enzyme *ptyalin* breaks the starches into simple sugars. Those that escape the saliva are later digested by the enzyme *amylase* in the small intestines.

The body cannot digest fiber carbohydrates like cellulose at all, although our intestinal bacteria will convert them for us to a limited extent into simpler components that we can utilize.

## Fats

*Lipids*, or fats, are water-insoluble macronutrients, unlike the carbohydrates. Despite their artery-clogging reputation, fats are absolutely essential to health. They are named according to function, chemical structure, physical characteristics or their associated body tissues:

*Phosphoglycerides* are present in all cells as major structural components of cell membranes (the cell's "skin") and are associated with fat storage. *Steroids* include cholesterol, the various sex hormones and adrenocortical hormones. *Prostaglandins* regulate hormone activity and metabolism in many tissues and organs. The notorious *triglycerides*, stored in fat tissue, insulate and cushion the body, giving women their curves. In excess, they contribute to cardiovascular disease and are the bane of the overweight. Nevertheless, triglycerides do provide a secondary source of energy when sugars and starches are unavailable, as during periods of fasting and weight loss.

Burning fat to produce energy does not metabolically stress the body to anywhere near the extent that protein burning does because fat is a clean-burning fuel source, its waste products being $CO_2$ and water. Burning protein to produce energy generates the additional waste products urea and ammonia, which are more taxing on the body to eliminate. The body therefore preferentially burns fats when glucose and its storage form glycogen are exhausted.

# What Cooking Does to the Macronutrients

All of the macronutrients are greatly denatured by heat, thereby becoming toxic to us. Let's look at how this happens.

## Fats

Cooked fats have been known to be toxic for some time. Fats heated above 96° F (36° C) create lipid peroxides, which are oily, oxidizing compounds —

proven carcinogens. Heating unsaturated fats (those liquid at room temperature) at high temperatures produces trans fatty acids, which create toxic free radicals in the body that result in cancer, aging, birth defects and liver toxicity.

The presence of heated fats in the bloodstream lowers blood cell capacity to carry oxygen and also blocks capillaries with fat globules. Fatty deposits then accumulate on the vascular walls and contribute to atherosclerosis and other forms of heart disease. Cardiovascular disease is currently the number one killer of Americans, with cancer coming in a close second.

Heated oils come loaded with mycotoxins, toxic byproducts of the microzymas discovered by Béchamp. (See Chapter 5.)

Processed foods usually contain hydrogenated or partially hydrogenated oils. Just read the labels. These oils are often found even in "health food stores." This type of cooked fat is solid or semi-solid at room temperature and was created by food oil refiners to make products like margarine in order to compete with saturated animal fat products like butter and lard.

The body responds to the presence of trans fatty acids by raising the "bad" cholesterol (LDL) levels while lowering the "good" cholesterol (HDL) levels, thus increasing heart disease risk. In fact trans fatty acids have proven to be even more atherogenic than the saturated animal fats they compete against in the marketplace. Those who think they are making a healthy choice by buying margarine instead of butter are gravely mistaken.

David and Annie Jubb write, "All cooked fat, and pig fat especially, is unable to combine with water, causing it to separate out and be stored in the body. Cooked fats are not miscible with water, so they travel separately making blood sluggish, eventually being stored" (*Secrets of an Alkaline Body*, p. 25).

## Carbohydrates

Cooked carbohydrates are also toxic. In the spring of 2002, Swedish officials were so alarmed by recent research findings that they decided to inform the public immediately rather than wait for them to be published in a scientific journal. Shortly afterwards, the World Health Organization held a three-week emergency meeting to evaluate the Swedish scientists' recent discovery. They learned that starchy foods, such as potato chips, french fries, baked potatoes, biscuits and bread, contain very high levels of acrylamides, chemicals that have been shown to result in genetic mutations leading to a range of cancers in rats.

Acrylamides are 1,000 times more dangerous than the majority of cancer-causing agents found in food. They have been directly related to the formation of benign and malignant stomach tumors, as well as damage to the central and peripheral nervous systems. The US Environmental Protection Agency (EPA) considers acrylamides so dangerous that it has fixed the safe level for human consumption of them at nearly zero, allowing for very little in public water systems. *Yet the amounts found in an ordinary bag of potato chips are 500 times the amounts allowed in a single glass of water by the World Health Organization.*

Briefly, there was even a law in force in California requiring potato chip manufacturers to put cancer warnings on their packages! Most did not comply with the law. There were also supposed to be cancer-warning labels on the food ordered most often at American restaurants: french fries! Had this law remained in force, would parents who fed their children fries and chips have been charged with child abuse?

Unfortunately, this law was superseded by national legislation that prohibits states from enacting food contamination standards and warning labels that are stricter than federal requirements. Lobbyists from food companies succeeded in getting Congress to pass this bill.

In addition, cooked carbohydrates contain glycotoxins, one of which is an "advanced glycation end product" (AGE). AGEs contaminate the body, making it vulnerable to cancer and molds, such as *Candida albicans* and other yeast infections.

The May 2003 edition of *Life Extension* magazine discusses AGEs, referring to a new study published in the *Proceedings of the National Academy of Sciences*. Eating food cooked at high temperatures was proven to cause the formation of AGEs, which accelerate aging. AGEs also stimulate the body to produce chronic inflammation, which leads to devastating, even lethal, effects directly involved with these diseases: diabetes, cancer, atherosclerosis, congestive heart failure, aortic valve stenosis, Alzheimer's and kidney impairment.

The article declares, "Cooking and aging have similar biological properties. The process that turns a broiled chicken brown illustrates what happens to our body's proteins as we age. As the proteins react with sugars, they turn brown and lose elasticity; they cross-link to form insoluble masses that generate free radicals (which contribute to aging). The resulting AGEs accumulate in our collagen, skin, cornea of the eye, brain, nervous system, vital organs and arteries as we age. Normal aging can also be regarded as a slow cooking process."

The glycation reaction cross-links the body's proteins, making them barely functional. Their accumulation causes enervated (exhausted) cells to emit signals that produce dangerous levels of inflammation. (See Appendix F.)

Several studies of diabetics who ate cooked foods producing AGEs confirmed that the AGEs definitely showed up in their blood and urine.

The book *Diet, Nutrition and Cancer* also cites studies in which the frying of potatoes and toasting of bread inspired mutagenic activity. The authors explain, "The browning of food results from the reaction of amines with sugars." They cite studies showing that "the increase in mutagenic activity with time paralleled the increase in browning" (p. 285).

## Proteins

Cooking meat changes the molecular structure of some of its proteins, rendering them unusable by the body and making cellular healing, reproduction and regeneration difficult, if not impossible. These heat-compromised protein molecules become bound, making them harder to digest. Up to 50% of cooked proteins that one eats will coagulate and cross-link. Cross-linking of proteins is associated with Alzheimer's disease, as shown in the first study presented in Appendix D.

Because of coagulation, cooked protein is 50% less digestible and assimilable than raw protein, as research showed at the Max Planck Institute for National Research in Germany. This means that a person need only eat half as much raw protein to get the nutritional benefit of the same protein cooked.

Even meat cooked at low temperatures produces mutagens. The book *Diet, Nutrition and Cancer* further explains that mutagens in beef stock have been found in temperatures as low as 154° F (68° C). Frying fish with heat as low as 374° F (190° C) also produces mutagens, as does broiling hamburgers at 266° F (130° C).

Cooking protein above 104° F (40° C) begins to produce toxins. Higher temperatures create even more poisons, such as heterocyclic amines (HCAs), which are caustic compounds that have proven to cause cancer in laboratory animals. Some HCAs are so toxic to the neurotransmitters and their receptors in the brain that the body eventually responds to the continual poisoning by developing brain diseases, such as Alzheimer's, Parkinson's and schizophrenia.

Grilling is one of the worst ways to cook meat. The high temperatures of charcoal broiling and grilling create polycyclic aromatic hydrocarbons (PAHs). PAHs have also been found in smoked meats and roasted coffee.

According to T. S. Wiley, author of *Lights Out: Sleep, Sugar and Survival*, "The average serving of barbecued or burnt meat imparts to you an amount of cancer-causing particles equivalent to what you would get from smoking 250 cigarettes" (p. 176). The next time you have your barbecued ribs, just remember, you may as well be smoking 12 packs of cigarettes!

Among the novel substances produced by cooking proteins are beta-carbolines. While the body produces its own beta-carbolines, the ones that result from cooked protein are toxic and imbalance the body much like taking foreign hormones imbalances the body, although the body produces its own hormones. Also, 99% of the exogenous (foreign) beta-carbolines are different from the natural ones and influence the brain in unpredictable and chaotic ways. This results in attention deficit hyperactivity disorder (ADHD) in children, as well as stress, apathy, aggression and distorted sexual behavior in adults. The web page www.youngerthanyourage.com/13/ADHD.htm is devoted to thorough documentation of studies confirming these findings.

It has long and often been observed by vegetarians that meat eaters are more aggressive, angry and violent than vegetarians. Perhaps this belligerent mindset is due not just to increased testosterone levels produced by meat or some ethereal density of consciousness, but also to the presence of exogenous beta-carbolines from heated meat. One way to test this theory would be to compare the behavior of raw meat eaters with that of cooked meat eaters. (See Appendix C.)

When you think about how toxic cooked food is, it is really a wonder that we are still alive and that mankind has survived for so many generations. This is only because humans, along with rats and pigs, are some of the most versatile and genetically hardy mammals. However, I wonder how long we will be able to survive as new toxic chemicals are introduced into our diet at faster and faster paces. (See Appendix A.)

Appendix D summarizes a number of informative studies published in professional scientific journals that demonstrate the toxicity of cooked food and support the claims made above in this section.

# Toxic Cookware

As if the poisonous byproducts of cooked food were not enough, there is ample evidence that cookware creates additional toxicity. Iron skillets are not recommended for people who have too much blood iron. Aluminum pots and pans may contribute to Alzheimer's disease.

The news program *20/20* once did an exposé on Teflon, which is so toxic that it often kills pet birds that breathe its fumes. Teflon also stimulates the body to produce flulike symptoms in people when the pan gets overheated, creating fumes. Some women who worked at the DuPont plant mixing the chemicals to make Teflon gave birth to babies with birth defects. Almost all Americans now have some detectable amounts of Teflon in their blood, and they are getting close to the level that harms lab animals. Pending review, the Environmental Protection Agency is now advising consumers to stop using Teflon products.

# Is Cooked Food Addictive?

We know that fermenting food sugars and starches into alcohol makes them addictive for many people. Would heating food do the same thing?

Raw fooders are convinced that cooked food is addictive. They base this conviction on the empirical (observational) evidence of both their own and others' subjective experiences. Raw fooders very rarely become addicted to a favorite raw food. They may develop temporary cravings but know that this is simply the body calling out for certain nutrients it needs.

Studies have shown that proteins heated by any cooking method contain harmful beta-carbolines that make a person want to eat more. The more protein in the food, the more beta-carbolines are produced. High protein foods include meat, eggs, nuts, seeds, fish, dairy, soy and beans.

Guy-Claude Burger states, "Cooking induces an intoxication that sets off a feeling of bogus hunger that impels us to eat even more. . . . Cooking has made men into compulsive eaters."

He says that an instinctive raw fooder (see Appendix C) might indulge in a bit of cooked food and find that his instincts go out the window. The person then finds himself completely overtaken by cooked food, which jams the instincts and makes initial foods (unaltered foods we are genetically designed to eat) seem less appealing. The person then goes on to compensate by eating even more cooked food, and an addictive cycle becomes habitual. When returning to 100% initial foods, one can require a rather long time, several days or even weeks, before fully regaining the pleasure of eating them.

Dr. Robert Sniadach explains in his Essential Natural Hygiene course that cooked food eaters get hangovers from eating cooked food. They also experience withdrawal symptoms when giving up cooked food, just as addicts of drugs, alcohol or tobacco do.

On the Internet, I once read a posting by a man who had been a heroin addict. He credited a 100% raw food diet as a major factor in his healing. Sometime later he decided to eat only 80% raw, 20% cooked. This went on for a while until he decided to go back to eating 100% raw. As he compared cooked food to heroin, his words were telling: "Cooked food is the *addictive tincture* of food in its natural form."

Victoria Boutenko worked with many people, teaching them to eat raw. Yet those who would not commit to a 100% raw diet would often backslide. For example, a friend of hers chose to eat 95% raw at the same time Victoria and her family switched to 100% raw food. Victoria and her family suffered cooked food cravings for only two months; her friend was still struggling *eight years later* with cooked food temptations!

For years, Victoria observed many people and wondered why they backslid. Some had even been completely healed of cancer and went back to cooked foods, only to die after they reverted to cooked foods. They had reintoxicated their clean bodies, redrained them of energy and redeveloped their cancers.

She wondered what the determining factor was until one day she attended an Alcoholics Anonymous meeting with a friend and realized that cooked food was addictive in much the same way that alcohol is.

Thus she began a 12-step support program to get people off cooked food, which worked wonderfully for nearly all her students. Her complete program is found in the book *12 Steps to Raw Foods: How to End Your Addiction to Cooked Food*. (Note: Most of the steps do not correspond to the ones found in the typical 12-step programs, like Alcoholics Anonymous.)

Boutenko emphasizes the need to go on a 100% raw food diet. That 1% of cooked food leaves the door open to temptation. She met many people who ate 99% raw and returned completely to cooked food months later. She urges people to commit to two months of 100% raw, avoiding temptation zones — restaurants, parties and potlucks where cooked food is served. Only then, she asserts, will the physical cravings disappear.

Before setting up the raw food 12 steps, Boutenko studied dozens of books on drug addition. She learned that the earlier in life the addictive substance is taken, the harder it is to stop. Since all of us began eating cooked foods as infants, this might explain why Boutenko noticed that only one person in 1,000 could stay 100% raw without support. She met only two or three people who remained successfully raw for one year by sheer willpower alone.

People tend to use cooked food like a drug to numb themselves when feeling bad. She concluded that cooked food was an addiction more difficult to overcome than even drugs because it is legal everywhere in our environment and socially acceptable, indeed strongly encouraged. People do not become ostracized when getting off drugs but may become social pariahs when getting off cooked foods.

In her book *The Raw Food Detox Diet*, nutritionist Natalia Rose declares that foods from mainstream supermarkets are especially addictive. "You must take the first step in healing your body by admitting that you are addicted to these unquestionably habit-forming substances that may currently rule your tastes and food impulses" (p. 14). MSG is just one ingredient sly food companies add to their products to create addiction. (See Appendix A.)

Morgan Spurlock, creator and director of the renowned documentary film *Super Size Me*, found that he became seriously addicted to the food at McDonald's. He would even suffer depression until he got his "fix" of fries, burgers and shakes!

One reason people on cooked diets experience so many cravings is not only addiction but also malnutrition. They are simply not getting enough nutrients, so they are constantly hungry. Obese people are often the most undernourished people in the world, which is why they are always hungry and always eating. The phenomenon has even been given a formal name, the overfed but undernourished syndrome.

When I was eating only about 90-95% raw, I personally noticed just how addictive wheat and dairy are. If I ate just a bit of either, I would crave it strongly the next day. Food manufacturers know this, which is why they manage to slip some hidden form of these addictive poisons into processed foods.

My body was so sensitive from eating mostly raw foods that when I ate wheat, I noticed that I would feel a mild stupor, somewhat like a drug-induced state in which I lost all alertness. If I had much of it, like a few pieces of bread or cake, I would fall asleep. For more information on the addictive nature of wheat and dairy, see the web site www.13.waisays.com/zombie.htm. (Also see Appendix A.)

The web site www.13.waisays.com contains much more information on the effects of food on health, all documented with scientific journal references. The writer even compares the toxicity of cooked food to that of cigarettes (see www.13.waisays.com/cigarettes.htm).

We've now learned the toxic truth about cooked food, so let's no longer be willing participants in the great cooked food experiment! Having discovered what's *wrong* with *cooked* food, let's next take a look at what's *right* about *raw* food.

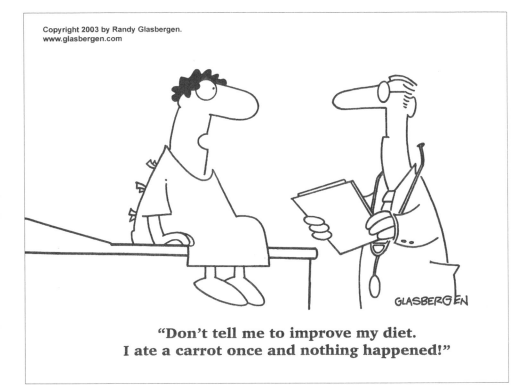

"Don't tell me to improve my diet.
I ate a carrot once and nothing happened!"

# 10
# The Raw Ingredients

So many people spend their health gaining wealth
and then have to spend their wealth to regain their health.
—A. J. Reb Materi, *Our Family*

It was once believed that the only concern with food was getting sufficient calories. The calorie paradigm, originated in 1789, is completely outdated, although conventional nutritional science is still influenced by it. Calories are the body's fuel supply, and they are not altered that much by cooking. But thinking that simply getting enough calories is enough would be like thinking that gasoline is the only thing you need to put into your car. How long would your car run if the only thing you serviced it with was fuel but neglected to add or change oil, brake fluid, radiator coolant, spark plugs and so on?

Raw food contains numerous essential nutrients that are either damaged or destroyed by heat. Most of them have been discovered only within the last century or a little more. This makes one wonder how many other important components might yet remain undiscovered in food that may also be destroyed by fire.

## Vitamins and Minerals

Dr. Ann Wigmore, founder of the Hippocrates Health Institute, determined that up to 83% of a raw food's nutrients are lost in the process of cooking. Each vitamin has a different ability to withstand heat: for example, about 50% of B vitamins are lost in cooked foods and 70-80% of Vitamin C. Overall, nutrient destruction is thought to be as high as 83-85%. Think of all the waste!

Jan Dries, who worked extensively with helping cancer patients heal using raw food, explains that cooking renders minerals inactive. "The electromagnetic field that is very important to minerals (because it makes their catalytic action possible) disappears when you heat them. Inactive memories of a mineral have a very disturbing effect on the kidney filters, which have to make sure they are removed" (*The Dries Cancer Diet*, p. 100).

In addition, some of the minerals may actually become toxic after cooking. Inorganic mineral elements are combined naturally in raw foods with molecules containing carbon, making them organic. According to Dr. Vivian V. Vetrano, "These [organic molecules] are the useful mineral compounds, and they are in the proper balance for human nutrition. When food is cooked, the minerals are separated by the heat from this organic combination, returning to inorganic molecules which recombine as toxic inorganic salts, such as sodium chloride, causing many health problems, such as arterial plaque, arthritis and Alzheimer's disease."

Don't fool yourself into thinking that taking vitamins and minerals in supplements will compensate for their depletion in cooked food! Such supplements are usually minerals extracted from rocks rather than from food sources (because they are cheaper) and are not easily absorbable or assimilable, if at all. The inorganic vitamin or mineral in a pill is rejected by the body and just becomes more toxic pollution. On the other hand, if one can find a food supplement that is a living food, such as low-temperature dehydrated greens, its nutrients could be more successfully absorbed, assimilated and utilized.

Review Professor Kollath's experiment described on page 149. He was unable to get his mice to achieve good health using supplements. Only a raw food diet worked.

Furthermore, there could be numerous nutrients yet to be discovered, making any multivitamin and mineral supplement incomplete. In fact in April 2003, Japanese scientists discovered the first new vitamin since 1948: pyrroloquinoline quinone, which plays a role in fertility. If someone had depended purely on supplements for vitamins, she may have found herself infertile without knowing why.

In addition, nature has everything combined synergistically such that all constituents work together in ways we do not yet understand. Professor Dr. Peter Schauder of the University of Göttingen in Germany says, "The various macro- and micro-nutrients influence each other and are able to strengthen or weaken each other during bio-chemical processes."

Dr. T. Colin Campbell, PhD, claims, "The whole is greater than the sum of its parts. Unlike supplements, fruit and vegetables contain a variety of nutrients which cannot be extracted."

For more arguments against using supplements as opposed to raw foods, see pages 338 and 373.

# Enzymes

Enzymes are protein molecules that act in specific ways, working in a "lock and key" manner with other molecules to facilitate chemical reactions in virtually every cell and every organ and every system in the body from digestion to elimination and everything in between. They play very specific roles in the body, helping it digest food, build protein in skin and bones, and aid in detoxification. They are catalysts that facilitate chemical reactions. Enzymes are what enable fruit to ripen and a seed to sprout and grow into a plant. Without enzymes, earthly life would be impossible.

Enzymes are the catalysts, the sparkplugs, of life. Mason Dwinell, LAc, even compares enzymes to "miniature suns." Perhaps this is why people who eat raw foods, full of enzymes, report feeling "switched on," as if a key has turned on the light and energy. But when they backslide into cooked foods, it's "power down."

We use three kinds of enzymes: metabolic enzymes to run our bodies, digestive enzymes to digest food and food enzymes in raw foods that enable the food to partially self-digest, thus conserving our bodies' limited enzyme-producing capacities.

Food enzymes are active, or "alive," in uncooked food. Once a food is heated, they chemically degrade, or "die." By conservative estimates, enzymes may begin dying at temperatures as low as 105° F. Within 30 minutes at 119°-129° F, all are dead.

Cooking alters an enzyme's "lock and key" configuration so that it can no longer perform its intended function. For all practical purposes, the enzyme is "dead." The protein molecule is still present, but its life force is gone, much like a battery that has lost its power or a spark plug that has worn out.

Dr. James B. Sumner, a Nobel Prize winner in 1946, claimed that the feeling of being easily fatigued in middle age or older is due to diminished enzymes as you add years to your life.

Dr. Edward Howell was the 20th century's foremost researcher on food enzymes and their significance to human nutrition. He discovered that food heated above 118° F for any extended period of time is devoid of active food enzymes.

If we eat cooked food, we force our pancreases to crank out more digestive enzymes than our bodies were designed to produce. By age 40, the average person has only 30% of his digestive enzyme production potential left. This is a major reason for increasing tiredness with age. According to Dr. Howell, "The length of life is inversely proportional to the rate of exhaustion of the enzyme potential of an organism."

In other words, the more cooked food you eat, the sooner you exhaust your limited digestive enzyme-generating capacity, and the sooner you begin to lose your spark, disintegrate and die.

Howell believed that there is no way to replenish this enzyme potential. Therefore, the best strategy is not to squander it with cooked food but to eat solely of raw food and no more of it than necessary.

Some raw fooders even take live enzyme supplements along with their 100% raw diet. Brian Clement of the Hippocrates Health Institute recommends doing so. Lou Corona does as well. Dr. Cousens also suggests that enzyme supplements, even on a live food diet, can be useful for increasing our enzyme content and energy.

Declining enzyme reserves are directly associated with aging. People who are 25 have about 30 times more starch-splitting salivary amylase than people in their 80s for example. Each child is born with an inherited amount of enzyme-generating potential. When it is used up, he will die of some degenerative disease that will correlate with his inherited predisposition and/or weak areas in his tissues and/or depleted and toxic condition. If he is a raw fooder, eating primarily or only raw, unheated food, he will more likely reach his optimal lifespan free of degenerative diseases. The more cooked food he eats, the shorter and/or more diseased will be his life.

It was formerly believed, with the "theory of parallel secretion," that enzymes were expendable, unimportant because the body could create them without limit and could waste them without concern. Later the "law of adaptive secretion of digestive enzymes" was shown to be true. This law states that the more digestion that is accomplished by food enzymes, enzymes inherent in raw food, the fewer digestive enzymes must be pumped out by the pancreas and intestine.

The body "knows" it has a limited amount of enzyme potential and secretes only the particular enzymes it needs at any given meal. It is as though the body has a limited bank account, a limited savings it can draw upon. Most researchers believe there is no way to make a "deposit," or to add to that limited enzyme-generating potential. We can only refuse to dive into our "savings" by eating raw food exclusively and no more of it than the body needs.

It was also formerly believed that eating cooked food was irrelevant to the enzyme question because enzymes were destroyed in the stomach upon contact with its hydrochloric acid and other gastric secretions during the digestive process. Starch digestion begins in the mouth with salivary enzymes. However, many of the enzymes lost in cooking are those that help further digestion in the "food enzyme," or cardiac, stomach (its upper section) for the first 30-60 minutes of the digestive cycle, before the hydrochloric acid and protein-digesting enzymes secreted by the lower stomach could destroy them.

Moreover, numerous meticulous studies on humans and animals have proved that some enzymes survive digestion and are reused. Some of them escape gastric breakdown and reactivate in the small intestine where they continue to facilitate further digestive processes. Extensive European studies (*Raw Energy*, p. 57) have confirmed the durability of most of the enzymes throughout the digestive process.

Dr. Howell's research revealed that the pancreas, being the main producer of digestive enzymes, grows larger when it is habitually overtaxed. The typical human pancreas is relatively large compared to those of wild animals when adjusted for body size. This hypertrophy indicates the pancreas is being overworked.

Dr. Howell also found that animals on cooked food diets had enlarged pancreases. For example, laboratory rats eating cooked foods had pancreases three times as big as those of the raw-fed ones. When their bodies were dissected, "An astonishing array of typically human degenerative diseases was revealed" (*Enzyme Nutrition*, Dr. Howell, p. 84).

In her video *Drugs Never Cure Disease!* Dr. Lorraine Day, MD, claims, "It takes the same amount of energy to make the enzymes for three meals a day of cooked food as it does *eight hours of hard labor*. Is it any wonder people are suffering from fatigue?"

Dr. Nicholas Gonzalez, who uses enzyme therapy, was influenced by the research of Howell, Pottenger and also Dr. John Beard, who first suggested that the pancreatic proteolytic enzyme trypsin could treat cancer. Gonzalez explains, "Our immune cells, our neutrophils and lymphocytes, use enzymes to attack and kill bacteria, viruses and fungi, as well as dangerous cancer cells that some scientists believe form every day in all of us" (*Eating in the Raw*, p. 10). He regrets that enzymes never get the press coverage they deserve and explains that without enzymes, DNA, which is always in the news, could do nothing.

Because eating raw food spares unnecessary depletion of the body's limited enzyme potential, the body is free to perform other vital, enzyme-mediated health functions. The body utilizes live, raw-food enzymes to enhance our vitality, body detoxification, tissue regeneration, metabolic function, scar tissue dissolution, excess fatty tissue autolysis (self-digestion) and dissolution of crystallized deposits in the tissues. In other words, our body has much greater capacity for housecleaning and self-repair if we ingest only fresh raw foods.

Dr. Rudolf Steiner, PhD, who wrote on anthroposophy, or spiritual science, referred to enzymes as "the bridge between the physical and the spiritual worlds." Perhaps this is because when eating foods rich in active enzymes, one frees up considerable energy that can be used for the body's more exalted energy centers and the mind's more exalted aspirations that require an abundance of energy to be made manifest.

# Phytochemicals

Phytochemicals found in plant foods have recently been discovered to play a role in nutrition that differs from that of other nutrients in that they are not assimilated by the cells nor used for fuel. Termed *phytonutrients*, these serve as antioxidants and modulators of the body's defense mechanisms, block carcinogenic substances from the cells, quiet and calm the nervous system and reduce cholesterol levels. Phytochemicals also help protect us from pollution, radiation and disease, along with performing many other functions.

Scientists are trying to genetically modify them so that they can be patented and thus be profitably sold in the form of "nutriceuticals," the technological food counterpart of pharmaceuticals. Of course it is immeasurably more healthful to eat nature's versions than man's.

Phytochemicals include resveratrol, which the body will use to switch on our antiaging genes, as mentioned in Chapter 1. Many red fruits and vegetables contain resveratrol. Rich sources include grapes, grape juice and red wine.

According to Dr. James Howenstine, author of *A Physician's Guide to Natural Health Products That Work*, 20 mg of resveratrol daily provides maximal health benefits. Red wine has 0.2 mg per glass. Since drinking 100 glasses of wine would prove toxic indeed, wine is definitely not the best source of this nutrient!

Phytochemicals also include flavonoids, lycopene and quercetin. To get the full spectrum of phytochemicals, you should eat from each of the colors of fruits and vegetables: green, yellow, red, orange, white and purple.

# Biophotons: Light Energy from the Sun

In 1982, German physicist and Nobel Prize winner Dr. Fritz Popp and his colleagues proved the presence of biophotons, biologically produced units of light, in vegetables. Biophoton emission can be thought of as a kind of biological laser light with a very high degree of coherence, capable of transmitting information, which ordinary, incoherent light cannot achieve.

One of the colleagues proved that these biophotons are stored in the DNA. Dr. Popp developed an instrument, the biophoton meter, to measure biophoton emission. Dr. Popp was able to demonstrate on a screen the luminosity of a fresh plant, contrasting that with the greatly reduced luminosity of a withered plant.

Dr. Popp's research went on to prove that the quality of a food is mainly dependent on the number of biophotons it contains. Cooking, adding chemicals, processing, preserving and irradiating all endanger the naturally intact biophotonic force of a food. Fresh, sun-ripened, organic food eaten straight from the vine, tree, stalk or ground contains the greatest number of biophotons.

We know that sunlight is essential to life. It is now known that the more light stored in food, the more nutritious that food is. Stored sun energy is transferred from the food into our body's cells in the form of biophotons. These "sun units" contain bio-information that has the power to assist in the regulation of all metabolic processes in the body, elevating the body's functioning to a higher order. Consequently, biophotons counteract the chaotic loss of structure in an aging body due to entropic degradation.

Dr. Popp found that healthy cells store light longer and radiate coherent light, whereas unhealthy cells radiate chaotic light. The biophoton energy of healthy people was observed to be much greater than that of people in poor health.

Wild foods were found to emit two times as many biophotons as cultivated organic foods. Organic foods emit five times as many biophotons as commercially grown foods. *Cooked or irradiated foods emit almost no biophotons.* Thus it follows that uncooked food is absolutely essential to good health, and wild food is best. Dr. Gabriel Cousens has even coined the term "malillumination," the counterpart to the word "malnutrition," to denote people lacking in the essential nutrient of sunlight. "We are human photocells whose ultimate biological nutrient is light" (*Conscious Eating*, p. 587).

Fruits are also very rich in biophotons. Fruits originate from flowers or blossoms. Because of their suitable structure, fruits are capable of accumulating vast numbers of biophotons.

# Electrons

German scientist Dr. Johanna Budwig found that live (raw) foods are rich in electrons that act as high-powered electron donors and solar resonance fields in the body to attract, store and conduct the sun's energy. Her research led her to conclude that the sunlight's photons are attracted by sunlike electrons, termed *pi-*

*electrons*, resonating in our bodies. Our bodies' pi-electrons attract and activate the sun photons, giving us an antientropy, or antiaging, edge.

She found that live foods, especially flaxseeds, were a particularly good source of electrons. The more we can take in solar electrons by eating live foods, the better we can attract and absorb solar electrons in direct resonance from the sun, thus enhancing our health and even our consciousness. Perhaps this is where we get the phrase "sunny disposition."

Dr. Hans Eppinger found that all cells are essentially batteries that seem to be charged up when people are healthy. Sick people's cells exist in a discharged state. Only uncooked foods are able to provide the body with the needed nutrients to restore and maximize the cells' battery potentials.

Dr. John Douglass theorizes that live foods have a "higher energy ability to awaken relatively inert molecules in our systems by either taking an electron or giving them one. This high-energy electron transfer ability is described as the 'high redox potential' of a particular molecule" (*Conscious Eating*, p. 575).

Dr. Douglass proposes that the high redox potential of living foods, which is destroyed by heat, is an important factor in their role of assisting the body to heal itself. Another raw food researcher, Dr. Chiu-Nan Lai, agrees that this high redox potential is a major reason for their usefulness to assist in the body's healing (*Raw Energy*, pp. 46–47).

A free radical is a molecule that is missing an electron, and since it wants to rebalance its electrical charge, it will try to steal an electron from wherever it can: molecules of fat, protein, DNA, etc. When DNA is altered, it can lead to cell mutation, possibly leading to cancer. Therefore, it is good to have spare electrons to give to these free radicals so that they don't wreak havoc.

A healthy, vital body contains lots of spare electrons. According to David and Annie Jubb, people who radiate, appearing to glow with light, are those with abundant spare electrons. Foods rich in electrons are raw fruits, vegetables, nuts, seeds and sprouted or soaked grains. Spirulina and flaxseed (also flaxseed oil) are especially high in the capacity to absorb solar electrons.

# Bioelectricity

Our bodies have a bioelectric potential. Human tissues and cells are electrically charged, working much like an alkaline battery. Brian Clement explains, "Just as an alkaline battery has a positive and a negative pole, a cell has a nucleus and cytoplasm. . . . The nucleus and cytoplasm of a cell attract opposite charges; the nucleus is the positive 'pole,' and the cytoplasm is the negative 'pole' " (*Living Foods for Optimum Health*, p. 35).

According to the bioelectric paradigm, a drop in this bioelectric potential is the first step of the disease process. Hence many people do not feel good even though their lab tests show no overt or diagnosable signs of disease. On a cellular level, these tired people are unable to properly dispose of toxins and absorb nutrients. Their bodies are enervated.

Kirlian photography has been able to visibly display the differences between the bioelectric field of a person eating dead food and that of a person eating live food. Kirlian photographers Harry Oldfield and Roger Coghill show such photos in their book *The Dark Side of the Brain*.

They also illustrate differences between the fields of cooked and raw plants. Their research indicated that the electroluminescence, the radiance seen in Kirlian photographs, is a measure of life force, and hence health, in the plants' cells.

European nutritionist Jan Dries researched along these lines beginning in the early 1980s. He found there was a specific bio-energetic value (BEV) for each food and that this value depended on the number of biophotons and also on the luminous intensity of light energy. He found that particular foods could be identified by their individual frequencies. A high reading indicated a high BEV.

Readings allowed for a determination of the medicinal properties of foods and herbs, linking specific foods to certain diseases. He found that certain people had what he called "cancer resistance," which differed from cancer immunity, and that certain foods had the same "cancer resistance" frequency. It was discovered that people ingesting these foods could develop cancer resistance.

Dries has been very successful in treating cancer patients with this diet. It is outlined in the book *The Dries Cancer Diet: A Practical Guide to the Use of Fresh Fruit and Raw Vegetables in the Treatment of Cancer*. The majority of the diet consists of tropical fruits, which vibrate at the cancer resistance frequency. Hence, people with cancer on his diet will eat primarily oranges, bananas, pineapples, avocados, melons, kiwi, persimmons, apricots, papayas and mangoes, among other foods.

His diet provides the body with the very thing it needs to activate its healing capabilities: increased bioelectric energy in the raw foods serves to stimulate the electrical potentials of cells, which leads to a depolarization of cancer cells and their consequent death.

Dr. Gabriel Cousens discusses the bioelectricity of live foods in *Rainbow Green Live-Food Cuisine* (p. 117). He claims that the nutrients in live foods supply the body with what it needs to increase the electrical potential in cells, between cells and at cellular interfaces. The electrical potentials of our tissues and cells directly result from our cells' aliveness, which is enhanced by live foods. In *Spiritual Nutrition* (p. 294), he explains that given the proper microelectrical potentials, cells are better able to expel toxins, assimilate appropriate micronutrients, oxygen and hydrogen into cell nuclei, and feed the mitochondria. These processes better enable cells to maintain, repair and activate their DNA molecules.

Dr. Hans Eppinger of the University of Vienna found that a live food diet resulted in raised microelectrical potentials throughout the whole body. He found that in addition to improving the intra- and extra-cellular excretion of toxins and the absorption of nutrients, live foods were the only types of foods that could help the body restore the microelectrical potentials of tissues after their electrical potentials and consequent cellular degeneration had begun.

It is believed that living foods get their electrical charges from the highly charged electrons sent to them by the sun.

# Hormones

The Pottenger cat study (page 151) was one study that showed that hormones are destroyed in cooked foods. Meat is a valuable source of hormones. This study indicated that hormones, such as the adrenal cortical hormone and insulin, among others, were definitely thermolabile, that is, destroyed by fire. They were even destroyed at the moderate temperatures of pasteurization. When given adrenal cortical hormone, the cats' adrenal glands were restored to normal function.

Curious to know why wheatgrass (in addition to a raw diet) had been so powerful in healing Eydie Mae Hunsberger, author of *How I Conquered Cancer Naturally*, of breast cancer, her doctor discovered that wheatgrass contained a plant hormone called *abscisic acid*. He found, doing tests on laboratory animals, that even small amounts of abscisic acid proved to be deadly to any form of cancer.

Finally, many a raw food woman who has gone through menopause *with few or no symptoms* knows how rich plant foods are in human hormone precursors!

# Water

Water is necessary to dilute toxins for their elimination, transport water-soluble nutrients to their destinations and perform a whole host of other functions. Water found in fresh food is superior to drinking water. Plants purify water by filtering it through their roots. Water from living plants is electrified. The best water is found in fruit. If one eats enough juicy fruits, one doesn't need to drink nearly as much water.

A young body is more than 80% water, but with age this can decrease to 60%. Getting old is often thought of as "drying up," "shrinking," or "withering away." These metaphors are not far from wrong. In fact an older body holds less water than a younger body. If we are to stay youthful in body, mind and spirit, we must be sure our source of water is the best and get as much of it as possible from raw food.

Cooking evaporates some of the water and also lowers the quality of the remaining water normally present in fresh foods.

# Essential Fatty Acids

The essential fatty acids (EFAs) linolenic acid and linoleic acid are necessary for healthy hearts, brains, skin, glands and hair. Most people are deficient in essential fatty acids because cooking destroys much of them. Foods rich in EFAs are flaxseeds, raw fish, avocados, nuts and seeds.

# Friendly Bacteria

People often think it is necessary to cook foods in order to destroy harmful bacteria, not realizing they are also destroying the necessary "friendly" bacteria that our intestines need for balance. A lack of good bacteria can result in yeast infections, intestinal disorders and other symptoms associated with weakened bodily defenses. Eating cooked food, especially cooked meat and dairy, causes putrefactive bacteria to proliferate and eventually dominate and replace the natural population of beneficial intestinal flora. This causes colon dysfunction and allows for the absorption of toxins from the bowel. This disease state is called *dysbiosis*, or *dysbacteria*.

According to Dr. Gabriel Cousens, some factors in raw foods stimulate production of healthy bacterial flora (*Conscious Eating*, p. 565).

# Oxygen

According to William Richardson, MD, "Heat processing reduces the oxygen found in fresh food — oxygen we need to resist disease." Cancer cells and AIDS viruses thrive in blood low in oxygen. Raw foods contain small amounts of hydrogen peroxide, which provides oxygen to kill these particular viruses.

Chlorophyll is what gives plants their green color. It has been likened to the "blood" of the plant. The chlorophyll molecule is almost identical to the hemoglobin molecule, which is the oxygen carrier in human blood. Therefore, when you eat plants in their living, unheated state, the chlorophyll actually feeds oxygen to your body. Cooked food does not contain this organic type of oxygen. This is why, when you eat lots of greens or drink wheatgrass juice, you immediately feel a surge of energy. Wheatgrass is an especially good source of oxygen.

Oxygen stimulates digestion, promotes better blood circulation in the body, promotes clearer thinking, protects against anaerobic bacteria, and nourishes every cell in the body. Without sufficient oxygen in the blood, the metabolism and digestion become sluggish. The body loses energy and is ripe for disease.

In addition to eating live plant food, other factors contribute to our oxygen supply: breathing clean, fresh air and exercising aerobically for at least 20 minutes, three to five times a week. Since plants breathe in $CO_2$ and give off $O_2$, it is also beneficial to have green plants in your environment.

Breathing exercises also help increase internal oxygen. According to Dr. Cousens, although 90% of metabolic energy comes from breathing, most people use only 10% of their breathing capacities.

Increasing our oxygen supply is especially necessary nowadays because, unfortunately, our air, especially the air in cities, where most people live, now contains less oxygen than it used to due to pollution. Since there is far less oxygen inside a building than outside, the Boutenkos even sleep outdoors in a gazebo to get that fresh air.

# Life Force Energy

In Oriental medicine, life force energy is referred to as *chi*. It flows through your body's energy meridians and acupuncture points. In India, this is called *prana*. Dr. Valerie Hunt of UCLA has proven the existence of such bioenergetic fields and their effects on health. There are now instruments that can measure them. Her book *Infinite Mind: Science of the Human Vibrations of Consciousness* describes these in detail.

Cooked food has no life force, no chi. Nutritionist Natalia Rose ranks raw foods in order of their vibrational life force energies from highest to lowest. Raw foods with high vibrational energies are fresh juices; organic, sun-ripened, fresh fruit; green vegetables; other vegetables, and honey. Raw foods with intermediate life force energies are organic nuts and seeds; organic sheep or goat dairy products; sprouted grains; organic, unsweetened, dried fruits, and agave. At the low end are other raw organic dairy products and raw oils.

In her book *Raw Food Life Force Energy*, Natalia prescribes high vibration raw foods, detoxification and deep breathing, along with yoga or dancing, to keep the energy flowing. I add acupuncture to the list since it is well known for unblocking energy obstructions.

# Suggested Reading

Some of the best books to read in order to learn more about these gems of wisdom pertaining to raw food diets are Dr. Edward Howell's books and Dr. Gabriel Cousens's *Conscious Eating* and *Spiritual Nutrition.*

# Coming Up...

People often wonder, "If this diet is so great, why did it take so long for us to find out about it?"

Section Three will show you that various groups of people in hidden niches of societies have actually known about this diet for thousands of years. There we shall discover the history of the raw food movement and its related, but much more comprehensive, movement known as Natural Hygiene. You will be introduced to modern-day leaders, some of whom relate their powerful personal testimonies, having miraculously healed themselves of "incurable" diseases by providing their bodies with the foremost condition of health they most needed: a raw food diet.

If you are already eager to start your new diet, you may choose to proceed to Section Four and return to Section Three later. But I do encourage you return at some point to this informative and inspiring history of these two parallel raw food movements.

# Section Three

# Raw Pioneers:

## History and Leaders

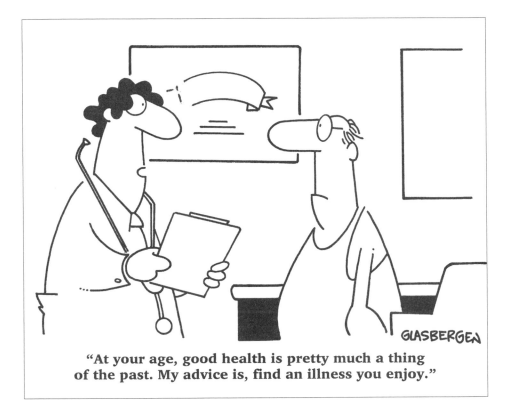

"At your age, good health is pretty much a thing of the past. My advice is, find an illness you enjoy."

# 11
# A Brief History of Raw Foodism

The disadvantage of men not knowing the
past is that they do not know the present.
—G. K. Chesterton (1874–1936), British author

This chapter presents a brief overview, by no means exhaustive, of the history of the raw food movement and its teachers. The inspiring stories of these leaders illustrate how passionate people are about the power of the body to thrive on a raw food diet.

The modern raw food and Natural Hygiene movements are essentially grassroots movements, receiving very little if any assistance from the media, medical establishment and government agencies. As mentioned earlier, part of the reason for their relative obscurity is that nearly all the books on the subject have been self-published and therefore have not been reviewed in magazines nor typically sold in chain bookstores. This is starting to change, however, due both to the diet's widening popularity and to its Internet presence.

For millions of years, mankind and his ancestors were raw fooders, as are all other animals currently on earth. Fire is thought to have been discovered some 400,000 years ago and put into widespread use for cooking around 10,000-20,000 years ago.

Thus man became the first and only animal species to experiment with chemically altering his food. No one knows why this came to be, although one theory is that a forest fire destroyed much of the food, forcing people to eat some of the cooked carcasses and plants that lay on the outskirts of the fire.

Another theory is that people found cooking destroyed visible parasites in spoiling meat. Further speculation is that people discovered that accidentally burnt food wafted an alluring aroma, thus leading them to start burning it on purpose.

In my opinion, the most credible explanation for the onset of cooking is one held by some anthropologists: as humans migrated to colder climates, the only way they could eat frozen food they stumbled upon or food left over from a kill was to heat it. Perhaps ice covered the meat, and fire thawed it out.

Any or all of these theories may be true. Once the practice of cooking began, however, the cooked food seemed to become addictive in a way similar to alcoholic beverages produced by fermentation.

Despite the many social pressures to partake of cooked food preparations, certain groups of people throughout history have rediscovered the power and pleasure of eating pure, unheated food.

One of the earliest known documents advocating a raw food diet may be the *Essene Gospel of Peace*. It is alleged to have been written over 2,000 years ago and indicates that Jesus was a member of the Jewish Essene sect, a group who advocated sun-ripened "Garden of Eden" foods.

The *Essene Gospel of Peace*, Book One, contains this revelation:

> And Jesus continued, "God commanded your forefathers: *Thou shalt not kill.* I say to you: Kill neither men, nor beast, nor yet the food which goes into your mouth. For if you eat living food, the same will quicken you, but if you kill your food, the dead food will kill you also. For life only comes from life, and death always comes from death. For everything which kills your food kills your bodies also. And everything which kills your bodies kills your souls also. Therefore, eat not anything which fire or frost or water has destroyed. For burned, frozen and rotted foods will burn, freeze, and rot your body also. Be not like the foolish husbandman who sowed in his ground cooked, frozen and rotted seeds. And the autumn came, and his fields bore nothing. And great was his distress."

The Essenes knew that the secret was to eat not only raw food, but also food as fresh from the vine as possible. Modern science has since proven that these two secrets were correct.

The Essenes established communities two to three hundred years before Jesus was born and were reported by historians to have lived an average of 120 years.

The Greeks also discovered the beauty of the raw food diet. The Pelasgians, a group of people thought by Classical Greek writers to have inhabited ancient Greece, ate only raw fruits, nuts and seeds. They lived on average to 200 years, according to Herodotus, acclaimed as the "father of history."

Pythagoras, who lived in Greece around 580–500 BC, was a famous Greek philosopher and mathematician, one of the earliest men in the Western world to formulate philosophical and mathematical theories.

According to his biography, Pythagoras studied with an earlier group of the Essenes on Mount Carmel. There he learned about live foods and took this knowledge back to Greece. He became a fruitarian and established a school of followers who also became fruitarians. He used raw food to help people with poor digestion. This knowledge was later passed down to Socrates and Plato.

In India, there have always been yogis and seekers of high spiritual development (enlightenment) who ate only raw food. One of these was Shivapuri Baba, who at the age of 50 went on a 35-year world walking tour. He even spent four years with Queen Victoria in England. Born in 1826, he died at the age of 137. He remained very vital until the last few years, when he aged rapidly due to eating the cooked food offered him by his hosts.

Paramhansa Yogananda, author of *Autobiography of a Yogi*, spoke admiringly of meeting a yogi who had been on a raw food diet for nine years.

In 1897, the Bircher-Benner Clinic of Zurich, Switzerland, became one of the first modern clinics using the raw food treatment approach. Founder Max Bircher-Benner, MD, discovered the writings of Pythagoras and began experimenting with live foods. He healed himself of jaundice with a combination of raw food and all the other healthful practices promoted at the clinic. He discovered that live food treatment helped patients recover from a wide range of ailments, no matter how serious their disease conditions.

In the USA in the 1920s, the Mormons, who numbered Joseph Smith and 25 of his followers, ate mostly raw foods because they knew that the diet served to increase spiritual awareness.

In the early 1900s, Max Gerson, MD, worked with raw foods, first healing himself of migraines and then proceeding to treat numerous patients, including those with lupus.

One of his patients was the famous doctor Albert Schweitzer, who recovered from diabetes with raw food, enabling him to stop taking insulin. Albert's wife recovered from tuberculosis while also on raw foods.

Gerson used raw food to treat cancer and wrote *A Cancer Therapy: Results of Fifty Cases*, which he published in 1958. There are several Gerson institutes in Europe and Mexico today. The Mexican clinic used to be in the USA but was chased out by our draconian laws persecuting anyone using alternative treatments for disease. (See Appendix B for more details.)

Also early in the 20th century, Professor Arnold Ehret of Germany was dying of Bright's disease, a kidney problem. All treatments failed him, including mainstream medicine and alternative approaches.

Remarkably, Ehret discovered hidden secrets about health quite by accident. Attempting to recover in a resort area by the ocean by means of rest and fresh air, he ran out of money while still quite ill. Discouraged, depressed and broke, he decided to commit suicide by starving himself to death.

Somewhere around the tenth or eleventh day of fasting, the depression and fatigue lifted. He suddenly felt healthy and energetic, regaining his will to live. He decided to take control of his health, researching on his own what to do. After fasting and taking on a fruitarian diet, not only did his kidneys heal, but he also obtained a level of vitality and mental health so superior that he termed it "paradise health."

He found that ill health is caused by the accumulation of toxins and "mucus" (phlegm) in the body and wrote several books and pamphlets, including *Rational Fasting* and *Mucusless Diet Healing System*. In the 1920s, he moved to Los Angeles, California, where he gave health lectures.

In addition to Ehret, Germany's heritage of raw fooders who influenced the California raw food movement was significant enough to warrant an entire book: *Children of the Sun*, a pictorial anthology edited by Gordon Kennedy. Many of these raw food leaders were actually forerunners of the natural healing, beatnik and hippie movements. These include Bill Pester, who influenced author Hermann Hesse, as well as Louis Kuhne and Adolph Just, who had a profound effect on Mahatma Gandhi.

Additional Germans made quite an impact on California's early raw food history. John and Vera Richter operated three live-food cafeterias in Los Angeles from 1917 until the late 1940s and published *Mrs. Richter's Cook-Less Book* (1925). Hermann Sexauer opened a natural foods shop in Santa Barbara. Maximilian Sikinger published a concise little booklet about live foods, meditation and sunshine, *Classical Nutrition*, in the Santa Monica Mountains (1943).

Iran has had a long history of raw foodism. A 20th century promoter of the diet was Arshavir Ter Hovannessian, who wrote *Raw Eating* in 1967 and founded the Raw Vegetarian Society.

He had been a sickly, middle-aged man, only able to work a few hours a day. After switching to a raw diet, he professed more energy than in his youth, able to run up mountains and work all day and late into the night.

He raised one daughter from birth on raw food and claims that it is easier to raise 100 children on raw food than one on cooked. His previous children, who were raised on conventional cooked food, were frequently sick, noisy and messy, with emotional tantrums, while the raw child was never sick and remained quiet and happy.

Arshavir also mentions in his book that in certain Asian countries, condemned prisoners were executed by giving them nothing to eat except cooked meat! They usually died within 30 days.

Ann Wigmore (1909–1993) founded the Hippocrates Health Institute in Boston in 1958 with Viktoras Kulvinskas, who is still active in the raw food movement. Dr. Ann was a pioneer in the development of raw gourmet cuisine, inventing such recipes as "energy soup," flax crackers and seed cheese.

Chased out of Boston by persecution from the authorities, she set up a clinic in Puerto Rico, where she successfully treated AIDS patients prior to her untimely death in a house fire. She was 84 at the time of her death and in such great health that she needed only two hours of sleep a day and had no gray hair. Laboratory tests proved that her hair had not been dyed.

Kulvinskas went on to author *Survival into the 21ˢᵗ Century* and *Life in the 21ˢᵗ Century,* both raw food classics. Since then Brian Clement has assumed the leading role at the Hippocrates Health Institute at their center in West Palm Beach, Florida. One of the happy clients of the Hippocrates Health Institute, Eydie Mae Hunsberger, wrote the book *How I Conquered Cancer Naturally* after recovering from breast cancer on a live food diet.

Arguably the most influential and well-educated leader of the 20th century health revolution was Dr. Herbert M. Shelton (1895–1985). Herbert Shelton became the most prominent leader of the Natural Hygiene movement, which advocates a nontoxic diet of primarily or exclusively raw foods, while also emphasizing a complete program of healthful lifestyle practices, including obtaining adequate sunshine, clean air, exercise, sleep and fasting, not to mention avoiding all drugs, vaccinations and supplements. Dr. Shelton called these the basic requisites of life. Victoria BidWell concisely summarizes them as "The Ten Energy Enhancers." (See page 107.)

Whether or not to advocate a strictly 100% raw diet has always been an area of controversy within the Natural Hygiene movement. Some authorities, like Drs. Vetrano and Zovluck, insist that true Hygiene requires strict adherence to a 100% raw diet, while others permit, or even advocate, the inclusion of some lightly steamed vegetables and/or starches.

Dr. Shelton became qualified as a chiropractic doctor in order to legally practice in the health field, although he never practiced that specialty. He studied and earned a number of other degrees in alternative health care paradigms. He dedicated himself to teaching Natural Hygiene exclusively, however, declaring it the most effective health care system of all.

He helped over 40,000 people regain health via fasting at Dr. Shelton's Health School. Only three people out of those thousands died under his care, even though many of the patients who came to see him had already been pronounced "terminal" by the medical profession! (To compare such a death rate with that of drug treatment, see Appendix B.)

When one such patient came to Dr. Shelton's (seventh and final) Health School, he came at a very late stage in his disease and died. After the patient's death, his wife sued for $890,000 and won, which bankrupted both Drs. Shelton and Vetrano and forced them to close the health school.

Dr. Shelton dedicated his entire life to promoting the truth about health. Not only did he run his school/fasting clinic full time, but he also researched, authored, and published a monthly health magazine for 30-some years. He traveled to give health lectures, became the prime mover in helping to found and establish the American Natural Hygiene Society (now the National Health Association), and wrote 39 books on the subject of human health and its philosophy.

He was often persecuted by the medical "authorities" and was in and out of courtrooms, enduring periodic incarcerations. He once spent 30 days in jail for "practicing medicine without a license" despite telling the judge, "I wouldn't practice medicine if I *had* a license!" He preferred to fast rather than eat the poor prison diet, using his time and energy to write. During this time, he even penned one of his book manuscripts.

Shelton was such a busy man that he did not take time to sleep or rest much, although obtaining adequate sleep was one of the health precepts that he taught. By skimping on sleep, he sacrificed his own health in order to get the word out about Natural Hygiene. Sleep is necessary for revitalization, especially of the brain and nervous system.

Consequently, Dr. Shelton died in 1985 at age 89 of Parkinson's disease. He was bedridden the last 17 years of his life. The total responsibility of running the health school fell totally on Dr. Vetrano's shoulders, though he was still able to advise and write for several of those years.

Though he worked himself to death and exhausted himself from the stress of constant battles with the authorities, he outlived all but three of his dozen siblings despite being the oldest child.

One of his students, T. C. Fry, became the world's leading activist in the Natural Hygiene movement. A gifted writer, he was the most enthusiastic promoter of raw foods during the '70s and '80s. He wrote books and magazines, lectured all across America, and developed a 2,200-page correspondence course that awarded health counseling certification diplomas upon completion.

The Life Science Health System changed hands twice in the 1990s. The three organizations in charge over the 25 years graduated and/or enrolled over 6,000 students. There are presently two revised and updated online versions of this course at the web sites of hygienic doctors John Fielder and Robert Sniadach.

T. C. Fry's most famous students were Harvey and Marilyn Diamond, who went on to write the all-time best-seller in diet and nutrition, *Fit for Life*, and its best-selling successor *Fit for Life II: Living Health*.

Fry encouraged his other students to become health counselors, proclaiming, "The health field is wide open — there's nobody in it!" meaning that all of the conventional and "alternative" doctors were not preaching true health practices.

Dr. Russell Trall, Dr. Sylvester Graham, inventor of the graham cracker, and Dr. Mary Gove were 19th century trailblazers of the Natural Hygiene movement. Dr. John Tilden and Bernarr Macfadden, who was Dr. Shelton's initial mentor, carried the torch into the 20th century.

Bernarr Macfadden (1868–1955) was a major force in the first half of the 20th century. Besides teaching Dr. Shelton about natural health, he also influenced Paul Bragg and Jack LaLanne. Macfadden was a bodybuilder and an astute businessman, building a health and fitness publishing empire. Always seeking publicity, he parachuted out of an airplane to celebrate his 80th birthday.

Victoria BidWell offers this more detailed history of the Natural Hygiene movement, adapted from *The Health Seekers' YearBook*:

In the early 1800s, medical doctors practiced the following more often than not. They indiscriminately bled the sick to get rid of "bad blood." They practiced burning at the site of diseased tissue. They prescribed purging, puking and poulticing to drive out disease. They fumigated the sick with gasses. They drugged the sick with poisons. They opposed any sunbathing and regular bathing with water. They strictly prohibited giving water to the sick when thirsty. They refused fresh air and sunlight into rooms of the sick. They cautioned against raw foods and prescribed cooked vegetables, grains, meat — in particular, meat broth — and alcohol in moderation. They ignored sanitary considerations and did not wash their hands going into surgery or from one surgery to another.

This milieu of ignorance for the natural, physiological needs of the human body and dependency on the medicine men and the belief that doctors knew better than their patients, the pain and suffering rampant and the rising disease records and death rates throughout the country had the American people frightened and despairing for themselves and loved ones.

In 1832, the Natural Hygiene movement was formally launched by Dr. Isaac Jennings of Ohio, a conventional medical doctor. The story goes that after having practiced the traditional drugging and bleeding and cutting out of diseased tissues and limbs for 20 years, and then having become thoroughly discouraged with the results, Jennings had gone undercover for 20 years while he conducted a personal experiment.

Finally convinced that the afore-listed medical practices were dangerous, if not deadly, Jennings began administering placebos of bread pills, starch powders and colored water tonics for his patients, while at the same time instructing them in healthful living habits. He assured his patients that they would get well if they would take his medicines.

He further prescribed a list of healthful practices which included the following: cleanliness, regular bathing, fresh air, pure water, complete rest with as much sleep as possible, fasting on water, sunbaths, a diet of mostly uncooked fruits and vegetables, exercise as ability allows, emotional equanimity and so on. For some 20 years, his many patients followed this regime. And they invariably got better.

By 1852, his fame extended far and wide, as his "get-well record" was remarkable. Upon becoming fully convinced of the efficacy of which he alternately called the "Let-Alone Plan," the "Do-Nothing Cure," and the "No-Medicine Practice," Jennings announced his discovery to the world. His teachings and writings reached other doctors and then the people. A very specific, alternative health care system, in direct opposition to conventional doctoring, was borne. Historically, Dr. Isaac Jennings is now credited with the prestigious title "Father of Natural Hygiene." The Natural Hygiene movement was thus formally planted as a grassroots protest against the pitiful recovery records and high mortality rates of the medical establishment.

Since my discovery of it in 1976, I have studied the history and specifics of this system and have been waving it under the banner of Natural Hygiene! — The Superlative, Alternative Health Care System! ever since. Historically, I can see where virtually all alternative health care systems, all raw food movement programs included, offered in America today have been either directly or indirectly influenced, in either huge or small ways, by what Dr. Isaac Jennings started. To further appreciate the history of these two parallel tracks, we could go back further to the Egyptians and Greeks and Romans in ancient times and to the Nature Cure movement from post–Dark Ages Europe and around the globe to modern times.

So many American doctors of the early to mid 1800s turned to the Natural Hygiene (then called *hygeotherapeutics*) care of patients that the movement boasted, up to the Civil War, a roster of more hygienic doctors than conventional. (I know this is hard to believe. But historical records prove it.) At least 100 hygienic schools, colleges, and sanitariums were erected all over "The Sweet Land of Liberty." Seventy-five water-cure institutions in the nation sprang up by 1853, and virtually all adopted most aspects of the hygienic system.

In 1858, Doctors Harriet Austin and James Jackson founded the largest hygienic institution in history; entitled "Our Home on the Hillside" in New York, it was a grand estate and boasted 250 beds. Many sanitariums dotted the Eastern seaboard and inward. Women were welcomed into the movement. Famous individuals aligned themselves with Hygiene: Baptist minister and physiologist Sylvester Graham (graham crackers), philosopher Henry David Thoreau, nurse Florence Nightingale, suffragette Amelia Bloomer, Seventh Day Adventist Ellen White, American Red Cross founder Clara Barton and Dr. John Harvey Kellogg (corn flakes), to name a few you may readily recognize.

The reform leaders effectively reached the masses with some 80 different, regularly published, hygienic magazines, leaflets and papers. And then there were the books — so many books. Think of it! Hygiene was so vigorously promulgated and so enthusiastically received among the people that practitioners of hydrotherapy and hygeotherapeutics actually outnumbered all the other doctors of traditional, allopathic and homeopathic medicine!

Most of the early leaders were Christians and presented the teachings in a scriptural format, along with temperance. Most famous for this combination of hygienic teachings and scriptural self-control was the minister Sylvester Graham. He lectured for self-discipline and against alcohol, often joining the women's temperance movement against liquor consumption. The nation's first vegetarian communes were established under hygienic influences. Farmers were supplying the nation with whole food, organically grown, in a form largely unpackaged and unprocessed and chemical free. The future health, happiness and longevity of the American people looked hopeful!

But when the Civil War devastated both North and South infrastructures, homes and farms, the hygienic revolution never recovered to its full glory. The torch lit by Dr. Jennings and his followers that burned so brightly, fueled by so many pre–Civil War hygienists, barely flickered in the darkness of Reconstruction.

The late 1800s witnessed the rise again of allopathic medicine, as well as the promotion of traditional doctors to a godlike status, the promulgation of the germ theory as the cause of disease, the technological progress of processed, cooked foods in cans and jars and the earliest beginnings of motivational advertising.

The powerful, mind-persuading techniques developed by psychologists and employed by advertisers would serve two primary purposes: (1) to even further elevate the status of doctors and health care professionals in the medical/pharmaceutical complex to all-powerful, all-knowing untouchables, thus instilling "The Medical Mentality" into the minds not only of the doctors, but of the people as well, and (2) to start the people eating cooked, toxic food out of boxes and cans and bottles rather than seeking fresh, whole, raw foods from gardens and produce shops and farmers' stands.

The forces that would bring about the health demise of the American people generations later, especially up to this very day, were building fortress foundations on post–Civil War soil: vast fortunes up to this very day were made from these strongholds; and the health, happiness and lives of the American people were to be sacrificed and bled out red onto this soil.

Dr. J. H. Tilden helped keep Hygiene alive and moving forward when he presented "The Seven Stages of Disease" paradigm and his landmark book *Toxemia Explained* in 1926.

Dr. Herbert M. Shelton followed Tilden and picked up the near-extinguished torch of 19th century Natural Hygienists, fully flamed it once again in the early to late 1900s and held it HIGH, calling — bold and loud, far and wide — for "a Natural Hygiene revolution" to wipe out the existing and rotten-to-the-core medical mentality at its worst.

Dr. Vivian Virginia Vetrano worked alongside him for some 40 years, up until his 1985 death, and then took up the Shelton torch on her own.

Throughout the late 1900s, Thunder Cloud Fry shot a bolt of lightning to Shelton's and Vetrano's by then fading TORCHES and lit up the world with followers of his "Big Course" (The Life Science Health System) and readers of his magazines and endless streams of affordable, easy to understand booklets and brochures. *Shelton*, *Vetrano* and *Fry* — these were the names of the 1940s to the end of the century to which we owe the most for getting the message and promise of Natural Hygiene out to the people.

My contribution has been to create new Natural Hygiene "contraband" and make available for the American health seeker and health seekers everywhere virtually every classic teaching that Dr. Shelton and T. C. Fry produced.

In the very late 1900s, many people began discovering the virtues of eating raw foods; but they were not exploring these virtues in the context of Natural Hygiene. These emerging raw food leaders began getting the raw word out: making DVDs and CDs, giving lectures, opening raw restaurants, constructing raw food web sites, writing raw food recipe books with basic teachings answering the question: Why raw foods. Thus, simultaneously with the resuscitation of the Natural Hygiene movement by Doctors Shelton and Vetrano and publicists T. C. Fry and myself in the early to mid to late 1900s, was laid down a parallel and very popular, very powerful group of raw food movement enthusiasts at the end of the 1900s and into the new millennium.

The happy ending to date is that a band of promoters and practitioners, teachers and students of the Natural Hygiene movement and the raw food movement alike around the world each now carry *his* or *her* torch . . . collectively lighting our global skies, dominating our cyberspaces and filling our home bookshelves. Their all-shining, mutual message is simple: "Eating mostly raw foods — even better yet, 100% raw foods — provides the body with the superlative nutrition the body needs." To make your life the best it can be, add the other nine energy enhancers.

---

Among Natural Hygiene's most prominent leaders today are Dr. Vivian V. Vetrano, Dr. Shelton's protégé, and Dr. Bernarr Zovluck, both of whom also suffered persecution at the hands of the authorities. Dr. Zovluck was forced to close his all-too-successful New York City clinic in the late '60s and now practices only by telephone consultations and his Internet presence.

Another 20th century figure, Dr. Norman Walker (1876–1985), became known for promoting raw juices and wrote several books on the topic. He invented the Norwalk hydraulic press, one of the premier juicers on the market today and the best of its day. He lived to be 109.

Naturopathic doctor Paul Bragg (1881?–1976) was crippled by tuberculosis as a teenager and developed his own version of the raw food diet, advocating 80% raw and a vigorous exercise program. He went on to become a health teacher to many, including famous people, like Jack LaLanne, Dr. Scholl, Conrad Hilton, J. C. Penney and others. He wrote 20 books, including the classic *The Miracle of Fasting*.

According to his daughter-in-law Patricia, Bragg remained very active and healthy until suffering a severe blow to his head while *surfboarding* at the age of

94 that culminated in his death a year later. However, there seems to be some controversy as to his exact birth year. While Patricia Bragg gives it as 1881, the US government's Social Security Death Index lists it at 1895, making him "only" 80 at the time of his surfing accident. The author hasn't been able to independently confirm either date.

Dr. Edmond Bordeaux Szekely (1905–1979) claimed to have treated 123,600 people over a period of 33 years at his clinic in Mexico, many of whom came to him with "incurable" diseases. His group had more than a 90% success rate using live foods together with the other important health factors. Unfortunately, Dr. Szekely himself didn't practice what he preached.

Other 20th century raw food advocates have included Dr. Bernard Jensen, Dr. Paavo Airola, comedian Dick Gregory and numerous others.

For more information on notable raw fooders, read *Blatant Raw Foodist Propaganda!* by Joe Alexander, one of the most inspiring books I read while transitioning to the raw diet.

The pioneers presented in this chapter laid down the foundations, started institutions and prepared the grounds for the blossoming of the live food movement into the 21st century. The next chapter will introduce you to some of the foremost modern-day leaders.

# 12
# Modern-Day Leaders of Raw Foodism

*To be a leader of men, one must turn one's back on men.*
*—Havelock Ellis (1859–1939), British psychologist*

The raw food movement and its variations are now growing by leaps and bounds, especially since the flowering of the Internet-based information explosion. It would have been an unending task for me to have profiled all of the movers and shakers in these grassroots movements, so I have included only those whose workshops I have attended, those natural hygienists Victoria BidWell has known personally, as well as Rev. Malkmus and Roe Gallo, whose personal healing stories are very compelling. Victoria and I were most impressed with all we have met — their high energy levels and radiant "raw glows." Most of them have also written books that I have quoted throughout this text.

## Elizabeth Baker: Active and Consulting in Her 90s

Elizabeth Baker wrote some of the very first books on the living foods diet, such as *The Uncook Book*, *The Unmedical Book*, *Does the Bible Teach Nutrition?* and *The UnDiet Book.* I saw her speak and lecture at the 2004 Raw Food Festival in Oregon, at which point she was 91 years old and still quite active! She said that her consultations kept her very busy. Her husband was also on the diet but died eight years previously after sustaining major injuries in a car accident.

## The Boutenko Family: Healed of Four "Incurable" Diseases

Victoria Boutenko writes that she and her family became raw after she was faced with a life-threatening illness. The whole family gained superior health: her husband became free of hyperthyroidism, her daughter of asthma and her son of juvenile diabetes. Victoria was healed of heart arrhythmia and also lost 120 pounds. The book *Raw Family: A True Story of Awakening* goes into much more detail. See her testimonial on page 62 also.

Victoria went on to teach classes in raw foods, as well as to cater raw food. She noticed, however, that her students would very frequently backslide. In fact, although she personally met hundreds who were healed of cancer by raw diet, she knew of 132 who reverted to cooked foods, developed cancer again, and died. It appeared that they actually preferred death to a raw food diet.

She kept wondering why this was happening, while her own family was immune to the temptation to backslide. Finally, she figured out that cooked food is addictive: unless one is eating 100% raw, as opposed to even 99%, one will be tempted to eat more and more cooked food. Victoria observed that it takes about two months of 100% raw eating to break the addiction. She explains all of this and much more in *12 Steps to Raw Foods*.

More than any other teacher I have read about or heard lecture, Victoria encourages a 100% raw food diet. She has witnessed in her clients the additive allure of cooked food to pull one back.

Her children, Sergei and Valya, also went raw perforce and improved in both their schoolwork and their physical health. But being children, they would fantasize about how they would celebrate their 18th birthday independence by going out to eat pizza, nachos and corndogs. Those SAD foods had been declared *taboo* since that auspicious day the family went raw.

Gradually such desires faded. Their love for raw food and its life-improving effects grew. They learned how to create raw dishes and published their own recipe book, *Eating without Heating: Favorite Recipes from Teens Who Love Raw Food*. In this book, they also discuss how their health became superior. Sergei even regrew some teeth, and his wisdom teeth grew in perfectly straight. They have also another book: *Fresh: The Ultimate Live-Food Cookbook*.

Most amazing was the improvement in the children's academic performance. Formerly below average in school, the two kids were able to complete two school years in one year after going 100% raw. High school then became boring, so they went on to college.

When I attended one of the Boutenkos' workshops, Victoria said that Valya was taking 27 units in one semester — which is a double load! — while also working 20 hours a week.

The Boutenkos were tested extensively for a scientific study being conducted in a university in Missouri on raw fooders. (See "Bone Mass in Long-Term Raw Fooders" on page 168.) The Boutenkos were found to be in extraordinary health. Victoria's heart was like "that of a baby," and her bone density was like that of a 17-year-old. The MDs performing the study were extremely enthusiastic about their health findings, asked the Boutenkos many questions, and gave them additional tests beyond what was required of the study.

Victoria's latest book, *Green for Life*, is sparking a new revolution among raw fooders who have reached a plateau, as well as among people who have never eaten a raw diet. See Appendix C for more information about this radical, yet wonderful, way of eating raw.

# Brian Clement and the Hippocrates Health Institute

For the past 27 years, Brian Clement has worked as director of the Hippocrates Health Institute founded by Ann Wigmore and Viktoras Kulvinskas. This is a 70-person, in-residence health facility. Clement does blood tests to see what residents need. I heard him lecture once and was especially impressed with his experimentation with wheatgrass. He found four ounces a day was the optimal amount for the average person. Any more than that did not seem to make a difference. His book *Living Foods for Optimum Health* was acclaimed by Coretta Scott King as a "landmark guide to the essentials of healthy living."

# Lou Corona

I have heard Lou Corona speak several times. He is radiant and dynamic. At the age of 53, he could pass for a 30-year-old. This is because he began the 100% raw vegan diet about 31 years ago! He had been very sick: badly constipated, plagued by severe acne and a tumor on his head, but he didn't want to have surgery because he knew of someone who died after surgery for such a tumor.

He prayed for guidance, and a white light presence told him to eat living foods and no animal products. He was told that he would receive a mentor, whom he later met: a man who looked *decades younger* than his chronological age. He immediately adopted the diet. Within six months, the tumor, acne and constipation disappeared completely. Lou gives workshops and is currently writing a book.

# Dr. Gabriel Cousens, MD: Seeking the Optimal Diet for Spiritual Growth

Dr. Gabriel Cousens, MD, is probably the foremost medical doctor promoting the raw vegan diet. He has done a great deal to verify its validity and usefulness through research. Because he has so much knowledge, Gabriel seems to have a hard time writing a book under 600 pages. But each page is packed with useful and interesting information.

Dr. Cousens was not satisfied with the results he obtained from the use of allopathic medicine. He began exploring various diets to find the right way to eat to enhance one's spiritual life.

After an amazing spiritual awakening experience, he was eager to find a diet that would reinforce that state. Eventually, he discovered the raw food diet and wrote about it in *Spiritual Nutrition and the Rainbow Diet* and again in *Conscious Eating*.

He established the Tree of Life Rejuvenation Center, a live food retreat located in Patagonia, Arizona. He now offers a university master's degree course in the study of live foods.

Gabriel wrote *Rainbow Green Live-Food Cuisine*, which explains how he has modified his raw food diet even more. He eliminated foods that push the "composting button," which means that they cause disease-promoting fermentation and putrefaction within the digestive system. The book starts with a scientific overview but is mostly a book of delicious recipes calling mostly for nonacidic, low-sweet live food that will not stimulate a rise in blood sugar.

Cousens has come out with a second book on the effects of diet on spiritual life: *Spiritual Nutrition*. In this book, he mentions that he has the same weight in his 60s that he had in high school. On his 60th birthday, he did 600 consecutive push-ups, whereas at the age of 21, he was able to do only 70.

He has a new book, *There Is a Cure for Diabetes: The Tree of Life 21-Day Program*, as well as a documentary on the same topic, *Raw for 30 Days.*

Also at the age of 60, he competed in the Native American Sundancing cycle. He completed three Sundance cycles of four days in the desert without food and water. No one else in the group of 52 people, which included dancers 40 years younger than he, was able to match his feat. He attributes this entirely to his live-food lifestyle.

According to Dr. Cousens, "The optimal diet is an individualized, live, organic, locally grown, vegan, highly mineralized, low-glycemic, well-hydrated diet of whole food prepared with love and eaten with consciousness and gratitude" (*Spiritual Nutrition*, p. 304).

# Roe Gallo: Allergic to the 20th Century

Roe Gallo's childhood was plagued by illness. She was likely one of those people who are "allergic to the 20th [now 21st] century" — hypersensitive to all the thousands of chemicals in our environment that have been synthesized only within the last hundred years or so.

She suffered asthma, constant colds and several bouts of pneumonia. One day she experienced a severe allergic response after eating pancakes. She was taken to an emergency room, where she reacted so badly to the medication aminophylline given her by the medical staff that her heart stopped. She ended up spending several weeks in the hospital growing weaker and weaker. Later she learned the doctors were recommending that she take a smaller dose of the aminophylline, though it had stopped her heart previously, because it was the best medication for her condition.

Intuition told her that taking this drug would only lead to a slow death as opposed to a fast one. While still in the hospital, she stopped taking the aminophylline, substituted certain visualization exercises, drank a lot of water to aid elimination of the drug residues, began eating only fresh fruits and vegetables her friends brought her, and slowly recovered. She didn't tell the medical staff what she was doing. Within a week, she had the physical strength to sign herself out and walk away against the doctors' wishes.

Later she resorted to the drug cortisone for pain, but it relieved the pain for only a few days. When the pain would return, along with difficulty breathing, the doctor would simply increase the dosage. After reading up on it in the *Physician's Desk Reference* manual, she discovered that cortisone was addictive and that it too would eventually kill her. When she confronted the doctor about her suspicion that the drug would shorten her lifespan, he warned her that she would die without it.

That's when Roe decided to take personal control of her health. She threw out the pills although, as she put it, "That was the most frightening thing I have ever done. I had always listened to doctors. I grew up on medications." She fasted for two weeks on water only, after which she felt better than she had ever felt in her 25 years of life. In her book *Perfect Body: The Raw Truth*, Roe describes how she attained super health on a fruitarian diet and exercise. She passed through menopause with virtually no symptoms! Her book includes inspiring testimonials of others she has helped with this diet.

Roe and Stephen Zocchi also wrote *Overcoming the Myths of Aging: Lose Weight, Look Great and Live a Happier, Healthier Life.*

# Dr. Douglas Graham and Training Athletes

Dr. Doug Graham is a chiropractor who focuses on Natural Hygiene diet counseling and writing. He has taken T. C. Fry's place in becoming one of the world's leading activists and proponents of Natural Hygiene, tirelessly lecturing to large and small groups. He has sponsored several Rawstock festivals, raw food events that draw large numbers of both seminar presenters and participants. He also organizes raw food vacation retreats.

A lifelong athlete himself, he especially loves to counsel athletes on the raw diet, most notably tennis star Martina Navratilova and professional basketball player Ronnie Grandison of the NBA. Olympic athletes from Aruba, Australia, Mexico, the USA, Canada and Norway have also sought Doug's counsel. His books include *The High Energy Diet Recipe Guide, Grain Damage, On Nutrition and Physical Performance: A Handbook for Athletes and Fitness Enthusiasts* and *The 80/10/10 Diet.*

Dr. Graham has been a pioneer in making raw fooders aware that they are typically eating way too much fat. He has done histories on over 5,000 raw fooders and found that they consume on average 65% of their calories from fat! (The usual American diet contains about 40% fat.) He works with people to get this down to 10%. Fat is very energy expensive to digest, he explains, and also prevents absorption of many nutrients. Read more about Dr. Graham and his controversial 80% carbohydrate, raw vegan diet in Chapter 17.

# David Jubb, PhD: Living on Little Food

David and Annie Jubb (no longer married) have written several books on the raw diet, including *LifeFood Recipe Book: Living on Life Force* and *Secrets of an Alkaline Body: The New Science of Colloidal Biology*. Annie Jubb has owned and managed raw, organic, vegan restaurants in San Francisco and Hawaii and is currently providing health readings, overseeing fasts, running corporate workshops, writing, filming and conducting health research.

David Jubb, originally from Tasmania, a southern Australian island grouping, gives health readings, writes and lectures both in the USA and abroad. David has eaten a pure, raw diet for over 30 years. He was the scientific advisor to live foods pioneer Ann Wigmore. (See Chapter 11.) David has written the book *Jubb's Cell Rejuvenation: Colloidal Biology: A Symbiosis*.

While I have never met Annie, I have seen David several times when he has lectured in San Diego.

Live foods form the basis of the Jubb diet. Live foods are full of life force, as demonstrated by Kirlian photography. This is a fascinating, sophisticated kind of photography in which an image is obtained by application of a high-frequency electric field to an object so that it radiates a characteristic pattern of luminescence that is recorded on photographic film. It is no surprise to see that a Kirlian photograph of cooked food appears dead in comparison to a Kirlian photograph of raw food, which reflects strength, height and liveliness.

David defines live food as meeting three criteria: its life force is present, being neither cooked nor irradiated; its preparation promotes easy digestion, and some semblance of it continues to grow wild in nature.

Hybridized foods having no wild counterparts are omitted because they are very low in life force. These hybrids are often bred to be high in fruit sugar and starch, which tend to stimulate the body to release excessive amounts of insulin during digestion. These high levels of carbohydrates promote hypoglycemia (a precursor to diabetes), fatigue, excessive weight gain and accelerated aging.

These hybridized foods include commercial bananas, dates, corn, rice, legumes, wheat and tuberous vegetables like carrots, potatoes and beets. Wild plants, such as burdock root, kale, bok choy, heirloom tomatoes, squash and dandelion are preferred. Oddly, this diet also includes raw, organic cheese, preferably goat's milk cheese, which is easier to digest than cow's milk cheese.

Using live blood cell analysis, David has seen how the blood turns bad when we eat hybrid food, even when it is raw.

I once asked David what he ate, and he said he almost never eats. He does drink, however, the drinks listed in his recipe book, such as sun teas and lemonade. Although he is primarily a liquidarian, consuming minimal calories, he is of medium build and not at all emaciated. He is full of energy and enthusiasm.

I spent three evenings in a row with him when he was here giving lectures, a sweat lodge event and a raw food potluck. I did not see him eat anything. Others have concurred that they don't see him eat. Apparently, he continues being a gourmet chef and just takes minimal nibbles to make sure that his food tastes excellent.

There do exist those who have cleaned out their bodies to such an extent that their food intake needs are minimal. David has eaten a pure, raw diet for over 30 years. Nutrient absorption increases with a clean system, and metabolism slows down when one fasts extensively. Moreover, cells do not die and need replacing as often.

# David Klein, PhD, and *Vibrance* Magazine

It was ulcerative colitis that prompted David Klein's interest in the raw food diet. His physicians had tried prednisone and Azulfidine drug treatments, which ameliorated the symptoms but ruined his health and had a "devastating effect" on his mental abilities.

He eventually discovered and studied T. C. Fry's Natural Hygiene course, adopted the diet and regained robust health within a few years. See his testimonial in Chapter 2.

He now publishes *Vibrance* (formerly *Living Nutrition*), the world's most-read raw food lifestyle magazine. Klein also wrote the book *Your Natural Diet: Alive Raw Foods*, which contains so many of T. C. Fry's teachings that David credited T. C. with co-authorship long after his death.

David has been director since 1993 of the Colitis & Crohn's Health Recovery Center, currently located in Sebastopol in northern California. His approach is holistic, based upon the principles of Natural Hygiene. He is both a hygienic doctor and a certified nutrition educator. Since 1992, he has counseled over 2,000 clients back to health via Natural Hygiene, occasionally teaching nutrition classes and giving health and nutrition lectures.

His book *Self Healing Colitis & Crohn's* is used as the teaching model for a course at the Canadian School of Natural Nutrition. He has led Raw Passion seminars and jamborees over the last 10 years and co-produced Rawstock health festivals in northern California with Dr. Graham. David was awarded "Honorable Mention — Best Nutritionist" in the *Share Guide* (www.shareguide.com) magazine's 2002 readers' poll.

David co-founded Healthful Living International, a leading Natural Hygiene organization. David is also a nutritional and healing advisor on the board of directors for St. John's Colonic Center in Bowie, Maryland. (He does not recommend colonics for inflammatory bowel disease however.)

He maintains the web sites www.livingnutrition.com and www.colitis-crohns.com. He may be contacted via e-mail at dave@livingnutrition.com or reached through the Colitis & Crohn's Health Recovery Center, P.O. Box 256, Sebastopol, CA 95473. Phone: 707-827-3469.

# Rev. George Malkmus:
# Why Christians Get Sick

A Baptist preacher, Rev. George Malkmus was diagnosed with colon cancer, "a tumor the size of a baseball," at the age of 42. Having already lost his mother to the recommended chemotherapy, he was determined to find something else that would cure him. So in 1976, he began researching health, nutrition and how lifestyle relates to health.

Another minister friend told him about the raw food diet, and it just seemed "too simplistic," but Malkmus decided to try it. After going on a raw food diet, he found that not only did his cancer go away, but also every minor complaint he'd had for years vanished. Gone were his hemorrhoids, hypoglycemia, allergies, sinus problems, high blood pressure, fatigue, pimples, colds, bouts with the flu, body odors and even dandruff.

Rev. Malkmus had always wondered why so many of the prayers for people's healings didn't seem to make a difference. He observed that the same percentage of Christians as non-Christians died of every disease under the sun. He began to realize that God had established certain universal laws that are perfect, eternal and unchangeable. When people violate these laws, they suffer the consequences. For example, if one jumps off a building, gravity will cause him to fall. If one eats denatured, dead or toxic food, she will slowly poison herself to death.

Malkmus came to realize that according to the Bible, mankind did not get sick after the fall from grace. No, man was quite healthy, living on uncooked fruits and vegetables and living an average of 912 years. It was only after the Flood that people began eating meat and cooked food. The lifespans recorded in the Bible were greatly reduced from that time on.

Malkmus proceeded to write *Why Christians Get Sick* and later *God's Way to Ultimate Health*. He also founded Hallelujah Acres, a healing and educational center. He found that eating just 85% raw would maintain most people in good health. He now eats that way himself, an 85% raw vegan diet, and has remained cancer-free since 1976. Pastors who have convinced their church members to adopt this diet claim they never have to pray for people's illnesses anymore!

Interestingly, George's wife Rhonda demonstrated that even a degenerated spine could be totally healed. Degenerated since age seven as a result of spinal meningitis, hers healed on the diet in less than two years!

George claims that in six months or less, over 90% of the diseases at his center are healed. In just three to five days, the person experiences increased energy. Only about 10% of the people suffer intense detoxification symptoms. On his staff are numerous medical doctors, registered nurses and other medical professionals who help supervise patients.

People from *all* spiritual paths can learn a lesson from this. Various highly spiritual or highly conscious people teach that we can avoid illness through prayer, meditation, visualization, hypnosis, positive thinking, intention and other spiritual practices. Yet many of these teachers themselves suffer heart attacks, strokes and cancer.

Using the mind and spirit is not enough. We must heed God's, or nature's, laws set up for the physical body. Eating uncooked food certainly is one of them. Just as we would not attempt to avoid the harm in jumping off a cliff by using prayer or meditation, we must also not think we can escape harm by tampering with the Garden of Eden diet.

# David Wolfe, Stephen Arlin and Fouad Dini: Nature's First Law

David Wolfe, his cousin Fouad Dini and his close friend Stephen Arlin collaborated on *Nature's First Law: The Raw Food Diet*. The interesting thing about this trio is that they began a 100% raw diet while still in their early twenties and already quite healthy, except for Fouad, who was obese.

They found that with raw diet, they were propelled into a state of superior health and vitality. Fouad lost 156 pounds. The fact that they started so young shows us that you can obtain vastly greater levels of health by going on a raw diet even if you are already relatively healthy.

Stephen Arlin is much more muscular than the average raw food person. In fact he is bigger than the average bodybuilder. People often cannot believe that he doesn't take steroids or at least meat. When people ask how he gets his muscular physique, he replies, "The same way a gorilla does!"

Arlin wrote the book *Raw Power! Building Strength & Muscle Naturally* to show how he is able to maintain such a muscular body on a 100% raw, plant food diet. He has repeatedly said, "A raw fooder is not something you become; it is something that you already are."

David Wolfe once said in an interview that his goal is to be the world's foremost promoter of the raw food diet. He has worked diligently toward that goal, traveling and giving lectures full time and also authoring several books: *The Sunfood Diet Success System*, *Eating for Beauty*, *Naked Chocolate* and *Amazing Grace: The Nine Principles of Living in Natural Magic*.

The notoriety of being a naturalist earned him spots on a reality TV show (*Mad, Mad House* on the Sci-Fi Channel), the Rosie O'Donnell show and the Howard Stern show. My favorite David Wolfe quote is, "We are tired of eating pesticide, herbicide, fungicide, larvicide, suicide, pasteurized, homogenized, cooked, boiled, glow-in-the-dark, pus-filled food."

David and Stephen established a raw food grocery called Nature's First Law, which can be found online at www.rawfood.com or www.sunfood.com — now called Sunfood Nutrition after a split between Wolfe and Arlin.

# Paul Nison: Healing Crohn's Disease

Paul Nison ate the SAD until age 19 when he was diagnosed with ulcerative colitis, a late stage of inflammatory bowel disease (IBD) and precursor to the deadly Crohn's disease. He suffered colitis flare-ups about six times a year that included ulcerations, sometimes bleeding, and spasmodic, frequent bowel movements. Although Paul's doctor told him that food had nothing to do with his condition, Paul's symptoms improved when he eliminated dairy, eggs, meat and sugar.

When Paul was 23, he moved to West Palm Beach, Florida. By coincidence, he was living near the Hippocrates Health Institute, where he learned about the health benefits of eating raw foods. He improved further after switching to an 80% raw food diet, but again Paul's physician warned that raw foods would only worsen his condition.

Later, after meeting a number of raw fooders and hearing their success stories, he progressed to a 100% raw food, vegetarian diet. It was only then that he completely overcame the ulcerative colitis.

Paul has since written *The Raw Life* and *Raw Knowledge*. Both books include interviews and photos of long-term raw fooders. He also has his own web site and online raw food store at www.rawlife.com.

# Dr. David J. Scott, DC, and Natural Hygiene

Dr. David J. Scott, DC, graduated cum laude from the National College of Chiropractic in 1950 where he was a member of the honor society. He has been in practice for over 50 years and has personally supervised the care of over 40,000 patients. He has fasted some 20,000 patients under his direct supervision, many of whom are of international origin. Raw foods, free of protoplasmic poisons, are the mainstay of his dietary teachings, although in rare situations of advanced disease, he sometimes recommends cooked foods until his patients are well enough to handle raw foods.

Dr. Scott is one of the most amazing men in the Natural Hygiene movement today! While the average age of death in America for men is now 74, Dr. Scott is 85 as of this writing. Yet he runs a full-time chiropractic office and directs or personally conducts all activities at Dr. Scott's Natural Health Institute. He attributes his great vitality to his strict adherence to the natural, physiological laws of life and most recently to his two fasts of 40 days each in the last two years.

Dr. David J. Scott's early interest was electronics. For this reason, he chose to enlist during World War II as an officer trainee in the then new field of radar engineering. During a courier flight over Nagasaki sometime after the bombing, he was awed firsthand at the sight of the ultimate capability of humans for mutual destruction. This exposure to human waste and suffering convinced Dr. Scott, both a Christian and a naturalist by conscience, to move into the field of natural healing.

He was seriously liver damaged by prescribed drugs during his military years and suffered many subsequent years of related chronic diseases. He gradually recovered his health with the help of chiropractic and Natural Hygiene. Consequently, he developed a strong persuasion in the inherent healing capacity of the living organism. Accordingly, he specializes in teaching an understanding of the consequences of a self-destructive lifestyle versus adopting a way of life that fosters nutritional excellence.

Dr. Scott has advanced into the space age of science with the latest technologies for demonstrating the status of human health using physiological parameters. He has a keen interest in the scientific demonstration of those physiological parameters that clearly reflect the inherent and progressive healing activities found within the organism. They are best described by his trademarked slogan Health by Design, which refers to the genetic blueprint for humankind laid down by the Creator. He monitors physiology carefully throughout the healing period and on into recovery.

He has lectured extensively throughout the United States and Canada for the American Natural Hygiene Society/National Health Association and the Canadian Natural Hygiene Society, teaching an understanding of the consequences of a self-destructive lifestyle. He also served the former society on its board of directors for a number of years. He was instrumental in formulating policies that have brought these educational societies to significance. He is also the founding president of the International Association of Hygienic Physicians. This is an international association of multidisciplinary primary care doctors specializing in supervised fasting.

Dr. Scott has been privileged to see his revolutionary ideas about natural health move from complete disdain by the scientific community to widespread acceptance and agreement during his own lifetime. This could only be made possible by his determination to pursue demonstrably exact science. The essence of Dr. Scott's philosophy and work is best capsulized by his lifetime motto — Profound Simplicity.

# Dr. Vivian Virginia Vetrano
# and Natural Hygiene

Dr. Vivian Virginia Vetrano is one of the world's leading health experts today. She has been a prominent leader in the area of research and application of Natural Hygiene's principles to healthy and sick alike for over 50 years.

She just turned 80 in November 2007. Still looking and acting like a woman in her 50s, she is a living example of the truth of this science, a science that can hardly be spoken of without reference to her name and her influence in the field. She exudes the vitality and extreme enthusiasm for life of a healthy, happy teenager.

Dr. Vetrano worked as manager and doctor at Dr. Shelton's Health School, saving lives by guiding people through long fasts and teaching the principles of

Natural Hygiene. She assisted Shelton in editing, writing for and producing his magazine, *Dr. Shelton's Hygienic Review*. Fluency in French has helped make her an internationally effective promoter of raw diet and the other health precepts of Natural Hygiene.

She received the Dr. T. C. Fry Fellowship for the Study of Natural Hygiene, becoming the first doctoral admittee of City University of Los Angeles (CULA). Though the formal presentation of Natural Hygiene dates back to 1832, and T. C. Fry's Natural Hygiene course has been taught in at least one medical school in France for more than twenty years, only CULA has offered a graduate degree program in the subject of Natural Hygiene. Though offered since the mid-1980s, this is the first time anyone has been admitted beyond the master's degree level.

Dr. Vetrano is one of the most renowned students, teachers, editors and doctors of Natural Hygiene. She earned her DC in 1965 and her MD in homeopathic science in 1977. Although she also completed medical school and received her MD degree, she has chosen not to use the title since she does not practice medicine.

Although Dr. Vetrano has been involved in numerous projects with Natural Hygiene, one stands out. In the early 1980s, when T. C. Fry was in South Korea buying persimmon trees, he boasted at the Tubercular Sanitarium near Seoul that he could have all their tubercular patients well within one month.

When the Koreans took him up on the offer, Dr. Vetrano agreed to take charge of the project. She started out with 50 patients as hundreds more called to see if they could be admitted to the project. Many became completely well within one month, while many of the others were well on their way to complete recovery by the time Dr. Vetrano left Korea. Both T. C. Fry and Dr. Vetrano were presented with awards and invited to come back and take charge of the entire sanitarium.

She is currently writing books on Natural Hygiene with Victoria BidWell as her editor and also does consulting for those who are writing on the topic. See her testimonial in Chapter 2.

# Many Others

As I mentioned before, this list is by no means complete. It includes some of the teachers who have made a major impact, although there are more and more appearing every year as this grassroots movement gains momentum.

Author and comedian Tonya Zavasta is carving her own niche in the raw food community by teaching how to stay beautiful on raw food. Author Frédéric Patenaude is reaching many aspiring raw fooders with his free online newsletter, "Pure Health and Nutrition," as is health educator Roger Haeske. Alissa Cohen and Cherie Soria have become famous for training many people to be live food chefs.

Numerous people have web sites and offer coaching in raw eating. Many of them are listed in the Resource Guide, which also lists restaurant owners and chefs who have contributed a lot. Many of these other fine raw food renegades and their stories can be found in *The Complete Book of Raw Food*, which is also a compilation of their favorite recipes.

Additionally, there are two controversial, *really radical* branches of the raw food movement that are so vastly different that they are not well accepted by the raw food mainstream, although their proponents embrace a 100% raw food diet. See Appendix C for more information.

# Let's Go!

It is now time for you, dear reader, to embark upon your own personal raw diet evolution or revolution. The next section of this book will answer any remaining questions or lurking doubts you may still harbor. Get ready for one of the most, if not the most, rewarding and exciting personal growth experiences of your life!

# Section Four

# Raw Passage:

## Your Journey to Raw Life

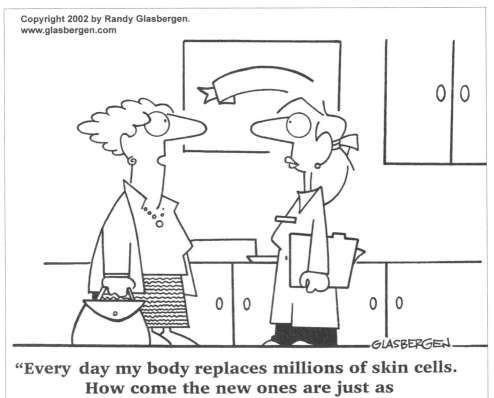

"Every day my body replaces millions of skin cells.
How come the new ones are just as
wrinkled as the old ones?"

# 13
# Getting Started

Now is the time to begin the work of restoring good health — not next week, next summer or next year.
—Dr. Herbert Shelton (1895–1985)

Do not wait; the time will never be "just right." Start where you stand, and work with whatever tools you may have at your command, and better tools will be found as you go along.
—Napoleon Hill (1883–1970)

The famous cultural anthropologist Margaret Mead observed, "It is easier to change a man's religion than to change his diet." The switch to a raw food diet may be one of the most significant things you will ever do in your life, opening up levels of energy and health you never dreamed possible. But this switch seldom happens overnight. It takes commitment, planning and education. Those who learn from the mistakes of others and those who take time to inform themselves about the reasons the raw diet is superior and what to expect during the transition period are the ones who most successfully stick to the diet.

## The Decision

"A journey of a thousand miles must begin with a single step" is a famous saying from *The Way of Lao Tzu*. The first step to going raw is to make up your mind to do it. For some, it may be easier to commit to a brief "experiment." A sudden decision never to eat another mouthful of cooked food in your life may be too disturbing to the ego. So some have simply resolved, "I will experiment and go 100% raw for a one-month period."

I know of one man who decided to commit to a one-year trial period. After each year, he would "renew the experiment." So far he has gone over ten years of eating 100% raw!

Do not say, "Oh, I want to go raw, but I am going to wait until all my canned, packaged, frozen and boxed food is finished." That could take weeks, or even months, by which time you may have lost most of the inspiration to go raw.

*Do it now!* Give all your SAD, processed food to a hungry neighbor or friend. Or donate the nonperishables to the Salvation Army, and get a tax write-off. Or keep some of it, the foods you know won't tempt you, for guests who want processed food.

Remember, it is not eating the raw foods that is usually the mental barrier. Most people find that changing the emotional and social associations with cooked food to be the biggest block. One must reprogram one's thinking and view food as good medicine and nourishment rather than as an object for emotional comfort, love, entertainment or social activity.

For all of the importance we give food, eating is nothing more than a few brief moments of savoring something that we chew and swallow, never to taste again. The "pleasure" of cooked food items is momentary and fleeting, but the negative effects linger on and on.

What the protesting cooked food addict never seems to understand is that once you have been raw long enough, the raw foods give *much more* pleasure in the eating than the cooked foods ever did. *Then it's not a matter of deprivation anymore!*

What we ingest ultimately makes us feel alive or moribund. The next time you are tempted to eat something you know is not good for you, ask yourself, "Is it worth being addicted, fatigued and poisoned for those fleeting moments of pleasure?"

# Methods of Transitioning

The easiest way for many people is to commit to a 100% raw diet without a period of dietary transition. The big danger in a slower transition is that while still indulging daily in cooked foods, you may lose your initial enthusiasm and inspiration, perhaps even forgetting the reasons you decided to go raw. How many of us have bought supplements that we stopped taking because we forgot why we started them in the first place?

During transition, the benefits may not come fast enough for you to see the superiority of the raw food diet. For some people, a slow transition results in backsliding into a diet of mainly cooked foods because of their addictive properties.

Some people nonetheless do find it psychologically easier and physically less disruptive to transition gradually into a raw diet. There are several ways in which this can be done.

## Transitioning One Meal at a Time

One way to transition is by changing one meal at a time. You can work out a plan in which you eat only raw breakfasts for a month. The second phase will consist of raw breakfasts and lunches. The third phase will have everything raw.

For some, this process may be too slow, and the results will not be dramatic enough to sustain positive feedback. They may wish to move on to the next phase on a weekly, instead of monthly, schedule.

Soon enough, after just transitioning two meals, you will be 60-70% raw. Most people eat more for dinner than the other meals. So if you eat just half of your dinner cooked, you will be eating about 75-85% of your diet raw. Many people feel so great eating this way that they stick with that plan as a way of life. This way they need not feel deprived of their favorite cooked dishes.

If you decide to eat 80-85% of your diet raw, I recommend saving the cooked foods for dinner. There are several reasons for this:

The first is well-being: you'll have energy all day, and the cooked food won't slow you down. At night, it's usually okay to wind down, but not at work.

The second is social: dinner is the one meal most people share with others, and the other people may be eating cooked food.

The third is pleasure: for many people, cravings for cooked food, or any food for that matter, arise more strongly in the early evening. Most of us are usually too busy and preoccupied with the day's activities to focus on the pleasures and comforts of food during the day. But we relax, unwind and crave food enjoyment in the evenings.

In my case, for example, I feel my tastebuds "open up" for more variety in the evenings. When I have eaten 90-95% raw, it has only been in the evenings that I have been tempted to eat something cooked.

# Food Elimination Transition

A second way to transition is to give up certain kinds of "bad foods" first. For example, one week cut out all sugar and table salt. The next week maintain the sugar and salt elimination while also cutting out pasteurized dairy. Next, omit cooked meat, then grains and later processed foods until everything cooked is substituted with whole raw foods or raw recipe dishes.

Again, for many, this process will prove too slow. Numerous benefits may be derived nonetheless from simply eliminating the "white evils" flour (wheat), table salt, sugar and dairy, even for those who have not determined to go 100% raw. (See Appendix A.)

Indeed, some people are so pleased with the health improvements obtained just by cutting out these four deadly whites that they never do make full transitions to raw diets.

# Reduced Temperature and Heating Time Transition

A third way to transition is to cook your foods at lower temperatures for less time. For example, if you typically eat your vegetables fried, steam them instead for five minutes, then three, then two.

This really only applies to vegetables because few people cook their fruits, and people who eat cooked nuts and seeds usually buy them that way. It is actually rather difficult to find truly raw nuts and seeds, especially because of companies' fears of salmonella poisoning and mold growth, but you can find stores that sell them in the Resource Guide in the back of this book.

This method could be used in conjunction with another method. For example, you could go cold turkey into raw foods but eat your broccoli and other vegetables steamed briefly at low temperatures for a while. This has worked for a lot of people.

## Instantaneous (Cold Turkey) Transition

Many have found that cooked food is so addictive, however, that it is simply better to take the plunge into 100% raw food to get the cravings and withdrawal symptoms over with as soon as possible.

One way to do this that will not frighten the ego so much is to think of going cold turkey as an experiment. You might commit to only one month of 100% raw foods at first, renewable after that.

This is the most sure-fire way to guarantee you will become hooked on a 100% raw food diet. After an entire month of eating 100% raw, organic food, the vast majority of people notice such profound health improvements that they find it impossible to return to old eating patterns. If you want to see dramatic results, stick with it for six months.

A huge advantage of jumping into a 100% raw diet is that you will not battle temptations as much as a part-timer does. After having gone "cold turkey" for a few months, you will no longer be seriously tempted by cooked foods. Even the aromas of coffee and cooking will not disturb you. I have heard a number of long-term raw fooders say that for them, cooked food looks like "plastic" or "pretty decorations" or smells like flower bouquets, but is not something they desire to eat.

Most people who are battling serious illnesses are wise to commit to 100% raw diets immediately, as this may be the only way to facilitate bodily revitalization and detoxification at a rapid enough pace and at deep enough levels to recover. When your life is in danger, you do not have time to waste.

Kristine Nolfi, MD, who healed herself of cancer with a raw diet, said, "The day I discovered I had cancer and had to face death — a painful death within about two years — it was not difficult for me to switch over to a raw food diet. I was grateful that something as simple as that could help me."

In her book *Raw Food Treatment of Cancer,* she explains her choice of this healing method over conventional drug treatment.

## Fasting Followed by Instantaneous Transition

For many, including myself, a brief fast or a diet of only freshly squeezed juice just before beginning an all-raw diet has proved very useful in moving from cooked to raw. I started with two weeks on raw juice, during which time I lost my cravings for salt, coffee and sugar. This made it much easier for me to stick with the raw food diet thereafter. After two weeks of not eating solid food, I was *thrilled* with just some salad and an avocado!

For more information on fasting, please see Chapter 15.

## Green Smoothie Transition

Victoria Boutenko, in her Roseburg Experiment (see page 167), found that when participants simply added a quart of her green smoothies to their daily diets, their cravings for cooked foods, including meat, sweets, alcohol and processed chocolate, disappeared. They began to crave raw food. By gradually replacing meals with green smoothies, many people would experience smooth transitions to raw diets. See "The Green Smoothie Diet" on page 503 for more details of this diet.

For more information, see her book *Green for Life.*

## Just Get Started!

Only you can determine which is the best transition method for you. I've always been one who gets impatient for results, but some like to take things slowly.

Carol Alt (*Eating in the Raw*) says that her athletic hockey-player boyfriend transitioned overnight, but she agrees that this way is not for everyone. She says you can start with baby steps, such as adding olive oil to pasta or other cooked dishes after they are cooked instead of before. Sauté in water instead of oil. Make your own salad dressings instead of buying the pasteurized ones in the store. Buy Ezekiel bread, which is sprouted and baked at low temperatures, though not truly raw, instead of regular bread. For some people, adding a few of these differences every week can build up momentum toward a mostly raw, or 100% raw, diet.

For those of you who are not in a great hurry, an excellent book on transitioning to a raw diet slowly is *The Raw Food Detox Diet* by Natalia Rose. Using her methods, you can transition over a period of years while still achieving many benefits and staying on track.

I once heard David Wolfe say, when asked about how a person could get started on a raw program, that just hanging out in a food co-op would help people get into the swing of it.

At first I thought that was very simplistic advice, but eventually I found myself driving all the way out to our local, organic People's Co-op more and more. I noticed how I loved to bask in the energy there, spending hours every weekend doing research for this book. It reminded me of my college days when I'd hang out at the library café and absorb the intellectual energy, getting inspired to study many more hours than I would normally have done on my own.

Even after publishing the book, I continue to enjoy the atmosphere and community of the co-op. I am certain that quantum physics would confirm the notion that by immersing yourself in the energy field of positive people, you absorb some of their thoughts and attitudes.

# Invest Time in Food Preparation during the First Months

People often remark that I have fantastic willpower to stick to a raw food diet. I tell them that I don't at all; I eat raw food meals that are so deliciously tasty I actually prefer them to cooked ones. Taking time to create wonderful dishes will definitely assist you on the road to raw. You will not feel deprived.

During the transition phase, you will want to take the time to prepare some elaborate dishes to satisfy your tastebuds. Just remember that these recipes, initially time consuming until you get the hang of them, will only be necessary for three to twelve months. Your tastebuds are used to dead foods that have been "enlivened" with intense spices, table salt and other additives, virtually all of which are toxic.

After some time, your tastebuds will become normalized. Live foods, without any sauces or complex chopping and blending, will then completely satisfy you. At that time, you will probably spend far less time in food preparation than you did as a cooked fooder.

Whatever plan you work out, write it down, commit, and stick to it! Give it a chance to see how the experiment works on you.

# (Un)Cookbooks

Although you can find many raw food recipes on the Internet, it is always nice to have several raw food recipe books. There are well over 20 raw recipe books at the time of this writing. I have 19 of them myself. Even if I get only one recipe that becomes a staple in my diet from a particular book, it was worth the investment. I find the books with color photos most inspiring. After a few months of food preparation, you may find yourself creatively coming up with your own raw recipes.

Your tastebuds take time to revert to normal. You have spent decades tantalizing them with spices, MSG — which by law does not have to be listed if it is mixed in with other spices (see Appendix A) — sugar and many other refined and unnatural "foods" or food additives. Once you have cleansed your body of those toxins, you will derive great pleasure from nature's food, our original diet. Then you will feel quite content to munch on olives, nuts or cucumbers. You may not even think in terms of "meals" but simply eat when hungry.

Until the time when you can eat as nature intended, however, you may want to take the time to prepare scrumptious food combinations from raw recipes. This will keep you from backsliding, as you will find raw recipe counterparts for nearly every cooked food you once enjoyed. For example, there are raw food recipes for hummus, pizza, spaghetti, Thai stir "fry," mock meatloaf, burgers, "mashed potatoes," corn chips, soups, tabbouleh and many more.

If you need photographs to inspire you, there are several books with plenty of color photos of raw dishes. Juliano Brotman's *Raw — The Uncook Book* contains some of my favorites. He owns a raw food restaurant in Hollywood and is also chef to some of the stars, such as Demi Moore. Some of the recipes are time-consuming, as they entail making two or three recipes in one. But the results are well worth it — truly gourmet eating.

Roxanne Klein and Charlie Trotter's *Raw* is also heavy-duty gourmet. I used to think Juliano's recipes were complicated until I saw this book. The recipes look intimidating, but once you get started, they are worth it. Each recipe is depicted in a stunning, full-color photo.

A book with simpler and faster-to-make recipes and plenty of color photos is Nomi Shannon's *The Raw Gourmet: Simple Recipes for Living Well.*

A more recent book with plenty of inspirational color photos is *Raw Food/Real World: 100 Recipes to Get the Glow* by Kenney and Malngailis.

As this becomes a more mainstream diet, even HarperCollins has jumped on board with Matt Amsden's recipe book *Rawvolution.*

A book with simple and fast recipes that kids would love is *Eating without Heating* by Sergei and Valya Boutenko. I recommend this to people who have kids since many of the recipes and color photos are of raw cakes, burgers and healthful raw versions of "junk foods" that kids love. It also has the then-teenage authors' story about how eating raw changed their lives and made them much smarter.

Other books that specialize in quick recipes include *Raw Foods for Busy People* by Jordan Maerin, *Raw in Ten Minutes* by Bryan Au, *Alive in 5* by Angela Elliott and *Raw Food Made Easy for 1 or 2 People* by Jennifer Cornbleet.

One of my favorite raw recipe books is *The Complete Book of Raw Food*, edited by Lori Baird. Although there are no photos, it is worth purchasing because it is a compilation of over 350 recipes from the world's top raw food chefs — often their favorites — so every recipe is a winner.

Three books that go into detailed information about each type of raw food and its value, i.e. each specific kind of fruit, vegetable, nut and seed, are *The Sunfood Cuisine* by Frédéric Patenaude; *Rawsome! Maximizing Health, Energy and Culinary Delight with the Raw Foods Diet* by Brigitte Mars, and *Living Cuisine: The Art and Spirit of Raw Foods* by Renée Loux Underkoffler.

One thing I liked about *Rawsome!* is that it contains recipes for raw Indian cuisine, a dining pleasure that I really missed after giving up cooked foods. It also contains many other raw versions of ethnic recipes as well as other gourmet raw dishes.

A recipe book that specializes in low-fat raw dishes is Frédéric Patenaude's *Instant Raw Sensations: The Easiest, Simplest, Most Delicious Raw Food Recipes Ever!*

Gabriel Cousens's *Rainbow Green Live-Food Cuisine* provides 159 pages of scientific and other information about the diet and about 300 pages of recipes.

If you intend to prepare simple recipes following strict Natural Hygiene with proper food combining and no toxic ingredients whatsoever, two books are excellent: Victoria BidWell's *GetWell Recipes from the Garden of Eden* and Dr. Doug Graham's *The High Energy Diet Recipe Guide.*

Don't buy Vonderplanitz's *The Recipe for Living without Disease* unless you are interested in raw animal foods, which make up the bulk of his recipes. (See Appendix C.) He has a lot of interesting scientific information before the recipe section, however.

Many other wonderful recipe books contain useful information or other educational material in addition to the recipes. See the Recipe Book Bibliography on page 575 for more recipe books.

There are also quite a number of videos that show how to make raw food dishes, but don't wait to get a recipe book or a video to get started! You can find dozens, if not hundreds, of raw recipes on the Internet. Simply search for "raw recipes" using your favorite search engine.

I have discovered many recipes on the Internet simply by inserting under Google (www.google.com) the words "raw recipe" along with the particular produce item I wanted to include or dish I wanted to mimic. You will also find many other free recipes at the web sites listed in the Resource Guide beginning on page 579.

# Educate Yourself

It cannot be emphasized enough how important it is to invest in books, especially recipe books, concerning the raw food diet to educate and inspire you. I suggest you read some of the books quoted or cited in this book, the ones that pique your interest. (See the Bibliography.) Go to the web sites referenced in the Resource Guide also.

When you study the health benefits of the raw food diet, you will become less likely to eat cooked food. You will realize that chewing something for a few minutes in your mouth and deriving pleasure for a short period does not come close to compensating for the detrimental effects.

When I was in college, I had a poster that read, "Short on the lips, long on the hips." Since I always put weight on my waist instead of the hips, I added, "Short to taste, long on the waist."

I remember how much I loved to eat at Kentucky Fried Chicken. I used to say, "The saddest moments are when I eat the last bite of my KFC!" Now I realize the highly touted "secret ingredient" was the MSG. (See Appendix A.) The pleasure of cooked food ends with the last bite and is often followed by painful indigestion, whereas the pleasure of radiant health continues throughout the day and night.

Reading, attending workshops and talking to other raw fooders will reinforce your knowledge and belief system, making you stronger in your convictions when you are tempted to give in.

For example, some people quit prematurely because they don't know that detoxification symptoms usually happen only at the beginning of the diet and are actually a good thing, a sign of cleansing. Victoria BidWell says that whenever a fasting patient complains of all the detox symptoms at any Natural Hygiene retreat, he is greeted by, "Wonderful! Something good is happening!" Victoria explains that with this attitude toward detoxification unpleasantries, you can "count it all joy!"

Some quit because they don't know that eating too many raw nuts or vegetables can result in indigestion. Consequently when they bloat, get gas or diarrhea, they think the diet is bad for them.

Others quit in despair because they spend so much time in food preparation. They don't know that after a few months, they will be content with simple, whole foods without needing complicated recipes.

Those who educate themselves on the raw food diet tend to be the ones who stick with it long term.

# Always Focus on the Positive!

It is much easier to take on a new, pleasurable habit than to stop practicing an old, somewhat pleasurable, but destructive, habit. So don't think of yourself as being deprived, having to stop eating the old way. Instead, view this as an adventure!

You will be substituting new, *brand new*, raw food dishes for every cooked dish you eliminate. *Think of all the exciting new dishes you will be tasting!* Take time to prepare raw gourmet dishes from recipe books or from the numerous raw recipes online. Or you might do as many experienced raw fooders do and eat mostly simple, whole foods.

Take time to hunt for ripe, mouthwatering, luscious fruit. There are thousands of different kinds of fruit. Although you may not have access to many varieties where you live, it is possible to mail order others from the Internet. Think of all the new foods you have never even tasted!

This is not a diet of deprivation. Many women who have been accustomed to limiting their fat consumption find that they can eat all the raw fat they desire and still lose or maintain their weight! Raw fat is wonderful, useful for the brain and nerves and required for beautiful skin. Raw fat also helps digest body fat by bringing lipase to it, the enzyme for fat digestion.

Get excited about how wonderful you will soon feel and how great the food you eat will be for perhaps the first time in your life! Inspire yourself by reading testimonials from raw fooders online or in books such as *The Raw Life* and *Raw Knowledge* by Paul Nison. Educate yourself for months reading about the benefits of the raw food diet. Join a raw food support group. If there is not one in your city, join an online one (see the list of chat groups on page 586), or get one started in your area by posting notices at your health food store.

# Kitchen Gadgets

If you prepare raw food that looks and tastes similar to cooked food, it will lead to an easier transition. The food will be so delicious that you will minimize any temptation to go back to cooked foods.

However, you will have to invest in a few gadgets if you don't already have them. Some are more important than others. For the budget conscious, I suggest getting the top brand of only a few, perhaps one at a time, such as the Cuisinart food processor and the Vita-Mix heavy-duty liquifier, or a slightly less expensive, but comparable brand, the Blend-Tec machine (formerly known as K-Tec). I have learned that buying the top quality brands saves money in the long run. You can also find them used in your local classifieds or online at Ebay (www.ebay.com).

If money is not an issue, you may even consider an "extreme kitchen make-over." Some people, for example, get rid of the stove altogether to create more kitchen space for the gadgets or for an additional refrigerator.

In preparing raw gourmet recipes, there are two indispensable kitchen tools: a food processor and a temperature-controlled dehydrator. The food processor will blend the food into a much creamier consistency than a simple blender will. Every week, it will save you hours of chopping, grating or stirring.

If you can afford it, get the Excalibur dehydrator. It dehydrates evenly throughout all the trays and makes it possible to remove some trays so you can put a pan or bowl in the dehydrator, thus making raw pies or warming up soup.

Whatever dehydrator you get must have a temperature control, or chances are it will heat up to 140° F or so, which is well beyond the point of enzyme destruction. You should generally not heat things above 105° F for maximal enzyme protection. I learned to tape the control down, as several times I accidentally bumped the temperature control button, causing everything to get heated up to 140° F. I had to give the food to a neighbor.

When first transitioning to a raw diet, you will love foods straight from the dehydrator the most because they will be slightly warm and crunchy or chewy, more like what you are used to. When first going raw, I found myself eating "garden burgers" or mock pizza straight from the dehydrator so they would not lose any heat!

Another item of great utility is a juicer. I recommend the Omega brand masticating juicer. Nowadays juicers can be found for very reasonable prices that do much more than juice. They may also homogenize soft-serve dishes like frozen fruits, make nut butter, grind seeds and nuts, and even make nut milk.

For most raw fooders, either the Blend-Tec or Vita-Mix is indispensable. The Vita-Mix is a blenderlike machine that has such a powerful motor that it can make cream out of celery in seconds. The motor goes 240 miles per hour, like a hurricane! The Blend-Tec machine is more powerful and a little less expensive than the Vita-Mix but carries a shorter warranty.

The advantage of these machines is that you can make wonderful, creamy soups. Using them, you can also make juice and nut or seed milk if you then apply a strainer. Without a strainer, you make "total juice," which still has the valuable fiber.

With the Vita-Mix, you can make silky-smooth milks without the bother of straining them; with the Blend-Tec, you need a strainer for such nut and seed milks.

The money spent is a lifetime investment in your health. If you use the cheap blenders instead, you will never be able to make the creamy green smoothies (Appendix C) that tear down the cellulose walls of the greens, releasing most of the nutrients.

Be careful not to blend things too long in these machines, as the food can actually become somewhat cooked if overblended. Some people add ice cubes to keep from overheating the food if it must be blended a long time. However, I have not found this to be necessary in the vast majority of cases.

If your juicer doesn't make nut milk, you can purchase a SoyaJoy, which has a nonheating option for making nut milk. Nut milk is great for getting calcium and for kids who are used to dairy milk. Milk from unhulled sesame seeds is also high in calcium. Be sure to use the calcium-rich cream skimmed off in another recipe, such as a soup. These milks look like cow's milk and taste great. You may add a few dates, a bit of agave nectar or unheated honey to sweeten your nut or seed milk a bit.

For just a few dollars you can get a sprouting jar, usually found at your local organic produce store. This is a jar with a wire mesh lid so that you can conveniently rinse the sprouts at least twice a day. In particularly hot, humid climates, the sprouts may need three rinses per day. Missing even one rinse, especially in hotter weather, can cause mold to grow on the sprouts. I once got a headache from eating moldy sprouts. I never forgot to rinse them after that! Another way to avoid mold is to rinse the sprout seeds with a solution of 0.3% hydrogen peroxide, which would be about one ounce of 35% food grade $H_2O_2$ per gallon of water.

A coffee grinder is useful for grinding nuts and seeds into a light, fluffy meal — something your homogenizing juicer cannot do. Be aware that ground nuts and seeds go rancid after three days and should be kept refrigerated even during those few days. The fresher they are when eaten, the better.

Many people like to grind flaxseed to sprinkle over their soups or salads. The "omega-3" fat that flaxseeds contain is great for the brain. Since it may be difficult to find truly raw flax oil that isn't rancid, this is the best way this fat can be absorbed.

The Saladacco, also known as a "spiralizer," is a fun and useful tool for making "spaghetti" strips from zucchinis, carrots, beets, spaghetti squash and yams. The texture of spaghetti is often missed more than the taste, so these make great transition foods. The spiralizer also makes flowerlike strips for garnishing, which truly add beauty and color to a dish.

A citrus juicer will save you a lot of time when you want to squeeze the juice from an orange or lemon and don't want to clean the juicer or take time to peel the fruit. You can get a plastic one very inexpensively or spend a bit more for an electric one. The electric one might be a better investment in the long run, as you will tend to extract even more of the juice.

Be aware, however, that juicing fruits wastes a lot of valuable nutrients. For example, oranges are naturally high in calcium, but orange juice has very little because the calcium is in the pulp. The soluble fiber is beneficial too.

Ice cream lovers may wish to purchase an ice-cream maker so that they can make raw ice cream. Even if you are a vegan, you can enjoy wonderful, delicious "ice cream" by using the cream left over from making nut or seed milk. (See the recipe on page 432.) Coconut cream and milk mixed with a sweetener also make great ice cream.

You will also be able to use many of the same things in your raw food preparation that you used for cooking: a spatula, a set of sharp knives, mixing bowls, measuring cups, a vegetable peeler, a cutting board, a strainer, cheesecloth and a salad shooter.

As for your old pots and pans, you may wish to donate them to a favorite charity or give them away. Keep a few for guests. Unplug your stove and cover it with a large board to give yourself more kitchen space. Throw your microwave out, as studies have shown that microwaved food is very toxic.

You may choose to hold on to your coffee maker. If you get involved in fasting, it is useful for making coffee enemas to aid in detoxification. This is part of the famous cancer cure at the Gerson Institute. Some people go through a mild coffee withdrawal after the cleanse, however. Yet many believe that coffee is a powerful way to detoxify the liver. Hygienists say it is too toxic to use. Some people trying to kick the coffee habit may not be able to endure the temptation to make beverage coffee with this gadget hanging around.

# Meal and Snack Planning

If you have been eating the SAD, you may be used to little or no meal preparation. You may have been eating out of cans, bags, microwave prepared dishes, restaurants and such. You may have gone to the grocery as infrequently as once in two weeks!

Going raw after spending so little time on food preparation can at first appear overwhelming. Suddenly, you realize you cannot depend on the freezer or cupboard to stash "dead" food that has no expiration date. Suddenly, you realize you cannot eat from vending machines or count on corner fast-food restaurants in times of emergency.

You will have to spend time planning meals, *but your health is worth it*. You may want to join a food co-op if one is conveniently located, as this will save on your grocery bill when you buy high quality organic produce.

You could also join a Community Supported Agriculture (CSA) farm and frequent farmers' markets for fresher produce than you will usually find at your grocery store — the fresher, the more nutrients.

You may wish to visit U-pick farms and rural roadside food stands, learn to grow your own food, even if from the balcony of your apartment, and purchase sun-dried fruits and truly raw organic nuts by mail order or online at some of the stores listed in the back of this book.

You can also save money by ordering produce by the case from the local organic supermarket. For information about where to find local farmers' markets, CSAs and food co-ops, visit www.greenpeople.com or www.localharvest.com.

You will need to pore through recipe books, planning which dishes to make for the week. Make a list of all the produce you will need, along with the corresponding dishes you will prepare. Make a list of all the snacks or lunch meals you will need. Then prepare enough food so that you will have leftovers the next day. This way you will not have to prepare food each day, although if you do have the time, fresh is always better in taste and nutrients.

You will need to pack lunches and snacks for work or school. Do this the night before to be sure that you will have them no matter how rushed you are in the morning.

Although going raw will temporarily mean more time for food prep, eventually you will become satisfied eating more simply. A plain avocado will have its own symphony of flavors. A burst of flavor will spring forth from a bite of raw walnuts.

There are now a vast number of good prepared raw snacks available online or in stores. They may appear somewhat expensive if you are used to buying cheap junk food like crackers or chips. Just remember that this is fresh food with a shelf life of weeks, not years, and that it is all organic produce. *You are worth it!*

Moreover, you will find that you will not need to eat as much since the food is so nutritious and satisfying. Once you have tried these pricey raw snacks, you might be inspired to create your own favorites at a mere fraction of the cost and keep them on hand.

As this diet catches on, more companies will produce more goodies because consumers will vote with their money and demand it. *In the meantime, don't let society's preferences set standards for you!*

## Stand Firm in Your Commitment!

If you decide to go 100% raw, you may want to inform all of your friends, or you may decide to wait until you've passed your first one-month hurdle so you don't look like a fool if you give up after three days.

Victoria Boutenko suggests that you decline all dinner invitations, potlucks or any social activities with cooked food for the first two months. Putting yourself in a "temptation-free zone" for two months will give you time to detoxify until most of your cooked food cravings are gone.

Why needlessly suffer by being around cooked food that you want but won't allow yourself to eat? After a few months, such food may not even be tempting. The physical cravings will be gone, at least. Some of the psychological cravings may take longer. For example, the smell of freshly baked cookies may remind you of your mother's love for you. But once you are free of addiction, the memory alone will no longer compel you to eat them.

One study, "Factors affecting adherence to a raw vegan diet," published in the February 2008 issue of *Complementary Therapies in Clinical Practice*, showed which factors make it more likely a person will stay raw. Some of these factors you don't want to have, like morbid disease, poor physical quality of life and few close friends and relatives! Others you can cultivate, such as belief in your ability to stay raw and higher education.

You can still enjoy friends and relatives if you go to social functions with your raw treats. You can increase your faith in yourself by behavior modification (see Appendix E), and you can educate yourself on the benefits of a raw diet even if you don't have a high school diploma.

# Foods to Stockpile

There are six basic kinds of raw plant foods: fruits, vegetables, nuts, seeds, sprouts and fermented foods. Sprouts include sprouted nuts, seeds, grains and legumes. Fermented foods include miso, tempeh, vinegar, sauerkraut and even wine.

Although some of these fermented foods are not technically raw, having been cooked prior to fermentation, the fermentation process imparts enzymes and makes them acceptable to many raw fooders when eaten occasionally.

However, Natural Hygiene teaches us that the alcohol content of fermented foods is poisonous and that vinegar, which is acetic acid diluted to 5%, is toxic to humans, even when consumed in small amounts. Purists shun their use.

From this palette of raw foods, a huge variety of soups, salads, salad dressings, crackers, breads, desserts, smoothies, pâtés and entrées can be prepared.

Some of the foods mentioned in this section may be hard to find, even at your local health food store. For this reason, some raw food stores that accept orders by phone or e-mail are listed in the Resource Guide.

You will want most of your food to be as fresh as possible. However, there are certain things you can store in your cupboard. Just make sure they are really raw, as the word "raw" means different things for different people. (See Chapter 18.)

Throw out your table salt, which is very toxic. (See Appendix A.) Some raw fooders invest in Celtic sea salt or the more recently popular Himalayan crystal salt, discussed in *Water & Salt: The Essence of Life* by Dr. Barbara Hendel. But Natural Hygiene considers all inorganic sources of sodium chloride to be toxic. Followers opt instead for foods naturally high in sodium, such as celery — juiced, shredded, chopped or liquefied — spinach, chard or sea vegetables: typically dulse, kelp and nori, which are the easiest ones to find in most health food stores.

Since you will not be using iodized table salt, you will need to make sure you get sufficient iodine. This is important in keeping the thyroid in good health. Low thyroid function is often a cause of fatigue and weight gain. Great sources of iodine include the following sea vegetables: dulse, kelp, arame, nori, wakame, hijiki and spirulina algae. I get liquid dulse and put some drops in my green juice. I sometimes sprinkle sea vegetables in with my salad.

Keep raw olive oil on hand for making salad dressings. Just mix it with raw apple cider vinegar and possibly unheated honey or raw agave nectar if you don't have time for a more elaborate recipe. The vinegar should be refrigerated once opened. Some have concluded that the oil needs to be refrigerated as well, whereas others, such as Aajonus Vonderplanitz, have decided that refrigeration destroys too many of its nutrients.

Another oil to keep on hand is raw coconut butter or oil. This is used in a lot of desserts and takes the place of dairy butter. I found out the hard way that raw coconut butter or oil shouldn't be used in salad dressings because if you refrigerate it, it congeals like butter. However, you could use it in a dressing if it's oily at room temperature and eaten right away.

Natural Hygiene teaches that we should exclude all refined oils: they are not natural foods. They are fragmented, highly caloric, too easy to overindulge and potentially addictive, which encourages overeating.

I suggest having several jars of raw, organic olives in the refrigerator. These make great snack foods and garnishes. Frédéric Patenaude suggests soaking olives that contain salt in pure water for 24 hours to release the harmful salt.

Nuts and seeds are items you can stock up on to a degree. If you buy them in a health food shop, and they have been sitting in bins for a long time, they may not be very fresh. You can purchase them from an organic food distributor, such as The Living Tree Community or Sunorganic Farm, both in California, and they will be shipped in thick plastic bags, which keep them very fresh. (See the Resource Guide for contact information.)

You can store some nuts and seeds in the freezer for up to six months. Freezing does destroy some enzymes, but not so much with nuts or other low-water-content foods. If you plan to use them soon, you may keep them in tightly enclosed containers or sealed thick bags. It is better to keep them in the refrigerator or freezer if they will not be eaten within a month or so.

Keep a few cups of flaxseeds around for making crackers. Sunflower seeds should be kept handy, as they are often required in raw recipes and are also good for sprouting, trail mix and sprinkling on salads.

Brazil nuts should be around your kitchen at all times. They are rich in selenium, an essential mineral depleted in much of our soils.

Keep a stock of pumpkin seeds, as they are high in zinc and tryptophan, an amino acid that the body uses in relieving depression and insomnia. If you wish to be a raw vegan, selenium and zinc are difficult to obtain in sufficient quantities without brazil nuts and pumpkin seeds.

Before eating nuts and seeds, make sure you soak them overnight and thoroughly rinse them to deactivate enzyme inhibitors. Even before doing that, it is good to soak them in a solution of $^{11}/_{12}$ water and $^{1}/_{12}$ food grade (35%) hydrogen peroxide in order to rid them of molds. Note that hydrogen peroxide purchased at drugstores, which is not food grade, contains toxic preservative chemicals.

According to Elizabeth Baker, this step is necessary because, as the oxygen is becoming more and more depleted in our environment, molds are increasing. Soak nuts and seeds for just eight to ten minutes, then drain the solution and rinse them very well. After that, soak them six to twelve hours in distilled or spring water. In a pinch for time, you can soak them two to three hours.

Most nuts and seeds nearly double in volume after being soaked. Soaked nuts and seeds not used right away should be kept in the refrigerator. Dehydrate them if you like them crunchy.

As explained in Appendix A, "Killer 'Foods' to Avoid," dairy is not the great source of calcium that it has been hyped up to be. You need to have a stock of seeds and nuts for calcium. Unhulled sesame seeds are the richest. Almonds are also high in calcium, but are now very hard to find *truly raw*.

Raw store-bought nut and seed butters are great to have on hand. They are used in quite a few recipes and are also handy to spread on a cabbage leaf or flaxseed crackers. Once opened, the jars should be kept refrigerated. The same goes of course for the homemade nut and seed butters.

Organic seeds for sprouting should also be kept on hand; they have a shelf life of ten years. They should be kept in tightly closed containers or bags.

Dehydrated or dried fruit is great to have around. If the label says "sun-dried," you know it is raw. If not, you must call the company to find out at what temperature it was dehydrated because it is typically over 118° F. Dehydrated fruit, such as sun-dried mangoes, apricots, apples, figs, prunes and raisins, can be kept on the shelf in tightly closed containers but should really be kept refrigerated unless eaten within a few weeks, as they often tend to ferment. These dried fruits can be used during the winter when fresh fruits are out of season. They can also be combined with nuts to make trail mix.

Make sure dehydrated fruits are organic and unsulfured. Sulfur nitrate and nitrite are chemicals used for preservation and color. For example, while orange-colored dried apricots may look more appealing to the eye than brown ones, the orange ones are sulfured and therefore toxic.

Dr. Harvey Wiley, former chief chemist of the United States Department of Agriculture (USDA), claimed that adding sulfurous acid to food is harmful to both the food and our bodies. It destroys vitamins in the fruit, degenerates the kidneys, and retards the formation of red blood corpuscles. If the label does not indicate unsulfured, assume that the fruit is sulfured.

Garlic, ginger, parsley, cilantro, onions, unpasteurized miso and lemons may always be kept in stock. They are used as seasonings in many raw recipes. Avocados and raw olive oil are commonly used as well.

Raw, unheated honey is a great food to have in your cupboard. It will last forever! Unprocessed honey has been known to last literally thousands of years. Jars of perfectly preserved honey were unearthed in the tombs of Egyptian pyramids. Honey is also very rich in enzymes.

Unheated honey can be purchased at farmers' markets or from local bee-keepers. However being an animal product, honey is neither considered vegan nor recommended by Natural Hygiene because of its formic acid content.

Stevia extract is a better choice if you are diabetic or hypoglycemic. Even when it is not raw, you need only a tiny bit since it is 200 times sweeter than table sugar. You can also grow your own in flowerpots.

If you do not like stevia's aftertaste, use agave nectar, which is low in its glycemic effect on the body and is plant based. Agave is a sweet liquid that comes from the cactus plant. If it is dark, it is not raw, but the light-brown-colored one is raw if so labeled.

Keep a tray of wheatgrass if you have a machine that juices wheatgrass. Dr. Ann Wigmore, founder of the Hippocrates Health Institute, experimented with feeding animals grasses and found that they instinctively preferred wheatgrass. She encouraged city dwellers to take two ounces thrice daily to protect themselves from air pollution and people with degenerative disease to take two ounces thrice also. I prefer to save time by keeping dehydrated wheatgrass on hand. If you do that, check with the company that processes it to be sure it has been dehydrated at less than 118° F. I sell such an item at www.livefoodfactor.com.

Always have mixed green leafy vegetables in the refrigerator. Putting them in the refrigerator inside a large plastic container with an unbleached paper towel on the bottom will help them last longer, as much of the moisture will be absorbed by the towel. You can also buy special green-plastic storage bags at a Whole Foods supermarket that have been shown to keep produce fresher longer.

By the way, don't toss the leaves from carrot, turnip or beet bunches. Put them in salads or in green smoothies. *The leaves are actually higher in minerals than are the root vegetables themselves.*

Always have a variety of fruits on hand. Fruits are foods that come from a flower and are the ripened ovary of the female flower. They typically contain seeds.

There are many different categories of fruits:

*Acid fruits* are mildly sweet and somewhat sour or tart. These include most berries, grapefruit, lemons, limes, oranges, sour apples, sour grapes and more.

*Subacid fruits* are also mildly sweet and sometimes carry a somewhat sour or tart punch. These include apples, apricots, papayas, peaches, pears, mangoes, plums and more.

*Sweet fruits* are very sweet and what we usually think of when hearing the word "fruit." These include bananas, cherimoyas, dates, figs, grapes, persimmons and so many more. Also included is all dried fruit.

Very few fruits have significant fat content. Those that do are *fatty fruits* and include avocados, olives and durians.

*Nonsweet fruits* are commonly mistaken for vegetables but are classified in botany as fruits since they bear seeds. These include tomatoes, cucumbers, okra, eggplants, bell peppers, zucchini and squash.

*Melons* include cantaloupe, casaba, crenshaw, honeydew, muskmelon, all other more exotic melons and watermelon (not a true melon).

See the food classification chart of each of these fruit categories beginning on page 557 for additional examples.

A common beginner mistake is to eat fruits before they have fully ripened. For example, bananas should have brown spots or streaks on the skins when they are ready to be eaten. Mangoes, persimmons, kiwis and various others should be soft with wrinkly skin. Papayas should have an orange, not green, skin. Eating unripe fruit can be a rather unpleasant experience. When in doubt, look for a tempting aroma to emanate from it before digging in.

# Techniques for Getting Off Cooked Foods and in Touch with Genuine Hunger

The following summarizes Victoria BidWell's teachings from throughout *The Natural Weight-Loss System*, a course published by T. C. Fry in 1986:

Although *weight loss* is in the title of this program, the text has helped thousands who were not overweight to overcome their cooked food addictions and/or eating disorders and stay on a hygienic program.

The process of relearning established patterns and replacing old, undesired habits with new, desired habits is called *behavior modification*, a social science popularized in the 1960s.

With this approach, the health seeker does not try to change a bothersome habit through deep psychological introspection, journalizing, affirmations and/or analysis. Rather, he or she focuses on the specific old *behavior* that needs *modification* and practices a new sequence of events to bring about the desired new outcome by means of a conditioned response. A system of punishments ("negative reinforcement") and rewards ("positive reinforcement") — disease symptoms and health benefits, respectively, in this case — helps condition the new response.

Studies show that consistent repetition of the new, modified behavior over a period of approximately 21-28 days leads to the automatic supplanting of the new, desired behavior pattern in place of the old, troublesome behavior pattern. This is why you have probably often heard that most self-improvement plans run for a minimum of 21 days, including many inpatient detox centers' programs.

The health seeker who unwillingly overeats time and time again can learn to systematically practice simple behaviors to get rid of compulsiveness by slowing down the time it takes to eat, thus increasing awareness of eating and also allowing time for genuine hunger to be satisfied and natural satiety to be reached. Each exercise, however simple-minded in appearance, helps to short-circuit that formerly "uncontrollable" urge to keep eating beyond the body's needs in order to serve the jaded appetite.

The following exercises restore controlled awareness, which makes impossible that craze-driven feeling that "no amount of food is ever enough." Of course these exercises work best not with cooked food, but with raw food since both the physiological and psychological addictiveness of cooked food reinforces the former overeating behavior.

## How to Slow Down Your Eating

- Take a few minutes or more of silence to relax before the meal.
- Take at least 20 minutes to eat the meal.
- Eat as a *pure activity* — no television, reading or other activity — or with light, pleasant conversation when with others.
- Put your utensil down between bites — or your food if no utensil is being used.

- Take time to chew the bite completely. In the mid-1800s, health promoter Horace Fletcher popularized chewing each mouthful a minimum of 32 times. The practice became known as *fletcherizing*.
- Take smaller bites.
- Use a napkin between bites.
- Stop eating completely for 5 minutes during the meal and relax.

## How To Finish Your Meal

- Stop eating before feeling the discomfort of abdominal distension and certainly before the pain of being too full.
- Stop eating when the taste of the food becomes less flavorful.
- Keep leftovers for second helpings completely out of sight. This will minimize your taking of second helpings.
- Leave just a little food on the plate to reinforce the idea that you do not have to eat everything all of the time.
- Leave the table or eating area when finished.
- Rest a few minutes after each meal if possible.
- Practice all behaviors with each meal for best results.

For more of Victoria's behavior modification program, see Appendix E.

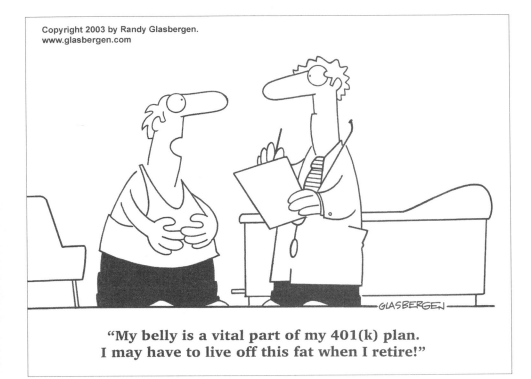

"My belly is a vital part of my 401(k) plan.
I may have to live off this fat when I retire!"

# 14

# Detoxification and Healing

When the elimination process is developed and toxic materials are ready to be thrown off by a strong body, we have literally earned a healing crisis. That healing crisis is what we need for nature's version of what we call a "cure."
—Dr. Bernard Jensen, DC (1908–2001)

Now that you are going raw, your body will conserve much of the energy that it otherwise would have expended to make the enzymes necessary for digesting cooked food. Your body will be free to use elsewhere the energy formerly allocated to the energy-expensive tasks of digesting, absorbing, assimilating and converting nutrients from cooked food into tissues and fluids. Your body will further conserve energy formerly used in having to eliminate — or store if energy reserves are low — the poisons in these cooked, processed, refined foods.

Victoria BidWell is fond of reminding me, "It's all about energy!" As a former stimulant addict, I now realize I was looking for energy in all the wrong places. Toxic food, drink and medications appeared to supply energy momentarily when my metabolism shifted into high gear to eliminate them. All the while, taking these protoplasmic poisons actually led to *wasted energy*.

I want to thank Victoria and Dr. Vetrano for their extensive contributions and editing running throughout this chapter and the next. In Chapters 14 and 15, we will be building on the foundational alternative health care science and teachings laid down in Chapters 4 through 7. Your review of these chapters would be most useful at this point. Victoria and Dr. Vetrano provide this summary:

---

If we want more energy, we must stop wasting it and start generating it. Real energy is generated while engaged in just one of the ten energy enhancers. Can you guess which one? It is during sleep primarily, as well as during other periods of rest, all forms of quiet meditation and/or fasting on water only. Energy is expended while engaged in all the other nine energy enhancers, but its use is minimized. The very biggest conserver of all the other nine energy enhancers is a clean raw diet. *When all is said and done, as health seekers, we are energy conservationists of our own body ecologies.*

All the energy freed up with the raw diet can now be used for cleansing, biochemical balancing, repair and other life-supporting, health-enhancing work. As soon as sufficient energy reserves are replenished, your body will proceed to de-

---

toxify and heal itself at the cellular and subcellular levels. As elimination of toxins proceeds, actual normalization of cellular structure and function at the molecular, atomic and subatomic levels will lead to repair and rebuilding of cells, tissues, organs and entire systems. These events have been likened to *natural microsurgery at its finest.*

Few people are at the pathological point of no return. Except for those rare cases, this cleansing and subsequent complete healing (for acute cases) and partial to near-complete healing (for chronic cases) is available to everyone. Learning and applying this knowledge is like winning the superlative health lottery! *And everyone who enters and stays with it is a winner.*

Although most people can safely go through toxin elimination and healing on their own, we are including a precautionary disclaimer from our *Health Seekers' YearBook*: "If you are ill or on medication, do not attempt this program without the supervision of a practitioner experienced in the dramatic effects of turning from a lifestyle that engenders disease to one that promotes health." We further advise, *"It is absolutely essential that you consult an alternative medical doctor before discontinuing any prescribed medications."*

The body is amazing in its ability to regenerate, repair and renew once the conditions for health are supplied! The natural diet for humans is composed of nontoxic raw foods, eaten in proper combination for ideal digestion, in moderate amounts and under conditions of emotional balance. This biologically correct food supplies the body with the nutrition it needs to optimize these processes. Also important are the nondietary forms of nutrition: clean air, pure water, sunshine and — especially — adequate rest and sleep. Well-supplied with these nutritive factors, the body will proceed to detoxify and heal tissues in its own chosen order and in its own sweet time.

The person in acute stages of illness who experiences a symptom flare-up or who just feels tired, uninspired and out of sorts all of the time, both situations being typical of the earlier stages of disease, will have an easier and speedier time of elimination of toxins and recovery than someone in the later stages of chronic, degenerative disease. (See "The Seven Stages of Disease" on page 548.)

For the individual who has been burning the energy candle at both ends, microscopic waste residues, exogenous chemicals and toxic endogenous byproducts of metabolism inevitably accumulate from years on SAD, cooked and poorly combined foods. Lacking the energy to keep itself clean, the body adapts with a process called *disease.* All endogenous and exogenous remote sources of toxemia including SAD, cooked food toxins end up in one of three places: they are deposited within cellular protoplasm; they are present in the fluids around cells and tissues, or they circulate in the bloodstream and lymphatic system.

Happily, all these poisons are mobilized for elimination just as soon as sufficient energy supplies are replenished! As elimination of toxins proceeds, they enter bodily fluids and exit through the primary organs and systems of excretion. The largest excretory system of the body is the skin, adding up to about 15 square feet. The excretory organ doing the most work, however, is the liver. The other primary organs of elimination are the lungs, kidneys, digestive tract and the circulatory and lymphatic systems.

Now we see the beauty and promise of going through detoxification and healing! Many people experience the process as episodes of healing crises recurring over various time intervals: hours, days, weeks, months or even years for the person in advanced stages of degeneration. *These episodes are invariably interspersed with periods of natural highs that eventually stabilize and become the permanent condition: clear-headed, euphoric well-being accompanied by physiological peace unlike anything experienced in recent years or past decades.*

Homeopathic pioneer Samuel Hahnemann, MD (1755–1843), observed that healing tends to proceed in reverse order from when the symptoms first appeared. Consider all the exogenous toxins of food-generated residues, the endogenous toxins of poor food combining and the ingested, absorbed and inhaled environmental pollutants, as well as drugs taken. These toxins are all retained and build up when there is an energy crisis in a toxic body. They typically detoxify in reverse order from when they were either taken into the body or created within the body and then accumulated.

In other words, you will probably detoxify from the lactic acid created from this afternoon's exercise routine before the toxins created and stored from last month's poorly combined meal. You will probably detoxify from the hamburger you ate yesterday before the grilled steak you ate last July.

What should you expect? As long as you observe a complete package of healthful living practices, especially adequate rest and sleep, then revitalization, cleansing and repair will proceed. Progress is more rapid for some than for others. *The pace is speediest while eating 100% raw.* The pace proceeds more slowly when you are only partially raw. Even when you are eating merely 5% cooked food, the process slows down.

So if you stay 100% or mostly all-raw and provide all the other conditions for superlative health in the right amounts, your body will eventually rid itself of virtually all toxins accumulated ever since infancy — the more raw the better! After revitalization, the processes of detoxification, renewal, repair and biochemical rebalancing take place simultaneously. The body's healing intelligence is awesome!

The bulk of this process usually completes within weeks or months for most people who are more tired than toxic. Dr. Vetrano realistically estimates it could take more than a year for the seriously sick person who is enervated, toxic and into latter stages of disease. For the very ill, the deepest levels of excretion of poisons and subsequent renewal can be expected to take years. Who cares? However long it takes, you are getting better, sometimes noticeably and dramatically better, every *week* if not every *day*!

Although it can never be proven scientifically, we go by a simple rule of thumb. For every year of eating cooked food, you need a strict month of doing everything right. This means especially eating a nearly all, if not 100%, raw food diet and getting plenty of rest, sleep and practicing all the other eight energy enhancers. The entire cleansing, renewal and healing process is greatly sped up by a period of fasting. Think of it as *fast*-ing.

# The Fatigue Factor

Many people going through detoxification complain of feeling "so tired all the time." In the following, Victoria explains this fatigue factor letdown as simply, "What goes up must come down!"

Reasons are two-fold why a health seeker, when going onto raw, wholesome, nontoxic, nonstimulating foods, feels especially tired, out of sorts and maybe discouraged and perhaps even lacking the mental/emotional wherewithal to continue.

First, the body is no longer continually stimulated with toxic food/drink. This leaves the detoxer to experience his actual state of extreme tiredness. The continual excitation and titillation are severely missed by the former stimulant junkie once they have been cut off. They had been delivering what felt like a genuine energetic boost. In physiological reality, the body had been overworked to expel the stimulants. You can only whip a tired horse so long before he can no longer respond with energy bursts and drops to his knees in agony.

Second, the body is working hard to detox existing poisons from fluids and tissues. This requires extra energy and leaves the detoxer feeling extra fatigued. (See the Law of Stimulation or Dual Effect on page 551.)

A person who cannot get going in the morning without coffee is *the* classic example of this drugging/stimulating effect in action. But that effect is also present within all toxic food/drink he ingests. This energetic boost is a *total illusion*. In physiological reality, it is a drain and not a boost! Stimulants in toxic food/drink are causing the body to go into an alarm mode. This squanders energy if the reserves are near-full, and the person feels energetic for the moment. This drains the last bit of energy if the reserves are near-empty, and the person crashes soon thereafter.

Dr. Shelton exclaimed, "We should get out of bed in the morning with a bounce!" Yet an estimated 90% of American adults have to jump-start with this dark brew. Drinking coffee is just beating your already tired body to get a little more mileage out of you before you collapse. (See the Law of Stimulation on page 551.)

What goes up must come down! When a person stimulates himself with a drug (cooked toxic food/drink) and feels up, he must come down with the inevitable drop in energy. Among health seekers who quit the poisons altogether and become bona fide detoxers, most experience this unpleasant fatigue factor. They dive into the physical, mental and emotional doldrums and can hardly drag themselves around. This is not the time to quit! *Revitalization is just around the corner.*

Since all foods/drinks on the Standard American Diet are toxic, ingestion of their exogenous poisons sets up a dangerous chain of events that leads first to exhaustion and finally to disease and untimely death. Certain foods and chemicals can be singled out as especially hazardous to your health — such as meat and dairy, refined sugar and flour, all excitotoxins, salt, all hot spices and caffeine. The fact is that all cooked and/or SAD food is stimulating, toxic, energy draining, and disease promoting. They all lead to an early grave.

These are the fatigue factor links in this health-robbing chain of events:

▶ Habitual ingestion of SAD food/drink, most of which is cooked, introduces exogenous poisons into the body.

▶ Digestion of poorly combined foods releases endogenous byproduct toxins into the body.

▶ Continual stimulation and irritation to the body's 75 trillion cells results in protoplasmic poisoning of tissues and fluids.

▶ Bodily toleration to poisons builds up while energy reserves drain down.

▶ Biochemical and psychological addiction sets in as the body reaches the upper limits of its ability to tolerate poisons.

▶ The SAD cooked food eater experiences constant stimulation boosts because his body is now in chronic activation of the fight-or-flight response as long as the food/drink poisons are ingested on a daily basis.

▶ The second-to-second drain of energy on the body to deal with SAD, toxic food/drink leads to energy fatigue, termed *enervation*, and to subsequent auto-intoxication.

▶ And the final fatal link? Once enervation sets in, the SAD cooked food addict has begun the descent into acute and then chronic disease and is well on his way to an early and miserable death. *No fun.*

Dr. Doug Graham summarizes the fatigue factor, "Most of what is called 'detox' is actually the reaction of a body that is no longer being irritated or stimulated — effectively 'forced' to function. The secondary effect of stimulation is sedation. Thus it is common to feel tired when [people] first [start on] the raw diet. It is not that the raw diet is making them tired; it is that they are actually 'coming down' off of the influence of coffee, refined sugars, meats and other stimulating foods" (*The 80/10/10 Diet*, p. 62).

# Possible Detoxification Symptoms

While serving as head instructor and exam corrector for many of the 3,000 students taking T. C. Fry's 2,200-page correspondence course, now a huge book entitled *The Life Science Health System*, Victoria BidWell prepared from it an overview of what symptoms to expect when providing your body the ideal conditions for detoxifying and healing. Our list lady Victoria alerts us to four certain and nineteen possible detoxification symptoms in the following:

You cannot make deals with your body or control its DNA-determined events. You can never know exactly what to expect. Every person is different, depending on inherited predisposition, available nerve energy supplies, amounts and kinds of toxins present and irreversible damage already done. How strict you get with the ten energy enhancers is the final determining factor. I can, however, preview for you what to expect.

Some health seekers undergo a lengthy, dramatic, troublesome and even miserable detoxification. Others notice no discomfort at all as they enjoy ever-increasing levels of higher energy and sharper mental clarity and higher Natural

Hygiene joy! Whether you experience one of these extremes or find yourself somewhere in between, be alerted to the more common detox symptoms. Ride on through them to get to the other side and reach your greatest state of superlative health and joy.

Next is a 23 point list of what to expect while fasting or eating a nontoxic raw diet. The first four describe initial and ongoing events common to all detoxing health seekers for the duration. The remaining 19 appear in no particular order. They may or may not be the detoxer's experience as revitalization, cleansing, repair and biochemical balancing take place simultaneously, or at least in stages and cycles, throughout the body's 75 trillion cells. I repeat: *Every detoxer's experience is different.*

1. *Nerve energy supplies revitalize.* This physiological event sounds too abstract to grasp. But we get it when we see firsthand or learn of health seekers who do revitalize. They start a fast while terribly tired. They remain terribly tired for days and even weeks. And then they revitalize so fully that many disease symptoms disappear. They move about energized and look bright-eyed and bushy-tailed — all without having eaten an ounce of foods for many days and even weeks! If we had a meter to measure nerve energy supplies for such detoxers, it would be obvious that while getting well, this meter's needle would have moved from *near-empty* to *near-full.*

2. *Body chemistry normalizes.* Dr. David Scott of Scott's Natural Health Institute in Strongsville, Ohio, has developed his own blood tests on about 100 different parameters that he works up on a weekly basis for patients at his facility. So useful in charting progress are these blood tests that he requires them before admitting his patients.

Most do fast during their visits, but some are simply eating raw and living the ten energy enhancers. Invariably, every patient with out-of-range initial readings shows blood chemistry normalizing, often after a healing crisis. If bodily reserves are adequate and time allows, a patient may fast to complete normalization on all parameters. If reserves are inadequate, refeeding commences with periods of detoxification, healing and body chemistry balancing taking place while feeding on nontoxic live food meals and/or drinks until reserves are built up.

While blood tests are seldom required at other alternative health care facilities, guests/patients can request them. Similar results of blood chemistry normalizing, with the health seekers going through healing crises that end in normalizing (whether fasting or living strictly on the clean raw diet) are virtually universal in all cases. Without the costly blood tests, we can only surmise that body chemistry is normalizing in ourselves too when we undertake to detox, whether it is during an at-home or in-clinic fast or by the slower route of eating raw foods and strict application of the ten energy enhancers.

I recently asked Dr. Scott if, in his opinion, a person in apparently good health, with no chronic, degenerative problems, a person who just wanted to start his or her own detoxing program by fasting and without going to a retreat, could safely undertake a short fast of seven to ten days. His response was a definite, "Yes. That should not be a problem under those circumstances, as long as the person is truly fasting, staying in bed, resting and avoiding stimulations of all kinds."

252

3. *Blood, fluids and tissues are cleansed.* At Dr. Scott's Natural Health Institute, prior to undertaking a fast and at the end of the visit, the patient may be invited to observe a sample of his or her own live blood under a glass slide and through a microscope. Dr. Scott's sophisticated technology allows you to view the microscope picture of your blood sample, greatly enlarged, on color television. Typically, prior to the fast, the blood is filled with unmistakable debris. But the blood is seen to be startlingly clear and clean afterwards. This is the scientific, impressive, astounding proof of Dr. Tilden's Seven Stages of Disease paradigm! (See page 548.)

4. The tongue gets coated and tastes bitter. The coated tongue may be light and barely white to heavy and furry. Depending on what is being eliminated, the coated tongue can exhibit any range of colors, from the most common white to greenish to reds and browns. This detoxer's tongue is the single, most visible sign that the body is cleansing. If a person fasts to completion, the tongue will turn pink and clean. The breath will smell pleasant. The bitter taste will disappear. These events occur at about the same time that a genuine and compelling hunger returns.

If a faster breaks his fast to begin refeeding without going to completion, the white and furry tongue will disappear, often within minutes or sometimes hours after that first bite of nontoxic raw food. But the telltale detoxer's tongue will just as speedily return between feedings as long as clean raw foods are taken. *This is the sure sign that detoxing is continuing.*

While eating the nontoxic raw diet and when elimination of toxins is not yet complete, health seekers will therefore experience the detoxer's tongue between meals and snacks, usually slightly. It is more dramatic upon awakening to break the night's fast/sleep with breakfast. With the morning meal, we are literally breaking a fast of the night's sleep: that is why the word elements = *break + fast.*

▶ Headaches are the nearly universal join-the-club badge of the toxic faster or detoxing raw fooder. They result primarily from withdrawals of the most notorious of the exogenous toxins: caffeine, nicotine, alcohol, sodium chloride, cooked food, SAD food and drugs.

▶ When resting nearly 24/7 and not eating, the faster needs less sleep. In fact the most common complaint of most fasters after the headache is the inability to sleep. Some speculate that while toxins are circulating in the bodily fluids in preparation for elimination, the poisons can stimulate the mental, emotional and physical functioning. Insomnia results.

▶ Nervous irritability and irrational emotional outbreaks can occur. These are also withdrawal symptoms, commonly experienced for 3-10 days and sometimes in cycles. Because of this unstable emotional/mental state, detoxers are forewarned not to make major, life-changing decisions until withdrawal is complete and stability regained. I have seen many people mess up their lives for years to come by not heeding this warning.

▶ Cleansing, and more so during periods of fasting than while eating raw, can bring about a unique physiological state with unique brain function. This state is often called *faster's high* or *detoxer's high*. Whether fasting or eating all nontoxic raw foods, this pleasurable altered state of consciousness is also called a *spiritual high* because the mind is so much sharper and clearer. Some even report being visionary in perception and thought.

This spiritual high is brought on by one or more events: by the detoxer's experience of deep rest and revitalization, by the lightening of the detoxer's toxic overload, by the detoxer completely letting go of emotional stresses, and by trusting completely in the healing powers of the body.

Finally, physiology explains the high. It is brought on when the 200 billion brain cells live not on glucose from daily food or stored glycogen, but on released and oxidized fatty acids from stored fat. This unique physiological state is called *ketosis*. The altered neuron and total body function from all of the above can result in extraordinary mental, emotional and/or spiritual experiences, especially if the detoxer has a big imagination and/or a mindset that enjoys transcending the material world.

▶ The kidneys increase filtration. The urine becomes foul smelling and dark colored. Kidney stones are sometimes passed.

▶ The liver undergoes cleansing, sometimes with virtually no symptoms, except for blood tests that show out-of-normal readings indicating a healing crisis in progress. A complete liver cleansing is typically followed by disappearance of any existing so-called liver spots or age spots on hands, legs, face and elsewhere.

▶ The gallbladder cleanses. Bile is sometimes vomited. Stones are sometimes passed.

▶ The mucous membranes throughout the length of the digestive tract and respiratory system are cleansed. Throughout every body orifice, phlegm is coughed up, sneezed out and otherwise eliminated by nearly every detoxer at some point. Phlegm is the sticky vehicle in which ride toxins for elimination. Phlegm appears in differing shades of whites, greens and browns.

▶ What the medical mentality calls the *flu* or *common cold* can occur. Symptoms include the following: cold sores, fever, shivering, sneezing, runny nose, coughing, sinusitis, inability to keep warm and more. In Natural Hygiene, the misnomers *flu* and *common cold* are always replaced with the physiological reality: the body has reached its upper levels of toleration for toxins and is conducting an elimination.

▶ The breath can become foul smelling. This is an olfactory indication of pollutants leaving the body in the form of toxic molecules in exhaled breath.

▶ Weight loss always occurs during the fasting detox and almost invariably occurs with the raw food detox as well. Such weight loss is temporary and should not cause concern. Body weight will normalize on the Natural Hygiene program.

To reach their desired weight, some health seekers will want to start a regular aerobics or weightlifting exercise program as needed for either weight loss or weight gain, respectively. But after a fast of more than a day or two, all health seekers will regain some weight immediately upon refeeding, as all fasters are in a slight state of dehydration. The body will quickly rehydrate itself and gain pounds upon eating juicy foods.

▶ The skin may become an avenue for elimination of toxins. Pimples, pustules, itching rashes or even open and ulcerated sores may come and go repeatedly. The body's orifices and pores may give off offensive odors, mild to strong. The mouth may have a foul or very salty taste as the body eliminates poisons and sodium chloride, respectively.

▶ Nausea, cramps, pain and/or unpleasant rumblings in the stomach and/or intestines can occur. These are signs of detoxing and healing. But they may be interpreted as hunger. This is always a false hunger.

▶ Genuine hunger is always a mild and pleasant urging to eat and is experienced in the mouth and throat. Most people have never experienced genuine hunger in their entire lives and cannot relate to this description experientially. We hope to change all that with these teachings. Being able to identify genuine hunger is at the crux of feeling satisfied on the live food diet and is therefore crucial to our success as health seekers!

▶ Pain may be experienced in localized areas where plaque, calcifications, tumors or some such toxic deposits exist. With continued cleansing and healing, especially during a properly conducted fast, the body breaks down these unhealthy tissues, cleans the toxic fluids and eliminates the morbidity. Such pain experienced is often simply a retracing impulse. Or this pain can be actually felt concomitant with structural or organic abnormalities during mending of past injuries.

▶ Weakness invariably occurs with fasting. The body's energies are being directed away from the musculoskeletal system and toward the cleansing of bodily fluids and tissues, especially tissues within the torso. Shakiness can also occur, with or without the weakness. Bouts of weakness and/or shakiness may also occur while eating raw and detoxing.

▶ The reproductive organs of both male and female undergo excretion of toxins and healing. This healing has led to restored capacity to reproduce in cases of sterility and to increased fertility in cases of limited fertility. *Many cases of men and women able to procreate, once detoxified, are on record.*

▶ Enlarged organs return to normal size if the induration, or hardening, sixth stage of disease has not yet been reached. Most prostate enlargements will reverse to normal if the gland has not yet fully enlarged and hardened.

▶ Swollen, edematous tissues normalize. All men and women experience swollen tissues normalizing as tendons in hands and feet appear and true facial features emerge. Puffy eyes, hands and feet are the first to normalize.

▶ Nervous system tissues of the eyes are cleansed. The reported cases of arrest and partial reversal of chronic degeneration in cases of macular degeneration, glaucoma and cataracts are few. Nervous system tissues are among the least responsive to correct themselves, even once the conditions for health are provided.

Many cases, however, of dramatically improved vision after a completed period of detoxification and healing are on record. Health seekers often report one or more of the following visual events: an upgrading of eyesight so that glasses are no longer needed, a downgrading in strength of prescription glasses, sharper and clearer vision with colors more bright and vivid, eyes that no longer burn or hurt when in use, dry eyes that rehydrate and otherwise normalize. Disappearance of annoying floaters, the misshapen black specks that move around on the surfaces of the eye lens and that can obstruct clear vision, also occurs.

▶ The arteries are cleaned out of fatty/cholesterol/toxin plaque. Blood tests during cleansing often show a rise in fats as they leave their arterial storage places and move into the bloodstream prior to elimination. Given sufficient time for healing, tests also show a normalizing of all body fat readings. With normalizing of cholesterol and triglyceride levels, the health seeker's pulse rate and blood pressure also move into normal ranges.

This last change is perhaps the most exciting to many people, since half of the American people die of a heart and/or vessel disease! Death by cardiovascular disease can be virtually eliminated as a possibility in the health seekers' lives who go through the cleansing and healing and who follow up with strict healthful living practices.

This long list of possible detox symptoms is far from exhaustive. For the complete story, we urge reviewing some of the many supportive materials in The FastWell & GetWell Library at www.getwellstaywellamerica.com. *Fasting for the Health of It: 100 Case Histories Selected from over 200,000 Clinical Records* by Jean Oswald and Dr. Herbert Shelton is a tremendous inspiration. *The Hygienic System, Volume III: Fasting and Sunbathing* by Dr. Shelton is the most detailed and complete text on fasting ever written. Dr. Vetrano and Drs. Tosca and Gregory Haag have also recently prepared over 30 live DVD lectures on what to expect while fasting and detoxifying on raw foods and on healthful living in general.

According to Dr. Bernard Jensen, a person must pass through three stages in getting well: elimination, transition and rebuilding. A healing crisis sometimes happens during the transitional stage. This is earned by good health habits and is accelerated during fasting. A healing crisis could last up to three days. The body is strong enough to throw off toxins at such a rapid rate that fever or past disease symptoms may appear, intensifying the detox crisis.

After the healing crisis subsides, dramatic improvements often manifest. In his book *Dr. Jensen's Guide to Diet and Detoxification*, he cites the case of a person who went from near blindness to reading the newspaper with ease (p. 65).

Depending on the toxicity of the drugs and the existing energy supplies of the body, the ingestion of toxic medications dramatically slows down or completely halts the cleansing process. A friend I once counseled to juice diet for three days experienced shakiness and headaches, for which she took a tranquilizer. To combine detoxing and drugging is a mistake that undermines and reverses much of the progress already achieved on raw juices and right living.

A history of drug use or abuse usually means a person can expect the body will go through an intense elimination of toxins as it revitalizes and heals. It doesn't matter whether the drugs were legal or illegal, prescription or recreational. After all, drugs don't know anything about the law. They don't reason, "I'm a prescribed drug, so I won't poison these cells." A drug doesn't decide, "This person is breaking the law, so he deserves my poisons and to get sick!"

In Chapter 6, we explained at length that our bodies have adapted to today's horrendously toxic drugs even less than to cooked food. To review, introducing these protoplasmic drug poisons to suppress symptoms will cause the body's alarm system to send out emergency signals to the rest of the body. This event halts the elimination and healing processes while the body directs its energies to eliminating these new poisonous insults. Taking drugs during detoxification just adds more toxins to your already toxic body.

You may feel weak at times while cleansing. Do not worry. You will regain your strength. Get plenty of sleep each night. Take at least one rest or meditation period during the day even if you don't feel tired. Even twenty minutes will help.

Victoria BidWell calls doing so a *rest insurance policy*. She explains:

> You may be running on near-empty energy reserves. You may be so over-stimulated by the day's activities and concerns that you are unaware of how tired you really are. Stop to take complete rests. If you are indeed running on near-empty energy reserves and fight-or-flight response adrenaline, you are a crash just waiting to happen. You have lost touch with your body. You are living in your head as you experience the excitement of an overstimulated mind and over-stressed emotions. I have seen many people get in terrible and costly accidents or make horribly unwise decisions when so enervated and overstimulated at the same time!
>
> Many a seemingly energetic health seeker has vivaciously arrived for a fast at a retreat's doorsteps and then absolutely collapsed into deep exhaustion. They had hardly the strength to get out of bed once they let go of stimulating substances, thoughts and emotions. I have seen this happen countless times in a matter of hours or just a day or two and always to the great surprise and chagrin of the novice faster.

So always rest while detoxifying, even if this means making time for several rests or catnaps a day. Even five or ten minutes will help, but twenty is ideal. While your body is undergoing major revitalization and reconstruction, it needs much recuperated energy for that cleansing and repair process.

You may also experience loss of sexual drive. It will come back but without an addictive quality. Many raw fooders report feeling freedom from sexual compulsion while having the ability to enjoy sexual activity even more as a matter of choice.

One explanation for an overactive libido is triggering of the reproductive impulse. When the body is toxic, especially with residues of drugs and stimulating cooked food laden with chemicals, the mind experiences an instinctive survival compulsion to gratify sexual urges. In the innate wisdom of its DNA, the mind senses that its lifespan is in danger of being foreshortened. Inordinate amounts of stress triggering this instinctive survival mechanism often manifest as deviant sexual behavior in both animals and humans. This extreme reproductive compulsion has also been observed in plants and animals stressed beyond normal ranges.

Don't worry about any weight loss. This is normal. If your body appears to lose too much weight too rapidly, it will be only temporary. Your body will regain weight as it rebuilds new healthier tissues. This regaining usually occurs and stabilizes within weeks or months to a year for most people.

On the other hand, the overweight will be delighted to lose excess weight quickly, almost effortlessly, and keep it off practically automatically with a biologically suitable raw food diet. This is one thing that distinguishes living foods from other diets. Excess fat is much easier to keep off long term because this diet is not fat promoting and is a permanent way of life. *This is the way your body was genetically designed to eat.*

One common sign that you are eliminating toxins is feeling chilled, especially in the hands and feet. Some people in transition may even wear sweaters in the summer. In most instances, these chills are primarily due to the body directing more of its blood flow inward to heal the most vital organs and tissues first. (See page 391 for more on this topic.) Victoria BidWell identifies the two extremes of what to expect while detoxifying:

> If a person experiences any detoxification symptoms whatsoever, she can rejoice! Cleansing is occurring! "Something good is happening!" is the comforting encouragement for all novice detoxers.
>
> If virtually no symptoms appear after fasting a few days or going raw for a week or two, and if the energy is good, it means the health seeker is enjoying a detoxification honeymoon.
>
> However, if a person does not experience noteworthy symptoms, if he or she is in an advanced state of chronic degeneration, and if the energy has been and continues to be low, especially terribly low, this is a red-flag warning. It means he or she is so weakened that very little energy has been recuperated for elimination of toxins and healing thus far. More patience and time are needed just to get the energy reserves up to even half-full. These health seekers need to be under the care of a qualified professional to monitor progress. Every person is different.
>
> Many people breeze through, riding on a detox honeymoon high. A very few others may need care every step of the way. Most people undertaking a serious cleansing and healing do experience themselves somewhere between these two extremes.

Be patient during the detoxification and healing period. It may be over in just a matter of days or a few weeks. Afterwards you will feel so much better than before you started, certainly better than you have in years and maybe better than you can ever remember!

Deeper cleansing and rejuvenation periods may recur cyclically after days or weeks once your body has stored up energy for another round of deep cleaning and profound healing. For example, Victoria Boutenko writes that after being raw for a significant length of time, she finally eliminated residues of the DDT her father had sprayed around their home when she was only three.

Some people report that their stools smelled like the very food from which they were detoxifying. Suddenly, in the bathroom, they smelled food or drugs ingested previously, even *decades* before.

Aajonus Vonderplanitz reports that after having eaten clean and raw for decades, his body revitalized enough to detoxify a substance a surgeon had used to glue Vonderplanitz's bone together when he broke his nose at age 15. When a rash broke out on his nose, he had the pus tested out of curiosity. The laboratory test came back positive for aerospace/dental epoxy!

Recorded case histories from natural healing retreats show that a very few people deep into pathology will only get well with a long fast or a series of short fasts, with lengthy periods of strict energy enhancing in between. These rare and exceptional cases do exist. These people need to complete their detoxification and healing under qualified supervision. We are not offering pie-in-the-sky promises or miracle cures, panaceas or other such irresponsible teachings here. We want people to know the science and the truth.

We offer this general detox rule: The more SAD and junk food a person has eaten, the more abuse to which he has subjected his body, the more he has depleted his existing energy reserves, the more drugs he has taken, the more sleep he has neglected to secure, the more toxic his fluids and tissues have become from a lifetime of endogenous and exogenous poisoning, the more energy he will need to recoup before the body can even initiate major detoxification and renewal processes, much less bring them to successful conclusions. Many relatively young and drug-free people in good health and with high energy reserves may experience only very mild detoxification symptoms or no noticeable symptoms at all when going raw.

Our follow-up general detox rule is just as important to heed: The more a person wants to remain cleansed, healed and highly energetic, the more strict must be the energy-conserving healthful living habits once the detoxification and healing period is complete. A key cornerstone to experiencing this feel-good, natural high is the 100% all-raw food plan, or close to 100% raw.

Be encouraged! Only discouragement can take you off the path to paradise health! To repeat, the most intense phases of detoxification and healing are usually over in a matter of weeks or a few months for most people. A few chronic, degenerative cases will take more than a year. Stay the course!

Whenever finding the cleansing process too intense to bear, you can always slow it down with added fats or extra starches. Aajonus Vonderplanitz has counseled elderly people whose detoxification processes remained intense after three months to eat one cooked meal a week in order to slow symptoms down and lessen their intensity.

# Are Enemas and Colonics Useful?

Whether making use of enemas or colonics is necessary or even helpful during detoxification is a controversial subject among various natural healing proponents. Both treatments involve the large intestine (also called the *colon* or the *bowel*) but not the small intestine. These two intestinal organs are basically long tubes. The passageway through them is called the *lumen*. The small and large intestines have entirely different structures and functions.

First, let's look at the small intestine. Before reaching it, food is first chewed and liquefied with saliva in the mouth into a mass called a *bolus*. The bolus is further liquefied with gastric digestive juices, swallowed down the esophagus, and churned by the stomach into a substance called *chyme*. The stomach's pyloric sphincter opens to permit the chyme passage into the lumen of the small intestine. The three sections of the small intestine process chyme further and are called the *duodenum, jejunum* and *ileum*. The duodenum receives alkaline pancreatic juice and liver bile to process the starches and fats, respectively, into an absorbable liquid called *chyle*. Now, absorption of chyle from the small intestine and into the blood and lymph streams is ready.

Specialized, fingerlike projections called *villi* line the folds of the small intestine. The villi are covered with microvilli, which are topped off with brushlike borders. All three structures provide enormous surface areas for nutrient absorption at these brush borders. From there, chyle is absorbed by the blood and lymph streams. It ends ultimately at the cells' doorsteps for assimilation into the cells and to be used for nutrition. The three sections of the small intestine add up to 18-23 feet in length.

At five to six feet in length, the large intestine is short by comparison. It serves primarily as the body's trash compactor and storage container once most of the food's available nutrients have been absorbed at the brush borders of the small intestine. Material in the colon consists of dead cells and other bodily waste, as well as plant fiber and other indigestible materials. Bacterial colonies proliferate and homestead in the colon according to the amounts and types of debris present. These bacteria decompose some of the cellulose and other bowel contents, producing their own waste material, some of which may either be nutritive or toxic to the body.

Lacking the villi of the small intestine, the cells lining the colon have virtually no absorptive capacity. Besides serving as a moving storage container and compactor, one of the colon's primary functions is to absorb water into the bloodstream so that feces are not watery and can take a normal shape and soft consistency. The colon cells also do absorb a minute amount of nutrients and other byproducts of bacterial decomposition while the feces pass through the bowels. Some of these byproducts may be toxic, particularly those that result from the putrefactive decay of cooked foods, especially of meat and other animal products.

Bowel contents passing through the lumen finally evacuate via the rectum and anal canal. Movement of food through the entire digestive tract is performed by *peristalsis*: autonomically controlled, rhythmic muscle contractions of the gastrointestinal walls. Although peristalsis is an energy-intensive process, little energy expenditure is consciously experienced by people eating three square meals a day.

Two reasons account for minimal awareness of colon activity. First, the digestive tract has relatively few nerve endings beyond the mouth and throat to send signals to the brain. And second, the person eating has become used to the digestive process since it goes on all day, every day, 24/7. Most fasters, however, become very aware of their digestive tracts and the lack of this day-in and day-out intestinal energy expenditure. And people deep into intestinal pathology are often acutely and painfully aware of the passage of bowel contents through their lumens.

Dr. Alec Burton stated in a lecture at the American Natural Hygiene Society's 1994 annual conference that the entire digestive process is estimated to be only about 10-15% efficient. That is, the body uses 85-90% of the energy contained in food just to extract the remaining 10-15% for its many other needs.

Dr. Vetrano and Victoria BidWell are quick to point out here:

> On raw foods, which require far, far less energy to process than SAD foods, the energy efficiency is much, much higher. Probably around 70-90% is extracted for bodily use. (See "Live Food — It's All about Energy!" on page 110.) We point out that raw foods in general require very little digestive energy. In fact T. C. Fry correctly promoted fruits as *predigested*, since all they need are chewing well and swallowing before absorption takes place. Vegetables and sprouts require more energy — nuts and seeds more yet.

Enemas and colonics both involve introducing water or other liquids into the colon for the purpose of forcefully loosening up and flushing out two kinds of matter: transit feces and surface debris resulting from recent wrong eating or from decades of eating processed food. These water treatments, as far as they reach, may loosen up and flood out virtually all of the transit fecal matter and much surface colon debris. But contrary to popular belief, these treatments are totally ineffective in loosening matter that has been built into the cellular structure of the colon tissue walls. Nor can the flushing water reach into and loosen up toxins that have been deeply lodged into any diseased tissues, including diverticular pouches, polyps and tumors.

Enemas employ the comparatively weak force of gravity. Enema flushing reaches only into the anal canal, rectum and descending colon. This treatment can easily be done at home by filling an enema bottle with about two quarts of warm water and by permitting the elevated contents of the bag to trickle into the body. The water can be spiked with wheatgrass juice or coffee to stimulate surface bowel nerve endings. The liquid is held within the body by muscular contraction for a period of time and then expelled into the toilet.

By contrast, colonics employ water pressure provided by a sophisticated machine. The colonic flushing reaches much farther. It goes not only into the anal canal, rectum and descending colon lumens, but travels through the transverse and ascending lumens as well. A treatment typically involves many repetitions using up to five gallons of water in total during sessions lasting 45-60 minutes. This treatment is performed by trained licensed colonic therapists or by hospital nurses. The therapist controls the water pressure according to comfort level and sometimes massages the abdomen.

A third treatment intermediate between an enema and a colonic involves a colema board. Like the enema bag, the colema board treatment can be done at home. The fluid reaches only as far as the descending colon. Like the colonic, the person may lie down while the lower bowel is filled, flushed and refilled many times, although the force is considerably less than with the colonic machinery.

Among the three, the choice for those who can afford it is usually the colonic. Many people enjoy the relaxed atmosphere of lying back and letting someone else take control of the process while listening to pleasant soothing background music. I have had many a colonic therapist tell me that clients unwind to such a degree that they confide their greatest joys, pains and secrets, just as when going to a counselor or hairdresser!

Victoria BidWell contrasts the *do-nothing intelligently* stance of hygienic care with hydrotherapies and other forcing measures in general:

> The rationale in rejecting all treatments is that the body will naturally cleanse and heal itself in its own sweet time and in the sequence it deems wisest as the energy reserves fill up. All we need do is provide the conditions for health. The order and timeliness of all cleansing and healing are built into our genetic code and governed in their expression by how strict we get with the ten energy enhancers.
>
> Forcing measures are self-defeating. They first stimulate, irritate and then enervate the body. This renders such treatments relatively inefficient. They deplete the very energy reserves the body needs to fill up in order to direct its natural detoxing and healing processes. This fatigue factor inherent in all therapies thus renders colonics and enemas not just harmless, but potentially damaging.

Further dangers exist with the enema and colonic habits. Their continued use while fasting may upset the body's electrolyte balance and deplete its enzyme reserves by flushing out bowel contents and thus preventing the recycling of electrolytically balanced water. People with the binge/purge eating disorder often become addicted to purging through their bowels and have messed up their electrolytic balance to a dangerous if not fatal degree. Yet another danger is that the colon may become lazy as peristaltic activity is checked in expectation of further forced evacuations. This results in an addictive habituation to the use of mechanical evacuation aids. Ironically, overuse of colonics and enemas may lead to chronic constipation, one of the very conditions these treatments are designed to eliminate. Moderation is the rule of thumb here.

A young Herbert Shelton closely monitored the recovery progress of numerous patients at Lindlahr College's healing facility where he apprenticed to earn his doctor's credentials. He observed that those who received the fewest treatments and therapies, and the fewest colonics, enemas, sweat baths, cold showers and other such enervating interventions, fared the best. They recovered more quickly and thoroughly from their ailments compared to those who underwent hydrotherapy and other treatments.

Many alternative practitioners nonetheless see advantages in these water treatments. These therapists and health educators, including myself, realize that these gadgets are not natural. Why not take advantage of technology designed to assist us in detoxifying our bodies as quickly as possible? These gadgets may be useful in many cases if not abused.

Enemas and colonics are deemed necessary by some alternative professionals in cases of severe constipation or other pathology when the body has not had time to adapt to the ten energy enhancers to achieve excretion of toxins and natural healing. Even hygienic doctors have been known in rare cases to use enemas and colonic therapy with patients experiencing excruciating pain when the do-nothing intelligently approach had failed to bring timely results.

After years and decades of toxic eating habits, the processed food eater may accumulate a thick, mucoid intestinal plaque buildup onto the large intestine's inner surfaces. Bowel impaction can result. Both have been observed by colonic therapists, physiologists, postmortem examiners and forensic pathologists. Their years of observations are documented with highly disturbing photographs and X-rays as diseased tissues and impacted waste fill the bowel lumen. The body constantly works to keep such buildups and obstructions from happening at all. But if energy reserves are low compared to the toxic load continually imposed by the energy-squandering individual, new layers of plaque inevitably build up within the various tissues as the bowel lumen fills.

The large intestine and arteries have a particular affinity for such buildup, although the substances attracted and stored differ. The arteries accumulate cholesterol and other fats. The colon stores primarily uneliminated food waste, mucus and putrefactive bacteria.

Early 1900s American natural health educator Dr. Harvey Kellogg, at his Battle Creek Sanitarium in Michigan, first popularized this phenomenon by warning the world, "Death begins in the colon!" A hilarious Hollywood glimpse into life at The Sans can be seen in the movie *The Road to Wellville*. The emphasis on keeping the colon clean is vividly portrayed in this turn-of-the-century trip to a fancy health retreat for the rich and famous!

If one genetically predisposed to bowel problems abuses his genetics by eating a toxic diet, intestinal pathology inevitably results over time. One or more of the following can develop: flatulence, odor, diarrhea, constipation, colitis, ulcerative colitis, spastic colon, diverticulosis, polyps, tumors, cancer and other conditions.

Some bowel disorders are merely embarrassing or annoying. Others bring life-threatening pathologies, fear, pain and misery. X-rays in life and autopsies in death have shown grossly misshapen colons. They are most often impacted with blackened, stiff and/or oily, gooey substances. How sad to see these results of cooked food addiction: starches and sugars fermented, oils gone rancid, proteins putrefied — all congealed over time, some nearly petrified!

Autopsies have revealed that in certain cases, the normal 2½-3" diameter colon tube has been distended to 6" or more. These diseased bowels have taken on winding, detoured, fallen, convoluted shapes. They are weighted down with pounds of toxic gunk. They no longer take the healthy and relatively straight courses and sharp right angles of the colon's ascending, transverse and descending sections.

Black mucoid and tarlike plaque has been deposited so thick onto the inner colon walls that sometimes only a pencil-thickness hole in the lumen is left for waste transit! Think of the strain it must take to force a bowel movement through such a blocked colon! If you go for a colonic, your therapist will be able to show you classic photos of this disgusting and pitiable situation, either on wall charts or in textbooks.

Upon autopsy, actor John Wayne, a real meat and potatoes man, was rumored to have held 35-40 pounds of fecal matter in his colon. This may just be an urban legend, but it is easy to believe. Cooked fooders, especially eaters of cooked meat, do indeed risk impacted and diseased colons.

A healthy colon weighs only 5-10 pounds when empty. Most Americans on the SAD are estimated to be carrying around 15-20 pounds of unhealthy colon weight. Two situations most often motivate a person to take a fast to empty his large intestine or to detoxify while on raw foods and/or to go through a series of colonics. One is the presence of toxic buildup, partially created by the unfriendly bacterial homesteading. The other is the presence of miserable disease symptoms. Some swear by colonics in the initial stages of toxin elimination. Their goals are to loosen up and flush out the surface toxic material as speedily as possible and to minimize autointoxication resulting from possible absorption of even the most minute amount of this undesirable material.

Some people who choose variations of the SAD take colonics on a regular basis. They know their low-fiber, highly intoxicating diets keep their colons polluted. These colonic regulars reason that standing treatments will help. If you do opt for enemas and colonics because you are still eating cooked foods, be sure to replace lost healthy intestinal flora by taking probiotic supplements. Dr. Vetrano notes, "Costly probiotics are absolutely not necessary and a complete waste of money on a raw diet. The natural flora will repopulate naturally while on raw foods."

# Eating Less and Enjoying More

Providing an overall healthy lifestyle is adopted, the small intestine is thoroughly cleansed while a person continues eating raw for several months to a few years. With improved bowel function, nutrient absorption becomes highly efficient. Consequently, much less food is needed for sustenance. This results in food cost savings, as every nutrient is squeezed out of each bite of food.

Victoria Boutenko reports in *12 Steps to Raw Foods* that her family members can each get by on a salad and some green smoothie drink a day. They discovered that the daily green smoothie habit takes the edge off cravings, even for raw foods. The family members simply do not obsess over food anymore. Even her teenage son reported snowboarding for 10-12 hours, after which two oranges were all he wanted or needed at day's end.

You may think, "But I want to eat more than that!"

Yes, now you do. But after being 100% raw or close to it for a few years, you might become totally in touch at all times with your genuine hunger and basic physiological needs at the cellular level. You may find yourself following the dictates of both automatically! You might become so busy doing good works and fulfilling your life's dreams that you do not give eating three meals a day much thought — unless genuinely hungry, that is. This is freedom!

# The Detoxified and Purified Body, Mind and Spirit

Christian evangelist and television personalities Elmer and Lee Bueno built a Mexican-American ministry in the 1980s and 1990s based on the promise of natural detoxification and healing. They taught the Garden of Eden raw diet compatible with the biblical prescription of Genesis 1:29 and often reminded their students, "There were no cook stoves in The Garden of Eden." They called their organization Born Again Body! This name not only celebrates being born again in spirit, but praises the feeling of complete purification and rejuvenation of the body as well.

Lee lays out the possibility of achieving a born again body in *Fast Your Way to Health*. While helping write and edit Lee's book, Victoria BidWell delineated 20 signs of a detoxified and purified body, mind and spirit via fasting and/or raw eating. The first 17 are a compilation from Dr. Shelton's work. The last three are from Victoria's oft-noted experiences as a Christian practicing the ten energy enhancers.

---

- ✓ Bright pink tongue
- ✓ Sweet breath and fresh, clean-tasting tongue
- ✓ Normalized temperature
- ✓ Normalized pulse rate and blood pressure
- ✓ Soft skin, free of irritation and other abnormalities
- ✓ Return of normal saliva flow
- ✓ Clear, light, odorless urine flow
- ✓ Odorless excreta
- ✓ Normal pink color under fingernails
- ✓ Increased rapidity with which blood flows back into the skin when forced out by pressure
- ✓ Disappearance of unpleasant body odor
- ✓ Return of genuine hunger
- ✓ Disappearance of any acute symptoms of disease
- ✓ At least arrest, if not partial to near-complete reversal, of chronic, degenerative symptoms, if the faster entered with the same
- ✓ Bright, clear, sparkling eyes
- ✓ Renewed strength and vigor
- ✓ Sharp memory and use of mental faculties in general
- ✓ Loss of inertia/laziness and a quickening of the flesh to move forward in useful and unselfish projects while fulfilling God's plan for one's life
- ✓ Heightened appreciation for God and gratitude for all creation: nature, animals, human beings, the planet and the cosmos
- ✓ Feeling of mild to high joy and a peaceful sense of well-being

---

# Detoxifying Your Environment

As your body grows cleaner and purer, it will become more sensitive to environmental toxins. You may want to wear natural fabric, such as cotton, preferably organic if possible. You may choose hemp, silk and wool instead of polyester, acrylic and plastic. You may want to use nontoxic cleansers, including natural dish soap, laundry detergent and household cleaners. You may want the most natural personal care products. You may eventually want to make your own shampoo out of natural ingredients.

The rule of thumb is this: Never put *on* your body what you wouldn't want *in* your body.

You may elect to get the mercury out of your teeth. I know of one man who went on a 100% raw diet. His body finally got around to detoxifying his oral cavity, including his teeth. He had a lot of problems until he got all the mercury out. Make sure a dental dam is placed in your mouth during the procedure to prevent swallowing the mercury that is being removed. If you are on a tight budget, you can have mercury removal done at a dental college for about 60%-70% of normal rates and possibly even less.

You will begin to notice how toxic and irritating common aerosols are. These include items like dry cleaning chemicals, the toxins from new carpets, plant mold, perfume, hair dye, cosmetics and many other unnatural substances that didn't bother you before when your body was polluted. To make your life more natural, you will want to detoxify your environment by getting rid of all exogenous sources of toxemia.

# Overcoming Cravings for Cooked Foods

Numerous cases histories kept by many health care practitioners report that a client or patient detoxifying a particular food sometimes craves that very food.

Consider the person who has eaten a great deal of commercial ice cream over the years. The retained residues of undigested pasteurized cream and the numerous chemicals typically used in ice cream preparation will seep out of their cellular storage sites into the lymph and bloodstream to be expelled through the body's various channels of elimination.

Someone may unconsciously sense the food while it is leaving his body and develop a craving for it. As this happens, he may sense the ice cream while its remnant molecules circulate through the brain via the bloodstream. The experience may evoke memories of the smell, taste, consistency, coolness and nostalgic ambience surrounding his past ice cream indulgences. He may even enter into a woozy state as he craves this favorite dessert of years ago while olfactory and taste chemoreceptors interact to create a sense of vicarious longing for the familiar. Entirely below the level of consciousness, this sequence of events may inspire a desire to reindulge in the dessert experience as a form of psychic comfort.

Victoria BidWell elaborates on this fascinating process:

The limbic system of the brain is located deep within the cerebral cortex. It is a fist-sized mass of neurons some have called the *reptilian brain* because its electrical activity bypasses neurons associated with rational thought and is more primitive and instinctive in quality. The limbic system is also called the *emotional brain*. It plays a key role in memory. It works in concert with multiple areas of the two cerebral hemispheres of the brain to give us the gamut of emotions: highs and lows and everything in between.

Limbic activity bypasses the conscious mind when stimulated by tastes and smells. Other environmental triggers, such as sights and sounds and touch, can also come into play. But taste and smell are the most powerful and the most seductive.

When food or drug memories are at play, the limbic system can conjure up memories and inspire cravings so vivid that they can be experienced as absolutely beyond rational control. This is when people so stimulated obsess over thoughts and act out what they call *irresistible compulsions*. Their lives are out of control. Physiological science and neuroanatomy provide keys that can give back that control.

During detoxification, poisons are being eliminated that have actually been built into the body's own cellular structures as a result of ingesting addictive foods and/or drugs. These retained toxins leave the cells, go into the lymphatic fluid and bloodstream and circulate through the brain in the process of reaching their various eliminative channels.

The brain is stimulated by these poisons. When this stimulation, especially highly pleasurable memories experienced through the tastebuds and olfactory nerves, reaches the limbic area of the brain — *watch out!* Wildly concrete images of sight, sound, touch, taste and smell can be conjured up! And equally provocative accompanying memories and obsessions/compulsions can be evoked! Substance abuse of recreational drugs and addiction to prescription drugs both employ this same limbic pathway as do toxic food cravings. The desire to relive the drug experience, therefore, can be just as irresistible as the desire to eat the toxic food.

This phenomenon of reliving a taste or a smell, a drug experience, an ache or a pain, a memory or even an obsession/compulsion during detoxification and healing is formally termed *retracing*. It occurs among detoxers with regularity. If not educated as to what is happening, these people may feel helpless and hopeless as they give in to the confusing and overpowering urges for the very chains from which they are about to free themselves.

They must understand the science of physiology and brain function behind the helpless feelings. They must work with their bodies, minds and emotions in order to claim that freedom. Understanding this retracing factor demystifies the compulsion, gets rid of confusion and allows the person to consciously override these addictive urges.

The good news is that with this understanding, most times we can just count slowly and deliberately from 1 to 15. Or we can count from 1 to 100, if that's what it takes to carry us well past the urge to indulge. Or we can just offer little prayers or say to ourselves, "This too shall pass." We can direct our attention to some mindless task, demanding chore or pleasurable activity to move us through and well past the cravings. This is employing behavioral modification techniques at their best. See Appendix E for some behavior mod and mind/body practices I have found most useful for health seekers.

If you can get through these brief retracing spells without succumbing to their urges, you will never crave those foods with such intensity again — unless you reindulge. Perhaps another layer of plaque in your digestive tract or elsewhere still retains some molecular remnants of certain foods or drugs. When they are detoxified down the road, you might get a very mild and whimsical memory for those items.

For most people when it comes to food, the most intense cravings are primarily at the initial stages of eating raw. After a period of eating nearly all-raw or 100% raw for weeks or months, your relationship with food will normalize. Virtually all cravings for cooked food will either be gone altogether, or they will have lost their addictive stranglehold. Your life will become manageable.

Some raw fooders have found that eating a particular food raw helps detoxify the same food formerly eaten cooked. For example, if you have eaten a lot of roasted peanuts or heated peanut butter in the past, it may prove helpful to eat raw, soaked or sprouted peanuts when you crave roasted peanuts in order to detoxify from them.

In fact you may find it easiest to get through the cravings by substituting raw versions of the same cooked foods whenever possible. Aajonus Vonderplanitz once counseled an obese woman weighing 280 pounds into going raw. She loved her commercial ice cream. He taught her to make raw ice cream consisting of unheated honey, unpasteurized cream and raw eggs, which she ate nearly every day, sometimes up to a gallon a day! Yet she lost 140 pounds in five months.

A more natural substitute would have been modest amounts of raw homemade banana ice cream made from blended frozen bananas and other fruits instead.

The most common food category many people miss when going raw is cooked starches. They have turned so many times to starchy dishes for emotional comfort. Many of these "comfort" foods are made of wheat, which contains addictive opioid chemicals. (See Appendix A.) Nongluten grains, such as amaranth, millet, buckwheat and quinoa, are more tolerable and do not contain the addictive opioid chemicals.

To enjoy healthful raw grain products, you can sprout grains into these adorable little plants and then fold or grind them into other ingredients, form the shapes you want, and dehydrate the recipe. This all takes time, but it can be very fun!

Essene bread is made of sprouted grains. Raw pizza can be made with a crust of sprouted grains. Delicious raw crackers without any protoplasmic poisons must be made at home, as all commercial raw crackers have table salt and/or hot spices. Croutons made of sprouted ingredients are also yummy. Mock burgers can have a sprout base.

Like the raw nuts and seeds, sprouted grains are more energy expensive to digest than fruits and vegetables. Second only to raw algae, which few people can bring themselves to eat, sprouts are the most nutritious food on the planet! Plus, whole meals can be built around sprouts, and they are super inexpensive! The Sprouting Serendipity Library at www.getwellstaywellamerica.com offers a complete range of sprouting information: how-to books, recipe books, a sprout wheel, charts and a business-sized card.

In the next chapter, we'll examine the scientific practice of fasting and when to fast as a means to bring about detoxification and healing of body, mind and spirit.

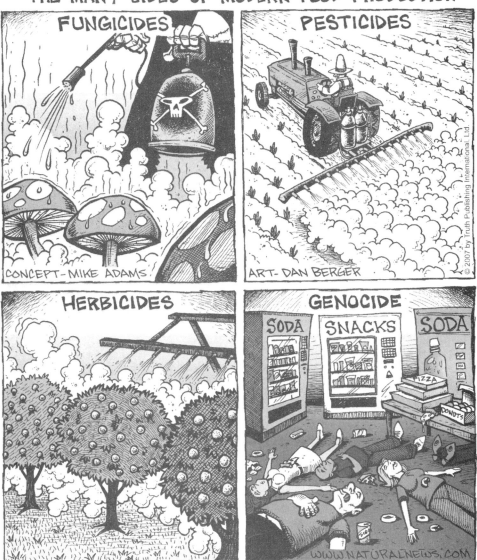

# 15
# The Fasting Factor

The philosopher is like a man fasting in the midst of universal intoxication. He alone perceives the illusion of which all creatures are the willing playthings; he is less duped than his neighbor by his own nature. He judges more sanely, he sees things as they are. It is in this that his liberty consists: in the ability to see clearly and soberly, in the power of mental record.
—Henri Frédéric Amiel (1821–1881), Swiss writer known for his masterpiece *Journal Intime*

Going on a fast refers to blocking out a period of time to be used by denying oneself something. *To fast* commonly means 'to abstain from something, usually food and/or drink'. People fast for different reasons: to cleanse the body and improve health, to lose weight, to break addictions, to increase spiritual or mental awareness or to take a social or political stand.

While many fast for the wonderful feeling of lightness and freedom it brings, most people fast because they want to get well. If the prospect of fasting doesn't sound particularly appealing, just be reassured that genuine hunger generally disappears in a few days. The physiological call for food is usually gone by the third day, although cravings and desire for food as entertainment may persist for some people.

Your body can cleanse and heal itself more rapidly while fasting or juice dieting, often referred to as *juice fasting*. Since the body doesn't have to spend so much energy digesting various foods and eliminating their residues, it can focus on revitalizing, expelling stored toxins and repairing damaged cells.

Dr. Paavo Airola explained why fasting is the "number one healer and rejuvenator" (*How to Keep Slim, Healthy and Young with Juice Fasting*, pp. 20–21). The body lives on its own substances by the process of autolysis, or self-digestion. The body breaks down and eliminates cells and tissues that are diseased or damaged, such as tumors, abscesses and fat deposits. Some of the protein of decomposed cells is recycled through what physiologists call the *amino acid pool*. The building of new, healthy cells is actually accelerated while on raw juices. Taking only juices provides a time of relative rest for the entire digestive system compared to taking whole foods. On raw juices, the nervous system is revitalized, mental powers are improved, body chemistry including hormonal secretions is normalized, and the entire body undergoes rejuvenation.

Many studies have proven the benefits of fasting. Among them are several by Dr. Mark Mattson, PhD, at the National Institute on Aging. His studies found that mice fasting every other day lived longer and were healthier than controls.

All living organisms make use of the extra rest during fasting to revitalize. This added rest serves to free up energy so that the body can normalize body weight, heart rate and blood pressure. The body can further make cellular upgrades as needed, establish overall health and prolong life.

Neurobiologists at Göttingen University in Germany found that the body, when put on a fast, reduces stress hormone levels and increases serotonin levels, thus creating the well-known *fasting high* people often experience several days into their fasts.

Dr. Gabriel Cousens notes that "youthing genes" are activated in fasting and has observed people experiencing *radical youthing* at his fasting retreats. Evidence of this is found in Paul Bragg, a health educator and frequent faster who often took long, labor-intensive mountain hikes while not eating. He enjoyed surfboarding with younger men well into his 90s, according to his daughter-in-law Patricia.

It could easily require several pages to list all the illnesses from which the body recovers when put on a fast. In the health by healthful living paradigm, fasting has proven to be the superlative method for accelerated healing and recovery from most diseases that run the gamut of acute to chronic.

# Fasting on Water Only versus Juice Dieting

One way to fast is on water only. Another way to abstain from whole foods is to take freshly made juices only. Juice dieters often dilute their juice with at least 50% water and maybe even more as the days progress. Some use juice dieting as a lead-in to fasting on water only. Some people even take a tiny bit of lemon juice and honey highly diluted with water, especially if they plan to be active while on juices.

Some people hold that fasting on water only is the only way to fast correctly and consider it superior to juicing. Natural Hygiene teachers consider *juice fasting* to be a misnomer that should be correctly termed *juice dieting*.

For elimination of toxins and healing, Dr. Vetrano explains the superiority of fasting on water only compared to juice dieting:

> Since the body has to cleanse itself [during a fast], the less interference it has, the better. That is, the less juice, the better. The body does not need to waste its precious nerve energy and stored reserves to handle quarts of juice every day.
>
> Perhaps the greatest detriment to the juice diet in comparison to fasting is that the juice diet does not force the body to rely solely upon its reserves for nutrients. Instead of forcing the body to break down its tissues for the vitamins, minerals, energy reserves, and proteins it needs, many of these nutrients are supplied by the juices.
>
> When juice dieting, the metabolism does not slow down as much as it does when abstaining from all whole or juiced food and taking in only water. Therefore, the more active physiological/nutritional situation set up by juice dieting causes a greater depletion of the body's protein stores than fasting on water alone.

On the other hand, Dr. Paavo Airola declared fasting on juices to be superior for many reasons in his book *How to Keep Slim, Healthy and Young with Juice Fasting*. For one thing, he maintained that the juice nutrients are easily absorbed directly into the bloodstream without putting a strain on the digestive system. Thus the healing and rejuvenating process of autolysis, or self-digestion, is provided freed-up energy due to the efficiency of absorption. He claimed that taking in the juice nutrients speeds up the healing and recovery.

Furthermore, Airola claimed that the juices provide alkaline minerals the body uses to alkalinize its fluids and tissues, since they contain abnormally high levels of acids during fasting on water only. The body uses the abundance of minerals from vegetable juices or broths to correct mineral balances and restore biochemical balance throughout the body.

Dr. Airola cited Dr. Ralph Bircher-Benner in claiming that raw juices contain an as yet unidentified factor that "stimulates a micro-electric tension in the body and is responsible for the cells' ability to absorb nutrients from the blood stream and effectively excrete metabolic wastes" (pp. 38–39).

Dr. Cousens also prefers juice dieting to fasting on water only. He points out that healing crises occur less often on juices. He maintains that the alkaline minerals of juices, especially in greens, provide the body with what it needs to neutralize its overacidic condition.

Dr. Vetrano's and Victoria BidWell's Natural Hygiene response to both Drs. Airola's and Cousens's juice dieting reasoning must be considered:

Think about it! To get well, the whole idea of fasting on water only is to *inspire the body to live off its own reserve nutrients in certain tissues exclusively*, healthy and unhealthy both. This is the most favorable setup for complete healing to take place in as short a time as possible. *If an ill person takes juices, however, he is living partially on juice nutrients; and this auspicious setup for exclusivity is sabotaged.* The possibility of inspiring the body to break down unhealthy tissues until they are completely autolyzed and the ill person is completely well is therefore less likely and certainly less speedy on a juice diet!

Their acid stance is also not correct. Both of these doctors consider an acidic condition pathological while fasting on water only and want to correct it by giving the sick person raw juices. When fasting on water only, the toxic body *is* more acidic. *But that is perfectly normal and as it should be!*

The stored wastes and poisons are all acidic. As they leave their storage sites for elimination, the body will be perfectly and correctly acidic! But the body will normalize its chemistry to alkaline in its own sweet time.

Of *course* healing crises do occur less often on juices! But a healing crisis is called a *healing crisis* because that is when healing occurs most efficiently and rapidly. That happens most thoroughly and expeditiously on water only. Is this not exactly what the sick person wants — complete and rapid healing? Besides, in some cases, full healing cannot even take place while taking in nutrients; for these health seekers, a fast on water only is the only route to take to inspire complete bodily healing.

When taking nutrients, the juice dieter's metabolism is not slowed down significantly, even if resting a great deal. If the juice dieter is active, it is not slowed down much at all. But the faster *on water only* goes into a deep state of complete rest, and metabolism is slowed down dramatically. In comparison, the juice dieter's needs for protein are much higher than those of the faster on water only. With anything over just a few days, therefore, the juice dieter is potentially creating a serious protein deficiency. With fruit and veggie juices, health seekers are getting the full spectrum of minerals for some detoxification and healing; but they are not getting enough protein. Nutrition becomes lopsided. With the fast on water only, nutrient conservation in general and protein conservation in particular take place. This is ideal for complete healing.

Fasting is commonplace in European clinics where 14-21 days in duration is customary. Supervised fasts of up to 40 days on water only and juice diets of up to 100 days are considered safe for most people seeking therapeutic fasting supervised by European experts. The general consensus among most European clinicians is that juice dieting gets superior results to fasting on water only.

Furthermore, with juice dieting one can go about daily business and even get moderate exercise. It is even possible to continue working if the person is relatively healthy.

Many people, myself included, have noted that they can still work while on a juice diet, although deeper excretion of toxins only comes with complete rest during a fast on water only.

# Fasting and Freedom from Addictions

Dr. Cousens likens the effects of fasting on the body to the effects of rebooting on a computer. Often when your computer acts up, a simple reboot is all you need to get rid of the problem. The body works more efficiently after a fast.

For many people without hard-core eating disorders, the cellular memory of — and cravings for — coffee, drugs and cooked food are either virtually erased or greatly diminished after a fast of a couple of weeks. Victoria BidWell is an expert on the obsessive-compulsive eating disorder. She points out the exception to this postfast phenomenon of losing interest in SAD, cooked foods:

The depths of a person's addiction to SAD, cooked food is often not revealed until he or she takes a fast and then starts on all live foods. Then the addictions surface — sometimes with a vengeance.

The new raw fooder may find himself, much to his despair, hopelessly hooked on cooked. Most hard-core food addicts will still struggle, even after taking a fast or juice diet. They will have to put out behavior modification, visualization and affirmation energy. They may need to get ongoing counseling to get completely free from their SAD food addiction. At the root of their problem is a self-image that needs radical changing from hopeless and unhappy to believing in new possibilities, choosing to do right and wanting high joy as a way of life!

> Certainly going all-raw, practicing the ten energy enhancers and taking a fast is the best route to help these far-gone addicts regain hope, get control of their lives and *get happy*.

Paul Bragg wrote of a woman he supervised on a fast. She had been smoking four packs of cigarettes and drinking a fifth of whiskey a day! She was also a heavy drinker of colas and coffee. Her nerves were so shattered that her hands trembled while writing. She suffered from insomnia, blurred vision, pasty and flabby skin tone and thoughts of suicide.

When Bragg put her on a fast, he allowed her to smoke a little and drink small amounts of alcohol and coffee. But on the third morning of the fast, these poisons began to nauseate her. Any time she began to drink alcohol, tea or coffee, she would vomit. For the next seven days of the fast, she had no desire for these poisons. Bragg put her on a raw diet another ten days, then on a fast for another ten.

Her skin tone renewed to perfection after that. She became happy and carefree, and she was *free from addictions*! Bragg reported, "She became one of the best writers in the Hollywood TV and movie world. Her income doubled and tripled. Her personal magnetism increased, and she attracted a handsome, wholesome man for a husband" (*The Miracle of Fasting*, pp. 110–111).

Through his experience in supervising fasts, Paul Bragg proved repeatedly that anyone with addictions can find the answer in fasting. When the body becomes clean, it will no longer tolerate poisons without taking action to expel them. Joseph Sarelli declared that he was freed from an addiction to four packs a day of cigarettes after a 27-day fast (*Naturally, the Hygienic Way,* August 1984).

German Professor Arnold Ehret maintained, "If an alcoholic were to be made to fast for a few days or eat nothing but fruit, he would soon lose his taste for beer and wine. This proves that the entire civilized mass of foods from beefsteak to seemingly harmless oatmeal creates a desire for these detestable antidotes: alcohol, coffee, tea, tobacco. Why? Because overeating makes man lazy, and consequently he has to pep himself up with stimulants" (*Rational Fasting*, pp. 40–41).

# Spiritual Benefits of Fasting

Spiritual benefits from fasting are well known in nearly every religion, though religious ritual fasts are sometimes very brief — a day or even less. Early Native American Indians fasted while going on vision quests and taking passage into manhood. Muslims fast from sunrise until sundown every day during their holy month of Ramadan, not even drinking water, despite living in the desert. Fasting is also practiced in Judaism and Christianity. The Bible mentions fasting 74 times. Moses, David, Elijah, Jesus and others mentioned in the Bible fasted for as long as 40 days and 40 nights, a length commonly referred to as the *master's fast*.

During the Golden Age of Greece, the great philosopher Pythagoras required his disciples to fast for 40 days before being initiated into the mysteries of spiritual teachings. Plato, Socrates and Aristotle also required their students to take fasts. They believed that only through fasting could the mind be purified enough to understand the deep teachings of life's mysteries.

After Mohandas Gandhi led the passive resistance movement of Indians against British imperialism and an independent India was established, internal strife between Pakistani and Muslim Indians broke out. Gandhi hoped people on both sides would respect his love for a free India and his efforts to make the dream come true. He further capitalized on the people's inability to distinguish between fasting and starvation by conducting personal protest fasts to inspire members of the two factions to restore peace in the new India.

His refusal to eat unto what appeared to be starvation was so effective and so well publicized that the fighting stopped. Gandhi, however, knew exactly how long he could safely fast, as Dr. Shelton had provided Gandhi with Natural Hygiene counsel and a copy of *The Hygienic System, Volume III: Fasting and Sunbathing*. Gandhi's fasts popularized social and political fasting. It is practiced to this day by leaders and protestors alike.

Many raw food teachers have also remarked on spiritual powers improving with fasting. Arnold Ehret considered fasting the master key to mental and spiritual evolution. It was said of Dick Gregory that after extensive juice dieting, he lost not only weight, *but also his anger*. He claimed that as fasting cleanses the body, poisons are thrown off, releasing hatred and other sick emotions.

Steve Meyerowitz writes, "You may even discover some psychic abilities as waste products from undigested food and other materials no longer interfere with nerve linkages and your vital energies are free to center in your upper chakras [energy centers] instead of your stomach. Conquering your appetite and desires allows you to focus your thoughts on the discovery of the 'heaven' within" (*Juice Fasting & Detoxification*, pp. 118–119).

Dr. Gabriel Cousens explains that fasting accelerates the purification of the body and thus allows the physical body to be a better conductor of the kundalini energy. Fasting "improves the alignment of the chakras and subtle bodies, which makes it easier for the cosmic prana to enter the body and increases the possibility of the awakening of the Shakti Kundalini."

Cousens goes on to describe in detail his own experience with a 40-day fast in which his mind "dissolved into the Light of God" and four hours of meditation seemed to go by in a few minutes. His crown chakra became one "whirling vortex of energy" connecting him with the dance of the cosmos (*Spiritual Nutrition*, p. 340).

Victoria BidWell explains why some Christians experience a spiritual high when fasting:

During a fast, the flesh is neither fed nor satisfied with lustful longings for food. The faster draws closer to God and can better listen to the Holy Spirit. I recall deep into my long fast at Dr. Scott's one day. I walked barefoot on the lawn and lay down to rest on the cool grass. Suddenly, I felt the whole property being lifted up into the cumulus clouds. Then the proverbial peace that passes all understanding flowed through me. It brought love, joy and gratitude into every cell of my body.

## Fasting and Mental Health

According to Dr. Shelton, mental powers such as memory, attention and association are quickened during fasting. Imagination is at its best. This is because blood flow increases, and nerve energy used to process food is freed up for use elsewhere in the body. He explained, "Large amounts of blood and nervous energies have to be sent to the digestive organs to digest a meal. If these energies are not required there, they may be drawn upon by the brain in thinking" (*Fasting and Sunbathing,* p. 67).

Brain tissues are also cleared of toxins during fasting. In fact many times Dr. Shelton saw mental health during a fast improve greatly among his patients. Depression and pessimism lifted. "Insanity is frequently overcome while fasting, and practically all cases are improved by the fast" (ibid., p. 68).

Dr. Yuri Nikolayev of the Moscow Psychiatric Institute and Alan Cott, MD, have also had great success in treating mental illness, including schizophrenia!

Michael Bobier reports that he had been obsessed with and almost suicidal over a woman who broke up with him for another man. By his 20th day of a fast on water only, Michael was not only free of his jealousy, but even felt compassion for her and her new companion because they were on a cooked diet and drank alcohol (*Living Nutrition*, Vol. 19, 2007, p. 59).

Stephen Buhner sheds some light into how the mind is affected by fasting. When the intake of carbohydrates is low enough, the body is forced to use fat stores for fuel. This change is called *ketosis*. "When in full ketosis, the mind simply works somewhat differently. Thinking can be just as acute, but it tends to be slower, more reflective, more studied and deeper, and aside from thoughts of food or ending the fast, less inclined to dwell on future plans" (*The Fasting Path*, p. 76).

Victoria BidWell now assists health seekers wanting to fast at her school named *Our Hygiene Homestead in The Woods* located in Concrete, Washington. She consults with Dr. Vetrano when hygienic teachings need clarification and with Dr. Zarin Azar (see New-Earth Medicine on page 595) when fasting supervision is needed. Victoria shares with us highlights of her experiences and knowledge about the Natural Hygiene fast in the next several sections.

## The Natural Hygiene Fast

I had the great education and pleasure of spending at least six years of my life, all totaled, at most of the Natural Hygiene retreats during the 1970s and into the 1990s. In my travels, I met, worked for and/or studied with most of the most renowned names of those times. These three decades spanned the great heyday of Natural Hygiene and fasting that T. C. Fry's publications, especially his *Healthful Living Magazine*, inspired among his 36,000 subscribers. At most of these places, the institutions were filled and overflowing with three-month-long waiting lists.

My longest fast on water only was in 1992 for 36 days at Dr. Scott's Natural Health Institute, followed by two weeks on lettuce and watermelon and another 18 days of fasting on water only. Most of the healing benefits in body, mind and spirit that I harvested then have lasted to this day.

Humans and animals alike have practiced fasting for thousands of years and for many reasons. Yet we never see advertisements for fasting on television. And medical doctors argue against fasting in the media and to their patients who bring the subject up. If the idea of fasting sounds too radical and tempts you to give up your conventional to alternative paradigm shift, just know that no one is forcing you to take a fast. The slower method with raw foods and juices also gets results.

Remember, *it's all about energy. Disease is an energy crisis in a toxic body.* Also, keep in mind that the high rate of disease arrest and partial or complete recovery among health seekers who undertake a fast is backed up by "The Natural, Physiological Laws of Life" presented on page 549.

Physiologists estimate that at least 75% of the energy the body uses on a daily basis for people eating conventional SAD foods goes not for body heat and movement and mental/emotional work, as you might think. Instead it goes for these supremely energy-expensive metabolic tasks: digesting food in the mouth, stomach and intestines; absorbing chyle from the small intestine into the blood and lymph streams; circulating absorbed nutrients through the liver for initial cleansing; moving nutrients to the cells; assimilating nutrients into the cells; converting nutrients into energy and/or using them as raw materials for reconstructing cellular matter, and eliminating toxic byproducts and metabolic and cellular waste.

These nutritive and eliminative processes feed, tear down, rebuild and keep clean the 75 trillion cells of the human body. These many processes — and not the combination of body heat, muscular contraction and mental/emotional activities — take up an estimated 75% of a person's energy generated during rest and sleep! (This estimate is much lower for people on clean-burning live food diets, however.)

So why fast? It's so simple. Abstaining from all food intake — and resting from virtually all physical activity and mental, emotional and sensory excitation while taking in water only — free up the body from all of the aforementioned demands for energy and provide the body with an extended period of deep rest on many levels. Nerve energy is generated and its reserves filled while the body subsists on its nutritive reserves. But this restored energy is not used on processing food. It is used for autolysis of unhealthy tissues and for cleansing and making fluid and cellular upgrades and tissue repairs as needed — all the while balancing body chemistry — all to the greatest extent possible.

In many cases, medical intervention may be absolutely necessary during a critical accident emergency or for an 11th hour disease crisis. Barring these cases, however, and always whenever the health seeker takes the holistic course of action in acute disease, and in most cases of chronic disease, this natural process of providing a sick person a time-out period for fasting and cooperating with the body's design gets better results and faster results than any other known method.

Indeed, this period of fasting provides time for the body to bring about the closest thing to a "healing miracle" possible. It offers a veritable fountain of youth! Fasting also provides a time-out period from cooked food addiction. When only small amounts of fresh raw foods and juices are taken to break the fast, they are enjoyed and welcomed by the health seeker with a relish indescribable! The 10,000 tastebuds have gone cold turkey for the duration of the fast. The mind, emotions, body and especially its tastebuds are ready and poised for this new radical dietary shift into raw foods and the other nine energy enhancers like never before!

## *Fasting* and *Starvation* — Defined

The idea and practice of going without food for an extended period of time is considered by adherents and proponents of the medical mentality to be the most unconventional, fanatical and dangerous of all alternative health care practices.

This is because these ill-informed medical doctors and their followers have mistakenly confused fasting with starving. They do not understand that a Natural Hygiene fast, properly conducted and supervised, provides a period of time for the most rapid and most complete elimination of toxins and healing known for the human body. They have a lot to learn and need a crash course on the Natural Hygiene fast.

To rightfully educate those misinformed and to get it really straight ourselves as well, we must start with three sets of basic definitions and distinctions.

First, the term *fasting* comes from an Old English verb that meant 'to make firm or fixed', while *starvation* comes from an Old English verb that meant 'to die'. Interestingly enough, these Anglo Saxon derivatives with their archaic meanings hold true even today. When a person fasts, therefore, he firmly withholds food, fixed in his resolve not to eat. When a person starves, however, he withholds food until nutritional reserves are exhausted and until the body begins to feed upon its essential tissues unto death.

When misunderstood, fasting conjures up images of Nazi concentration camp victims — waiting to die. No wonder the uneducated are horrified at the idea and practice of fasting! This horror is compounded by two facts. First, the alternativists, who by conventional definition are to be mistrusted by the medical doctors, have largely taken over the practice of fasting as their domain and area of expertise. Second, fasting is wholeheartedly condemned by virtually all conventional medical doctors.

By the end of this chapter, however, you will be so well informed on the idea, practice and benefits of the Natural Hygiene fast, that you will see it for the blessing it has been in the past for others and could be in the future for you. "This fasting knowledge will put you among the elite Natural Hygiene intelligentsia!" Dr. David Scott once proclaimed to me.

# What the Natural Hygiene Fast Is and Is Not

The second set of distinctions to make clear to the uninformed is to define just what the Natural Hygiene fast is and what it is not. Following are seven parameters. Let me emphasize here as a Natural Hygiene health educator that these seven parameters are speaking strictly of the Natural Hygiene fast as practiced and popularized by Drs. Shelton and Vetrano while supervising over 80,000 fasters combined and by those who stay within those boundaries.

Now, here are the seven parameters in a nutshell that distinguish the Natural Hygiene fast from both other alternativists' versions of fasting and from the dreadful practice of starvation:

---

**1.** The Natural Hygiene fast occurs only with complete abstinence from all food/nutrients in any form while taking only distilled water according to thirst and while the body safely lives on its totally adequate reserves.

Starvation may occur even while taking in insufficient and nutrition-deficient amounts of food or may occur in the complete absence of food over an extended period of time.

**2.** Once underway and in a matter of a day or two, the Natural Hygiene faster almost always experiences a distinct lack of hunger.

During starvation, the individual almost always experiences a compelling sense of hunger.

**3.** The Natural Hygiene fast represents a peaceful period of complete rest, willingly entered into and always marked by a genuine calm once the faster cooperates with his body.

Starvation represents a tortuous period of turmoil for a person that is forced upon his body by himself or by someone else and is marked by extreme distress.

**4.** The Natural Hygiene fast is always undertaken for beneficent reasons: mental, emotional, spiritual and/or health-related.

Starvation is often undertaken for social, spiritual or political agendas and coercions.

**5.** The Natural Hygiene fast is properly prepared for and properly supervised by a trained practitioner who daily monitors the faster's vital signs, eliminations and subjective experiences.

During starvation, a person is never properly supervised.

**6.** The Natural Hygiene fast represents a process of the body utilizing its nutritional reserves and autolyzing morbid tissue while abstaining from eating.

Starvation represents a process of the body, exhausted of its nutritional reserves, slowly breaking down its vital tissues essential to life functions.

---

A key noun in literature on fasting is *autolysis*. The verb is *autolyze*. (The prefix *auto-* means 'self', and *-lysis* means 'digesting'.) During fasting, the body is very busy doing just that: autolyzing, or self-digesting.

As soon as energy is regenerated, the body eagerly autolyzes excess body fat and morbid tissues, such as tumors and cholesterol deposits in arteries. *Autolysis* is thus an exciting word to add to our health-seeking vocabulary!

7. The Natural Hygiene fast is always followed by proper refeeding and a feeling of increased well-being and improved health.

Starvation is always followed by learning to live with irreversible tissue damage if one survives, and if not, by dying.

# The Five Kinds of Rest Taken on the Natural Hygiene Fast

The third item above is so very important to the Natural Hygiene fast, it needs further emphasis for the health seeker who is mildly interested in studying more on the subject. The third item is also what distinguishes the Natural Hygiene fast from those of other alternativists who advocate their forms of fasting.

During the Natural Hygiene fast, the faster must, by definition, secure complete rest. She must not be going on hikes and swims, driving around, spending hours on a computer or seeking other such distractions and entertainments. Doing so is not fasting: it is just *not eating*!

The Natural Hygiene faster is a *complete rester*. Her sole focus is to revitalize her nervous system. Revitalization only occurs during rest, sleep, fasting and other forms of complete stillness, as in meditation and prayer. The revitalization, however, is accelerated while resting or sleeping and fasting! *Remember, it's all about energy.* During the Natural Hygiene fast, the health seeker increases energy levels by securing rest on five levels:

✓ **Rest from physical activity**
The faster makes as few demands on her musculoskeletal system as possible and takes as much bed rest as possible. She goes to bed to rest, relax and/or sleep. Or she lounges around during a minimum of her waking hours. She secures as much physical rest as possible, sleeping in, interspersing her day with naps and then retiring very early. A leisurely slow walk or brief period of mild stretching may be allowed for all but the very weak faster and according to the supervisor's orders.

✓ **Rest from physiological duties of processing food**
During a fast, the tremendously energy-expensive processes of digestion, absorption, assimilation and elimination of food are brought to an end with the processing of the last meal. To repeat, physiologists speculate that 75% of our nerve energy is spent on the daily processing of food. During fasting, however, the entire gastrointestinal tract rests. The basic metabolic activity is at a healthful restful minimum.

The energy normally used to process food while eating is thus freed up to repair, restore and renew the body, mind and spirit. Deep physiological rest is secured during fasting for most of the body. But some organs and systems are working overtime carrying out the many eliminating and healing activities. The more toxic the health seeker, the more energy is needed to carry out these activities, thus the importance of securing physiological rest.

✓ **Rest from sensory input**
During a fast, the health seeker retreats from the sensual sensorial onslaught of sight, sound, touch, taste and smell that makes up the excitations and fabric of daily life. The faster should use her eyes, ears and other sensory systems as little as possible and stay in a quiet place to secure a rest and respite for all the senses.

✓ **Rest from emotionalism**
Ideally, the faster retreats to a Natural Hygiene school and sanctuary setting, away from all the emotional input and output of daily life. Experts estimate that upwards of 90% of all illness has a stress-related factor. Therefore, this emotional rest is truly beneficial for minimizing psychosomatically induced diseases.

✓ **Rest from mental activity**
The faster puts away concerns and projects that demand mental effort and concentration or that present distractions. The brain is the center for all mental activity. It is also the housing for nerve energy regeneration. In order for the revitalization that brings health and energy, the brain and entire nervous system need this mental time-out period of rest, sleep and fasting.

Obviously, the Natural Hygiene faster is not watching television, not on the phone, not at the computer, not reading, not at hobbies, not taking regular exercise, not exchanging recipes with other fasters all day and night, and not engaging in endless conversations. Ideally, the health seeker is securing deep and complete rest on all five of these levels, taking part in any of the above activities minimally or only because of emergencies.

To so abstain is very hard for the thrill-seeker. Even the health seeker who is more relaxed and not a stimulant junkie can get very fidgety. But your knowing just what a *properly conducted fast* is now can help you prepare mentally and emotionally for a fast you may decide to undertake later. It is best to get your affairs in order before checking out from daily routines to fast. Ideally, you want to be able to let go and enjoy complete rest with a brain that is flat-lined into peacefulness and pleasantness!

## The Natural Hygiene Fast versus the Juice Diet

The third set of definitions needed follow. The phrase *to go on a fast* has been misunderstood. To use the phrase correctly, when a person *goes on a fast*, he is abstaining from one or more items. Thus, a *water faster* refers to a person who is taking in everything and anything but water. *The juice faster* refers to a person who is taking in everything and anything but juice.

Once these distinctions are made, a person who is taking in only water and fasting from everything else is correctly said to be *fasting on water only*. Among the Natural Hygiene intelligentsia, therefore, when we speak of *taking a fast*, it is always a fast on water only.

Likewise, when taking in juices only, the novice incorrectly says that the person is *fasting on juices*. But since taking juices, or food nutrients in any form, for that matter, is actually eating as far as the digestive system is concerned, the Natural Hygiene-educated person correctly states that one taking in juices is on a juice diet.

The term *Natural Hygiene fast* is defined very strictly, and it is a *water-only* and *complete-rest endeavor*. Let me repeat this very important distinction: the body does not differentiate between metabolizing juices and whole foods. Either way, the body is eating, digesting, absorbing, assimilating food nutrients and eliminating waste. To drink juices is the same as to eat, as far as the body's metabolic processes are concerned. Juices, being devoid of fiber, simply require less energy to process. Being on juices only, therefore, is not properly defined as 'juice fasting'. Rather, *being on juices only* is properly defined as 'fasting from whole foods and juice dieting, both'.

Following are 12 distinctions between the Natural Hygiene fast on water only and the juice diet on 8-ounce glasses of raw juices only, three to four times a day or more as needed or directed.

1. During fasting, eating and digestion halt. But during juicing, eating and digestion continue but with the nutrients simply in a liquid form. Juice dieting, therefore, is not fasting in any sense of the term in the Natural Hygiene paradigm.

2. During fasting, hunger is absent after two days, more or less. But during juice dieting, hunger continues.

3. During fasting, revitalization, cleansing, body chemistry balancing and repair processes are an estimated three to five times greater than during juicing.

4. During fasting, sodium chloride is rapidly eliminated. But during juice dieting, sodium chloride elimination is less dramatic.

5. During fasting, weight loss is an estimated three to five times greater than during juice dieting.

6. During fasting, nutritional balance is maintained. But during juice dieting, one or more nutritional imbalances can occur within days or weeks.

7. During fasting, deep physiological rest is secured. But during juice dieting, the deep physiological rest secured is more than when eating solid foods but much less than when fasting.

8. The longer fast of 7-10 days, and more requires retreat and supervision when the faster has a condition that requires monitoring. But a period of time spent juice dieting, in most cases, does not.

9. During a longer fast, energy levels invariably drop; this necessitates complete bed rest. But during juice dieting, energy levels normally allow modest activity and even a modest workload, as long as breaks to rest are allowed.

10. After a fast, an equal number of days feeding is required to regain full strength. But after a juice diet, fewer days are required to regain full strength.

11. The fast is not necessarily superior to juice dieting. The two physiological modes of Natural Hygiene care are employed for different reasons and in different cases to achieve different results.

12. It should be noted that in certain disease situations, the health seeker cannot get well on juices only and will need a long fast or a series of short fasts before health is recovered. These special cases are rare, but should nevertheless be noted.

## How to Break the Natural Hygiene Fast

Dr. Scott once warned me, "You can undo all the good of a long fast in just a few days by doing all the wrong things." He was of course referring to going right back to the ten energy robbers, and especially to large servings of cooked, SAD food. No one goes on a fast with the intention of doing wrong immediately afterwards! To end the fast on the right track is absolutely essential.

All Natural Hygiene doctors select fresh raw fruit or fruit juices in small amounts and typically six servings a day for breaking a fast. After a few days of whole fruit on this frequent feeding schedule, larger amounts and more variety of fruit and just three times a day are served. Raw vegetables, nuts and seeds are typically added within a week of a fast or sooner.

Except for special situations, and with Drs. Shelton and Vetrano behind me, I start health seekers with the following break-fast schedule:

### Breaking the Fast

**DAY 1:** Whole fruit six times a day, four ounces starting at 8 AM and every two hours until 6 PM.

**DAY 2:** Same as Day 1, only serving eight ounces of fruit each time

**DAY 3:** Three meals of 12 ounces total, serving tomatoes, cucumber, celery, lettuce and red bell pepper

**DAY 4:** Same as Day 3, only serving meals of 16 ounces total

**DAY 5 and onward:** Regular meals with veggies, nuts, seeds and avocado as well as the other fruits are given, as presented in *The Health Seekers' YearBook*'s Chapter Nine: The Year in Live-Food Menus.

Melons are the preferred break-fast fruit! They are the very easiest to digest, since most are 92-98% water. Dr. Scott not only breaks virtually all fasts at his institute with watermelon, but he also serves watermelon with lettuce for virtually all breakfasts! The mild sweetness of the watermelon does not set up too much excitement for the post-faster's tastebuds and does not entice him to drink or eat beyond genuine hunger. Other juicy fruits are also favorites used by other practitioners: oranges, sweet grapefruit and grapes.

I remember Dr. Vetrano breaking my very first fast of 17 days on a four-inch-square piece of heavenly watermelon. It took twenty minutes to eat. It knocked me out! Full of energy when I sat down to eat this little block of red melon, I immediately passed out into a two hour deep sleep and then became exhausted for the day during the refeedings. I was *so impressed*. This was proof of how the body uses so much energy for the digestive process!

All break-fasters are encouraged to take a long time to drink their juices or eat their meals. If breaking your fast on juices, a teaspoon at a time or slow sipping with a straw is ideal. It takes as much as ten to twenty minutes to get the digestive system reactivated. Likewise, eating the whole food slowly will get the live food connoisseur off to the best start.

Some fasters have gone through hell during some point in their fasts. Now breaking those fasts can be a heavenly delight of sight, sound, touch, taste and smell! Dr. Vetrano teaches health seekers to learn to "eat sensationally." A better time never presents itself to do so than upon the break-fast!

## Questionable Candidates for the Natural Hygiene Fast

Most people in acute and chronic disease are prime candidates for fasting to get well. Dr. Vetrano and I must caution health seekers who are not prime candidates for the Natural Hygiene fast.

Although each health seeker's condition is different, it is questionable whether certain patients should fast on water only, even under the best of monitoring. Certainly these questionable fasting candidates should never fast on their own. Self-conducted, extreme fasts outside the boundaries of proper supervision can be extremely dangerous! Since proper care observing the ten energy enhancers, including refeeding and exercise schedules, is crucial to getting well, the following health seekers in their special situations need guidance with these post-fast activities as well.

Dr. Vetrano next presents her list of those who are questionable candidates for the Natural Hygiene fast, prepared for the *Health Seekers' YearBook.* She points out, "Every case is unique, and whether or not an individual should fast is up to the doctor to decide. Without question, if a health seeker is on this list and the doctor recommends a fast, the patient must be closely supervised from beginning to end."

---

### Questionable Fasting Candidates

✓ **Those who are extremely thin and undernourished**

These people may go on short fasts of 1-3 days with definite benefit. And with getting strict with the ten energy enhancers between fasts, these people may be restored to health.

✓ **Those who are in extreme weakness, depending on its cause**

✓ **Those who are in extreme stages of chronic, degenerative disease**

---

✓ **Those who have some cancers, especially of liver and pancreas**

✓ **Those with inactive kidneys accompanied by obesity**

✓ **Those with difficult breathing due to cardiovascular disease**
 Caution and supervision must be taken with any abnormal rhythms of the heart.

✓ **Those taking insulin**
 Insulin-dependent health seekers must be fasted under competent supervision. A fast provides time for the body to eliminate the toxins that impair normal function of tissues and organs and time for the pancreas to repair the beta cells so that metabolism of carbohydrate, fat and protein is normalized.

✓ **Those who are afraid to fast**
 They should not undergo a fast until they have well educated themselves and lost their fears.

✓ **Pregnant women who are in a state of good health**
 They may safely fast but should limit themselves to just three to four days.

Doctor Vetrano and I conclude this crash course on the wonderful benefits of the Natural Hygiene fast with a primary caution:

*In cases of many acute and most chronic diseases, for the fullest rest and greatest healing to take place, a longer fast is almost always required, making the retreat setting essential. For any health seeker deciding to take a fast of significant length, therefore, proper supervision by a trained specialist is necessary.*

Fasting in acute and chronic disease is serious. Fasting is not a toy for playtime, nor is it a time for novices and the ill-informed to monitor themselves and decide their own care. Most people in relatively good health with no serious complaints can fast safely seven to ten days. But even these less serious conditions in health seekers can develop into very serious situations once a short fast progresses into a longer fast and as cleansing and healing crises become intense and heretofore unknown disease symptoms in progress surface.

If you are in reasonably good health and intend to fast for more than a week, it is best to consult with your Natural Hygiene, holistic or naturopathic physician or a qualified health educator. Second best is to read up on fasting so you'll know what to expect and how best to break your fast correctly. If, however, you are in poor health, if your energy is low and you have chronic, degenerative symptoms, you most certainly should get consultation.

Since Dr. Shelton's most famous book, *Fasting Can Save Your Life,* is now out-of-print, Dr. Vetrano considers our crash course on the Natural Hygiene fast and how to break it the next best thing for do-it-yourselfers.

I now turn our fasting chapter back to Susan.

# Natural Hygiene Fasting Case Studies

The first six reports are real case studies from fasting clinics, taken from the book *Fasting for the Health of It: 100 Case Histories Selected from over 200,000*

*Clinical Records* by Jean Oswald and Dr. Shelton.

Among the 100 health seekers whose conditions improved or who healed completely after fasting are case histories on the following acute and chronic diseases: abdominal tumors, alcoholism, bursitis, breast tumors, varicose veins, headaches, back pain, ovarian cyst, brain tumor, eczema, hemorrhoids, osteoarthritis, angina, glaucoma, Hodgkin's disease, spinal meningitis, overactive thyroid, multiple sclerosis, rheumatoid arthritis, ulcerative colitis, schizophrenia, appendicitis, lupus, anemia, snoring, drug addiction and more.

# Kidney Stones Passed

[Therese, age 44, fasted under the supervision of Dr. Scott for 10 days in 1977 and 14 days in 1978.] After Therese's first fast, she returned to the same X-ray specialist who stated that two kidney stones were clearly visible on her X-rays. On her new pictures, no remnant of the stones remained; the stones had crumbled and passed.

In 1978, Therese and her "health nut" son, as she called him, returned to Dr. Scott's Natural Health Institute. Both fasted two weeks.

Therese told me her improved health was worth the effort to overcome her former bad habits. She eats no dairy products, fried foods or meat and is still changing other dietary habits, such as proper food combining, to prevent the formation of more kidney stones. "Rome wasn't built in a day," Therese said to me.

# Cataracts Gone

[Helen, age 54, fasted 14 days in 1979 under the supervision of Dr. Scott.] Helen put away her honey, aspirin, and Darvon after the fourth day of her fast. She discovered there was no use trying to mix the hygienic system with the drug system; it was like trying to mix oil with water. Helen discovered that the fundamental principles of the two systems are the exact opposites of each other, just as their means of care are opposites. If she attempted to use both systems and relied upon drugs for part of her remedial resources, she would fail to make full use of hygienic means.

After Helen developed full confidence in Hygiene, in her body's own power to both restore and preserve health, she recovered. After fasting twelve days, her eyesight had improved tremendously. And the cataracts were gone. The eyes are just as much a part of the body as the skin, lungs or heart. Helen had to change her former toxic habits to change the health of her eyes. "The disappearance of the cataracts seemed like a miracle," Helen said to me.

# Woman Finally Carried a Fetus to Full Term

[Rachelle fasted under the supervision of Dr. Shelton for 10 days in 1932.] There are different reasons for sterility; many respond favorably to the fast, others do not. In this particular case, Rachelle had 28 spontaneous abortions. After a

10-day fast and a four-month diet of raw fruit and vegetables, she became pregnant and later gave birth to a healthy boy.

## Insanity Reversed

[Mr. S. A., age 35, fasted 39 days under the supervision of Dr. Shelton in 1940.] Hygienic care greatly improved Stan's mental condition. I have used fasting in cases of mental disease and have no doubt that fasting is distinctly beneficial. I am convinced that when the insane person refuses food, this is an instinctive measure designed to assist the body in its reconstructive work. Many people have lost their abnormal mental conditions while fasting. All who have had extended experience with fasting have seen cases of insanity recover health while on the fast and many others make great improvement while fasting.

## Parkinson's Tremor Gone after Several Fasts

[Monica, age 39, fasted three times under the supervision of Dr. Shelton: 30 days, 14 days and later another 14 days in 1941.] The developments in this case are typical with the exception that Monica completely recovered. Full recovery is not the general rule. The majority of fasters make sufficient progress to become useful again but retain part of the tremor.

Monica was at the health school for nine months and had previously suffered with Parkinson's disease for six years. After she had fasted 30 days, the tremor immediately recurred, but not as severely as before the fast. After the second fast, the tremors were less. After the third fast, the tremors were gone. For more than 10 years, I remained in contact with Monica. She has had no recurrence of the tremor.

## Deafness, Impotence, Enlarged Prostate and Sinus Congestion Gone

[Mr. A. B., age 70, fasted 42 days in 1960 under the supervision of Dr. Shelton.] On the 36th day of fasting, Art regained hearing in his deaf ear for the first time in six years. His prostate gland had shrunken to nearly normal size. After he fasted, he spent three weeks on a raw fruit and vegetable diet. He was no longer impotent, his sinus congestion was relieved, and the recovery of hearing was permanent.

I have conducted a number of fasts in people from 70 years to over 85 years of age, and I have found no reason to consider aged people to be in a class by themselves. Adult animals of any species, including *Homo sapiens*, can fast much longer than the young of the same species. Old people actually stand fasting best. Growing children stand it least, although they stand it well. People do not get too old to use fasting as a method for healing.

The regenerating effects of fasting are especially apparent in the old. So I do not hesitate to place old people upon a fast, but I watch them more closely than I do younger people not because they do not stand fasting well, but because they are often possessed of hidden weaknesses that render it inadvisable to carry the fast to great length.

## Ankylosing Spondylitis Healed

Vern Caloudes wrote his miraculous fasting account in the June 1984 issue of the journal *Naturally, the Hygienic Way*. A very athletic young man in his 20s, he got early warning signs of ankylosing spondylitis, a disease in which the body slowly fuses together the spinal vertebrae, creating pain and extreme immobility. Initially, Vern lost flexibility, had a choppy gait, collapsed after running, and experienced a great deal of pain.

He received the official diagnosis of ankylosing spondylitis at the age of 29, by which time he was practically bedridden. It took him 20-30 minutes just to move across the room, always on his hands and knees. He was warned to lie as straight as possible to be able to stand straight, and he took the drug Indocin to ease the pain.

Since medicine offered no cure, Vern desperately sought the answer in alternative health and read Dr. Shelton's best-seller, now out-of-print, *Fasting Can Save Your Life*. In 1981, Vern went to the California Health Sanctuary where he fasted for 30 days on water only. Although he was still experiencing some discomfort in parts of his body, he writes, "But a miracle was occurring elsewhere in my body. Mobility in my neck and hips began to return. This was the first sign that my life was turning around."

Three and a half months later Vern returned for another fast. Since, as a runner, he had eaten an excess of candy bars (25 in a day!), he went through sugar withdrawal. Later he went on to do two more fasts. Director Arthur Andrews wrote the following in his case file:

> April 30, 1984. 100% hygienic raw diet. . . . No pain anymore. Can basically do whatever he wants. In the past year he has participated in 10-15 road races (running) for pleasure, not for competition. . . . Doesn't push to exhaustion, nor does he run anything longer than 3 miles to 10 kilometers. He has done a few training runs of up to 10 miles. . . . Feels comfortable and getting stronger. Says if he didn't ever get any better, he'd be happy with what has been accomplished.

Vern went on to affirm his life commitment to eating only raw foods and to practicing Natural Hygiene's ten energy enhancers. Vern vowed, "Even though not all my movement has returned, I do everything with great joy because there is no more pain."

## Baby Healed from Whooping Cough

Joe and Cindy D., friends of your author, once took their 9-month-old son to Dr. Shelton's fasting retreat in 1979 because the boy had whooping cough with nonstop coughing. Much to their surprise, Shelton advised that the infant fast on water only! These parents were at first concerned because he was so young, but Dr. Shelton assured them their child would be fine. After five days of ingesting only water, the baby was well!

By contrast, some friends of theirs took their own baby with whooping cough for conventional treatment with medications. He took over a year to heal!

## Extreme Emaciation Resolved via Fasting!

Dr. Shelton related the story of one young man who was so emaciated that the medical and naturopathic doctors attending him for months while getting no results were at their wits' end. Dr. Shelton was called in for consultation as a last resort.

To the astonishment of the doctors, Shelton recommended a fast, to which they reluctantly agreed. Following the young man's fast, his digestive capacity returned. He went on to achieve a complete recovery.

# Further Fasting Cautions

Note that not all of our raw food friends are enthusiastic about fasting. Some of those mentioned in Appendix C believe it is better just to eat properly. Instinctive eaters believe that one should fast only when nothing smells or tastes good, which is the body's only true call for a fast. This is what animals instinctively do, fasting only when sick and refusing food until well.

Educate yourself first if you do decide to fast. If a fast on water only is to be longer than a week or so, especially if it is your first fast, consider using the guidance of a doctor or health educator trained in fasting supervision.

How you break a fast is critical, especially if the disease process has not been fully reversed. There is one infamous account of a man deep into chronic degeneration who undertook a long fast and broke it improperly without supervision on meat and potatoes. It killed him!

When one is fasting on water only, the digestive system shuts down and needs time to reactivate. So break the fast with fresh juice or fruit. A juice diet should be broken with whole raw fruit. One day of juice or whole fruit for each day of fasting on water only is the standard recommendation.

Most people consider the fast fully broken when their prefast strength and vitality have returned. They are then ready to return to live food meals of fruits, vegetables, nuts, seeds and sprouts in proper combination at that time.

## The Details of Drug Withdrawal

If you have been taking recreational, prescription or over-the-counter drugs — your body doesn't know the difference — you could go into a more intense elimination than would happen on the raw diet or juices alone. It is therefore often not advised to fast while on drugs or immediately after quitting drugs, unless under proper supervision.

Dr. Vetrano cautions, "Natural Hygiene doctors cannot take people off meds. They must ask their clients to have their medical doctors tell them how to get off prescriptions. Only after several weeks of quitting medications should a fast be taken. With steroids, however, it is best to wait a year before fasting. This permits the adrenal glands to return to full function. A crisis could occur, and with too little cortisol, death could result unless the client took his steroids again at the onset of the crisis."

Legally, an MD is the only health professional who can tell you to stop taking drugs or reduce your drug dosage. Holistic physicians, such as chiropractors, acupuncturists, homeopaths and naturopaths, know how bad these drugs are but cannot tell you to cease taking them at the risk of being taken to court for practicing medicine without a license and being hauled off to jail. (See Appendix B for more on how the medical system works.)

Therefore, we can't advise you to stop your prescription medications either. We do recommend consulting first with a naturopathic doctor or other doctor trained in fasting supervision from among those listed in the Resource Guide. Some even offer supervision and guidance by phone.

# Fasting for a Heart Attack — A True Story

Lest the fasting information presented herein make you too fearful of pursuing fasting as a means of health recovery, just be aware that even some people falling into the questionable categories listed above have achieved remarkable fasting recoveries under proper care or even their own care.

This case history is presented to show you what can be accomplished, even in life-threatening emergency situations. It demonstrates the power of the body to heal when simply resting and conserving energy, even when ideal conditions are not provided. The story dramatically portrays the remarkable restorative powers of the human body under conditions of nearly total physiological rest.

Please note that this represents an extreme case in fasting, since most people don't wait until a life-or-death situation to begin fasting! Also, most people do not have mystical, near-death experiences while fasting. It happened in this case only because the storyteller was so close to death. People in hospitals sometimes report such near-death accounts. They correlate with being near death, not with fasting.

In July 1998, Leo Duerson of Wasco, Oregon, wrote the following account of his recovery from a near-fatal heart attack, entirely at home without any medical intervention at all, merely by means of complete rest and fasting under the telephone supervision of hygienic doctor Bernarr Zovluck.

Had Leo called 911 instead, he most likely would have been given drugs and subjected immediately to a heart bypass operation or other invasive coronary procedures. He may not have even survived such an operation. Most certainly had he survived, he would have been handed a medical bill numbering tens of thousands of dollars.

Leo had been advised to exercise only in moderation due to his heart condition. His heart attack resulted from not monitoring his exercise. He also had long been going against his doctor's advice by ill-advisedly partaking in his beloved wife's nonhygienic cooking.

Leo's amazing story is reprinted here in his own words with permission, edited only slightly for clarity, from the August 1998 issue of *The Natural Health Many-to-Many*:

I exercised for 5 days. Believing the body was strong enough to endure short periods of work, with the idea I would rest after 10-15 seconds in much the same fashion as in lifting weights, I decided to use a weed-eater (a small machine used for cutting weeds). The problem was, I forgot to monitor the time. Feeling faint, I decided to lie down, but then came the near-fatal mistake.

After resting, I decided on another attempt — again not monitoring the time. It felt like somebody hit me over the head with a 2x4. I had all I could do to maintain consciousness with my arms, legs and eyes totally out of control and focus. After a period of time, I was able to walk 40' to my pad on the ground, where I rested until able to get to my bedroom and later to the couch to be close to my wife, who was knitting in the living room.

That night I had an out-of-body experience. It started with the pounding of my heart, then hyperventilation until I thought my heart would explode. Recalling Bernarr's often-repeated recommendation, I closed my eyes and concentrated upon the symptom. Almost immediately the hyperventilation ceased, and my heart slowed.

Each time I started to breathe normally, my heart started to pound harder, so all I could think of was to concentrate on my breathing until I entered a trancelike state in which I was not sure that I was breathing. I sensed my body was floating with my legs above me. I passed by a door with a bright, shining light to the left and underneath the door. I asked the Lord God within, "Are you going to take me now?"

I got the answer, "No!"

I then passed another door that was totally black. I'm not a devil-thinker, so I did not even think to ask the same question. I do not know how long it was before my breathing returned to normal, but I was then able to get up from the couch and walk to bed.

Throughout the above [17-day] fast, Bernarr was always available — 24 hours a day, 7 days a week, for both my wife and me. My fast and recovery period was particularly rough on my wife, who was instructed under no circumstance to call 911. When I was in a trancelike state, or when going into or coming out of, she was totally helpless to do anything and in fact was on occasion told to leave the room because I realized that I had to do it totally on my own.

Again Bernarr's recommendation to "close eyes, concentrate on the symptom" always cut through the discomfort of the symptom, which occasionally was somewhat scary. My body at times was like a 4th of July celebration, with flashes of heat, pains, aches from leg to arm, to leg, to chest, to groin — the whole 2,001 parts.

It was not long before I began to look forward to the next happening. One in particular was an event which I looked forward to: a bubbling sensation in arteries leading from the heart toward the left and right shoulder and another from the base of the neck on the right side up to my temple. I sensed that blood was finding new pathways to various parts of my body.

I terminated the fast before I wanted, as I sensed that my wife was having a more difficult time than I. I do not think that I would go on a long fast again at home. She upsets herself more than I wish to tolerate. During a fast, I become supersensitive to other people's reactions. . . .

Once again the heart started *banging*, and once again I had to concentrate on the pounding until reaching a trancelike state — a condition which was becoming very disagreeable [to my wife] but the only means I knew of survival. She then became very upset and refused to leave until once again I was breathing normally, and even then under protest. She thought that I might die while she was not there for me. I had to reassure her again and again that the body would not self-destruct while in a state of complete rest.

After the near-fatal mistake and the out-of-body experience above, I decided to return to the fast for another three days — terminating for those reasons given. I had one hell of a time on fruit, as I had a hypoglycemic reaction. In fact I do not recall . . . just how I terminated, but it took 3 days of experimenting. And once I did terminate, it took several months before I could eat fruit without cloves or cinnamon without getting a reaction like that of hypoglycemia.

Immediately after breaking the fast, I proceeded to exercise, lifting very light weights until out of breath or until I had a heavy chest, always increasing repetitions, speed and weights, resting as needed.

I notice that if I slack off, I immediately have less energy and seem to lose strength. I'm inclined to think I'll be on an exercise routine for the rest of my life.

[You] might ask — "A longtime natural hygienist (since 1981) having a heart attack and/or heart condition at age 70? What gives?"

Bruno Comby, in his book *Maximize Immunity* . . . states something to the effect [that] it is not the fruits and vegetables that make you healthy; it is the cooked food that makes you sick.

Note Lou's confession at the end. Though he had been practicing most of the principles of Natural Hygiene for 17 years, he hadn't let go of cooked food — hence the heart condition. He went on to live another seven years.

The occasion of his death was equally instructive. He eventually died at the hands of the medical profession in the aftermath of an accidental fall that left him with a brain hematoma (swelling or tumor) and a severe, continuous headache. Instead of seeking Dr. Zovluck's counsel, which would have been the same as for his heart attack — complete physiological rest — he sought medical diagnosis and treatment.

The "learned" MDs recommended brain surgery to relieve the pain and swelling and to excise the hematoma. When the first surgery proved unsuccessful in relieving his pain, they performed a second brain operation, which killed him.

Dr. Zovluck teaches that meditating, or focusing attention intently, upon any symptoms that may appear from time to time throughout the fast will accelerate the healing process by directing the healing energy to those areas of the body.

Victoria BidWell, a student of Dr. Hans Selye's fight-or-flight work, explains the fear response and wisdom of calming down:

When the body goes into the alarm mode because something is perceived as terribly wrong in the body or in life circumstances, every cell in the body is affected by the nervous, glandular and circulatory systems. In fact all systems are readied for extreme action. The body is mobilized to fight or flee the situation so it can get back to normal. Skin vessels constrict, and goose bumps appear. Sweat glands pour out sweat. Secretion of digestive enzymes and insulin stops. Digestion halts. The mouth goes dry. Adrenaline and other stress hormones and neurotransmitters flood the body. Bowels and the urinary bladder relax, and their control is often lost. Blood flow to the heart and muscles increases. Voluntary muscles dilate to accommodate powerful action. Blood vessels to the brain constrict. Muscles of the head constrict and cause headaches and fear for some and euphoria and fearlessness for others. Much more is going on in the body's 75 trillion cells, but you get the idea. Emotional balance for all who do not possess self-mastery is completely lost.

All of this heightened neurophysiology throws people without coping techniques into a state of great fear. They start trembling and entertaining dreadful thoughts. Dangerous decisions can get made. They can actually see things and hear things that are not there and act upon them. Paranoia can kick in. If these fearful imaginings and poor choices are allowed and acted upon while in this unique physiological state of alarm, the situation can be made much, much worse. This is why knowledge of how the body, mind and emotions work and self-control are so important. While fasting or in emergency situations, knowing yourself and practicing self-mastery are all-important. Keeping cool and maintaining emotional balance could save your life.

# Our Final Fasting Farewells

Fasting should be a complete rest for the entire mind and body — rest from food, drugs, emotional stress, mental tasks, excitement of the five senses and all but the most mild and limited of physical activity. It's even best to stay in bed sleeping with eyes closed 24/7, or as close to that as you can manage, for the duration of the fast. This permits the body to focus as much of its attention and energy on revitalizing, cleansing and healing as is humanly possible.

Yet what good does it do to detoxify and heal if you simply go out and reintoxicate yourself? Next we will look at how to stay raw in a world that caters to cooked fooders. The answer begins in changing the doors of perception through which we pass. It all begins in the mind.

# 16
# How to Stay Raw
# in a Cooked World

*When I have finally decided that a result is worth getting, I go
ahead on it and make trial after trial until it comes.*
—Thomas Edison (1847–1931)

*Edison failed 10,000 times before he made the electric light. Do
not be discouraged if you fail a few times.*
—Napoleon Hill (1883–1970)

Eating raw on a tropical island where natural foods abound would be very
easy, but as the saying goes, no man is an island. So how do you remain on your
raw food diet in a world so biased in favor of the "killinary" art of cooking? How
do you stay on a raw food diet in a world of cooked food?

## Staying Raw in Social Situations

Undoubtedly, the most difficult thing about going raw is that it is virtually
unheard of in every culture. Society simply does not make staying raw convenient. We are swimming against the current when we cease to eat cooked food.
We are defying cultural norms no matter what country we are in. It is truly a
cooked food world. Ironically, we appear "radical" when we revert to the original, natural human diet.

Making advance arrangements for social situations will help you stick to
your diet. If someone invites you over for dinner, explain what you are doing and
why. If you want to decrease social resistance, place the blame on your doctor:
"My doctor has me on a restricted diet."

Offer to bring your own food, and ask that the host not take this personally.
Request that you be allowed to contribute a dish so that you know there will be at
least one raw dish there. I often use this as an opportunity to share with people a
mini-lesson on the virtues of a raw diet.

Remember that you are not socializing with your friends just to partake of
the same food. The real reason you are socializing is to enjoy communication and
love, not food. Partaking of food with others simply heightens the pleasure of the
get-together. True, breaking bread with others is an ancient custom. But some

customs, such as eating cooked food, need to be changed for those who care about their health.

The worst situations may occur in the rare event of traveling to foreign cultures or perhaps cultural pockets within your own borders where dietary pleasures are not associated with health consequences at all. In such cases, you may politely explain that you are "allergic" to cooked food (you are!) or that your doctor has given you strict orders to eat uncooked food only. Just don't mention the fact that *you* are your own doctor! Where there is a will, there surely is a way to back out of established eating customs politely, either at home or abroad.

When I first went raw and visited out-of-town family and friends, I brought my raw recipe books and made meals for everyone. This was my way of advertising that raw dishes are delicious, and it also gave me a gracious way to avoid eating their food. Sometimes they would joke that they couldn't wait for me to leave so they could have "real" food. I would point out the irony. What is real food? Food designed by nature or food denatured by technology?

When going to a cooked potluck, eat beforehand and take a small bag of sun-dried fruit with nuts (trail mix) or sprouts in a little bag in case you get hungry so you won't be tempted to eat the ever-present cooked food. For your contribution, bring a raw food dish. Unless it is a plain lettuce salad, your new treat will probably be the hit of the party. So you had better take the recipe along too!

Some dishes are so tasty nearly everyone asks me for the recipes (see Chapter 21), so I have gotten into the habit of writing them on cards that I tape to the dishes. Your friends will appreciate your raw dish, especially if it contains raw fat, which is very delicious. Most likely, it will be a novelty, especially if it is a gourmet or dehydrated raw dish.

Eventually, all your friends will understand and accept your raw food "fanaticism" to some degree. They will be prepared for it and get used to it. Some will look forward to it with mild curiosity. Furthermore, you will eventually help those who are open-minded enough or physically sick enough to follow your lead. These true health seekers who do take their own raw journeys will be grateful to you forever!

If you live in a big enough city, you will eventually connect with other raw fooders through postings on the health food store bulletin board or the Internet, and you will join them in raw food potlucks and gatherings. Have you been to www.meetup.com? Put "raw food" and a zip code into their search engine in order to find registered raw food groups nearby. The social situation will improve in time.

Find support by joining raw food Internet chat rooms. Go to www.yahoo.com and click on "groups." Under "search," type in "raw food" or "living food." To find a local group, add the name of your city and state. You will find numerous groups of people with whom you can share experiences, recipes and advice, even if they are not local. Many are listed in the Resource Guide at the back of this book.

The social life situation is often a major stumbling block to going all-raw. But as Dr. Doug Graham points out in an interview with Frédéric Patenaude, "I want to know how a person can have a social life when sick. How does a person go out and have a good time when not feeling good?"

Graham further points out that one's social life may also be impaired by lack of confidence owing to poor skin or overweight from a cooked diet. He goes on to remark that the social life issue is especially a problem for young people who are single. He advises them to seek out others with similar values. He tells them, "It's cool to be different. It's cool to be healthy."

# Eating Out

As you might suppose, most raw fooders do not eat out as frequently as most cooked fooders. After all, you pay restaurants to cook your food. Almost all restaurants are geared only towards cooked food. Even the salads in a mainstream restaurant will have some cooked ingredients: croutons, bacon bits, cheese, chicken or shrimp (which jack up the prices), as well as salad dressings with pasteurized oils.

So what about the times you want to, or are more or less forced to, eat out? This happens often in social and business situations. It can be done. One can actually eat in a restaurant and remain totally raw.

One strategy is to know of every buffet-style eatery and salad bar in town. Select a place where you are allowed to pick from an array of both cooked and raw foods. Such buffets typically offer at least ten completely raw, totally unsalted, condiment-free fruit and vegetable serving bowls at the salad bar. The items may not be organic, but they are still relatively nutritious and full of flavor if you arrive with genuine hunger.

Sometimes my husband and I even "smuggle" food into an all-you-can-eat buffet, bringing our own raw salad dressing, sunflower seeds or other trimmings.

Create a stunning fruit salad, or prepare yourself a vegetable plate. By bringing along a ripe avocado and dicing it into a vegetable mix, you can create a feast! If you want to follow proper food combining, bring a little bag of nuts or raw nut butter in a small container instead of the avocado to have with nonstarchy vegetables or acid fruits.

A second plan, used when more formal dining with private seating is desired, is to call ahead and make sure that a vegetable salad or fruit plate is offered. This assures that you will not end up where there is absolutely nothing on the menu to eat. Pack the avocado or nuts regardless.

Victoria BidWell claims that in all her years of bringing her own food to a restaurant, she has upset restaurateurs only a few times and was asked to put her own food aside. She explains, "Wait staff don't care if you bring your own food, especially if you are charming and leave a tip on the table prior to ordering."

Victoria Boutenko manages eating out by handing the waiter or waitress a card that states she eats only raw food and requests a salad of various raw fruits or vegetables. She states that the chefs must derive great pleasure from the opportunity to exhibit their creativity because the resulting salad she receives is always remarkably beautiful.

Another strategy is to eat ahead of time, or later when possible, simply joining your friends and associates for the company they offer. This method may not work for business lunches or with people you don't know very well, as it often makes them feel uncomfortable to be eating when someone else in their party isn't.

If you are the engaging, outgoing type who loves to entertain, you may be able to keep them so enthralled that they hardly notice you are simply sipping on orange juice or perhaps not eating at all.

Finally, some restaurants permit one member of a party to consume a brown-bag lunch, sometimes asking a small service fee for the place setting, while the others order. It's always best to inquire about this possibility with the restaurant in advance since you can't count on brown bagging to be allowed. Also make sure brown bagging is acceptable to your dinner companions.

One lunch that I often bring to work is a raw salad of mixed greens with dressing or avocado, along with a snack of dried fruit and raw nuts or raw olives. I also pack an emergency snack of fruit in case I get stuck in traffic on the way home.

Those of you who eat out for lunch breaks on a regular basis will need to begin packing lunches. Just for brown baggers, Victoria BidWell and Shirlene Lundskog have prepared *Brown BagWell & StayWell!* This book presents 90 lunches, either vegetable or fruit based, most served through Shirlene's former catering service in Logan, Utah. Nearly all of them are raw.

Originally inspired to appeal to children and to help parents prepare school lunches that follow proper food combining dictates, the book conveys a contagious enthusiasm for brown bagging.

# Traveling

What about when you are on the road or flying to a destination? How can you remain raw while traveling? In such cases, it is necessary to plan ahead, as is the case always with the raw food diet. You simply cannot count on restaurants, be they on the road or in the airport, to cater to raw fooders. Remember, you are paying them to cook the food, which is a service you no longer want.

Therefore, you must be proactive and plan ahead so that you do not backslide due to hunger. Come armed with nature's "fast food": raw munchies. Such raw snacks may simply be whole, live foods: apples, pears, cucumbers, celery, carrots, sun-dried fruit and nuts. Others may require preparation: homemade trail mix, nut butter, flaxseed crackers, homemade banana nut-bread and raw cookies. See the recipes in Chapter 21 for some of these delicious dishes.

The point is to be prepared. The word is not yet out enough for the world to cater to raw fooders. Since the media focus is on high-profit, SAD foods, our live foods get little attention. There is simply not yet a big enough market for the food giants to commercialize raw food products, and dedicated live food entrepreneurs are few. However, thanks to the Internet, raw food authors, teachers and a few openly raw celebrities, the word is now spreading at a faster pace.

If you are fortunate in your travels, there may be fresh juice or smoothie stands for you to order a drink, even if nonorganic, but never count on it. Never leave the house without an emergency snack to tide you over until you can reach a supermarket or other produce vendor.

In fact you may wish to leave some dried fruit, raw nuts or flaxseed crackers in your car for such cases, rotating the unused ones every few weeks or so. When worse comes to worst, always carry handy bottled water to live on until you can get to your closest live food supply.

# How to Avoid Backsliding

While still experiencing frequent and intense cooked food cravings during detoxification and transition to a raw diet, avoid putting yourself in temptation zones: restaurants, parties, potlucks, dinner invitations and so on. Select and practice appropriate behavior modification techniques that will see you through those moments and places that are unavoidable.

When you are shopping and see free samples of cooked food, don't give in to the lie that "one little bite won't hurt." Anything you put into your mouth that doesn't *add* to your health *subtracts* from your health. Once you start giving in to indulgences, you will find yourself SADly "enjoying" daily bites and samples. Before you know it, you will descend gradually and inevitably into old food addictions.

"Just one bite won't hurt" is the attitude that creates bad habits. In Overeaters Anonymous, this is called "the first compulsive bite." That first bite of cooked food could set you off on a cooked food backslide.

If you do backslide into cooked food addiction, which is easier to do if eating only partially raw, don't get into guilt and self-condemnation. Never give up! Just get back onto raw foods with the aid of fasting on water only, juice dieting or monomeals if necessary. It is usually easy to get back on the program if you fast for a day or, better yet, a few days.

A brief period of fasting or light eating, especially with plenty of rest and sleep, will permit your body to quickly detoxify from the poisons in the cooked food you have recently eaten, as well as lessen your cravings for it. This will provide the revitalizing boost you need to quickly give you the light, clearheaded feeling that keeps you hooked on raw.

However, don't get into the habit of bingeing on cooked food, thinking that it will be easy to get rid of the toxins and cravings later by fasting! This kind of thinking could set up the binge/purge syndrome characteristic of eating disorders. Yo-yoing back and forth between the worlds of cooked foods and live foods could also greatly weaken your self-esteem and willpower. Mustering up the determination to get back onto a raw diet may become more difficult or seemingly impossible if you feel you have repeatedly failed.

Some people yo-yo like this for decades, making themselves miserable with illness, guilt, self-loathing and discouragement, trying to do what they know is right but without the key factor of a 100% raw diet. As Mark Twain (Samuel Clements) joked, "It is easy to stop smoking. I have done it hundreds of times!"

My new friend Victoria BidWell confesses that this has been her own worst error since 1976. Even after having gone all-raw for one three-year "Hygiene honeymoon" coupled with all the other healthful practices, she confides, "One of the dozens of reasons that I have stepped forward to involve myself and Dr. Vetrano in your *Live Food Factor* to help make this second edition even better was because I saw that your teachings and experience, combined with our teachings and experience, could help me and countless others get off the raw/cooked yo-yo, waste-of-time-and-energy syndrome, once and for all!"

To avoid falling into this quagmire of repeated failure, it may be wise and beneficial to start out committing to a shorter period of 100% raw, such as a few weeks or a month, rather than promising yourself you will never eat another bite of cooked food for the rest of your life. After the initial period is up, you can re-assess and hopefully renew your commitment for a longer period the next time.

Three to four weeks of an all-raw diet is a good minimal goal to set because psychological studies have shown that 21-28 days is how long it takes for a new habit to be formed, but don't set a goal you know you can't keep. Although it may sound silly, it actually helps to draw up a written contract with yourself and sign it. If you don't feel you can trust your own word, you can even add a penalty clause, like committing to make a donation to your least favorite charity or political party upon failure.

Despite that, if you discover that your initial goal was too ambitious to complete, you may need to renew your commitment for a shorter interval, like a week. Or you may need to approach the new diet by committing yourself to one day at a time. That may be how some with eating disorders will need to start raw, counting the days and renewing the commitment on a daily basis. Only you can decide which method is best for you.

Finally, if you do backslide into cooked foods, don't beat yourself up over it! Renew your mind by reading more about the benefits of raw food and healthful living practices. Reprogram your left brain with all the audio lectures, DVD presentations, books and Internet support material now available. Reprogram your right brain with positive affirmations. It's easier and much more enjoyable to keep commitments when you truly understand why you are making them and when your subconscious is in synchrony with your conscious mind.

Counteract feelings of deprivation by finding pleasurable ways of pampering yourself that exclude all processed foods. Treat yourself to some great gourmet raw recipes or your favorite organic melons. Reward yourself with a hot tub session, a dip in the swimming pool or a relaxing massage.

Use the Smart Recovery method, a rehabilitation program for overcoming addictions. Basically, it teaches that if you yield to a temptation to indulge in something that is negative to your health, observe it. Detach yourself so that you can analyze the experience. See how you felt just before backsliding, and remember the aftermath consequences. Keep a journal. Take notes. Read the notes the next time you are tempted. Use the rational analytical left part of your brain to make the decision to return to healthful living practices. See Appendix E for more behavior modification techniques and right-brain strategies to help you stay on track.

# Enhanced Sensitivity to Cooked Foods

After persisting with raw eating for a time, you will notice that if you do begin to backslide into cooked foods, you may feel so momentarily terrible that it will be easy to get back to the pleasures of the raw diet. If you return to raw right away, your body will not have had time to build up a tolerance to the protoplasmic poisons inherent in cooked diets. Your body will have cultivated an enhanced sensitivity to all unnatural foods and will have retained sufficient energy reserves to carry out an immediate cleansing crisis.

Someone who smokes his first cigarette will usually react violently with expulsive symptoms because his lungs are still relatively pure. These symptoms may include coughing, nausea, racing heart and sweating.

After he has smoked even just one pack within 24 hours, his body has already given up reacting so strongly and begins its adaptation process to the toxins by suppressing those energy-draining self-defense measures, but the damage that continued smoking causes will persist below conscious awareness at the cellular level as greater degrees of toleration are reached.

Habitual exposure to any toxic substance that is not instantly fatal results in a gradual buildup of tolerance. Cooked food, nicotine, alcohol, chemical aerosols — it's all the same. Habitual exposure leads to tolerance, which leads to addiction, which leads to disease. The body is simply following the Law of Vital Accommodation. (See page 551.)

A clean body is more sensitive and efficient at eliminating any reintroduction of toxins because it has high energy levels and thus low tolerance for poisons. For example, a raw eater given novocaine may find that it has worn off during the middle of the dental procedure because his body so efficiently and swiftly eliminates the drug.

This has happened to both my husband and me. Pain is more muted when you're eating raw. There seems to be a higher tolerance for it. Some raw fooders don't even accept painkillers during dental work, not wishing to add more toxins to their bodies.

Toxins that used to go unnoticed may suddenly elicit strong reactions. As a former eater of processed foods, I often unknowingly consumed MSG. (See Appendix A.) After going raw and unwittingly eating some, as I did when buying guacamole with "spices" listed among the ingredients, I would not be able to sleep until about 3 AM and would feel itchiness all over my skin. Sometimes migraine headaches resulted.

If you do decide to go 100% raw or nearly so, people will tell you, "Oh, but you have to eat at least *some* cooked food," or "You are too fanatical, too obsessive, and this is not healthy."

Just remember, if you do give in to that one compulsive, toxic bite, your enhanced sensitivity may leave you feeling temporarily much worse than when your body had built up a tolerance to the poisons in that food.

As Frédéric Patenaude puts it, "You will be much more affected by small doses of poisons than most people. A cup of coffee could have the same effect on you as five cups on your neighbor" (*The Raw Secrets*, p. 54).

David Wolfe joked at a workshop that his uncle used to preach, "Everything in moderation!" David would reply, "Yes, *especially* moderation!" What he means is that there is a time and a place not to be moderate, and certainly this applies when your health is at stake.

Dr. Shelton used to declare that there is no such thing as moderation when it comes to poison. He mocked those echoing the advice of those who advocated "moderation in all things" by asking, "Would such people advise moderation in adultery or moderation in murder?"

You might wonder, "Well, if my body has adapted to the toxins in cooked foods, what's the big deal?"

It is important to recognize that the body builds *disease* as it builds toleration — one bite at a time. As Shelton warned in *The Hygienic System, Vol. I: Orthobionomics*, "Toleration to poisons is merely a slow method of dying."

# The Glorious World beyond Temptation!

At last, after an extended period of months to a year or more of consistently applying the ten energy enhancers, including 100%, or close to 100%, adherence to a raw food diet, you will enter the *glorious world beyond temptation*. Cooked food set before you will neither smell nor look edible. It will appear as mere "plastic," "pretty decorations" or "fake food." At this promising point, you may stop in gratitude to marvel, "How in the world did I ever eat and even enjoy that?"

The odors of some cooked foods will be utterly repulsive: dead animal flesh and hot grease, for example. Other aromas, like that of freshly baked bread or cooked spices, may continue to smell pleasantly nostalgic, stimulating your brain's limbic system that associates those smells with pleasant memories. But in the glorious world beyond temptation, you will neither swoon nor salivate for such unnatural foods.

Being on a raw diet at that point is an absolute joy, definitely not self-sacrifice. You are free of those old addictions. In fact if someone paid you to do so, you would still not consume those cooked "treats."

Indeed, the reality TV show *Wifeswap* advertised a $20,000 offer to find a committed raw food family that would exchange diets with a cooked family for a week. It took them weeks to locate a volunteer. The buzz around the Internet raw chat groups was, "No way!"

The show eventually did find a volunteer family, but the kids got so sick after one cooked meal that the father cried and begged that they not be forced to eat another one.

Re-entering the world of cooked food, with its deadly sights, smells and tastes, would make you absolutely miserable. You have no temptation to back-slide whatsoever. You know it would be painful and enervating to readjust. Even one serving of cooked food would leave your purified body, with its heightened sensitivity, in a toxic state of alarm — inducing sleepiness, heaviness, depression, constipation and/or other acute symptoms of poison rejection.

Your body is now operating so perfectly, so sensitively, that life is indeed glorious! But be forewarned that in this grand physiological mode, the slightest bit of ingested toxin will be propelled swiftly outward, potentially leaving your body in momentary pain or with a sense of sluggishness and mental fog for hours or even days.

Congratulations! You have now become as our ancient ancestors, a truly natural, raw food eater! You know you are completely healthy at this point in your raw journey back to nature because you feel so good! You know you are totally free of addiction when you feel no temptation whatsoever to indulge in today's perverted, cooked, adulterated, processed foods. You know you are happy when your every movement is an effortless pleasure, when you wake up every morning *with a bounce*, just glad to be alive!

The saddest thing about being in the glorious world beyond temptation is to watch the sick people of the world get sicker. Either they do not know about the principles of health by healthful living, or they know but refuse to apply them. The saddest thing of all is when our loved ones know them intellectually but will not apply them in practice.

# Paradise Health

As explained previously, Professor Arnold Ehret coined the term *paradise health* to describe the condition of one who has reached a state of total detoxification and purification of body, mind and spirit. In appreciation and gratitude for his trailblazing example, I conclude this chapter with a description of this extraordinarily wonderful state of health potentially achievable for most of us, given sufficient time and effort.

Victoria BidWell calls this natural high *superlative health* and *Natural Hygiene high joy*. Dr. Vetrano calls it *Hygiene euphoria*. Arnold Ehret called it *paradise health*. You may come up with your own favorite term to name how marvelous you feel when you get there.

Some argue that paradise health is no longer attainable without periodic fasting and consuming extremely high quality food, including super foods, supplements and only organic food, due to all of the unavoidable environmental toxins and emotional stresses to which we are constantly exposed in everyday life that drain our vital energy reserves.

Considering these secondary sources of toxemia laid out in Chapter 4, this argument may very well be true. But compared to living in the same toxic world while eating a steady diet of refined, adulterated, cooked food, you can achieve a level of health on an 80%-100% raw diet that will astound you!

Your health and energy levels will surprise you once you have gone through revitalization, detoxification and healing. Adding the other nine energy enhancers to your daily life, especially adequate rest and sleep, will further enhance your energy levels. You will rediscover your childlike joy and awe of life!

After you have been eating as closely as possible to a 100% live food diet for several years, if not just several weeks or months, you will find yourself in exceptional health. What were formerly minor complaints that you viewed as nuisances are now gone: things like athlete's foot, acne, mild headaches, grogginess after meals, bouts of constipation and mild aches and pains.

You will likely experience much less thirst. Cooked foods are water-deficient. The body needs a lot more added water to digest them. Cooked food contains toxins, especially table salt, that must be diluted so as to be kept out of harm's way and close contact with all cells in the body.

Virtually all overweight people are carrying around 10-20 pounds of edematous water weight that is eliminated swiftly on raw, salt-free food. With plenty of fresh fruit and vegetables in your diet, you may need to drink only *half as much* water as formerly — or *even less* — and you will carry around no waterlogged tissues!

*Body odors may vanish* or drastically reduce, proving that they originate from the internal poisoning of cooked, processed or otherwise poorly digested food. Some long-time raw fooders can go days, even weeks, without a shower. Yet no one notices. A totally pure body on a biologically suitable diet does not have bad breath or body odor. Unwashed feet will not stink. Even sweat, sputum, vaginal discharges, stools and other bodily emissions may become odorless.

Note: If an occasional odor manifests even though you have been internally clean for years, it may mean your body has been digging deeper to expel toxins from earlier years. It could also mean that you are eliminating some pollutant to which you were recently exposed or that you aren't digesting your food well due to overeating, emotional stress, contaminated food or poor food combining practices.

Digestion and elimination that once took up to 100 hours to complete on a cooked food diet will take only 18-36 hours. To check your transit time, eat some beets. Red appearing in the stools will indicate elimination of the beet residues, allowing you to calculate transit time. New raw fooders, including myself once, are sometimes a tad alarmed upon seeing this for the first time, thinking it to be blood!

Other foods you can use to check transit time are whole sesame seeds, flax-seeds or fresh corn, some of which will remain intact in the stools and be visible. Charcoal supplements obtainable from health food stores are yet another substance that can be used for this purpose.

Your stools will likely be softer and more frequent, passing without strain, quite unlike those on fiber-poor diets that leave most cooked fooders chronically constipated, diarrheic and/or laxative dependent. You may find yourself eliminating after every meal. You will no longer have time for your favorite bathroom reader.

Your sinuses and lungs will no longer be clogged with phlegm. Your tongue will taste clean and fresh. With high energy and a clean diet, your absorption and assimilation of nutrients will be much more efficient. You will thus save on grocery bills.

As you approach paradise health, detoxification syndromes commonly called by the medical men "colds" and "flus" will pay increasingly infrequent visits to your body until they vanish altogether — despite exposures to sick people. If symptoms do occasionally appear, they will be much milder than formerly and disappear more quickly, particularly if you take a day off to rest and fast in bed.

You will usually know immediately what health mistake you made that led to the occurrence because of your body's enhanced sensitivity to toxic exposures. Consequently, your fear of germs and catching disease will vanish. You will now feel in near-total control of your health!

As your body becomes more alkaline, your mood will improve. Because of increasing well-being and energy, your confidence will soar. Your dreams appear vivid, possible and achievable. Your desire to reach out and grasp all life has to offer impels you forward with courage and strength! You step forward full of energy, creativity, focus, gratitude, love and willingness to extend yourself to help others.

So many raw fooders have reported finally taking up that one passion in their lives they had been denying themselves and then discovering their true missions in life. They change addresses, career paths and surprisingly often even their names. Every day becomes a marvelous new adventure!

You rediscover your childhood sense of curiosity and wonder at the everyday miracles of life. You have been lifted out of your former toxin-induced mental fog. You find yourself gravitating toward other positive-minded people and releasing former toxic, dead-end relationships. You tell them of the live food factor and the other nine energy enhancers.

Now that you are feeding your body with live food, you will feel more alive and joyful than you ever dreamed possible!

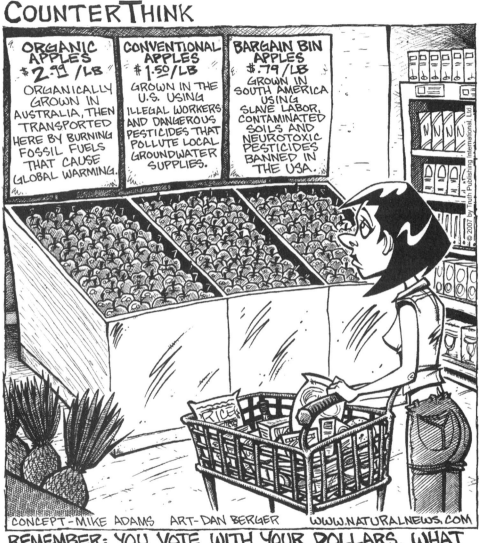

# CounterThink

**ORGANIC APPLES $2.99/LB** — ORGANICALLY GROWN IN AUSTRALIA, THEN TRANSPORTED HERE BY BURNING FOSSIL FUELS THAT CAUSE GLOBAL WARMING.

**CONVENTIONAL APPLES $1.50/LB** — GROWN IN THE U.S. USING ILLEGAL WORKERS AND DANGEROUS PESTICIDES THAT POLLUTE LOCAL GROUNDWATER SUPPLIES.

**BARGAIN BIN APPLES $.79/LB** — GROWN IN SOUTH AMERICA USING SLAVE LABOR, CONTAMINATED SOILS AND NEUROTOXIC PESTICIDES BANNED IN THE USA.

CONCEPT - MIKE ADAMS    ART - DAN BERGER    WWW.NATURALNEWS.COM

REMEMBER: YOU VOTE WITH YOUR DOLLARS. WHAT YOU BUY IS WHAT YOU ENCOURAGE.

# 17
# Nutritional Controversies

A veteran USDA meat inspector from Texas describes what he has seen: "Cattle dragged and choked . . . knocking 'em four, five, ten times. Every now and then when they're stunned they come back to life, and they're up there agonizing. They're supposed to be re-stunned, but sometimes they aren't, and they'll go through the skinning process alive. I've worked in four large [slaughterhouses] and a bunch of small ones. They're all the same. If people were to see this, they'd probably feel really bad about it. But in a packing house everybody gets so used to it that it doesn't mean anything."

—Gail Eisnitz, *Slaughterhouse*

There are various nutritional recommendations and guidelines that not everyone agrees with. In this chapter, I present some of these differing points of view, especially when they appear convincing. You must ultimately do your own research and find out what makes the most sense to you.

This chapter's purpose is to inform you about choices you will have to make if you go raw. Please don't use these issues as excuses not to change your diet! *Most of these controversies are things you need to consider even if you do not go to a primarily raw diet. Ignorance is not bliss when it comes to your health.* Get informed, and don't stop with this book!

## Vegetarianism vs. Meat Eating

There are several aspects to consider in deciding whether or not to include meat in your diet.

### Design/Nature Considerations

Many people think humans are vegetarian by nature, or design, though most of us are omnivorous in practice, eating both plants and animals. The clues that we are biologically vegetarians include the facts that we have a relatively long digestive tract through which meat putrefies before leaving. We also lack claws and fangs with which to tear up meat.

Dr. Doug Graham lists 31 comparisons between carnivores and herbivores, clearly putting humans in the vegetarian category (*The 80/10/10 Diet*, pp. 16–18).

Robert Young argues, "All the longest-lived and healthiest cultures on the planet are almost exclusively vegetarian, and I have yet to see any culture using animal food come remotely close to their healthy longevity" (*Sick and Tired?* p. 116).

In *Are You Confused?* author Paavo Airola pointed out that the longest-lived people around the world — the Bulgarians, Hunzakuts, East Indian Todas, Yucatan Indians and Russian Caucasians — were either vegetarians or consumed very little meat.

Our genes and digestive tracts are most similar to chimpanzees, especially bonobos, which share 99.4% of our DNA sequences. Chimps in the wild eat a mostly fruitarian diet of fruit, green leaves, vegetables, nuts and seeds. But a small volume percentage of their diet is insect matter and even 2-5% meat by some estimates, since they kill and eat colobus monkeys occasionally when their customary foods are unavailable. As stated earlier, many scientists have concluded that we are biologically frugivores, like chimps and apes.

Some anthropologists believe that Cro-Magnons, who lived 40,000-20,000 years ago, ate meat. Yet Robert Leakey, a highly esteemed authority on the evolution of the human diet, has stated that Cro-Magnons did not have canine teeth. He concluded that they were not equipped to eat wild game and likely ate a primarily vegetarian diet, as did chimpanzees.

The popular diet book *Eat Right for Your Type* claims that those with blood type O cannot be healthy without meat. Yet three prominent raw fooders who have the O blood type do not eat meat. Dr. Cousens has been a vegetarian for over 20 years, Lou Corona for 31 years and David Wolfe for over a decade. I have met them all personally and can say they are all very healthy and energetic.

## Health Considerations

Meat is among the most toxic of naturally occurring foods. Eating raw meat presents some potential dangers to one's health, as discussed in Appendix C. The occasional contamination of raw meat by parasitic bacteria and worms has been recognized for many years, but cooked meat creates mutagens that have been directly linked to cancer. (See Chapter 9 and Appendix D.) The fat in commercially sold meat contains 10-15 times the pesticide concentration of that in plant tissues. Animal fats store toxins. Animal fat tissues are toxin storage depots, a characteristic not exhibited in plant tissues.

*The China Study* documents that a diet high in animal protein promotes cancer and other diseases of affluence, such as heart disease and gout. A diet high in plant protein does not have these adverse effects. It was documented that consumption of animal-based foods results in increased tumor development while consumption of plant-based foods results in decreased tumor development and even tumor regression.

Furthermore, it was found that anyone interested in obtaining optimal body size, height, weight and muscle development can achieve maximal potential on an exclusively plant protein diet. It may take longer to build muscles with plant protein than with animal protein, but musculature developed on plant foods is superior. Slow and steady wins the race.

Another concern with meat consumption is the modern practice of rendering, whereby whole dead animals are boiled in vats of acid. Then the remaining hooves, fur and bones are removed and the acids neutralized with lye to create a "food" for farm animals. So livestock animals are fed dead animals — oftentimes diseased livestock carcasses, roadkill and euthanized pets, whose remains contain the poisons that were used to euthanize them.

This nightmarish "food" is fed to animals that are natural vegetarians, such as cattle. Sometimes animals are even fed animals of their own species, which is totally unnatural. This is what is thought to have caused mad cow disease, the human variant of which is expected to kill many people in the next 15-20 years, due to its long latency period. Will we see "mad chicken disease" emerge in future years as well, since many livestock chickens are fed dead chickens?

These poor livestock animals are also drugged with steroids and antibiotics in addition to being forced to eat an unnatural diet of inferior food full of pesticides and herbicides. Some of the pesticide and herbicide residues from all the plant food the animal ever ate are concentrated in its fats. All of those pollutants reach the body of the person consuming animal products, thus injuring him or her also.

Most meat is laden with harmful ingredients. It is high in nitrogen compounds that are metabolized into uric acid. Our bodies lack the digestive enzyme uricase to break this acid down, which then ends up being deposited in our tissues if we eat more than a few ounces of meat a day.

Dr. Gabriel Cousens stated in a lecture that according to studies, 3-13% of what is diagnosed as Alzheimer's is actually mad cow disease. We also have "mad fish disease," "mad deer disease" and even "mad squirrel disease," although none of this is being reported officially.

# Spiritual Considerations

Many people have chosen not to eat meat at all because they believe they can expand their consciousness by eating vegetarian diets. Living food indeed seems to have a higher spiritual vibration, imparting a vibratory advantage to the one who ingests it. These vegetarians believe that dead animal food products lack the life force that living plant food provides.

The Jubbs write, "Life force is the electric energy a living animal has between its nerves and blood. When the animal is dead, this force is no longer present. Yet in vegetation, the sun's light (life force) remains within it after it has been harvested. Each cell of the plant stores the energy of the sun within it" (*LifeFood Recipe Book,* p. 2).

When you eat meat, even raw meat, you are losing much of the advantages of a raw food diet, as discussed in Chapter 10. As Dr. Cousens explains in *Spiritual Nutrition* (p. 222), the sunlight energy is stored as activated electron energy in the carbon/hydrogen bonding we find in organic live plant foods. These foods boost our electrons and oxygen. They contain biophotons from the sun. When animals metabolize this food, they too get these benefits of direct sunlight plant energy.

Furthermore, most animals in the USA are raised in very cruel conditions and slaughtered in such a horrific manner that anyone seeing it would be repulsed into vegetarianism. By purchasing such meat, we are voting with our dollars that these brutalities continue. Recent research has shown that animals, like people, have a wide variety of emotions, such as playfulness and love. They even exhibit their own forms of laughter.

Unless we purchase kosher meat, we are also ingesting the adrenaline and various fear molecules that were flowing through their bodies when they realized they were being killed. Many believe there is bad karma (an energy that brings back to you what you put out, good or bad) in eating such meat.

## Ecological Considerations

In addition, not eating meat benefits the planet because of the vast resources saved that would otherwise go into feeding and watering animals compared to growing plant foods. As discussed in Chapter 1, we are literally robbing water from future generations with every hamburger we eat.

According to Dr. Cousens, *a vegan saves about 1½ million gallons of water per year when compared to a flesh and dairy eater.* Some may argue that water is recycled anyway, so it doesn't matter. However, there is a real shortage of unpolluted fresh water. Some say wars will be fought over water in the future. *Even now such water costs more than oil in some locations since it has to be transported large distances using oil.*

A second resource wasted in raising animals for food is land that could be used to grow plant food for people. Fourteen vegans can live off the land that it takes to feed one meat eater. According to John Robbins in *Diet for a New America, if meat eaters in the USA would reduce their meat consumption by a mere 10%, the resources saved could feed the 60 million people who starve to death annually.*

A third wasted resource from raising livestock for food is oil. According to Cousens, for each calorie we derive from consuming beef, 78 calories of fossil fuel are used, compared to less than four calories of fossil fuel burned for each calorie of plant food consumed.

In addition, a report by the United Nations (2006) concluded that cattle-rearing *generates more global warming greenhouse gases than even transportation.* Anyone who has seen the documentary film *An Inconvenient Truth* is aware of the serious repercussions of this environmental issue.

Finally, raw plant food simply *tastes better*! Even if it were discovered that raw meat were definitely healthful and better for the ecology, I would remain a vegetarian because of the sheer pleasure of eating fresh raw fruits, vegetables, nuts and seeds.

Some raw fooders, after remaining raw vegans for several years, have nonetheless concluded that they needed to add some raw meat to their diets (most likely to get Vitamin $B_{12}$). You may not agree with this, but it was nonetheless their experience, and they certainly did not wish for that to be the case. Perhaps we are not all genetically alike in regard to this controversial issue.

If you are interested in learning more, there are more pro and con arguments relating to eating raw meat, as well as other raw animal products, such as dairy and eggs, in Appendix C.

# Vegans and the Vitamin $B_{12}$ Issue

There are over a dozen studies showing that it is very difficult for some vegans to satisfy their Vitamin $B_{12}$ needs dietarily or via internal bacterial production. While gut bacteria make it chiefly in the large intestines, it is absorbed mostly from the small intestines, so we cannot profit much from this source.

Some people get enough of this vitamin by eating unwashed green leafy vegetables since bacteria that make it cling to the plant surfaces, but most of us do not have our own gardens. Furthermore, if you have ever eaten unwashed greens straight from the garden, you are also likely to be eating insects and their eggs. This is what our primate cousins do, but this idea would be rather disgusting for most of us. Nonetheless, 80% of all humans eat insects deliberately, and the rest of us do so inadvertently at times.

Some people think they can get $B_{12}$ from sea vegetables, such as blue-green algae or spirulina. But recent studies have shown that the $B_{12}$ in sea vegetables is often an analog form of $B_{12}$ that cannot be used by the human body. Since analog $B_{12}$ competes for the same receptor sites as the truly usable $B_{12}$, it may in fact create a situation in which you have *less available $B_{12}$.* But with raw nori, $B_{12}$ levels in the blood were shown to be neither increased nor decreased.

The liver can maintain a storage depot of up to ten years' supply of Vitamin $B_{12}$, but more typically 2-5 years. This is why many vegans take years to feel the effects of $B_{12}$ deficiency. The longer one has been a vegan, the greater the chance of suffering $B_{12}$ deficiency. This is especially true of raw vegans since many "cooked vegans" eat foods fortified with $B_{12}$, such as nutritional yeast or soy milk. I have talked to and read about long-term raw fooders who have experienced this.

$B_{12}$ deficiency results in one or more of these neurological symptoms: extreme fatigue, achy joints, depression, numbness and painful tingling in feet and hands, nervousness, paranoia, impaired memory and/or behavioral changes. $B_{12}$ deficiency can ultimately result in death if clear warning signals are not heeded, and sufficient $B_{12}$ is not supplied in a timely manner.

Some of this damage can be almost irreversible, according to Dr. Gabriel Cousens, if it becomes chronic. In *Spiritual Nutrition*, he cites three cases in which large groups of people went on a fruitarian diet devoid of $B_{12}$: Johnny Lovewisdom's vegan community in Ecuador, a fruitarian community in Australia and a group of African Americans who migrated to Israel. Each group suffered severely, especially the children, whose nervous systems were still developing.

$B_{12}$ deficiency is especially problematic for a growing fetus or even a growing child, as it can permanently arrest brain and peripheral nerve development. Most health professionals agree that every pregnant or nursing woman, *regardless of the diet she is on*, should consider taking $B_{12}$ supplements to avoid this possibility.

Dr. Cousens found that in his clinical experience, even meat eaters have a high rate of $B_{12}$ deficiency. There are other causes of deficiency, such as malabsorption, oral contraceptives, fungal infections, tobacco smoking, Vitamin $B_6$ or iron deficiency, emotional stress, liver or kidney disease, pancreatic tumors, failure of the small intestine to contract and move food, or exposure to radiation, drugs or other toxins.

Cousens has done extensive research with vegans and $B_{12}$ and has concluded that about 80% of the vegan and live-food population are $B_{12}$-deficient. He points out a high homocysteine level in the blood is associated with a lack of $B_{12}$. Diseases associated with high homocysteine levels include heart disease, Alzheimer's, age-related hearing loss and many more.

Although supplementation with $B_{12}$-fortified nutritional yeast, which is next to impossible to find raw due to FDA regulations, may help, Dr. Cousens does not recommend it because it increases internal acidity. Instead, he advises taking $B_{12}$ supplements, saying, "This is the first time in history that we can be completely successful live food vegans. What I mean by being successful is completely healthy, including no $B_{12}$ deficiency and no elevated homocysteine levels."

When he made that statement in a lecture, I asked Cousens if he thought that genetically we were meant to be vegans. His reply was that we probably were originally, but when we got kicked out of the Garden of Eden, things changed (perhaps a DNA mutation). Now we are trying to get back to the Garden of Eden, so we should be vegan, especially if practicing yoga. He explained that yoga opens up the 72,000 nadis (the spiritual nervous system). If we eat animal products, we take in the animals' experience of cruelty, suffering and misery. The energy of death literally permeates our inner being.

Others would argue that modern agricultural methods have utterly destroyed the bacteria that produce this important vitamin at the same time that air pollution has also placed excessive demands on our bodily supplies of it.

There are several schools of thought on the whole veganism/$B_{12}$ issue. Some are strict vegans due to philosophical or ethical reasons, believing it is very bad karma to eat any animal products. When you see how badly animals we eat are treated, as depicted in some of the videos like *Meet Your Meat* or *Eating*, it doesn't take much to convince you that this is the case. Even if veganism is not the way our ancestors ate, the technology of supplementation may help us remain healthy vegans. Another reason to be vegan is spiritual, as stated above. A vegan diet enhances one's prayer, meditation and yoga practices.

Another school of thought is that it is neither genetically natural nor healthful to be strictly vegan. Vegetarian species often eat eggs, insects, small vertebrates or soil. This includes gorillas, another primate closely related to humans in DNA structure. We might not be genetically suited for veganism — vegetarianism, yes, but maybe not complete veganism. Or perhaps in an environment of high quality food grown in cobalt-rich soil and unwashed greens, we could be truly vegan without supplementation.

Adherents to the no-supplement philosophy point out that vitamins have only been discovered within the last century or so. New nutrients are being discovered all the time. You may take a $B_{12}$ supplement, but what if scientists discover down the road some other nutrient you are missing because you are eating true to your philosophical code but not to your genetic code?

Many people believe that it is safer to eat your nutrients in whole foods for this reason. Nutrients work together synergistically. The whole is greater than the sum of its parts. Therefore, it is always optimal to obtain missing elements from natural foods in order to get the as-yet-undiscovered nutrients. (See page 373 of Chapter 19 for more discussion of this topic.)

Brother Nazariah, a leader of the Essene Church of Christ, had been a raw fooder for five years when he became very weak, with painful feet and hands. His central nervous system became damaged from running low on $B_{12}$. He added fermented raw dairy products (yogurt and kefir) and eggs to his diet. The symptoms disappeared.

In the 30-some years of his raw food experience, Nazariah came across many vegans who were suffering similar symptoms of Vitamin $B_{12}$ deficiency. Yet they would stubbornly cling to the idea of veganism because it was theoretically best, and they didn't want to violate their philosophy.

In an interview with Frédéric Patenaude, he addresses the issue of veganism. He points out a study published in *Ahimsa Magazine*, a pro-vegan periodical, that actually concludes that vegans have a high incidence of degenerative brain diseases, such as Alzheimer's, dementia and others. He says that in the 1990s, the magazine *Vegetarian Times* published the results of a study claiming that lacto-ovo-vegetarians (those consuming dairy and eggs) lived longer than meat-eaters, but meat-eaters actually lived longer than vegans.

Dr. Stanley S. Bass is one modern-day hygienic doctor who would agree with Nazariah. He discovered empirically that the vegan diet could lead to deficiencies, especially of Vitamins $B_{12}$ and D. He experienced inflamed gums, loosened teeth, paleness and excessive weight loss. He has also counseled numerous raw food clients, including raw diet authors and lecturers, who complained of anxiety attacks, panic attacks, depression and various muscle tissue problems.

Dr. Bass spent years testing various diets on mice. He found that fruitarian mice became so nutrient deficient that they engaged in cannibalism! His studies nevertheless confirmed that raw diets are nutritionally optimal so long as they include some fermented dairy, eggs, bee pollen or other animal products to provide sufficient $B_{12}$ and D.

Along the same lines, Professor Jared Diamond, author of the Pulitzer Prize winning *Guns, Germs and Steel*, speculates that the lack of animal protein in the diets of traditional highland New Guineans was the root cause of their widespread cannibalism!

An interview with the late hygienic doctor Christopher Gian-Cursio, ND, DC, is posted on Dr. Bass' web site entitled "With Three Generations of Vegetarian Hygienists" (see www.drbass.com/generations.html). Dr. Cursio observed nearsightedness, inadequate skeletal development and undeveloped musculature among third generation raw vegan family members.

It appears that perhaps some people may feel a need for small amounts of raw animal products, such as eggs or meat, for at least limited times under certain conditions. My theory is that perhaps some people are poor assimilators of Vitamin $B_{12}$ and perhaps other plant nutrients yet to be discovered, or they may live in far northern climates that provide insufficient sunlight for making Vitamin D at certain times of the year. Everyone has his own biochemical individuality and needs consistent with his present health status and inherited predispositions to consider also.

Some people want to be raw fooders for optimal health and don't care about being strict vegans. I know someone who eats about a pound a month of raw liver, where $B_{12}$ is stored, from cattle naturally raised on pasture. Most the time he is a raw vegetarian. He began doing this only after eating raw for years, once he began exhibiting $B_{12}$ deficiency symptoms.

Another solution is to mix raw egg yolks into smoothies, but it might take several eggs a day to get enough $B_{12}$. (See Appendix C for how to make sure your eggs come from healthy chickens.) Some people find egg whites to be so toxic when ingested and metabolized that the body produces phlegm in which to carry the toxins for expulsion.

If someone already extremely healthy wishes to follow the vegan philosophy, he can supplement with nutritional yeast even though it isn't raw. Researcher Michael Donaldson of Hallelujah Acres performed a study he called "Metabolic vitamin $B_{12}$ status on a mostly raw vegan diet with follow-up using tablets, nutritional yeast, or probiotic supplements" (*Annals of Nutrition & Metabolism*, 2000, Vol. 44, pp. 229–234, PubMed ID 11146329). It showed that the use of one tablespoon a day of Red Star Vegetarian Support containing 5 mcg of $B_{12}$ was enough to keep 85% of the vegans with a serum level of 200 pg (that's picograms, billionths of a gram!) of $B_{12}$ per milliliter of blood.

Though a serum level of 200 pg keeps most deficiency symptoms at bay, Dr. Cousens now thinks 340-405 is optimal since it keeps the homocysteine level within the normal range. Other researchers have suggested a value above 500 pg is even better.

In any case, if a person is still struggling with health issues, he should not add more acidity or fermentation with eggs or yeast. In that case, one could take $B_{12}$ sublingual supplements, the methylcobalamin form of which is often recommended as the best. Injections are another option, but their toxic preservative chemicals sometimes induce "side" effects, up to and including sudden death! Note that individual $B_{12}$ supplement pills typically contain much more than what is needed on a daily basis, but one may need to take a pill at least every three days or so since only about 1% is actually absorbed.

Victoria Boutenko is convinced we can get sufficient $B_{12}$ if we eat large amounts of greens. She often eats about two bunches of kale a day for many of the health benefits such a diet provides. The greens must be organic. Pesticides probably destroy $B_{12}$-producing bacteria. I have read, however, that washing the greens removes $B_{12}$, and many stores also spray their greens for bugs. Perhaps buying organic greens from a local farmer who doesn't wash them would solve that matter.

Another concern of great significance, however, is that today's soil is severely depleted of minerals, including the cobalt upon which $B_{12}$ production depends. The main reason vegans are having such a tough time getting $B_{12}$ — and minerals such as zinc and selenium — might not be a sign that we are meant to eat animal products but rather that our soil is so seriously depleted of minerals. Another factor is that while the supply of $B_{12}$ is down, the body's demand is greatly increased by mercury from dental fillings, auto exhaust and other environmental pollutants.

Several studies have been published which discuss the need for $B_{12}$ supplementation in raw vegans. One is "Vitamin $B_{12}$ status of long-term adherents of a strict uncooked vegan diet ('living food diet') is compromised." It was published in *The Journal of Nutrition* (Oct 1995, Vol. 125, Issue 10, pp. 2511–2515, PubMed ID 7562085). Another is "Metabolic vitamin $B_{12}$ status on a mostly raw vegan diet with follow-up using tablets, nutritional yeast, or probiotic supplements," published in *Annals of Nutrition and Metabolism* (2000, Vol. 44, Issue 4–5, pp. 229–234, PubMed ID 11146329).

# Restrict Your Calories for Longer Life

UCLA researcher Dr. Roy Walford discovered that by reducing caloric intake by about 30%, one might extend his middle years by up to 40% toward the longest possible lifespan. He wrote about this in *Maximum Life Span*. Since the publishing of that book, his rat research and conclusions have been duplicated on primates.

One's diet must not only be restricted in calories, but also rich in nutrients. Thus Walford recommended nutritional supplements.

According to Gabriel Cousens, MD, there has never been an incident in the history of medicine when such effects in so many different species could not be applied to humans as well.

Unfortunately, Dr. Walford himself died at 79. According to research on animals, his diet may still have extended his remaining years even though he started it so late in life. You can still turn on the youthing gene even if you start the calorie-restriction diet in middle age.

Walford died of ALS, or Lou Gehrig's disease, which is thought to be genetic. He believed his disease was exacerbated by exposure to nitrous oxide during a research stay in Biosphere 2 but that his practice of calorie restriction slowed its progression. He certainly exceeded the life expectancy of someone with ALS, but he missed an important piece of the puzzle by continuing to eat cooked food. Another question about his diet arises: in his quest for low calorie intake, did he consume a lot of mercury-laden fish, leading to his ALS?

Raw fooders like David Wolfe often combine reduced caloric intake with raw foods for maximal health and longevity. He is fond of saying that he eats less in order to live longer so that he will be able, in the long run, to eat more.

Man has intuited this simple health secret throughout the ages. An ancient Egyptian transcription translates, "Man lives on one quarter of what he eats. On the other three quarters lives his doctor."

Benjamin Franklin wrote, "To lengthen thy life, lessen thy meals." It just makes common sense. No one who is obese lives to 100. Toxins are stored in fat; whoever is overweight thus carries around a life-threatening toxic accumulation.

The longest living societies, such as the Hunzas, ate diets low in calories.

Dr. Cousens pointed out in a lecture that eating raw enables us to cut our calories in half since so many micronutrients, and even the macronutrient protein, are deranged or destroyed by cooking. Cooking ruins up to 100% of the enzymes, 50% of the protein and 80% of the vitamins and minerals. Much more than that is destroyed, as pointed out in Chapter 10.

By eating raw foods, Cousens claims, we can get complete nutrition *even on a diet of 50-80% less food* (*Spiritual Nutrition*, p. 301). He cites research by Stephen Spindler showing that calorie restriction turns on the antiaging genes and that such a diet can reverse age-related degenerative changes and thus reverse the aging process to some degree. Caloric restriction promotes the self-suicide of cancer-producing cells.

Research at Harvard Medical School and BIOMOL Research Laboratories has shown that taking the supplement resveratrol may even turn on the antiaging genes, much like a low-calorie diet. If you prefer to get this phytonutrient in whole foods, it is found in organic grapes, red wine, pine tree bark and other plants, such as Japanese knotweed (*polygonum cuspidatum*). Of course cooking will destroy this nutrient.

Tonya Zavasta is on the cutting edge of combining eating raw with minimal calories. In her book *Quantum Eating*, she reveals her beauty secret. And this woman of 50 years could easily pass for 25! She combines 100% raw eating with CRON (calorie restriction with optimal nutrition).

On top of that, she dry fasts every day from 2 PM until 7 AM. *Dry fasting* means not only *not eating*, but also *not taking in any fluids*, including water. She explains that for every 6,000 drops of water, one of those drops is "dead" water, or $D_2O$ instead of $H_2O$. Deuterium replaces the normal hydrogen in those water molecules. This toxic water can only be replaced by dry fasting.

# Food Combining

Natalia Rose emphasizes that proper food combining allows food waste to quickly exit the body, thus conserving energy. Slow-exiting foods and poor food combinations drain your energy and enzymes and result in gas, bloating, fatigue and body odor. Hygienic author Dennis Nelson summarizes the usefulness of food combining as an energy enhancement in his book *Food Combining Simplified: How to Get the Most from Your Food* (p. 5):

> The term *food combining* refers to those combinations of foods which are compatible with each other in digestive chemistry. The goal is to aid the digestive process. By applying these principles, your nutrition will be enhanced, as only food that is digested is capable of nourishing us. And we avoid the poisonous by-products of indigestion, along with the unpleasant symptoms (gas, gastritis, bloating, acid reflux, diarrhea, constipation).
>
> Rather than use drugs to suppress the symptoms of indigestion, it would be wiser to remove the causes. Simple meals of compatible combinations maintain good digestion. Efficient digestion also has a beneficial influence on the body's energy level.

Way behind the times, most mainstream nutritionists still consider the theory on which the practice of food combining is based to be nonsense. By contrast, nearly all mainstream physiologists acknowledge that the human body does have digestive limitations. The teachings of Natural Hygiene explain the solid biochemical and physiological foundation for the principles of food combining that may be employed to conserve energy, maximize digestion and minimize the creation of endogenous toxins so that discomfort/disease repercussions do not result.

Good oral, gastric and small intestinal digestion of nutrients leads to their proper absorption and nearly complete assimilation into the cells. Proper food combining is therefore absolutely fundamental to good health.

Comprehensive information on the endogenous toxins created by bodily and microbial biochemical reactions when poor food combinations are eaten can be found in a lengthy article in Victoria BidWell's *Common Health Sense: Issue I, Volume 1* by Dr. Vetrano entitled "For Superlative Digestion, Practice Superlative Food Combining." Following is the long list she has compiled of these endogenous toxins: ptomaines, which include cadaverine, agmatine, tyramine, histamine, muscarine, neurine, ptomatropine, putrescine; toxic gases, which include $CO_2$, methane, hydrogen, nitrogen, ammonia and hydrogen sulfide; acidic poisons, which include acetic, lactic, propionic and butyric, and toxic amino acids, which include indole, skatole, ethyl mercaptan and methyl mercaptan.

Many newcomers to raw foods have never even heard the term *food combining*. Once they run across it, they soon realize that their favorite taste treats are digestively incompatible, and they are reluctant to give them up. Once they understand that these "treats" compromise health, most start observing at least a few of the proper food combining basics with most meals.

Generally, fruit should be eaten at least 30 minutes before other foods. This is because it passes into the small intestine quickly, requiring very little stomach digestion at all. Otherwise, fruit would sit in the stomach and ferment if mixed with denser foods that take longer to digest. This is why such combinations often result in gas, bloating, acid reflux and/or upset stomach. The exception is greens, which combine well with most fruits, especially when blended. (See Appendix C.)

A hydrotherapist of 30 years' experience found that many people actually need up to two hours to digest fruits before they should eat other foods. She saw quite a few give up on the raw diet because they didn't know that this was their problem.

Melons should be eaten alone, not even with other fruits. However, since melons are rapidly digested, other food may be eaten 20 minutes later.

It is also considered inadvisable to mix together in the same meal starches, which require alkaline digestive juices, and proteins, which require acidic digestive juices. If they are to be consumed together, the starches should be eaten first.

Victoria BidWell and Dr. Vetrano list Dr. Shelton's food combining rules and a classification of individual food items into proper food combining categories in *The Health Seekers' YearBook*. They are reproduced here beginning on page 555 of Appendix F.

At her web site www.getwellstaywellamerica.com, Victoria carries an extensive line of food combining materials, including several books, placemats, a food combining wheel, wall charts, a wallet card, DVDs, Dr. Shelton's booklet *Food Combining Made Easy* and Dennis Nelson's *Food Combining Simplified*.

Some people even experience that proper food combining becomes less important when eating 100% raw since the body does not have to use as much of its own digestive enzymes. Eating only one type of food at a time is easiest on the digestive system nonetheless. Therefore, some advanced raw fooders eat *monomeals* consisting of only one type of food at a time, perhaps followed slightly later by a second kind of food. This is also how instinctive eaters eat. (See Appendix C.)

## Nuts and Seeds: Hard to Digest?

Nuts and seeds contain enzyme inhibitors that make them difficult to digest. The enzyme inhibitor keeps the nut or seed from sprouting before conditions are right for the baby tree to grow. Dry nuts and seeds should be soaked in pure water for eight to ten hours and then rinsed and drained before eating. Many people like to soak them overnight, then rinse them in the morning and store them in the refrigerator covered in pure water.

Seeds can also be sprouted in a sprouting jar or sprouting machine over the course of several days. If you do not like the light, "sprouty" taste of sprouted seeds or soaked nuts, dry the soaked nuts for a few hours in a temperature-controlled dehydrator. They will also keep longer in the refrigerator if dehydrated. If you don't have a dehydrator, let them dry on unbleached paper.

Even after soaking, nuts and seeds are energy expensive and sometimes difficult for some people to digest simply because they are high in fat, with a high density and low water content. Macadamia nuts are about 90% fat! So you should limit your intake of them. Most people do well eating up to 2-4 ounces of nuts and/or seeds a day. However, if you eat a lot of the gourmet raw dishes, you may end up consuming more than this. If the body cannot use more than this, it will just end up converting the surplus calories into fat.

One factor that contributes to the difficulty of digesting nuts is that many of them, even those purchased from health food stores, are not really raw. Most have been heated somewhat to dry them to inhibit mold growth. Since a salmonella infestation in some almonds a few years ago, many nuts are heated beyond the temperature that destroys enzymes despite having labels that boast "raw." It is often necessary to ask the distributor if the nuts are truly raw.

Many raw fooders are finding greater health by making nuts and seeds only a small part of their diet. Victoria Boutenko found that by making greens and fruit the vast majority of the diet and allowing only 5% or so of our diet to come from nuts and seeds, we match our diets to the natural diets of our closest relatives, the chimpanzees. (See Appendix C.)

For more on this topic, see Dr. Vetrano's article "Genuine Fruitarianism" at the end of this chapter.

# Organic Food: Is It Really Necessary?

One thing people tend to become more aware of when they switch to raw diets is the superiority of organic produce. It costs more because it is not government subsidized like that grown by conventional agribusiness that depends on chemicals. *Government officials, receiving campaign contributions from agribusiness, pass laws subsidizing only toxic commercial farming and cattle ranching practices! In other words, your tax dollars are assisting in poisoning you.*

Because of the higher retail cost of organic produce, the advice to go organic is often met with resistance. When most people think of organic produce, they think it simply means "pesticide-free." But there is a whole lot more at stake.

## Nutritional Value

You might buy a pound of organic apples for $2.29 or a pound of commercial apples for 99¢. While you may save double the money on the commercial variety, you may get only half the nutrients plus a number of unwanted toxins that accumulate in your body and slowly poison you over the years.

Organic foods appear to contain on the average twice the amount of micronutrients as commercial produce, but in some cases it is three or four times as much. David Jubb (*LifeFood Recipe Book*, p. 5) points out that in at least one study, organic spinach was found to have twice the calcium, four times the magnesium, three times the potassium, 69 times the organic sodium, 117 times the manganese and 80 times the iron of its commercial counterpart! Note, however, that this was just one small study. There are great variations in nutritional value among different crops of both commercial and organic produce.

Organic berries were found to have up to 58% more antioxidants than those grown conventionally, according to another study published in the February 2003 issue of the *Journal of Agriculture and Food Industry.*

A 1993 study published in the *Journal of Applied Nutrition* proved that over a two-year period, organic foods contained up to four times the amount of trace minerals, 13 times the selenium and 20 times the calcium and magnesium of commercially grown food. They also had less of the toxic metals lead and aluminum.

A four-year study begun in 2004 in Europe called the Quality Low Input Food Project has found that organic food contains 40% more antioxidants. This is the biggest study yet done on organic food. Complete results have not yet been published at the time of this writing.

As Dr. Cousens points out, these remarkable differences, based on a fresh-weight (not dehydrated) basis, are not as obvious on a dry-weight (dehydrated) basis. Consequently, scientists hired by chemical-based farming companies will report dry-weight comparisons.

Besides inferior nutrient content, commercial produce lacks in bio-energetic values. (See Chapter 10.) European tests on the bio-energetic values of foods proved that chemically grown foods are inferior to those cultivated organically.

It boggles my mind that so many people go to all the trouble of buying organic produce, even growing their own, only to cook out so many of those nutrients for which they are paying so much extra or working so hard to grow.

## Toxins in Commercial Produce

If you do not buy organic food, you may save a little money in the short run, *but you will pay much more in the long run when your health, clarity of mind and emotional balance suffer.* For one thing, the standards for commercial produce are very low. The food could have been sprayed with any number of toxic pesticides, fungicides and herbicides.

Some of the insecticides sprayed on commercial produce, such as DDT, are even banned here in the United States but are sold to countries in Latin America. So if you save a few dollars to buy the commercial melon imported from Mexico instead of the organic one grown here, you may be ingesting toxic DDT that was banned here decades ago! Even among the pesticides legal in the USA, over 20% have been linked to cancer, birth defects, developmental harm and central nervous system damage.

Toxic limits are set for adults, not children, which means infants and children are getting 2-10 times of the alleged "safe" limits, sometimes more.

Before the widespread use of these poisons, high rates of cancer in children were unheard of. Since most pesticides and herbicides are neurotoxic, they are also directly linked to hyperactivity and attention deficit disorder in children. According to Dr. Cousens, children put on organic diets show a 50% recovery rate from just this one change. Imagine if a drug could boast this rate of recovery — it would be front-page news!

Some studies have shown IQ reductions in children reared on commercial produce. One study done in Mexico involved 33 children. It was called "An anthropological approach to the evaluation of preschool children exposed to pesticides in Mexico" (*Environmental Health Perspectives*, Vol. 106, Issue 6, June 1998, PubMed ID 9618351). The study found a drastic reduction of intelligence compared to those eating food without pesticides.

There is only a certain amount of pesticide deposition that a person can retain in his tissues without observably ill effects in a lifespan of seventy-five years. One study showed that in North America, *most one-year-old babies have already acquired that seventy-five year maximum* ("Can environmental estrogens cause breast cancer?" *Scientific American*, October 1995, Vol. 273, Issue 4, pp. 167–172, PubMed ID 7481720).

Even for adults, this accumulation of toxic pesticides can lead to horrific effects, such as cancer, reduced mental function, decreased mental clarity, poor concentration, attention deficit disorder and Parkinson's disease.

In *The Weight Loss Cure "They" Don't Want You to Know About* (p. 33), consumer advocate Kevin Trudeau reveals, "One board member from the Mayo Clinic, whose identity must be kept secret, shared with me the data showing that virtually all cancerous tumors are loaded with pesticides and herbicides used in the production of most commercial food!"

Meanwhile, many of the pests these chemicals are intended to kill are growing resistant to the pesticides, so farmers are forced to use greater quantities. In the past forty years or so that pesticide use has been commonplace, farmers in some areas of the country have increased their per-acre saturation levels fivefold. Yet the crops that have been destroyed by insects have nearly doubled.

Currently, 500 species of insects have become pesticide-resistant. Since their lifespans are so much shorter than those of humans, they can spawn offspring genetically resistant to these toxins much faster than we can. This is because it takes many, many generations for a species to adapt genetically to something new in the environment — if it is even biologically possible to do so fully.

As Howard Lyman points out in his book *Mad Cowboy*, pesticides and other toxins used on produce represent a huge industry. Interestingly, the same companies that produce toxic chemicals for pesticides, herbicides, fungicides and industrial and household products also produce prescription drugs! *Thus they profit at both ends: poisoning the people and providing the drugs that reduce the symptom severity of those poisons.*

This circle of profit is no conspiracy theory, but an easily provable fact. For example, Monsanto, a leading company of pesticides and genetically modified seeds, was owned by the Pharmacia Corporation, which sells prescription drugs. Merck is a pharmaceutical company that also produces chemicals and precursors for pesticides and other neurotoxins.

Remember that these pesticides, herbicides and fungicides kill farm workers, who experience high cancer rates. Why would you want to support such an industry?

A friend of mine who traveled to South America says the locals in the country he visited don't eat the food that has been grown under agribusiness contract and sprayed with costly pesticides. Locals can't afford that produce, as independent growers don't have the money to buy pesticides. The big farming operations use pesticides only on export crops.

Ironically, the common populace is saved by poverty: they don't have enough money to buy poisoned food. Thus we rich Americans are "privileged" to eat only the most toxic stuff!

In addition, commercial produce is often covered with chemical waxes and preservatives to prolong shelf life and improve its appearance. Brenda Cobb, author of *The Living Foods Lifestyle*, mentions seeing some plump, luscious-looking nectarines that were still packed in the box at a grocery store. She read the ingredient list and recognized only two: varnish and shellac. "I don't know about you, but where I come from, we use these products on furniture. They're certainly not something we'd consider eating. If we're going to eat varnish and shellac, why not just go to the hardware store and buy a pint or gallon of each and turn it up and drink it?"

Unfortunately, even some of the organic produce has been covered with wax for longer shelf life. The organic label refers only to how it is grown and not what is done to it later. The only way to know for sure is to ask the store manager. One of the advantages of shopping at the local farmers' market is that the produce is very fresh and rarely covered with wax.

But wait, there is more! If the toxicity in commercial produce and the lack of nutrients are not enough to make you go organic, *read on*!

# Genetically Modified Organisms (GMOs)

Commercial produce may have been grown from genetically modified seed, whereas organic produce, by definition, may not. So, if you are eating commercial produce, especially corn or soy, there is a good chance it was genetically altered, and there is no law in the USA requiring that this be stated on the label.

Genetically modified organisms (GMOs) have been found to be much less nutritious and even poisonous. In a study by Dr. Arpad Pasztai at the Rowett Research Institute in Scotland, animals fed diets of GMOs were found to have smaller organs than those fed with traditional foods. *Their hearts, livers and even brains shrank after eating genetically modified potatoes for only ten days.*

Companies like Monsanto have developed GMOs so that they could patent seeds, as selling unpatentable seeds has not been particularly profitable. Also, since GMO plants do not reproduce once the "suicide" gene has been inserted into their DNA, farmers must purchase new seeds every year, resulting in a potential food monopoly akin to the oil and banking cartels.

This practice institutes a sneaky form of monopoly that will only get worse and worse until a small elite cartel controls our entire food supply.

The way the monopolists try to persuade us that this is ethical is by claiming that we need this technology to feed the world's hungry, but the truth is that GMO crops actually yield 4-10% less than heirloom varieties (*Spiritual Nutrition*, p. 506).

Furthermore, since they have genes spliced from other sources, GMOs may contain any number of allergens that are not listed, thus inducing allergic responses in some people. For example, according to Jeffrey M. Smith, author of *Seeds of Deception: Exposing Industry and Government Lies About the Safety of the Genetically Engineered Foods You're Eating*, a gene from a brazil nut inserted into soybeans made the soy allergenic to those who normally react to brazil nuts. This type of thing happens a lot, and the vast majority of corn and soy is now grown from GMO seeds.

Some GMOs combine genes from both plant and animal species! In fact the FDA and EPA even classify as insecticides certain corn and potato strains that were designed to produce toxins to kill insects. So when you eat commercial corn or potatoes, you could be unsuspectingly eating an insecticide!

GMOs accelerate aging. Ingesting unnatural, toxic, genetically modified foods introduces still more poisons into our bodies. GMOs thus add to disease progression. Because GMOs are unable to reproduce, their life force is weak. Dr. Cousens said in a lecture that *GMOs deregulate our cells' DNA into premature aging*.

Instinctive eaters claim that they cannot notice a proper taste change when eating GMO-altered food because our genes simply aren't programmed to recognize them.

Europeans are much more informed about these "Frankenfoods" than Americans are. In Europe, by law, they must be labeled as such. Most Europeans refuse to eat them. In the United States, no labeling whatsoever is required. Companies are certainly not doing it voluntarily because they know a lot of people wouldn't buy the produce if they did.

GMOs are helping to destroy our eco-structure. Since the wind blows pollen from these plants, they combine with natural plants. Animals eating these hybrids have been harmed. Farmers have had their natural, organic seeds contaminated as well.

For more information, see the web site www.cqs.com/50harm.htm, which hosts the article, "50 Harmful Effects of Genetically Modified Foods."

As people wake up to the dangers inherent in GMOs, many are uniting to fight back. On August 3, 2004, Trinity County in California became the second county in the nation to ban the production of genetically engineered crops and animals. There have been several more since then.

Meanwhile, pressure from agribusiness has resulted in legislation being introduced in Congress to outlaw counties from banning GMOs.

Undoubtedly the most disturbing consequences of food sprayed with pesticide have been the damage done to the natural defense mechanisms of bees. Bees are disappearing from all over the world, and we are in grave danger of losing them. According to experts, colony collapse disorder is caused by bees having their natural defense mechanisms destroyed by pesticides and genetically modified foods. They are unable to fight against the viruses that are destroying them. Without bees, there will be fewer fruits, vegetables, flowers and no honey.

In parts of China where bees have already died out, people have tried to pollinate by hand but can do only a tiny fraction of the millions of plants that bees pollinate for free. If this problem is not corrected, only the wealthy will be raw fooders. In fact only the very well off will be able to eat much of anything but rice, corn and wheat.

# Organic Foods Even Taste Better

Moreover, organic food tastes better, in addition to being more nutritious. It usually tastes richer for having been grown in soil with more minerals and nutrients.

Animals can tell the difference between organic and commercial produce. In 2002, the Copenhagen Zoo began to feed its animals at least 10% organic produce. "For one reason or another, the tapirs and chimpanzees are choosing organically grown bananas over the others," keeper Niels Melchiorsen told the magazine *Økologisk Jordbrug* [Ecological Agriculture].

"Maybe they are able to instinctively tell the difference, and their choice is not at all random. ... The chimpanzees are able to tell the difference between the organic and the regular fruit. If we give them organic and traditional bananas, they systematically choose the organic bananas, which they eat with the skin on. But they peel the traditional bananas before eating them."

# In a Pinch...

Sometimes you might find yourself in a city where there is no organic produce available. In such a situation, it may be necessary to eat commercial produce — or fast.

It is good to keep in mind that produce covered with a shell or peel generally contains less pesticide and herbicide residue provided you don't eat the peel. So you could buy bananas, citrus fruit, nuts or corn on the cob with husks or avocados. Figs, cauliflower and peas are also relatively safe.

Studies have found that the produce items containing the greatest amount of chemical residue are strawberries, dates, carrots, grapes, peaches, nectarines, apples, raisins, cucumbers, celery, spinach and unpeeled potatoes.

It is worth mentioning here that Victoria Boutenko said in a lecture that her family was healed on a 100% raw diet that did not consist of organic food. They didn't know about organic food when beginning their raw diet. However, that was over a decade ago, and commercial produce has undoubtedly become much more contaminated since then. As soon as they found out about organics, they made the switch.

Keep in mind that toxins accumulate in your body. You wouldn't consider eating "a pinch of arsenic" on a regular basis. Cultivate the same attitude with pesticides, herbicides, fungicides and all the more than 10,000 chemical additives in our foods.

If Codex Alimentarius takes effect (in 2010), I would recommend that children and teens especially eat *absolutely no food with pesticides*. The toxic levels will become much higher than they currently are. Please see the Internet video clip "Nutricide" with Dr. Rima Laibow, MD.

## And a Final Warning...

The organic food industry is growing by 20% a year in the United States. Anything with that much economic potential attracts a lot of attention. Therefore, the federal government, influenced of course by big, greedy food corporations, has assumed control over the definition and use of the word *organic* under the guise of standardization.

This is not good news. It means that lobbying efforts by commercial agriculture are well underway to gradually dilute these standards over time. Already, an "organically fed animal" can be fed merely 70% organic feed. In October 2005, Congress voted to weaken organic standards still more by allowing numerous synthetic food additives and processing aids to be included in processed foods labeled "organic."

The consumer needs to keep on top of these changes in order to know the current meaning of "organic." Soon, growers and consumers may have to come up with a totally different label, something like "super" or "pure," if we are to maintain high standards.

Sadly, all of the expense, pain and suffering from pesticides are neither necessary nor financially efficient in growing healthy crops. Studies have shown that when crops are high in minerals, bugs don't eat them! It is nature's balance for bugs to prefer unhealthy crops, so efficient farmers could simply add minerals to their soil.

To find where you can purchase organic food locally, visit www.greenpeople.org and www.rawfoodplanet.com.

An excellent documentary film on what is happening to our food is *The Future of Food*.

# Nuking Our Food by Irradiation

The process of irradiation exposes food to a dose of ionizing radiation that is equivalent to millions of chest X-rays. The explanation given to pacify consumers is that this destroys the "harmful bacteria" in meat and imported produce.

*As always, the real reason for nuking the food supply is economic*: the increased shelf life of hermetically sealed irradiated food allows for long-distance shipping and storage so that large agricultural corporations can grow food in countries with much lower environmental and worker safety standards. As a result, smaller local farms will suffer economically, and unsuspecting consumers will suffer physically from the radiolytic byproducts of this process.

Another reason is political: to assuage our fears of germs and "predatory" insects while protecting these companies from related lawsuits.

When industrialists find their waste products, like fluoride and chloride, too expensive to dispose of, their lobbyists convince government officials that this toxic waste has potentially "healthful" uses so it can be sold for huge profits. Why *not* put toxic fluoride and chlorine in the water? Why *not* sell radioactive waste, the byproduct of nuclear energy production, for irradiation of meat, grains and other foods at a profit of $50,000 a pound?

Irradiation kills not only bacteria, but also most nutrients. The food is left with no energy, no life force. It doesn't even ripen properly. According to Dr. Cousens, between 20% and 80% of the vitamins are destroyed, along with all of the enzymes and biophotons (*Spiritual Nutrition*, p. 507).

The irradiation process also creates the known toxins benzene and formaldehyde in the food, as well as unknown chemicals that are potentially toxic. According to research, animals consuming irradiated foods have suffered early death, stillbirth, genetic damage, cancer, stunted growth, organ malfunctions and vitamin deficiency. Germany experimented with irradiated food and has decided to ban the process.

Dr. Gabriel Cousens cites a study in India in which researchers fed irradiated wheat to children. After a month, leukemialike changes occurred in the children's white blood cells and chromosomes. When they stopped eating the irradiated wheat, their blood parameters reverted to normal.

Cousens cites five studies that claim irradiation is safe, yet all have been found to be invalid studies (*Spiritual Nutrition*, pp. 507–508). Two of the studies were found to be flawed. A third study found that the animals eating irradiated food lost weight and had miscarriages, and two more studies used irradiated foods well below the FDA-approved levels. In spite of all this, the FDA approved the use of irradiation in our food supply!

There is a special symbol on some food packaging, the *radura*, to indicate irradiation. This looks a bit like a flower with two leaves surrounded by a circle. No labeling is required on processed foods or spices, so we cannot always know if something is irradiated. To see what the radura looks like, go to <u>www.fsis.usda.gov/news_&_events/fsis_images/index.asp</u>.

Recently irradiated foods have been permitted in school lunches. Severen Schaeffer predicted that as irradiation of fresh produce becomes widespread, city dwellers will have access to no fresh food, and new forms of pathology will appear.

Sadly even organic food might become irradiated. This is because organic laws pertain only to how the food is grown, but not to what happens to the food later. The best way to prevent eating irradiated food is to speak to the manager of the store.

Find a food co-op of politically aware and health-conscious people who would never allow such food to enter their store. Purchase organically grown food from the local farmers' markets. Ask the merchants how it is grown and treated. Some of them use organic growing methods but cannot use the organic label due to the red tape and expense involved in the certification process. It is highly unlikely that local farmers irradiate their food, as the equipment required is so costly.

Even if you have never been politically inclined, the shocking information on Codex Alimentarius may jolt you into action. The UN started this plan in 1963, and their aim is to have *all food irradiated by December 31, 2009*. In addition, supplements and other natural health modalities will be illegal to buy unless people take action. Go to www.healthfreedomusa.org for more information and sign the petitions there. Also see the half-hour documentary on the Internet *We Become Silent: The Last Hours of Health Freedom.*

# High vs. Low Glycemic Index Food

High glycemic index (GI) food is food that is high in fast-digesting sugars that cause the body to release excessive insulin, resulting in fat storage, fatigue and accelerated aging. If one consistently eats a lot of it, he or she will not feel good at all.

These symptoms, however, are more typical of people consuming refined sugars and grain products on the SAD diet and not so typical of those eating raw diets with an abundance of fresh fruit as staples.

Some sweet fruits, melons in particular, score high on the GI scale; most others are in the mid-range. Root vegetables, such as potatoes, beets and carrots, are often considered high, although testing is usually done on the cooked versions of these foods. Raw starches are actually low GI foods. Note that *cooking* approximately *doubles the glycemic response* of a food in many cases! This is yet another reason to stop eating cooked food.

Hybrid plants (see next section) tend to have higher glycemic indices than their heirloom counterparts. Promoters of eating according to the GI scale stress minimizing high GI produce, which includes melons, cooked root vegetables, cooked grains, honey and dates. However, Dr. Gabriel Cousens has found that carrots, traditionally thought to be a high GI food, are not a problem when eaten raw.

As stated earlier in this chapter, Dr. Douglas Graham believes the glycemic index to be the least reliable of nutritional indexes. He says that this issue is less relevant on his 80/10/10 diet. I have found that on days when I eat only fruit until dinner, including lots of high glycemic fruit (with the exception of dates), I seem to experience no negative effects, just as Graham has stated.

Hygienic doctors consider fruits to be perfectly good foods. They even break fasts with watermelon, a high glycemic fruit. As Dr. Vetrano points out, "To outlaw these wonderful fruits on the basis of some abstract chart prepared by people without years of experience in breaking fasts and feeding sick people into health is absurd!"

An illustrative glycemic index chart for selected food items is presented on page 330 for those of you who may be interested nevertheless.

Technically, the glycemic index is a measurement of the type or quality of carbohydrate in a food and how much 50 grams of it raises blood glucose levels over a two-hour period, with the consequent release of insulin from the pancreas as the food is digested.

There are some variances in the figures depending on the soil in which the food is grown and the particular plant variety, so these numbers are approximations only. You will find somewhat different values given in different charts and databases because of these variations.

A high GI is defined to be over 70. Medium is in the range 56-69. A low GI is 55 or under. These numbers correspond to a reference standard that is arbitrarily assigned the glycemic index value of 100. To further confuse matters, some researchers use white bread as the reference standard; others use glucose.

I constructed the GI chart for raw foods, but reliable data is sparse. Those items marked with an asterisk are either definitely or likely cooked.

# Hybrid vs. Wild Produce

For centuries, farmers have applied the known technology of their time to improve crops to make them taste and look better. This earlier upgrading via crossbreeding was a relatively primitive kind of genetic engineering that did not involve artificially mixing genes of different species in test tubes.

Through the methods of selection, grafting and cross-pollinating, farmers hybridized foods to make them taste sweeter. Hence, we now have foods that taste very sweet compared with their wild forebears, as with beets, carrots and bananas. Farmers also made hybrid plants for other commercial purposes, such as cold-resistance, few or no seeds, ease of harvesting and transportation, longer shelf life, fewer imperfections in shape and other aspects of appearance, including color variation.

There are hundreds of varieties of potatoes. Yet as a result of hybridization and standardization, we are able to find only a few at the grocery. The same goes for most other crops.

The downside of this trend has been that most of our commercial produce is much less nutritious. For example, hybridized fruits without seeds cannot even reproduce themselves. Such seedless foods have reduced life force. From a bio-energetic point of view, hybridized crops have not been an improvement at all. Biophotons are stored in the DNA. (See Chapter 10.) "Upgrading" crops means altering their DNA, which creates a serious loss of bio-energetic value.

This is why wild food is superior to cultivated or hybrid food. Dr. Popp of Germany found wild organic foods gave off twice as many biophotons as cultivated organic foods.

Exactly which foods are not good for you is a matter of debate, however. David Jubb highly recommends avoiding bananas and carrots, among other things. But Dr. Doug Graham is a big believer in bananas, even hybrid sweet ones. Dr. Cousens has concluded that even hybrid sweet carrots are great, as does Rev. George Malkmus.

No one disputes the value of eating wild plants, however. You may wish to experiment with eating wild plants, which are much more potent in biophotons and other nutrients. A book by Bradford Angler, *Field Guide to Edible Wild Plants*, can guide you as to which are safe to eat. Just be careful. Go out into the countryside, as plants in the city will probably have been sprayed or otherwise chemically polluted by mutagens.

Read the *Field Guide* carefully! Victoria BidWell knew a woman who was looking for wild carrot tops without any guide or experience. She chose hemlock and died. Chris McCandless, subject of the book and film *Into the Wild*, also made the fatal mistake of failing to distinguish between two plants.

Aajonus Vonderplanitz describes eating a mushroom he thought was safe only to fall extremely ill, requiring eleven years to fully recover! He figured that the plant mutated from its original form, which is why he was unable to properly identify it. It wouldn't hurt to stay away from wild mushrooms altogether.

A friend of mine got sick immediately after eating four ounces of a wild tuber that later turned out to have been pokeweed, a poisonous plant. He fasted for a few days, which relieved most of the problem, but didn't feel completely normal again for a couple of weeks. I asked how he could have avoided the experience. He said he should have tasted just a nibble and then waited to see how it affected him.

Nibbling and then waiting awhile, even a whole day, may be the best solution when in doubt. This is what wild animals do, and this is what Igor Boutenko did when out in the wild with his family.

The Boutenko family, Victoria, Igor and their two children, went on a hike for several days and ran out of food. After fasting several more days, they became very hungry and realized that various animals were surviving on food in the forest, so why couldn't they?

They each gathered plants that looked good but didn't eat any. Then they all got together and rubbed the plants, smelled them, and tasted tiny bits under their tongues. Igor, as head of the family, got to try a full test of the plants that had passed every preliminary test of all four family members. They then waited thirty minutes after he ate. When he did not get sick, they all ate that plant sprinkled with the olive oil and sunflower seeds which they had brought with them.

If you are not that adventurous, you may wish to grow your own crops from heirloom seeds. One company that sells these seeds is Seeds of Change in New Mexico. (See their contact information on page 589 in the Resource Guide.)

You could also sign up for an herb or wild-plant walk with an experienced guide in your local area.

And if you have a garden, eat the weeds! The lamb's-quarters and other weeds you once pulled are higher in nutrients than many of the things you are intentionally growing.

# Glycemic Index Chart

| Sweet Fruits | | Vegetables and Greens | |
|---|---|---|---|
| Apple | 38 | Bean sprout | 25 |
| Banana | 52 | Beet* | 64 |
| Cantaloupe | 65 | Cabbage | 10 |
| Cherry | 22 | Carrot juice | 43 |
| Date* | 103 | Carrot | 16 |
| Fig, dried | 61 | Celery | 0 |
| Grapefruit | 25 | Corn* | 37 |
| Grape | 46 | Lettuce | 10 |
| Kiwi | 52 | Mushroom | 10 |
| Mango | 55 | Onions | 10 |
| Orange | 43 | Parsnip* | 97 |
| Papaya | 58 | Peas* | 48 |
| Peach | 42 | Spinach | 15 |
| Pear | 38 | Squash | 0 |
| Pineapple | 66 | Turnip green | 15 |
| Plum | 39 | Watercress | 15 |
| Prune | 29 | Yam* | 37 |
| Raisin | 64 | **Nuts** | |
| Strawberry | 43 | Almond | 0 |
| Watermelon | 72 | Brazil nut | 0 |
| **Nonsweet Fruits** | | Cashew* | 22 |
| Avocado | 0 | Hazelnut | 0 |
| Bell pepper | 10 | Macadamia | 0 |
| Cucumber | 15 | Peanut | 14 |
| Red pepper | 10 | Pecan | 0 |
| Tomato | 15 | Walnut | 0 |

*definitely or likely cooked

# The Acid/Alkaline Balance

A very important factor in health that is discussed very little in mainstream medicine is the acid/alkaline balance of the body. Yet in 1931, German cell biologist Dr. Otto Warburg received the Nobel Prize for discovering that cancer cells thrive in a high-acid, low-oxygen biological terrain. In a speech, he claimed that nobody could say we do not know the prime cause of cancer. And that was 75 years ago!

Since then acidity has become associated with numerous other diseases. As Victoria Boutenko asks, why aren't medical doctors routinely checking for our acidity levels when this is such a crucial health factor?

On the pH scale of 0-14, seven is defined to be neutral, whereas anything above seven is alkaline, or basic, and anything below seven is acidic. When we eat too much food that leaves an acidic residue, the body must draw upon its limited alkaline reserves to keep the body from overacidifying. According to Robert Young, PhD, our blood pH is ideally maintained at 7.365, mildly basic. According to Brian Clement, urine and saliva should test at an average of 6.5 in a healthy body. To maintain optimal health, we must eat at least 80% alkaline-residue foods and not more than 20% acidic-residue foods.

Acidic residue elements include sulfur, phosphorus, chlorine, bromine, fluorine, copper, silicon and iodine. Processed and artificial food products, foods high in protein (such as meat, seeds, nuts, eggs), drugs (prescription and recreational), soft drinks, tobacco, all refined sugar and flour products, air pollution and coffee are some of the main exogenous factors in swinging us toward acidity. Excess emotional stresses from positive or negative experiences create endogenous factors that likewise promote acidity.

Alkaline residue elements include potassium, sodium, calcium, magnesium and iron. Not all authors are in agreement as to which fruits and vegetables leave an alkaline ash residue once the body metabolizes them. There is agreement however that most all *do* leave an alkaline ash. Perhaps there is some disagreement because each individual piece of produce can vary vastly from its kin, depending on the soil in which it grew. However, everyone agrees that greens and especially sea vegetables are very alkaline and help us balance our pH. Note that citrus fruits, such as lemons, are initially acidic in the mouth and stomach but leave alkaline residues in the body upon being metabolized.

To envision what body acidity is like, think of the calcifications that form on your car battery, and imagine the same thing accumulating in your digestive, nervous and circulatory systems! An acidic body at first leads to minor health complaints and later to major diseases and depression. If one becomes too acidic, he or she will die of acidosis.

The body must compensate for acidity in order to save the life of the organism by mobilizing important alkaline minerals, such as calcium, from the bones to neutralize the acidic condition and create a tolerable blood pH. Therefore, an acidic diet eventually leads to more serious complications, such as osteoporosis.

An acidic environment in the body is also conducive to the growth of health-destroying microorganisms. Dr. Theodore Baroody points out that acidic wastes have an affinity for the connective tissues of the joints. As toxic depositions are made, arthritis results (*Alkalize or Die: Superior Health through Proper Alkaline-Acid Balance*, p. 20). As they accumulate in the muscles, the irritation results in muscle aches. As toxic deposits accumulate in glands and organs, disease results there as well.

Normal alkalinity in the body is characteristic of great health, leading to a blissful "high" feeling. The reason people self-medicate with recreational drugs is to feel this normal, natural, alkaline high. But the effect is a counterfeit: it is fleeting, ultimately leading to a much more acidic state — hence the big crash after the high.

It is best to eat raw fruits and vegetables, especially green leafy vegetables, to achieve a sustained alkaline high and superior health. Sprouts are also good.

Other factors that will increase your alkalinity are positive thinking, kundalini yoga, sunlight, fresh mountain air, laughter, joy and long, slow, deep breathing.

To learn more about this complex topic, read *The pH Miracle: Balance Your Diet, Reclaim Your Health* by Robert Young, PhD, DSc, and *Alkalize or Die* by Dr. Theodore Baroody.

# Drinking Water

For years, mainstream nutritionists have been telling us to drink eight glasses of water a day. Some raw fooders recommend drinking most of the water for the day in the morning, such as routinely drinking six to eight glasses upon rising. Some of these notions have been based on the false idea that water flushes out toxins. By now, however, we have learned that only the body does the acting. (See the Law of Action, defined on page 549.) Water is used by the body, among other things, as a replenishment of internal fluids that provide a transport medium for nutrient delivery and waste removal: water does not do any "flushing" out of toxins whatsoever.

Dr. Vetrano cautions that drinking excess water creates an extra energy burden on the waterlogged tissues since the body must expend energy to eliminate the excess water. Dr. Shelton and Dr. Vetrano have advised to drink according to thirst: "A pleasant mouth and throat sensation, with the tongue seeming to get double and triple its normal size as you experience an actual yearning and quickening for water: that is thirst."

This contrasts with Dr. Fereydoon Batmanghelidj's teachings in *Your Body's Many Cries for Water*. Dr. Batmanghelidj spent time in the Middle East as a doctor to prisoners of war with thousands under his care, many of whom were sick. He found that many of the sick were severely dehydrated, and that if they were given sufficient water, their disease symptoms ceased completely.

This led him to more study and observation and to write his popular book. The simple theme of this book is this: if you wait until you are thirsty before drinking water, your body is already in an alarm mode, and the fight-or-flight response is already activated — the body is crying for water! To avoid this pathological condition, people are urged to drink water throughout the day without waiting for thirst. His book gives great advice to cooked fooders, but raw fooders simply don't need that much water.

Victoria BidWell illustrates how salt and cooked food addicts can actually misinterpret the need for more water as the need for more food:

> Some people with compulsive eating disorders in particular have been conditioned to misinterpret what is true thirst for water as false craving for food and will enter into a binge episode when misinterpreting simple thirst. If these people are eating cooked food — or even salted and condimented raw food — they will soon experience intense false hunger again and develop the "bottomless pit" syndrome, eating until it hurts and still feeling hungry, when they were really just thirsty and when sufficient water would have satisfied their false hunger cravings completely! Having partaken of salted, water-deficient foods, they are extremely dehydrated at this point. Demoralization, despair and fear of being out of control with their food set in next. This activates the fight-or-flight response, to which they have been conditioned to respond by eating! Natural Hygiene offers a way out of this vicious cycle for many reasons, primary of which is that the hygienic foods keep the body naturally hydrated. They are water-sufficient.
>
> The fruits are, generally speaking, 75-95% pure water (melons being up to 98%), while the vegetables are 60-90% pure water. Nuts and seeds are 5%. On this water-sufficient diet, the health seeker will seldom be thirsty. Most "hardcore hygienists" actually drink little more than a few quarts of water in a month. If, through periods of intense exercise when living in hot climates and/or while transitioning to the 100% raw, water-sufficient diet, you still get thirsty, drink pure water only or fresh juices — or just eat melons! But when not yet in touch with his or her sense of genuine hunger, the health seeker should first drink some water to see if that satisfies the bodily needs and to avoid attempting to appease a false hunger. In a nutshell: You may not be hungry at all — only thirsty!

Other raw fooders also estimate that we do not need eight glasses of water a day. Gorillas and other apes in the wild drink almost no water relative to their massive sizes. The usual eight glasses a day is for cooked fooders, not raw. Cooked food is already relatively dehydrated and contains exogenous toxins that need to be diluted so as not to cause harm to the body's delicate tissues. Furthermore, a highly processed diet contains huge amounts of sodium chloride (table salt). Once ingested, the sodium chloride must be diluted with water by the body. This results in water retention and inordinate thirst.

My own experience is that I drink probably half as much water as I did when eating cooked foods. One may nonetheless still need eight glasses a day during the detoxifying transition period in order to dilute toxins and provide a fully hydrated transport system within the body to facilitate the detoxification process.

For some raw fooders, drinking water can even deter cravings. Frédéric Patenaude, in his book *The Raw Secrets: The Raw Vegan Diet in the Real World*, refers to a friend experiencing this. His friend felt that cravings were his body's way of crying for water to help eliminate the toxins of the food craved. Raw fooders have observed that as the body detoxifies something, one will crave that very thing. As explained previously in Chapter 14, this phenomenon is known as *retracing*.

Drinking water within an hour of eating (before or after) is thought by many raw fooders not to be a good idea, except for maybe a few sips, because it dilutes the stomach's digestive juices already at work in their optimal concentrations as needed for proper gastric digestion.

However, on the other side of the controversy, both Roman Devivo and Antje Spors, authors of *Genefit Nutrition*, recommend drinking water right before eating. Dr. Batmanghelidj writes that drinking water an hour after eating food actually aids in its digestion.

Everyone who is educated on the topic agrees that tap water, contaminated by fluoride, chlorine, lead and numerous other toxins are out of the health arena. Anyone who still believes fluoride belongs in the drinking water should read *The Fluoride Deception* by award-winning investigative reporter Christopher Bryson or *Fluoride the Aging Factor* by John Yiamouyiannis.

To mention just a few things, fluoride was used in Nazi Germany's concentration camps to pacify the prisoners. It permanently damages that part of the brain that has to do with willpower. It results in lowered thyroid function, which is why cities that have it in their drinking water tend to have higher obesity rates. A Chinese study on the effects of fluoride on the nervous system found that fluoride contributes to a higher incidence of learning disabilities, including attention deficit disorders, and can be a danger to the fetus if a pregnant woman consumes it (*Neurotoxicology and Teratology,* Issue 17[2], 1995).

Chlorine is also toxic and causes scarring of the arteries, which then sets up the scarred artery tissue to attract cholesterol. This kills living organisms, including people. Both fluoride and chlorine are toxic industrial-waste byproducts. Companies that were looking for cheap disposal methods found ways to make waste disposal actually profitable: convincing people that these toxic chemicals would be healthful to have in their water! Since taking a shower in toxic water is the equivalent of drinking around five glasses of water in terms of exogenous toxins absorbed through the skin, one should have a water filter on the shower.

At the very least, one needs a reverse osmosis filter for drinking water. Yet many prefer to drink water that is even closer to its natural state, such as spring water.

There is a controversy among raw fooders and other health-conscious people about which water is best: distilled, spring or some other water. The argument for distilled is that it contains pure water molecules with almost no toxins included. Rainwater is naturally distilled by solar evaporation, but it absorbs acidic pollutants from the air as it falls. The argument in favor of spring water is that this is what people have traditionally drunk, water from springs and streams from melted snow coming down mountains and/or fed by rainfall. Such water picks up inorganic minerals as it travels through the ground into the groundwater.

Some maintain that drinking distilled water alone can even be dangerous, as it can cause the body to lose minerals by osmosis. Promoters of distilled water claim that the only minerals released are toxic, denatured and not absorbable by the body and therefore needed to be removed.

Promoters of spring water, on the other hand, claim that it contains minerals the body can use, while those who promote distilled water argue that these minerals are not assimilable and are present in nutritionally minuscule amounts anyhow compared to what fruits and vegetables contain.

Dr. Joseph Mercola advises us to "avoid distilled water, as it has the wrong ionization, pH, polarization and oxidation potentials, all of which damage your health and drain minerals from your body" (*The No-Grain Diet*, p. 151).

On the other hand, Dr. Baroody, who has a PhD in nutrition, claims that the idea that distilled water causes the body to leach out minerals is a myth. He claims he could not find even one reputable source for this information. In his book *Alkalize or Die* (p. 123), he claims, "Only distilled water produces a completely negative ion reaction in the system. And negative ions are alkaline forming. All other forms of water contain varying amounts of positive (acid-forming) ions, except alkaline-restructured water."

He goes on to claim that distilled water helps the body to create a more alkaline internal environment. He does not recommend spring water because of the heavy pollution it contains, explaining that toxic wastes have been buried in the earth for many years, contaminating the ground water. There is evidence that detergents, farm chemicals — and even radiation — have contaminated many spring sources. He also recommends water filtered by reverse osmosis, as well as electronically restructured alkaline water.

Yet although Baroody claims that distilled water is negatively charged, it too takes on a positive charge in the presence of polluted air, which includes virtually all indoor and outdoor urban air. This is why ionized (negatively charged) water is becoming more and more popular. First it is distilled and filtered, then ionized.

In contrast, True Ott, who has a PhD in nutrition, claims that water alkalinizers or ionizers are based on junk science. When my husband and I developed arthritis from using one, we called him after noticing he had written about this topic. He explained, "These machines strip electrons from the contaminants themselves, and this creates hydroxyl ions which are harmful free radicals. The $OH^-$ ions attack cells and stimulate adrenaline, which is why there is a short-term buzz, but in the long run it creates a condition that breeds cancer. It can also cause arthritis."

Gabriel Cousens agrees that alkaline water is toxic: "The alkaline water's hydroxyl ions are electron takers, not donors. The alkaline water, however, may give you a feeling of energy because, as cells are destroyed from free-radical oxidation, they give off energy. Unfortunately, this is short-term energy" (*Spiritual Nutrition*, p. 478).

In a lecture, David Wolfe condemned well water for having too many minerals, rainwater for being aggressive and pulling out minerals (as he says people in Hawaii have found) and distilled water for being "corrupt, dead and dangerous." He claims that spring water is "intelligent" and has information in it. He says he has researched this so thoroughly that he cannot settle for less and actually goes directly to springs and fills up bottles.

Another issue of vital importance is that with all this bottled water, we are ingesting toxic amounts of xenoestrogens, which leach from the plastic water bottles — and other plastic food containers, for that matter, including the ubiquitous Saran Wrap. These lead to cancer, especially of the breast and prostate. The solution is to get a reverse osmosis filter for your kitchen and carry your water around in a food-grade stainless steel container such as that found at www.enviro productsinc.com.

Consuming cruciferous vegetables, especially raw broccoli, kale and cauliflower helps protect us from these carcinogenic particles that mimic estrogen.

# Controversial Foods and Seasonings

The tastebuds of people transitioning to the raw food diet are accustomed to the intense flavors of chemical-laden, processed foods filled with MSG, salt, refined sugar and spices. They therefore find it easier to transition by using strongly seasoned, raw gourmet dishes. Most of them are also improperly combined. Many feel they have given up enough already, so why not use a little unpasteurized soy sauce or Celtic sea salt to enhance the flavor of their soups and salad dressings? Some people keep eating these transitional dishes for years.

Hygienists and other purists assert that raw diets should be kept simple. Anything that does not taste good enough to be eaten in its raw state *alone in a monomeal* should not be eaten at all. Once tastebuds are cleared of all the toxic taste stimulators in processed foods, the natural flavors of whole foods can be sufficiently intense to satisfy: celery tastes wonderfully salty; a carrot can taste more delicious than the finest chocolate cake!

These purists also point out that some foods are toxic even when raw. The rationale here is that if people want to heal from disease or want to achieve optimal health, these protoplasmic poisons will slow down the body's ability to cleanse and heal itself. Any item that is even the slightest bit toxic should be excluded despite its ability to enhance flavor. Therefore, foods omitted from the purist diet, despite their appearance in many raw food recipes, include nama shoyu (unpasteurized soy sauce), garlic, onions, cayenne pepper, jalapeños, black pepper, chili peppers, mustard, salt in any form, vinegar in any form, unpasteurized miso, cold-pressed oils, refined oils and alcohol.

This list includes any foods that are so hot that they burn the tongue. It also includes foods that contain stimulants, such as raw cacao. In addition, purists believe in eating foods as close as possible to their natural, unrefined state. Hence, the use of oils (refined fats) is discouraged.

Hygienists counsel against the use of any fermented foods whether raw or not, such as miso, tempeh, kombucha and sauerkraut, because they contain alcohol, a protoplasmic poison. The other school of thought is that these foods are so rich in enzymes and beneficial bacteria that this more than offsets the drawbacks of the small amount of alcohol they may contain. Even fermented cooked foods, like most misos, are rich in bacterial enzymes.

Nearly everyone is aware of how bad table salt can be. Entire books have been written on the topic. Its health hazards have long ago entered mainstream knowledge. (See Appendix A.) Still, some raw fooders debate whether Celtic sea salt, Himalayan rock salt and other forms of natural salt are healthful. Some believe we should avoid them altogether. Others claim they are a great source of trace minerals.

According to Dr. Cousens, a vegan diet tends to cause the body to wash out chlorine, the natural chlorine found in plant foods and needed by the body, not the harmful form found in tap water and swimming pools. He says we can utilize the chlorine and sodium salts contained in Celtic sea salt and Himalayan salt.

Even Celtic and Himalayan salts are composed primarily of toxic sodium chloride molecules. Consumption of even these natural salts in amounts sufficient to season foods on a daily basis still contributes to pathologies such as edema (water retention), cardiovascular disease, overeating and high blood pressure.

# Eating Foods in Season

It is always best to eat locally grown foods in season. For one thing, produce purchased in season and locally is always marketed at the best prices. For another, this can help you make sure you are not eating highly pesticided food. If you eat melons when they are out of season, and they are not labeled organic, they could have been imported from a third-world country where they are in season but where laws for pesticide use are very lax.

Moreover, eating foods in season encourages you to eat local foods. One advantage of that is supporting the local farmer. When you support your local farmer, you not only profit by eating food that is fresh and in season, but you also help reduce the profits of giant food corporations that care more about profits than your health.

In addition, seasonal food grown locally is also fresher and thus higher in nutrients and biophotons than food that has been trucked or shipped from far away. Studies have shown that the sooner one eats something after picking it, the higher its nutritional value. It is always best to eat your foods freshly picked — the fresher, the better.

Finally, another advantage of eating foods in season is sparing the planet from more air pollution and oil usage due to the vast amounts of fossil fuels burned up in shipping food hundreds, or even thousands, of miles to the market. This issue is growing in political significance, as many believe we have reached, or are on the verge of reaching, "peak oil," after which oil prices will skyrocket.

# Supplements and Super Foods

No one disputes the fact that most of our farm soil is minerally deficient. Even a study done as early as 1936, reported in Senate Document 264, 74th Congress, second session, found that 99% of Americans are minerally deficient. It announced that our soil is severely deficient in minerals. According to this document, "Our physical well-being is more directly dependent upon minerals we take into our systems than upon calories or vitamins or upon precise proportions of starch, protein or carbohydrates we consume. . . . Disorder and disease result from any vitamin deficiency. It is not commonly realized, however, that vitamins control the body's appropriation of minerals, and in the absence of minerals, they have no function to perform. Lacking vitamins, the system can make some use of minerals, but lacking minerals, vitamins are useless."

More reports followed: The 1992 Earth Summit Report indicated that the mineral content of the world's farm and rangeland soil had decreased dramatically. In 1993, the World Health Organization reported that our soil is 95% depleted of basic survival nutrients. These reports also explained the danger to our health and lives. Despite both public reports, nothing has been done. It is up to each of us individually to educate ourselves to find out how best to fully mineralize our bodies and then collectively to join forces to revolutionize and reform health education among the wider public.

A common theme in fruitarian circles is the contention that if the soil does not contain enough minerals to grow the fruit, it will simply grow a plant without bearing fruit. People adhering to this erroneous belief have gotten themselves into serious health difficulties due to nutrient deficiencies.

If you purchase an optical refractometer, one with a range of 0-36° brix, you can get some indication of your food's mineral content. Manual refractometers are cheaper than digitals and don't require batteries. By squeezing a drop of liquid from a piece of produce (with a garlic press if necessary) onto the viewing plate, you can observe the density of the plant's juice, which correlates with its nutritional content. This procedure is explained further at www.crossroads.ws.

With the use of this tool, you will soon realize that the mineral content of our soils and thus the plants grown in them have been radically depleted. Our produce, including much that is grown organically, is lacking nutritional richness. This may explain some of the reports of dental problems among raw fooders who eat primarily fruit, the least mineral dense of our natural foods.

I heard David Wolfe state in a lecture that he believes the lack of minerals in our soil has not been corrected intentionally. The government and "powers-that-be" would like us to remain mineral deficient as that makes us easier to control. Raising the amount of minerals in your body, according to Wolfe's research, will increase your consciousness level, taking your awareness and aliveness to a higher level than the raw food diet alone will do.

One way to correct a mineral deficiency, if you live near the ocean, is to water your plants with diluted ocean water, which is mineral rich. Read the book *Sea Energy Agriculture* by Dr. Maynard Murray in order to learn about this. If you don't dilute the sea water enough, it will kill the plants, but you need a certain amount in order to remineralize the soil.

Some raw fooders say we should not take any supplements in the form of pills, as these are not natural. In fact some of them, especially when not coming from a reputable company, may have toxic fillers. Instead, one can replenish his minerals with "super foods." These super foods include bee pollen, goji berries (also used in Chinese medicine), sea vegetables like dulse and nori, spirulina, noni juice, blue-green algae from Upper Klamath Lake, Peruvian maca, sprouts and wheatgrass juice.

David Wolfe claims that the top three super foods, in terms of their association with longevity, are goji berries, royal jelly and cacao beans.

There is controversy among raw fooders as to whether cacao is a healthful food or whether it is even possible to eat truly raw cacao due to its bitterness. David Wolfe cleared up the latter issue in an interview by stating that he has plucked it from the plant himself, sun dried it and enjoyed eating it. Wolfe claims in his book *Naked Chocolate* that cacao is one of the most powerful antioxidant foods and a great source of nutrients, including magnesium. Others feel that its antioxidant value does not offset the anxiety and insomnia it creates.

David Jubb encourages the use of bee pollen, claiming that two tablespoons of this food contains more nutrients than two weeks' worth of eating at fast-food restaurants.

Other raw fooders say we need additional supplements. Many recommend additional enzymes. I heard Brian Clement say in a lecture that he takes 20 enzyme pills per day.

Lou Corona, a prominent raw fooder who has been on a raw diet for more than 30 years, promotes the use of enzymes and takes 30 enzyme pills a day. He also recommends probiotics, which help us maintain healthy intestinal bacteria.

He traveled all over the country, talking with many organic farmers, and learned that the demand for organic food was increasing so fast that many of them did not have time to grow the food properly. He also claims that the raw fooders who do not take supplements, while being free from disease, are not experiencing their maximal health potential.

Dr. Gabriel Cousens says that he has observed in his clinical practice that the healthier a person becomes, the less supplementation he has to take. This is probably because as one becomes cleaned out at the cellular level, especially in the small intestines, nutrient absorption is enhanced.

Victoria BidWell and Dr. Vetrano have this to say on the supplement/super food controversy:

Concerning supplements, the vegan whole food diet is nutritionally sufficient provided foods are eaten raw, organic and with enough protein to meet one's unique needs. The need for exogenous $B_{12}$ may be the sole exception in rare instances and can be determined by blood tests if a person feels unwell on this diet. Concerning "super foods": Fruits, vegetables — including greens and sea vegetables — nuts, seeds and sprouts are the *true* super foods, so long as the ingredients are raw and organic and consumed in proper food combinations according to dictates of genuine hunger and under conditions of emotional balance.

Many so-called super foods are merely unconscionable marketing scams: enterprising profiteers promote exorbitantly priced, toxic quasi-foods that give a stimulating poison buzz but are promoted as nutritional boosts promising to provide extra energy, healing and/or a spiritual high. Spending good money on good foods instead of on designer protoplasmic poisons will save the supplement/pseudo-super food addict hundreds, if not thousands of dollars a year. The *true* super foods will bring superlative nutrition to the table for body, mind and spirit.

For further discussion of supplements, see Chapter 19.

# Fiber: How Much Is Necessary?

The average American eats about 10 grams of fiber a day, although around 30 is recommended. Fiber is essential for gastrointestinal health. Uncooked fiber is like a sponge that absorbs toxins. Victoria Boutenko discovered in her research that wild chimpanzees, our closest relatives, eat 300 grams of fiber a day! She has concluded that we should be getting around 70 grams per day. Most people don't get that much, even eating 100% raw, if they are juicing a lot and eating refined vegetable oils.

*Dietary fiber* is by definition 'the indigestible part of a plant.' The body extracts its usable nutrients from food via mastication in the mouth and then the processes of digestion which occur within the stomach and intestines. Peristaltic action pushes the fiber and food remains slowly through the intestines. The fiber contributes to intestinal health as it travels by carrying along excretable bodily wastes. The fiber is eventually evacuated in the stools. The water-insoluble fiber of vegetation is stiff, whereas the water-soluble fiber of fruit is soft.

The word is even out to all SAD eaters that their favorite "foods" lack necessary fiber. Its relative absence from their diets has resulted in shelves full of various remedies for diarrhea and its flip-side disease, constipation.

Virtually all cases of diarrhea and constipation that haven't advanced into degenerative bowel disease can be completely stopped within days or a few weeks by getting off SAD foods completely and practicing high-fiber eating habits. Advanced cases of chronic bowel disease may require a period of fasting first. Certainly no pricey bulk tablets or high-fiber cereal will be needed ever again once a person turns to a plant-based diet emphasizing raw fruits, vegetables, nuts and seeds. These foods all contain wonderful fiber!

Even when drinking raw juices for one or even two meals a day occasionally, the very last thing you have to be concerned with is getting enough fiber! However, the raw fooder consuming refined oils is not getting fiber in those oils. We can get more fiber with less chewing by using the Vita-Mix or Blend-Tec machines, which completely liquefy foods without separating the fiber from the juices. You can always add ground flaxseeds and/or psyllium husk powder to your meals for even more fiber.

Victoria BidWell shares "The Fiber Facts" from *The Health Seekers' Year-Book* to show us the benefits of fiber-rich natural foods:

---

**1.** Excluding juices, the Natural Hygiene/raw diet is 100% fiber rich, typically containing 60-90 grams or more of fiber, while the SAD — with 70% of the fiber refined out — contains only about 10 grams. Mainstream nutritionists recommend getting a minimum of 25-30 grams a day.

**2.** The raw diet has none of the fiber broken down by cooking, while the SAD has most of the remaining 30% broken down by cooking.

**3.** The raw diet insures a high nutrition-and-nontoxic quotient, since it eliminates refined sugar, salt and condiments to add flavor, while the SAD insures a low quotient, requiring refined sugar, salt and condiments to give back flavor lost in cooking natural foods.

**4.** Raw food fiber acts as a peristalsis stimulant to the muscular walls of the digestive tract and inspires 2-4 bowel movements a day so that raw foods pass through the entire digestive system within 18-36 hours, while fiber-deficient foods do not stimulate peristalsis and take 48-96 hours and even more before the typical one bowel evacuation a day, if that.

**5.** Raw foods provide a fiber-rich bed for the growth of friendly bacteria, which help in the formation of the larger, bulkier, softer stool and their easy, regular passage, while the SAD foods contribute to unfriendly bacterial homesteading and formation of smaller, harder stools and their difficult, irregular passage.

**6.** A high-fiber, raw diet promotes light feelings of tranquility and well-being while a fiber-deficient SAD promotes heavy feelings of distress and discomfort.

**7.** The Natural Hygiene foods are not associated with the diseases of civilized foods. Epidemiological studies clearly show that populations on high-fiber diets escape virtually all the diseases associated with refined, low-fiber foods: coronary heart disease, gallstones, diverticular diseases, appendicitis, hiatal hernia, varicose veins, hemorrhoids, colon cancer, colitis, obesity, constipation, diabetes and others.

---

Fiber authority Dr. Denis Burkitt substantiates all Victoria BidWell's "Fiber Facts" in *Don't Forget the Fiber in Your Diet*: "The food component that has changed the most with adoption of Western dietary habits is the amount of indigestible fiber. The most harmful change that has occurred in Western diets over the past century has been the partial replacement of natural carbohydrate foods by an increased consumption of fat and animal foods and refined sugar and flour."

This change led Dr. Burkitt to conclude that fiber is the single most important nutritional element in our foodstuffs. We are in agreement about one thing: if the food is eaten live, it will have all of its fiber intact.

# The Proper Dietary Proportions of Carbohydrates, Fats and Proteins

Definitions of the macronutrients — carbohydrates, fats and proteins — are found in Chapter 9, along with some comments about standard daily recommendations.

Research by modern diet authors Dr. Robert Atkins and Dr. Barry Sears, advocates of low carbohydrate diets, has indicated that the ratio of macronutrients in the diet can play an important role in one's health and feeling of well-being.

However, mainstream nutritionists disagree about the optimal dietary ratios of each of these macronutrients, thus the raging controversy that leaves people in dietary confusion and makes dietary programs a multibillion-dollar business worldwide.

Controversy surrounds the optimal ratio of macronutrients *even within raw food circles*. Some contend that certain people are genetically predisposed to need a lesser amount of carbohydrates than the average American eats and function better with a combination of nearly equal caloric percentages of these three macronutrients. Eating a high percentage of carbohydrates can cause the pancreases of some people, especially those with prediabetic conditions, to secrete excess insulin, which has been found to be implicated in accelerated aging. Excessive insulin secretion may also induce fatigue, brain fog, weight gain and mental confusion.

According to this view, everyone must find by trial and error what the approximate ratio is that makes him feel best. Some people do well on a high carbohydrate diet that includes a lot of fruit, while others need a lot of protein along with the fat that typically accompanies it. Some people have intermediate requirements for each.

Although the book is not about raw diets in particular, *The Metabolic Typing Diet* by William Wolcott and Trish Fahey provides tests and explanations that enable one to determine which metabolic type he is, and the corresponding ratio of macronutrients he needs. They found three main types: the carbo type, the protein type and the mixed type.

Another guide to macronutrient ratios that also includes a great deal of information about the raw food diet is *Conscious Eating* by Dr. Gabriel Cousens. This comprehensive nutritional book includes a thorough analysis of the topic and provides information for determining your own individualized dietary needs.

David Wolfe also deals with the macronutrient ratio issue in his book *The Sunfood Diet Success System*. In years of talking with many long-term raw fooders, he found that all of them had the three macronutrients in their diet most of the time: raw fats (nuts, seeds, avocados, olives), raw carbohydrates (fruits) and raw proteins (green leafy vegetables).

At times, these raw fooders would go for brief periods omitting one group, but after some days or weeks, they would again return to a balance of all three groups. He refers to "the sunfood triangle" and points out differing macronutrient ratios for various purposes, such as losing weight, gaining weight, detoxifying, overcoming candida infection, enhancing mental clarity, gaining the competitive edge in athletics and enhancing spiritual clarity.

He stresses that these are to be used strictly temporarily, or else an imbalance would result. For example, minimizing fats to 0% or close to it enhances both spiritual clarity and the detoxification process. This is why a diet of fruits and vegetables only, especially in juice form, is potent in freeing up energy for cleansing while greatly enhancing spiritual inspiration and insight as well.

# Dr. Graham's 80/10/10 Diet

Dr. Doug Graham's 80/10/10 diet consists of 80% carbohydrates, 10% protein and 10% fat. He has interviewed thousands of people on several types of diets: omnivorous SAD, vegetarian, vegan and raw food. He found that everyone ate too much fat, according to studies by Dr. John McDougall, MD. The average intake for most groups was 42% fat, 16% protein and 42% carbohydrate. But raw fooders ate even more fat, often averaging in excess of 65% of their calories coming from fat! He found that some ate double the fat of the fast-food-eating mainstream!

The reason is that some raw fooders are convinced that the only way to get enough protein is to eat a large quantity of nuts, often consisting of 80% fat calories, and seeds, which are about 70% fat. They also tend to eat a lot of salads with salad dressings that contain purified, refined fat. Most would never dream of taking in refined carbohydrates (sugar and flour) or refined protein (protein powder). After all, these do not occur naturally and are highly processed. Yet most love to consume large quantities of refined fat (oils)! Dr. Graham refutes claims that oil can be a "health food," saying that this is why the raw food community is being "laughed out of the scientific community."

Raw fooders in transition are especially prone to overeating fat since they make their gourmet raw dishes to simulate cooked entrées. Doug explains how in the back of their minds, they may recall that these are supposed to be "transition" dishes, "but today they are still celebrating their transition . . . and what a party it is!"

Many question, "So what? Aren't raw fats good for you? A lot of the harm from fats is because they are cooked. Also, aren't plant fats much better than animal fats?"

While raw plant fat is far superior, too much of it is nonetheless harmful. Dr. Graham personally knows two raw fooders who have undergone open-heart surgery because their high-fat raw diets resulted in near-total blockage of their coronary arteries!

He bases much of his theory not only on his own clinical results, but also on studies of long-lived people with low fat diets that were close to the 80/10/10 he prescribes. In his book *The 80/10/10 Diet*, he even cites five studies that link high fat diets with diabetes, exploding the myth that this disease is caused by high sugar diets.

Cooked or raw, a high fat diet leads to heart disease; reduced oxygen-carrying capacity of red blood cells, which predisposes us to cancer, and increased demand for insulin, leading to insulin resistance and later diabetes.

In his book, Dr. Graham lists 31 differences between humans and carnivores, making it quite clear that meat should not be a staple in our diet, if eaten at all. He further makes a compelling case against our being any other kind of -vores, such as graminivores or omnivores. He elaborates on the relative difficulty we have in digesting starchy roots and tubers, legumes, fermented foods and dairy.

According to Graham, we are frugivores. A *frugivore* is one who eats chiefly fruit and tender greens. Our staple food should be fruit. Fruit is delicious in its simple, natural state. Furthermore, humans don't make Vitamin C, and fruit is our main source of it. Perhaps most significant of all, fruit sugars enter the bloodstream rapidly and exit just as rapidly. Their ease of digestion makes fruit the "perfect food for human consumption." He also emphasizes that we should eat fruit in its fresh, whole state, rarely juiced or dehydrated.

The popular idea that we shouldn't eat much fruit if we want to be healthy just doesn't make sense from the viewpoint of a naturalist. Since eating mostly fruit didn't lead to cancer, candida, chronic fatigue and diabetes in times past, why should it be avoided today in someone with those conditions?

Graham says we can eat nuts, seeds and high fat plants in moderation, but eating them in excess causes digestive difficulties. We should also have plenty of green leafy vegetables in our diets in order to obtain minerals and other nutrients.

You may partake of this diet and eat nothing but low-glycemic fruits and vegetables of course, but then you would have to consume considerably larger amounts of produce since higher glycemic fruits are also higher in calories. Sweet fruits are much more calorific than nonsweet fruits and vegetables, so you will likely need to include some of them in the diet.

Fruit has gotten a bad rap in nearly all diet plans partly because it is so high in carbohydrates. According to Graham, we need high-carbohydrate diets. We don't need more than 10% fat and 10% protein. Much of the protein we get can come from fruit. Gorillas are the strongest animals on the planet, and they build their muscles on greens and fruit. He also figures that if you make an average of the ratios consumed by other primates, the figure you come up with is almost exactly 80/10/10 (p. 71).

As Dr. Graham explained, when we eat high-fat diets, which he defines as being above 10-12%, the fat lingers in the bloodstream. It coats the sugars and slows down their assimilation by interfering with insulin's ability to latch onto them. He says that when we overeat fat, "a thick coating of fat lines the blood vessel walls, the cells' insulin-receptor sites, the sugar molecules, as well as the insulin itself. These fats can take a full day or more to clear from the blood, all the while inhibiting normal metabolic activity and preventing the various structures from communicating with each other." He states that *sugars you eat today* can mix with *fats you ate yesterday.*

The resulting accumulation of sugar causes several things to happen: the pancreas sends out more insulin to attach to the sugar, which also gets coated by fat. After years of this, when the pancreas becomes exhausted, diabetes can result.

The microbe *Candida albicans*, which is beneficial at normal levels since it consumes our excess sugars, also proliferates to unhealthful levels. On a low-fat diet, sugar gets processed and redistributed, causing yeast levels to drop since there is no longer any sugar stuck in the blood for the yeast to feast on.

In addition, the oxygen-carrying capacity of each individual red blood cell is reduced when blood fat levels rise, and the actual number of viable red blood cells diminishes. This makes one experience fatigue and even brain fog after eating fats. When on a low-fat diet, people notice a heightened mental clarity and zest for life.

The proof of his theory lies in the results Dr. Graham gets. He has successfully treated people with Type I, as well as Type II diabetes. They have gotten off insulin within *weeks* or *days*. People are freed from *Candida albicans* infections. Athletes, including Olympians and professionals, get maximal performance results on this diet.

Dr. Graham disagrees with the idea that there are significant differences in the ratio of macronutrients that individuals need, according to genetics. He explains this in a web site article called, "Half Fast Test." (Get it?) According to his research, sports physiologists have found only a plus or minus 5% difference between the very slowest oxidizer, who would need more carbohydrates, and the fastest oxidizer, who would need more protein. Therefore, he concludes that everyone should get between 80% and 85% carbohydrates.

Doug also claims that the glycemic food index is the least reliable of nutritional indexes. He laughs at many of the other diet variations we come up with, challenging us to find any example in nature of a species whose individual members eat foods from completely different categories, based on their blood types, metabolic types or any other biochemical factor. Do goldfish, cats or dogs change their dietary requirements when they move to different parts of the world? We all descended from people who ate tropical fruit, and that is our ideal diet.

Note: This diet may seem easy to follow at first glance, until you realize how little of the nuts, seeds and fatty fruits, such as olives, avocados and durians, you would be allowed to eat. To illustrate this, Graham offers a hypothetical diet consisting of four pounds fruit, one pound lettuce, 1¾ pounds vegetables, two teaspoons olive oil and a modest three ounces nuts — just over a handful. In this diet, fat makes up 35% of the calories!

Other raw fooders besides Doug Graham say they have found through experience that fat and sugar, when either is taken in large quantities, are incompatible. If you are going to eat a lot of fruit, go easy on the fat and vice versa.

Live food expert David Jubb concurs that our diet should be slightly less than 10% fat, slightly less than 10% protein and the rest complex carbohydrates.

He is also very adamant about avoiding hybrid produce, which contains "runaway sugars" that can upset the liver and pancreas. (See more on that topic on page 328.)

Certain fruitarian authorities maintain that such extreme all-fruit or nearly all-fruit diets as those T. C. Fry promoted and others espouse don't provide enough protein. For many on this diet, a lack of minerals and/or protein has resulted in a loss of some, *or even all*, teeth!

Impressed by T. C. Fry's literature, Ken Rose, a young marathon runner from Los Angeles, adopted an all-fruit raw diet. When his teeth began to loosen in their sockets, he called Fry for advice. T. C. assured him that it was just a temporary detoxification reaction and that he should continue doing what he was doing. Unfortunately for Ken, he then proceeded to "detox" all of his teeth right out of his head. He ended up with a full set of dentures! (See the section on overeating fruit on page 359.)

While some people may have dental and B$_{12}$ issues on this diet, others apparently thrive on a mostly fruit diet. Fruit is considered a *sattvic* food, which means it nourishes the consciousness. Its alkaline ash contributes to calmness. When people move in the direction of making a diet lighter and lighter while on the path to eating less and less, they often progress through the stages of omnivore, vegetarian, vegan, raw vegan, fruitarian and then liquidarian, consuming only raw soups and juices.

Dr. Vetrano has carried on Dr. Shelton's recommendation that vegan diets should include two to four ounces of raw nuts and/or seeds daily. The following section is a condensation of a much longer essay written by Dr. Vetrano, the full version of which can be found in the second part of *The Health Seekers' Year-Book with The Best of Common Health Sense*.

# Dr. Vetrano's "Genuine Fruitarianism — Eat Your Veggies, Nuts and Seeds, Too!"

A common pitfall of those who have chosen "nature's way" is to eat only fruit and few or no nuts or seeds, with few vegetables. They have been advised by some "authority" on nature against everything, basically, but fruit.

However, the fact that we instinctively eat nuts and some seeds, just as we eat anything that in its natural, raw state, looks, smells and tastes good in the as-is condition would seem to mean that these items should be in our diet.

Nuts and seeds, when fresh, are some of the most delicious and satisfying foods! They are packed full of bone-building minerals and proteins and, like other fruits, are truly God's demonstration of love to humans presented through nature. It would be a genuine sensory, emotional, mental and physiological deprivation to avoid fruits.

The practice and philosophy of fruitarians abstaining from every food except sugary fruits is incongruent with the correct definition of *genuine fruitarianism*, as I am defining it herein. Advocates of the all-fruit diet imply that *fruitari-*

*anism* means 'eating exclusively of fruits'. *Genuine fruitarianism* is most properly defined as 'eating chiefly of fruits, with the inclusion of nuts, seeds and vegetables'.

Botanically, nuts and seeds are also fruits and therefore belong in the diet of the fruitarian, as well as some vegetables, which are not fruits. A great misdeed is done when the word *fruitarian* is used erroneously to fit some particular hypothesis about human nutrition. I disapprove of the misuse of the word *fruitarian* because it leads people down a dangerous path to a deficiency of protein.

Unfortunately, most individuals are easily misled because they think fruits are only those succulents that have a high sugar content and that are produced by trees; whereas many foods we casually call *vegetables* are actually classified botanically as fruits. Nuts and seeds are also classified as fruits. The error in these individuals' ideals and ideas has caused much weakness, sickness and suffering among so-called fruitarians.

Superlative health can be maintained on a diet of fruits only, providing nuts and seeds, which are fruits, are included. However, most individuals do better by the addition of raw, leafy vegetables to the fruit and nut diet.

There is no denying that fresh fruits and vegetables contain nutritionally adequate proteins. However, a diet composed chiefly of those fruits that have a high-sugar and low-protein content absolutely does not supply proteins in adequate quantities for most people's needs. Most people can't eat enough of these foods to supply their protein needs.

The proteins in fruits are of good quality, but the quantities contained therein are inadequate to maintain nitrogen balance in most cases. We need nuts and seeds, which contain proteins in higher concentrations, to supply our needs.

Our Creator endowed us with an elaborate digestive system, capable of secreting large quantities of all types of protein-digesting enzymes because these are needed for the digestion of protein foods. The addition of nuts and seeds to the fruit and vegetable diet makes the diet *genuine fruitarianism* and will prevent the development of a primary protein deficiency and the diseases which build upon this deficiency.

The one finding from experimental research that stands out most is that for most nutrients, the amount needed for any individual varies greatly. Each individual is unique, having his/her own metabolic and biochemical differences; the amounts of proteins, vitamins and minerals needed are quite varied.

So great are the differences in requirements of protein from individual to individual, and under the varying circumstances of life, that some who eat only fruits and very few nuts or seeds develop a protein deficiency after a year or less on this diet; yet others may continue for several years before showing a protein deficiency.

A great emotional problem, illness or other great stress of life may cause a prior subclinical deficiency to surface quickly and abruptly. Because of the great variability in protein requirements of individuals, the Recommended Daily Allowance (RDA) of protein is set at 30% over the daily consumption that is necessarily allowed. Most hygienists, with cleaner systems and better digestion from proper food combining, on an all-raw or mostly uncooked diet, should not need a 30% excess of high protein foods because of their increased digestive and assimilative capacities.

Those neophyte health seekers on "only fruit" who develop protein-deficiency symptoms usually also develop an array of other symptoms not directly attributable to a dietary deficiency of proteins. The symptoms of protein deficiency are mingled with symptoms of toxicity, caused by excessive fruit eating and from other wrong ways of living not yet cast off.

They have an unrecognized protein hunger that keeps them ravenous and gorging on fruit all day long — yet never feeling satisfied even after a large meal. These individuals don't know what is going wrong. Here they are feeling worse and worse when they thought they were eating a health-giving diet! Under these conditions, any disease can develop, according to the individual's diathesis ('inborn tendencies', or 'genetic predisposition').

When protein is lacking and fruit is eaten in excess, nutrition is poor. Metabolic processes are impaired because nutrition is impaired. All the functions of the body become impaired, including digestion and the elimination of metabolic wastes. As these metabolites (bodily wastes) caused by poor elimination increase, they add to the wastes absorbed from the intestinal tract.

The excessive fruit eating continues because of a driving hunger, thereby increasing the toxic wastes absorbed from the gut. Then organs begin to function less efficiently. Digestion becomes more impaired, and internal secretions are inadequate.

Because of the endogenous and exogenous toxicity and insufficient protein for normal function of the internal organs, the endocrine glands diminish their secretions and begin to atrophy; thereafter, the body goes downhill rapidly.

Because there is insufficient protein to form digestive juices, as well as insufficient protein for continuous repair of the lining membrane of the intestinal tract, many symptoms frequently relate to digestion and the digestive tract. Toxic products of indigestion are absorbed and can cause problems elsewhere in the body, in addition to the protein deficiency syndrome.

Both protein deficiency and starvation diminish the rate of cell division of the mucosa of the gastrointestinal tract which, in health, is obligatorily renewed about every three days. Besides the impairment of digestion, there is less mucus to protect the stomach and intestines from the fermentative products of bacterial decomposition and the acidic gastric juice. Ulcers are very likely to form. When they do, they heal very slowly because the rate of cell division is very slow.

When excess fruit is eaten, it can't all be properly digested or absorbed; consequently, it ferments in the digestive tract. This is the "green light" for bacteria! If food is not digested, it lingers in the digestive tract; and the bacteria are forced to do their duty, which is to decompose organic matter wherever it is found. So they decompose it in the gastrointestinal tract just like in a warm, wet garbage pail, forming the various highly toxic alcohols that irritate the lining of the stomach and intestines.

Thus, in conjunction with other wrong ways of living, overeating on fruits can lead to inflammation, the 4th stage of disease, and eventually to ulceration, the 5th stage. Some of these highly toxic, alcoholic products are absorbed and cause problems elsewhere in the body, thereby masking and compounding the protein-deficiency syndrome.

The poor results which I have seen in people who have tried eating only fruit for prolonged periods strengthen my view that the ideal diet for health-minded people must contain ample nuts and seeds, as well as fruits and some vegetables — especially the leafy greens, the foods to which we are constitutionally adapted. In other words, these are the foods that God designed for us to eat and has provided via nature and in a natural state.

The early symptoms of an excessively low-protein diet are functional in character and are often missed by the layman. The body's ability to make the best out of a detrimental situation, by using the body's reserves of protein and calories, masks the nutritional deficit for quite some time before cellular and then anatomical degeneration occurs.

A protein-calorie deficit may not manifest for years because the body slows down its metabolism and learns to live on fewer needed nutrients. Additionally, the individual lacks energy and of necessity slows down activities. Therefore, the decreased metabolism and diminished activities permit the conservation of all nutrients.

This is a definite and purposeful, conservative effort of the organism, aimed at the prevention of pathological deterioration. It is successful because the cellular and anatomical damages from protein-calorie deficits may be postponed for years. This is a portrayal of the "fearfully and wonderfully made" design and the physiological intelligence of the living organism. The body gives you ample time to discover your problem and to correct it before serious damage can occur.

When people are eating only fruit, they develop protein-deficiency symptoms, plus an array of other symptoms not attributable to a dietary deficiency of proteins. The symptoms of protein deficiency are mixed with symptoms of toxicity that develop from excessive fruit eating and from other wrong ways of eating and living. Under these conditions, any disease can develop, according to the individual's diathesis.

Consequently, the early symptoms of chronic protein deficiency may be merely listlessness or apathy. More revealing symptoms are many: slow healing of wounds, low energy, fatigue, weakness, loss of weight and skin, nail and hair problems. The list continues: diminished secretion of the glandular part of the pituitary gland (adenohypophysis), causing a low basal metabolic rate; growth failure in the young; diminished adrenal cortical secretion; permanent anestrus (sexual inactivity), and suppression of lactation.

Anovulation with absence of menstruation is common, especially in those females who have lost a lot of weight. Irritation increases, and endurance decreases. Edema develops when there is insufficient albumin in the blood to hold the fluids in the vascular system. Low-grade, long-standing cases develop "flaky-paint" areas of hyperpigmentation. Teeth often thin and go bad.

One or all of these above warnings must be heeded. Adding nuts to the all-fruit diet has often brought about a quick return of energy and strength and a disappearance of the many aforementioned disturbing symptoms. A happy health seeker is the result!

You may wonder why all this fuss about proteins? Well, they are so important that they are associated with all forms of life. We are literally made of proteins. About 75% of the body solids are proteins. I would like to assure everyone that it is not because of a vegetarian diet that a deficiency of proteins arises, but because of unwise fruit-eating practices that exclude ample vegetables, nuts and seeds!

I have composed diets for many patients. For most of those health seekers, I successfully used nuts and seeds as the sole concentrated source of protein. After returning home from my health school, these individuals continued eating according to my instructions; and not one of them ever went into protein deficiency.

Actually, everyone consuming cooked meat would be deficient in protein were it not for the fresh vegetables and fruits in their diet. Cooked proteins have lost much of their value, and some of the proteins have been deaminized and have become indigestible, toxic substances. The deficiencies of the meat diet have to be supplied by vegetables and fruits anyway!

Where do hygienists secure their protein? Where does anyone secure protein? They are in all foods, except they are more concentrated in grains, legumes, animal flesh, eggs, milk, cheese, nuts and seeds. Hygienists use fruits, nuts, seeds and vegetables. Do these foods contain adequate and good proteins? Yes, they do. There are some vegetarian hygienists who still use cheese and grains and legumes in addition to, or rather than, nuts and seeds. The most ideal concentrated proteins for humans, however, are found, not in grains or cereals, but in the raw nuts and seeds.

## A Case History of Protein Deficiency

A perfect example of how a protein deficiency can arise in a hygienist follows: This woman patient was going through a divorce; hence, she had emotional problems, one of the conditions which create a need for more protein. She had taken a thirty-day fast the same year, which depleted her reserve proteins. These were only partially replenished due to absence of appetite because of her emotionally draining situation. The body readily soaks up and rapidly assimilates all the proteins in the diet immediately after fasting.

Because she did not eat any concentrated proteins after this fast, she consumed only adequate protein to take care of her obligatory protein needs. After a long abstinence, the body's needs for protein approach those of the growing child, almost twice as much as that which an adult woman would usually require.

She was not replenishing her reserves. She wanted to stay thin; so she kept her diet very low in calories, eating mostly fruits, such as melons, and vegetable salads. At certain seasons, she consumed only honeydew melons or watermelon.

Very seldom were nuts eaten. She exercised occasionally when she was strong enough.

Since her emotionally charged situation was not one that could be solved overnight, she expended huge amounts of nerve energy in hyperemotionalisms, going from jealousy, anger, hurt and depression to rage. These circumstances and life conditions caused further depletion of her protein reserves.

Consequently, she was unknowingly in negative nitrogen balance for almost a year and a half. Sure enough, as anyone could have predicted, she developed a pure protein deficiency, not complicated or caused by any other illness, such as infections, burns, cancer or tumors. Edema was the sole visible symptom which caused her to seek my care. It took a year and three months for the edema to develop.

Other signs and symptoms of protein deficiency were apparent, but she did not realize their significance. The enamel was being dissolved off her teeth. They were getting so thin you could see through them; the edges were sharper than normal, and then they began to just chip away, forming little notches. She had very dry skin and loss of her hair. She complained of being so sleepy all the time that she could barely hold her eyes open. She also complained of weakness, lassitude and a feeling of not being nourished.

It was like a "deep-seated hunger," she said. In conjunction with all that, she would wake up at night with a mouth so dry she thought she had slept with her mouth open. She had to drink water to wet it.

In spite of all the protein-depleting conditions, it still took a year and three months to get to the point where edema showed up because there are proteins of good quality in fruits and vegetables, just not enough to take care of emergency situations where more than the obligatory loss is necessary. The body's protein reserves were finally used up to the point where the albumin of the blood was low enough to permit the plasm to leak out of the blood into the tissues. This woman was advised to eat at least two ounces of nuts a day, and the edema subsided within one week.

An explanation of the cause of her symptoms follows. The edema was a late development because the body tries to maintain normal plasma levels of albumin as long as possible. She was using slight amounts of her reserve protein daily for a year and a half. The enamel of her teeth was slowly wearing away because of insufficient, high quality saliva to re-enamel her teeth after each acid fruit meal, which usually takes place in normal physiology.

She loved citrus fruit and would eat it frequently. Had she had sufficient protein, the enamel would not have been dissolved off by the acids. The nightly dry mouth indicated diminished salivary gland secretion. The dissolution of the enamel of her teeth showed the inadequate composition (lacking protein) of the salivary secretions. Dry skin was due to low thyroid secretions from endocrine imbalance due to protein deficiency. The loss of hair is also due to protein deficiency, as well as low thyroid hormones. The sleepiness, lassitude and weakness are all protein deficiency symptoms.

Physiologically, it has been discovered that there is a genuine, instinctive call for protein in humans. It is difficult to distinguish; nevertheless, with practice, some people have felt it. This woman would eat a meal and be stuffed with food, yet still be hungry and unsatisfied. Yet her emotional problems muted her appetite, especially for concentrated protein foods. She gained weight, but it was low-grade fatty tissue and not good muscle.

Since she began eating nuts and seeds daily — all these symptoms are subsiding. Her energy, strength and vitality are returning. She quit wasting her energy by excessive emotionalisms and has almost fully recovered.

## The Protein Needs of the Body

Those who calculate the protein needs of humans calculate it too high — purposely — to make allowances for individual differences and for the varying conditions of life which may call for more protein, as is shown by the foregoing case history. The RDA for protein is too high to begin with because it is based on the essential amino acid needs of the fast-growing animal such as the rat, and the scientists' premises and theories are erroneous.

However, modern life seems to be packed full of stresses, worries, anxieties, emergency situations, emotional hurts and problems to solve. Eating sufficient calories in the form of fruit and vegetables, without a concentrated protein source such as nuts and seeds, may provide for all the essential amino acids and protein needed under ideal conditions. But when one is under stress, or is highly emotional, and undereating on only fruits and eating almost no nuts, there finally comes a time when the body's reserve proteins are depleted. They then must be replenished.

## The Digestion of Nuts and Seeds

At this point, we need to cover a little more thoroughly the digestion of nuts and seeds. It is well understood that the benefits of nuts and seeds will be derived from their proper digestion. They must be broken down by the process of hydrolysis to the various amino acids and other nutrients contained therein. If nuts and seeds cannot be digested, and if they putrefy in an individual's gastrointestinal tract, they cannot provide that individual with the amino acids and other nutrients which are needed. Those people who really cannot digest nuts and seeds will have to find alternative sources of vegetable proteins.

Most people digest nuts and seeds better than they think. Many people read scare stories about the enzyme inhibitors in nuts and seeds and then become frightened and refuse to eat them. Others get "knots" in their stomach when they eat nuts and seeds. Some say their stomach never seems to empty if they eat nuts.

Of the many who complained about nuts and seeds and who came under my care, most of them have been able to digest nuts and seeds. There were very few people who had gastrointestinal problems that were unable to enjoy nuts and seeds. After a fast of sufficient duration, many of those who could not digest nuts and seeds previous to the fast did very well on them after the fast — and they were very pleased with the situation. It is important for you to remember that there is nothing wrong with nuts and seeds. The problem can be found in the individual's digestive system. Once this is corrected, there will be no problem with the digestion of nuts or seeds.

Some people love nuts and seeds so much that they invariably overeat on them. Naturally they find that they cannot digest them. When they cut the nuts and seeds down to smaller portions, taking them twice a day instead of all at once, they do much better.

If you find that you cannot digest nuts and seeds presently, do not become discouraged. If you live properly and secure all the needs of life with extra rest and sleep, you will soon be able to digest nuts and seeds very well. Meanwhile, you can use other foods for concentrated proteins. This does not mean that you should choose meat, eggs, cheese, milk or milk products, however.

What do you do if you temporarily can't digest nuts and seeds? I use the word "temporarily" because nuts and seeds are highly digestible, in spite of what you may have heard about the protease inhibitors. It has been said that Cabeza de Vaca lived from autumn through early winter using pecans as his sole food throughout that entire time.

The foremost principle to which you should adhere is to search for foods that you can digest in the uncooked state. This is the most health-promoting alternative. Eating uncooked vegetables and fruits will permit you to recover your health more rapidly so that in the future, you will be able to digest all types of nuts and seeds. If this fails, then try something else, still not using animal or cooked foods.

Here are a few suggestions. First, try eating nuts in smaller quantities. You may start with a half-ounce portion of sunflower seeds or some fresh, unroasted nuts with fruit in the morning, with your salad at noon and with your evening meal, whether it is fruit or vegetables. After a week or two, if and when you feel you can handle more nuts and seeds, increase them in half-ounce increments until you are securing the amount necessary for your strength and health.

I have often had to vary the way I feed nuts and seeds, as well as fruits, to sick individuals. Some people handle nuts and seeds very well when they eat them completely alone, as a meal. Then I have found the opposite to be true. However, more people digest nuts and seeds better when eaten with very juicy vegetables or fruit. It depends upon the state of health of their particular digestive system. Try eating nuts and seeds alone or combined to see which way suits you most.

If splitting the servings of nuts or seeds or eating them alone does not work, then try perhaps soaking them for a short time first. I do not approve of soaking them so long that they become a sprout because many of the proteins are thus lost in the manufacture of the sprout. I do approve of soaking them just long enough to make the seed or nut less crispy and less dry.

Again, start out with small amounts and increase very slowly. Do not give up. Give your body time to become adjusted to nuts and seeds. Don't let others convince you that you cannot digest nuts or seeds for some unfounded reason. Just because others tell you that you cannot digest nuts and seeds should not keep you from trying.

Experiments on dogs have shown that it takes approximately one month for them to adapt to either proteins or starches. For instance, the dogs were put on a biologically abnormal diet of starches to see how they would react. It took them one month to fully adapt their digestive secretions to handle this diet. Then an abrupt switch was made to feeding them a more natural meat diet. It again took one month for the meat to be optimally digested. Human digestive adaptation is similar. It takes time for people to adjust to new diets and new foods.

# It's Up to You to Decide!

Ultimately, it will be up to you to decide which macronutrient ratios work best for you. Factors to consider might be age, workloads, exercise programs, stress levels, possible pregnancy, lactation and so on.

Perhaps more important than the ratio of carbohydrates, fats and proteins is the ratio of fruit, seeds and greens. For more details, see Appendix C.

In the next chapter, we'll take a look at many of the common mistakes made by raw fooders. Maybe you know of people who say, "Oh, I tried that diet, and it didn't work!" or, "I just couldn't stay on that diet." We'll examine these failings and find out where those people fell down.

# 18
# Common Pitfalls to Avoid

*We are living in a world today where lemonade is made from artificial flavors and furniture polish is made from real lemons.*
—Alfred E. Newman

Numerous common pitfalls typically await people trying to implement the raw food diet, at least at first. Some of these make it harder to stay on the raw path. The purpose of this chapter is to make you aware of them so that you may take precautions.

## Assuming a Food Is Raw When It Isn't — Although It May Be Labeled "Raw"

Anything heated above 118° F (48° C) is not considered raw by our standards, as enzymes have been destroyed. It is preferable not to heat anything above 105° F (40° C), if possible, in order that all enzymes may be preserved because some of them will be destroyed between 105° F and 118° F.

Arguably, certain enzymes remain intact at higher temperatures than 118° F because their unique molecular structures can withstand somewhat higher temperatures. Unless you are sure, it is best to err on the side of caution. The extent of destruction also depends on how long the foods are heated.

The word *raw* means different things to different people. For several cheese companies, for example, "raw" meant that the cheese was pasteurized at lower than the usual temperature. Raw fooders were purchasing this "raw" cheese until, after calling the manufacturer, they discovered it had actually been heated to 135° F.

I used to think dehydrated fruits were always raw until I called a company that sold dehydrated fruits and asked which raw fruits they had. I eventually learned that some they classified "raw" had been heated from 120° F to 140° F!

Thus it is crucial not to assume an item is raw by our definition but rather to call the processor to find out the exact temperature to which the food in question is subjected. The retailer is not likely to know, nor often the distributor.

In her recipe book *Hooked on Raw: Rejuvenate Your Body and Soul with Nature's Living Foods*, Rhio explains that she called numerous food suppliers to research whether their food was truly raw. She discovered that figs, dates and prunes are often steamed. Sometimes, "raw" tahini has been heated to 150° or 160° F in processing. "Raw" groats are often preheated as well.

Rolled oats are sometimes thought to be raw, but the intense pressure applied to the oats by the rollers effectively creates enough frictional heat to render them nonraw.

Nuts can also be deceptive. If you find a bag of commercially grown nuts or seeds at a grocery store, chances are they have been fumigated at temperatures above 118° F in order to destroy molds, often in the country they were imported from.

Therefore, nuts should be purchased in bulk from a reliable vendor and kept in the freezer to remain fresh. Freezing causes little damage to their enzymes because nuts have such a very low water content. You can also buy them in bulk at a health food store, but they will not be as fresh and may not even be raw.

Cashews are almost never *truly* raw, though labeled so, because they have to be heated to 156° F in order to get them out of their shells while neutralizing the poisonous sap that surrounds them. There are, however, a few raw food vendors who guarantee their cashews to be truly raw. These are listed in the Resource Guide. Their suppliers painstakingly and carefully separate their cashews from their shells by hand. Because this process is so time-consuming, truly raw cashews are expensive.

Most of the almonds grown and consumed in the United States and Canada are grown in California. In 2007, the Almond Board of California, the oversight body that regulates the California almond trade, implemented a rule requiring all California distributors and retailers to sell only almonds that have been pasteurized. Moreover, they are being falsely and misleadingly labeled "raw." This rule applies both to organic and commercial almonds.

For now, it is still possible to skirt this regulation by buying directly from growers. However, the USDA is proposing to extend this requirement to all almonds sold nationwide.

Oils are nearly always pasteurized. Unless their labels specify the temperature at which they have been heated, they have been heated above 118° F. Even those labeled "cold pressed" are generally heated to at least 160° F. A very strict raw fooder would not even use such fractionated, refined foods, preferring whole foods instead.

If you do choose to use them, you may have to shop online (see the Resource Guide) or in a health food store to find truly raw oils. They can only remain so without going rancid if the vendor sells them in dark containers from the refrigerated section. However, olive oil is stable enough to keep for a time unrefrigerated.

Maple syrup is never raw. Sometimes you may be able to purchase the raw tree sap directly from a grower, but it will be much less sweet than the concentrated syrup.

The jarred honey in commercial distribution has nearly always been heat processed, even when labeled "raw." The best sources of truly raw honey are health food stores, local farmers' markets and beekeepers themselves.

Even then you must determine whether the honey was extracted by the more modern heat method (140° F) or by the old-fashioned centrifugal method. Sometimes, truly raw honey might be labeled "unheated" or "really raw." You can always ask the store for the beekeeper's telephone number, call him, and ask which extraction method he uses.

Better yet, go visit him and buy your honey directly from the beekeeper. Not only will you save money, you might also get an education in beekeeping. Beekeepers love to talk about their bees. Keeping your own small hive is always an option, especially if you live in the country.

If you buy your honey still in its comb, then it is truly raw.

Juices can be very deceiving, appearing to be raw when they are not. People new to the raw diet might assume that bottled fruit juices are raw when they are almost invariably pasteurized.

Due to regulations that reflect a phobia of *E. coli* bacteria and potential lawsuits, it is now nearly impossible to find raw juice. It has usually been at least flash-pasteurized. The surest ways to get truly raw juice are to have the store make it right in front of you or to make it yourself.

Even then at many of the juice bars, you have to make sure they are not adding "extras" to your fresh-squeezed juices. For example, some add yogurt to smoothies. I once had fresh-squeezed lemon juice at a juice bar. My husband said I acted "spaced out" later. Then he realized they probably had added sugar to the lemon juice. Also, don't let them add ice if you want the full flavor.

I once ate some raw wild rice at a raw food restaurant that was simply divine! I went home, sprouted a bunch for myself and got constipated. Upon researching it, I learned that wild rice is always dried at 150° F for an hour or so. Thus it is never raw. When soaked, wild rice appears to sprout, but it is actually just tearing. I went looking for sources of wild rice that were truly raw and could find none.

Another word that can be deceptively misjudged for "raw" at times is "fresh." If you go to a restaurant and ask for what the menu calls "fresh guacamole," for example, it may mean that the powdery mix was actually only *freshly made* that day rather than *made from fresh* raw avocados and other raw items.

Finally, because of our country's obsession with germs, you can safely assume that most imported, packaged or bottled foods have been pasteurized.

# Judging the Diet
# before You Give It a Chance

*Genetically the raw food diet is for everybody.* Oftentimes, however, people try it awhile and decide it is not for them because they run into some of the following problems and are not educated enough about the diet to realize what is happening.

First, many are frustrated by detoxification symptoms, such as diarrhea, extra sleep requirements, colds, fever, flulike symptoms and headaches. Some people say, "I cannot do the raw diet because it gives me diarrhea," blaming the diet for the detoxification symptoms that result when the body is actually cleansing and healing itself.

These detox symptoms may come and go, and it is important not to try to stop them with medications. Doing so will not only stop the body from detoxifying but also add to the body's toxic burden, further polluting bodily fluids and tissues and resulting in further symptoms of illness. Just keep eating raw, and review Chapter 14. The symptoms will go away, and you will feel better than you ever have if you persist with the raw food diet.

Second, many believe they cannot digest raw vegetables. Some people, unaccustomed to such large amounts of fiber in their diets, get bloated a lot in the beginning. If this is the case, you may juice the vegetables or blend them into soups or purées. This will make them much easier to digest. The bloating will pass as the body cleanses itself and gets accustomed to a steady high-fiber diet with all of its superlative nutritional benefits.

Some raw fooders believe we are not even meant to eat very many raw vegetables. They claim that only herbivores, with their three or four stomach compartments and digestive tracts twice as long as ours, can digest them well. Plus, herbivores have specific enzymes that we don't have, and a much higher bacterial population than do we, for cellulose processing.

Others say that we can digest raw vegetables but must adapt to some degree, as we have eaten so many foods low in fiber for so long while on cooked diets.

Dr. Cousens acknowledges that through so many generations of eating meat, some people may no longer have the digestive power to assimilate all their nutrients from a vegetarian diet immediately and may require months or even years to transition.

Victoria Boutenko believes that through eating so much cooked food, we have lost our ability to make sufficient hydrochloric acid in the stomach. She has researched her theory that we can correct this deficiency by eating large quantities of green leafy vegetables, which are much more nutritious than other vegetables. (See Chapter 8 and Appendix C.)

Third, many, especially men, find that they lose too much weight. This is only temporary and will pass. You may need a year in which to lose weight and then regain until you achieve your ideal weight. When you rebuild, it will be with much healthier tissue since the building blocks are richer in nutrients.

It is important to realize that the weight lost is almost entirely fat and that to build healthy muscle mass requires more than diet. It requires persistent resistance training exercise.

Fourth, many people find nuts, often a major protein source on a raw diet, difficult to digest. Excessive nut consumption can even cause constipation or bloating in some people. So don't overdo them. Two to four ounces a day is plenty for most people. Also, be sure to soak nuts and seeds for about eight hours, then rinse thoroughly in order to rid them of enzyme inhibitors that impair digestion. Grinding the nuts before eating them also aids digestion.

Some raw fooders who have found nuts difficult to digest have concluded that they shouldn't eat very much fat. Actually, that is not the case; raw fats are very good for us. People eating a lot of raw olives, avocados or coconut cream often won't get that sluggish feeling that some do from nuts and seeds.

Fifth, many are frustrated over the preparation time required for some of the complicated transition recipes in which everything must be made from scratch, such as salad dressing, barbecue sauce, mustard and so on. They don't realize that after just weeks or months to a year, they will become very content with raw food in its simplest form. At this point, preparation and cleanup take five minutes at most per meal!

Sixth, many feel chills and, because their bodies feel cold, they interpret that to mean their bodies are crying out for cooked food. This is simply a temporary phase in which the body is sending a great deal of its energy and blood inward to cleanse and heal vital organs, leaving less heat to warm the extremities. This condition will pass in a matter of weeks or months. Experienced raw fooders actually tolerate temperature extremes much better than cooked fooders do.

See a lot more information on these topics in Chapter 19.

# Overeating Fruit or Not Brushing after Acid or Dehydrated Fruit

A number of raw food experts believe that humans are genetically frugivores, as are apes. This means that their primary food is fruit. Gorillas and chimps do eat principally of greens, but primates often prefer fruit when given the choice. In theory, we humans are also frugivores that can subsist on a diet mainly of fruit, or fruit and greens. (See Appendix C.) Humans don't make Vitamin C like most other animals, and fruit is our best source of Vitamin C.

One of the most unforgettable moments of my life was when, in a forest in India, I took dozens of bananas to feed the wild monkeys. I envisioned them shyly begging. Instead, they came down from the trees in droves and aggressively snatched the bananas from me. I was so scared I dropped the six or seven bunches that I had left. It was like something out of a Stephen King movie!

Jan Dries writes, "The famous paleontologist Richard E. Leakey has proven that [we are frugivores] beyond a doubt. Why else does the digestive tract of modern man — if we study anatomy and physiology — still resemble that of the chimpanzee? There have been hardly any mutations" (*The Dries Cancer Diet*, p. 12).

A diet of nearly 100% fresh fruit has worked for some well-known raw fooders and was highly touted in the earlier days of the movement. Entire books, such as *Fruit: The Food and Medicine for Man* by Morris Krok, heralded the health benefits of fruit. Joe Alexander tells about a time he spent 56 days eating only juicy fruits: no bananas, avocados or vegetables. He claims he never felt stronger in his life.

On the other hand, it has been observed that habitually overeating fruit can lead to the ruination of one's teeth. The strong acids in dried and acid fruit can wear away enamel, leaving teeth so thin they chip or break. In fact a diet excessively high in fruit can cause demineralization of the teeth with resulting serious dental problems. Victoria BidWell tells of a two-month period when she sucked on exceedingly tasty grapefruit sections nearly every evening because the grapefruits were on sale. It cost her $2,000 in two new front teeth crowns!

Certainly one should brush her teeth after eating citrus fruits or dried fruits because their acidity may destroy the enamel. The tips of the teeth may become translucent, and then they start to chip. Bits of dried fruit can get stuck between the teeth, and you learned as a kid that bacteria love to eat sugar.

Yet there appears to be more going on than this. Our soil is dangerously depleted of minerals. (See Chapter 17.) Sugar binds to minerals, and there are no longer enough minerals in the soil to yield sufficient minerals for the fruit. This means the body will be forced to pull minerals out of the bones and teeth in order to digest the fruit sugars and to neutralize the resulting acids. Our modern, hybridized fruit trees may also fail to extract enough soil minerals.

This phenomenon has been verified in an experiment summarized in an article entitled "Dental erosions in subjects living on a raw food diet," published in *Caries Research* (1999, Vol. 33, Issue 1, pp. 74–80, PubMed ID 9831783). Over a period of many months (median duration 39 months), 130 people eating a diet at least 95% raw were compared to 76 control subjects eating a standard mixed diet. It was found that those on the raw diet had significantly more dental erosions. They were eating 25-96% fruit (median 62%), and the daily ingestion of citrus fruit was 0.5-16.1 whole fruits (median 4.8).

Regarding teeth, if you notice that they are becoming translucent or feeling rough to the tongue instead of smooth, they are demineralizing. In that case, reduce the amount of fruit, especially acid fruits like lemons, limes, oranges and grapefruits, and eat more of the vegetables or the highly mineralized super foods mentioned previously in Chapter 17 that you should be eating every day anyway.

Dr. Doug Graham's theory of the reason behind the fruit/erosion connection was explained in his lecture "Fruit or Fat?" He clearly placed the blame on overeating nuts and seeds, which are high in fat and very acidic in their digestion. The body must neutralize these acids or face death, so it removes alkaline minerals from bones and teeth to do the job. Indeed, a diet high in fruit but low in fat seems to work well for serious athletes, according to his research.

On the other hand, Dr. Cousens and other raw fooders place the blame on fruit. Dr. Cousens points out that although a diet high in fruit may have been excellent fifty years ago, we now need to shift to a diet lower in sugar content, which would create less fermentation and therefore not feed mycotoxic bacteria (*Rainbow Green Live-Food Cuisine*, p. 9). He attributes this need to lessen our fruit consumption to increased physical, mental, emotional and spiritual toxicity in the world and in ourselves.

As mentioned previously, he pointed out that several small groups of people who ate primarily fruit had to stop the practice and alter their diet due to numerous health problems. Dr. Cousens is quick to note that just because something feels good in the short term, such as a primarily fruit diet, doesn't mean it's good in the long run.

Another perspective on why eating a high percentage of fruit is no longer viable is that fruit is picked before it is ripe nowadays for commercial reasons: to lengthen its shelf life and to make it easier to harvest and ship.

Fruit that is not vine or tree ripened tends to be lower in minerals than fully ripened fruit. Fruit picked prematurely tends to be more acidic than fruit that is vine or tree ripened. In addition, as mentioned previously, the depleted soil in which most fruit grows lacks sufficient minerals. The extra acidity of unripe and/or minerally depleted fruit is at least part of the cause of dental problems. Lack of minerals also makes fruit taste much blander, less sweet and flavorful, which is why fruit grown in mineral-rich soils tastes so much better.

In her book *Errors in Hygiene?!!?* Dr. Vivian Vetrano partially blames a sugary diet high in fruit and low in protein for the premature death of health educator and publicist T. C. Fry. He died at 70 with symptoms of $B_{12}$ and protein deficiency because he refused to eat more than a very few nuts and seeds on his mainly fruit diet. She objected when he kept offering to share his delicious, sweet fruits with her, "Sure you can stay off nuts, but look what it makes you do: overeat on sweet, dried fruit!" He also suffered from bad teeth and gums, perhaps partly from overeating fruit, although jaw injuries from a near-fatal car accident had certainly resulted in lost teeth and dental trauma.

Another problem with overeating fruit is that it may cause a hypoglycemic reaction from too much insulin secretion. One may experience fatigue, irritability and excessive hunger and thirst.

On the other hand, as we saw in Chapter 17, Dr. Graham says that eating too much fat with the fruit is the cause of the problem! I have found personally that by reducing my fat intake, I can now eat a lot more fruit and not experience hypoglycemic reactions.

Before, when I ate considerably more fat, I would often experience low blood sugar symptoms after eating only a small amount of high glycemic fruit. I experienced fatigue, lethargy and sometimes cravings for more sugar.

# Overeating Nuts, Seeds and Dehydrated Fruits

Some people actually gain weight on raw food diets by overeating nuts, seeds and dried fruits. While transitioning to raw, these easy gainers want to keep that stuffed, heavy, full feeling they used to get from cooked foods. This may be okay for the first six months or so, but one expects to sustain increased energy after a time. As discussed in Chapter 17, overeating fats or sugars, even raw fats and sugars, fatigues in a variety of ways, primary of which is the energy expenditure of the body to process excess food. Consider also that fats are energy expensive to digest, more so than sugars, and that digesting excessive amounts taxes the adrenals and the pancreas.

You wouldn't overeat nuts or seeds if you were out in the wild and had to crack their shells by hand. It would be too much trouble. You wouldn't even find them except in the fall season. But they can be very easy to overeat once shelled.

Likewise, if you were eating fresh fruit, it is unlikely you would eat five mangoes at a time. Most fresh fruits are 90-98% water. Their water content would make them too filling, and peeling them would be too troublesome. Yet it is easy to sit and eat five sun-dried mangoes. They are prepeeled and less filling without the high water content.

Water from fruit is about the best, purest water you can get. If possible, eat your fruit fresh. Dehydrated may sometimes be necessary for traveling or for storing out-of-season fruits — and certainly for enjoying certain recipes.

# Not Getting Sufficient Protein

There is a danger of not getting sufficient protein if you eat a diet of fruit alone and omit sufficient quantities of nuts, seeds, sprouted grains, sprouted legumes and/or green leafy vegetables.

For more information on protein, see pages 342, 381 and Dr. Vetrano's article beginning on page 346.

You absorb more of the protein as you continue to eat raw, so you need a lot less than the recommended daily allowance. But if you don't get enough, you will experience some of the symptoms listed in Chapter 19.

# Eating Too Much Fat

Often there is a great sigh of relief when switching to a raw diet because now you can eat formerly forbidden fatty foods, such as olives, nuts, avocados and seeds. Raw fat is wonderful for you. Most of the bad reputation of fats comes from cooked and rancid vegetable fats and from eating a diet so very high in cooked animal fats. These cooked fats are dangerous to the cardiovascular system, much more readily stored as fat rather than metabolized, and contribute to numerous disease states. However, *raw* fat is actually good for you, enhancing hormone production and supplying the nutrients needed to improve your skin. Some raw fooders hold that eating raw fat helps you metabolize or eliminate the stored cooked fat residues deposited within tissues or circulating in fluids.

Traditionally, Eskimos ate a diet of up to 80% fat. Since it was raw, they remained very healthy. This is often used as an example that we need not limit our fat intake, or at least the ratio of fats to carbohydrates and proteins, on a raw food diet. However, traditional Eskimos did not combine fruit with their fat either, since fruit was unobtainable.

As discussed in Chapter 17, when transitioning to a raw diet, raw fooders often eat way too much fat. This invariably leads to negative consequences. They indulge in fat because they want that heavy, satiated feeling in their stomachs. They eat too much of the raw gourmet counterparts to cooked food, like raw crackers, cakes, pizzas and so forth, as well as refined oils, nut butters, nuts and seeds.

Even on a raw diet, which is vastly superior to standard cooked diets, over-consumption of fats will slow down weight loss or cause weight gain, increase the likelihood of hypoglycemia when you eat high glycemic fruits the same day (according to Dr. Graham), and increase your need for sleep so that the body can deal with the overload. Although, to my knowledge, no studies have been done on people who overeat raw fat, Dr. Graham's clinical observation is that it is not good for the heart.

# Overeating and Undersleeping

Raw diet promoter Paul Nison claims that the most common mistakes raw fooders make are eating too much and sleeping too little. Overeating and/or not getting enough sleep most often results in fatigue. Some beginners may mistake this for a detoxification symptom. Just remember that for most people, for those not deeply descended into serious pathology, the main symptoms of detoxification will be over in one to six months. For those individuals already fairly healthy, any significant fatigue after that is due to overeating, not getting enough sleep and/or nutritional deficiencies, especially of Vitamin $B_{12}$.

If you eat too much fat, especially from nuts, you may get tired due to its relatively long, energy-intensive digestive process. I have noticed that when my fat calories are only 20% of my total intake, I need only six hours of sleep instead of eight.

Also, overeating in general (cooked or raw, fats or fruits) causes the pancreas to release excess insulin, resulting in fatigue. The resultant enervation always increases the rate of aging. Therefore, be careful not to overeat!

Eating anything close to bedtime stimulates the entire digestive tract and will result in insomnia for most people. Eating fruit, especially sweet fruit, close to bedtime stimulates the pancreatic insulin response, which further induces insomnia. Garlic, spices, onions and condiments eaten day or night may also disturb sleep. Drinking wine in excess of a glass or two is a great sleep-interrupter, especially if it is not organic and contains sulfites. None of this concerns the purist, who has given up these protoplasmic poisons.

The old adage that the sleep hours before midnight count for double has great merit. If you need to catch up on sleep, try going to sleep at 9 or 10 PM. You will be amazed at the results. Before the widespread use of electric lighting, people usually went to bed shortly after sunset, rising at dawn. An excellent book on how the invention of the light bulb has contributed to modern-day health hazards is *Lights Out* by T. S. Wiley.

One great bonus about the raw diet is that if you do miss a good night's sleep, you won't feel nearly as fatigued as you did when eating cooked foods. Even if you sleep for only a couple of hours, you can still feel great the next day! You will still need to catch up on missed sleep eventually. Sleep deficits are bad for every cell of the body and for mental/emotional health.

After years of being 100% raw, you will find you need less sleep, as your body will be energized, cleansed, healed and high in nerve energy.

## Succumbing to Social Pressure

People often feel snubbed if you reject their food offerings. It is considered extremely offensive in some cultures. On the other hand, in places like California, people are used to seeing a myriad of diet variations and are seldom surprised by any of them.

Victoria Boutenko reminds us to say "thank you" in at least three different ways if someone goes out of his way to prepare cooked food for you. Then politely explain why you won't eat it. People need to feel appreciated and acknowledged more than they need you to eat their food. Victoria reminds us that if you went to Russia, and someone offered you a bottle of vodka, you would likely find some way to excuse yourself from drinking it. Therefore, you could find a way out of eating the food too. For more information on handling social situations gracefully, see Chapter 16.

## Trying to Gain Weight with Raw Foods Only and No Weight Training Whatsoever

Victoria BidWell takes the lead to help health seekers leap over this pitfall with teachings endorsed by Dr. Vetrano and published in *The Natural Weight-Loss System*:

Most people want to look good, perhaps even more than they want to feel good! Most people are far more concerned with losing weight than with gaining weight. Nevertheless, over my 25 years as a Natural Hygiene health educator, many health seekers have complained of their "skeletonlike" silhouettes and have begged me for help in gaining weight. Getting skinny can get scary, as the thriller movie *Thin* so graphically portrays.

The weight Susan, Dr. Vetrano and I want to see health seekers gain is in the form of healthy muscle tissues and necessary fatty tissues and not in the form of just excess, morbid and unattractive fat. In the following, therefore, we bring you guidelines for getting well and for gaining weight, if needed. Please refer to the Law of Vital Accommodation detailed on page 551. When you challenge the body to accommodate itself to an added exercise routine, your body will, by natural law, lay on muscle tissue so that it can do that which you ask of it.

## The GetWell Weight-Gain System

✓ Undertake a short fast to improve digestion, absorption, assimilation and elimination of nutrients. After a fast and when you commence eating, your body will be in the very best position to build the healthiest of tissues with the best of foods and to wring every bit of nutrient out of every bite you eat. Remember: It's all about energy! And fasting is a time for the body to re-energize. *Remember, also: It is not only what you eat but what your body uses that builds superlative health!* Finally: It is systematic weight-training exercise that inspires the body to accommodate by building muscle tissue and gaining the sought-after weight in the form of sculpted, well-defined, attractive muscles with a minimum of fat for curvature and good looks.

✓ Change to the ideal diet of raw, nontoxic foods, eaten in proper combination.

✓ Maximize all fruit, but especially all the caloric dried fruits, sweet fruits and avocados.

✓ Take an extra fruit meal a day, even when genuine hunger is not present. But do not overeat yourself into sickness.

✓ Emphasize the caloric starchy veggies: corn, mature peas and carrots; sprouted lentils and garbanzo beans; shredded turnips, beets, potatoes, yams and sweet potatoes. Shredded and cut up underground veggies, instead of whole veggies, offer far more exposed surface areas, far more cell walls broken at those surface areas and far more sweetness and calories liberated from veggie cells. Cut out the non-starchy vegetables completely for 1-2 weeks at a time to maximize weight gain.

✓ Maximize the caloric, high-protein nuts and seeds, as they hold the amino acid building blocks for increased muscle tissues. Instead of the standard 2-4 ounces of nuts and/or seeds a day, take 5-6, especially when highly active and under stress.

✓ Take 4-6 ten-ounce glasses of fresh-made juices, smoothies or nut-based beverages, a day between meals. When smoothie and nut-based beverages are prepared in the Vita-Mix and thus thoroughly liquefied, they will be easier to process and will require less digestive energy for the person whose digestion is weakened.

✓ Undertake the GetWell weight-gain exercise schedule as follows:

• Aerobics: Days you do not weight train, just take leisurely walks. Avoid calorie-burning, aerobic exercise for 1-4 weeks at a time.

• Stretching: Do a stretching routine daily for 20-30 minutes.

• Weight training: After eating right, the building of muscle tissue with weight training will be your greatest weight-gain maneuver of all! If your health condition allows, weight train for 30-60 minutes every other day. If you are too ill or weak to go a full 30 minutes, start with 5 or 10 minutes. Train 3 times a week, and take one full day each week for complete rest. Weight-training sessions should consist of the following: first, a 5-minute warm-up of stretching; second, the weight-training session itself; third, a 5-minute cool-down of more stretching.

✓ Get strict with all of the ten energy enhancers, especially extra sleep and rest. The body especially needs extra sleep and rest in order to accommodate to all these lifestyle changes with a healthy weight gain.

✓ Do note that extremely weak or bedridden health seekers need to recover their energy and become strong enough to undertake even the least demanding of these weightlifting exercises.

# Buying and/or Preparing Too Much Food

One of the biggest mistakes I made at the beginning of my raw food adventure was buying too much produce or preparing too much food. Much of it went to waste. All of my food-preparing life, I was used to the mentality of saving time by whipping up huge batches of food and storing it in the refrigerator or freezer to reheat later.

On the raw diet, food will keep in the refrigerator for about a week, but you do want to eat it as fresh as possible. Cutting and chopping it makes it lose some of its nutrients, as does storing it too long. Besides, fresh food always tastes best.

I encountered this problem while feeding only my husband and myself. Of course if you are feeding children or others, this will probably not be a problem.

As cooked fooders, we were used to storing vast quantities of food. If some emergency came along, no problem: I always had at least a month's supply of pasta, grains, beans, canned goods, frozen entrées and such.

As a raw fooder, you won't find that many staples you can stockpile. Basically, you have to let go of the hoarding mentality. The only food items I stockpile now are jars of olives, raw nut and seed butters and nuts and seeds that I keep in the freezer. If dehydrated fruits have been dried thoroughly enough, they may also keep for a long time, even when unrefrigerated. Seeds for sprouting can be stored for two years or even longer in some cases.

# Not Eating Enough Greens

I attended a workshop by Victoria Boutenko in which she outlined the seven most common mistakes made by raw fooders. She mentioned many of the things I have already written about here, including something else — not eating enough greens. She explained that chimps and primates in the wild thrive on greens. She and her family felt something was missing until they started eating more greens and adding them to smoothies with fruit. Greens are the main foods that supply the body with what it needs to alkalinize itself. (See page 331.) They are extremely important for our physical health and sense of well-being. You will find more about her recommended green diet in Appendix C.

# Failing to Study the Raw Food Diet

Those who don't study the raw food diet may lose their inspiration or even forget why they went on it. When the going gets tough, they may cave in to cooked food. (See "Educate Yourself" on page 234.)

# Failing to Plan Ahead

Because raw, organic food is not found everywhere, as cooked food is, you will need to pack some food or plan ahead when traveling or even going to work or shopping. The Boy Scout motto *Semper Paratus*, which means 'always pre-pared', is absolutely essential to your success as a raw food eater. I have met a lot of raw fooders who, at least temporarily, fell out of the living foods lifestyle for the simple reason that they did not plan ahead, taking raw food with them on trips or while visiting others. (See Chapter 16.) Remember, where there is a will there is a way.

# Neglecting Other Areas of Health

Some raw fooders conclude that since they are now eating healthfully, they no longer need to exercise or go out for fresh air. There are many other factors in maintaining superior health besides proper food choices.

First of all, anything that goes into or touches your body will affect your health. You need to remove all toxic shampoos, soaps, make-up, moisturizing lotions, household cleaning supplies and the like. Don't put anything on your skin that you wouldn't eat! (See "Detoxifying Your Environment" on page 266 for more on this topic.)

Stagnant, polluted air is another source of toxins. Since air inside the house is usually even more toxic than the polluted urban air outside due to plastics and other unnatural products used in the home, it is advisable to spend more time outdoors and to buy an air purifier of good quality for use indoors.

Don't buy synthetic carpets, which emit toxic fumes for at least the first year, and avoid common paints. One company that sells nontoxic paint can be found at www.afmsafecoat.com.

Water is another source of toxins. You need to drink pure water (see page 332), not unfiltered tap water. You also need a good shower filter, since the toxin equivalent of several glasses of tap water are absorbed through the skin during a shower.

You need to exercise at least half an hour a day. Exercise should vary and include stretching (as in yoga), walking and anything else you find fun. I also recommend a mini-trampoline. The antigravity exercise it provides stimulates blood circulation and lymphatic flow, benefiting every cell in the body.

A proper amount of sleep, as mentioned earlier in this chapter, is certainly critical for health. Sleep is when the body regenerates nerve energy and heals.

Everyone needs to go out into the sun for about 20-30 minutes a day, longer if you are of African descent. Most of us are deficient in Vitamin D. The sun is the source of all life and energy.

Don't let all the talk of skin cancer scare you. One of the main causes of skin cancer is sunscreen, which is full of chemicals! Sunscreen also blocks out the absorption of the beneficial aspects of the sun, including the rays we use to produce Vitamin D. People deficient in sunlight often become depressed.

A good book on the topic is *The UV Advantage: The Medical Breakthrough that Shows How to Harness the Power of the Sun for Your Health* by Michael F. Holick, PhD, MD. He has published hundreds of studies on the beneficial aspects of the sun, claiming that they are not advertised because no one can make money from the sun! Another is *Into the Light — Tomorrow's Medicine Today!* by Dr. William Campbell Douglass, MD.

And what good does it do to stop eating cooked food if you are cooking your brain with cellular phone radiation? Cell phones are so bad, especially for children and teens whose brains are still developing, that studies in Europe indicate that massive numbers of these young people will have Alzheimer's in their 30s! In the US, cellular service providers protect themselves from future litigation by printing disclaimers in fine print in their manuals or contracts.

One reputable company that has devices to help keep radiation from the head of cell phone users is Biopro. For information, contact Dr. Dan Harper at 858-259-5945, ashuharper@hotmail.com or www.mybiopro.com/drdan.

Finally, negative thinking, including worrying, reacting, resentment and anxiety, creates an acidic condition within the body. Work on dealing with stress without triggering the fight-or-flight response, and create a positive attitude and an alkaline effect.

Gratitude for whatever you have is a powerful and fast route to positivity. Victoria Boutenko says, "Gratitude inevitably leads us to becoming aware of the unlimited wealth that life holds for every one of us. Grateful people tend to be happier, more optimistic, more satisfied with their lives than their less grateful counterparts" (*12 Steps to Raw Foods*, second edition, p. 176).

In fact researchers such as Bruce Lipton, PhD, in *Biology of Belief* and Candace Pert in *Molecules of Emotion* hold that on a quantum level that much disease may actually begin with the mind. A good DVD on this is *What the Bleep Do We Know?*

In her set of four CDs, *GetWell ♥StayWell Affirmations for Americans*, Victoria BidWell summarizes the body/mind research as follows:

> The immaterial thoughts/feelings that come through the immaterial mind and that then activate the material 200 billion brain cells create material molecules called *neurotransmitters* that communicate with the rest of the material body's 75 trillion cells. When a person experiences a happy thought/feeling (a nonmaterial event), the 200 billion brain cells create corresponding, concrete polypeptide molecules released at the synaptic clefts of the brain neurons (material events).
>
> These *chemical messengers* instantaneously flood out from the top of the head to the tips of the fingers and toes to communicate with every cell in the body (material events) and to "tell" the body cells to function in the happy mode. In other words, entertaining a specific thought/feeling (a nonmaterial event) creates a corresponding, biochemical, neurophysiological, cell-to-cell mode of functioning (material events).
>
> In other words, the immaterial determines the material. What we think/feel at the quantum level determines what will become of us. We are what we think and feel! And behavior changes accordingly! Now tell me, dear readers, is that "a fearfully and wonderfully made body" — or what?

For more on the other essentials of health besides diet, see "The Ten Energy Enhancers" presented on page 107.

# 19
# Frequently Asked Questions

He who does not know food,
how can he understand the diseases of man?
—Hippocrates (460–377 BC), the father of medicine

## Isn't a raw food diet boring?

A common misconception about the raw food diet is that it must be horribly boring. Even I, months before trying the raw diet, asked a long time raw fooder, "Don't you get tired of eating the same things all the time?" I envisioned a life of eating nothing but salads and fruit, maybe an occasional smoothie or some trail mix.

The truth is, when you switch to a raw diet, you will discover a vast number of totally new food combinations and taste sensations, not to mention all the recipes now available in books prepared by raw chefs. Raw eating has enjoyed renewed popularity long enough that at the time of this writing, there are dozens recipe books out, with new ones coming out every year. Just about any native or ethnic food you now enjoy has a raw counterpart. I enjoy raw versions of Thai, Indian, Chinese, Italian and Mexican dishes, although at this point, I am quite content to savor simple salads or whole food menus.

Cooking renders food's color spectrum pale, dull and lifeless. Raw food is bright, colorful and extremely attractive. Much of cooked food becomes mushy, whereas raw food comes in many different textures varying from crunchy to soft. Cooked food has lost the fresh, original flavors of live food. Cooked food is so bland that spices and condiments, often toxic and addicting, must be used in its preparation; otherwise, we would not find it at all interesting.

After your body has detoxified itself of spices and condiments, including table salt, plain raw food will begin to taste much more satisfying. For instance, a piece of celery will taste much saltier than it did when you were eating salt.

Victoria Boutenko was eating 100% raw plant foods when she wrote, "There are thousands of different tastes in natural food" (*12 Steps to Raw Foods*, p. 75).

George Malkmus concurs, "Each of the living foods has its own unique and vivid taste, whereas the dead foods share only three basic tastes: *sweet*, *salt* and *fat*" (*The Hallelujah Diet*, p. 96).

Fresh, unaltered, raw foods offer vastly distinct flavors. As Victoria points out, no two apples taste alike. Biting into one that is especially high in nutrients, and thus flavor, is a delightful surprise. If you eat two different Snickers bars, they will taste alike. You know what to expect. But if you eat two different dates, they may taste perceptibly different.

My friend Marie Tadič, whose testimony appears in Chapter 2, says that people often ask her if she gets bored on the raw diet. She replies, "No, I got bored eating all the same cooked foods all my life. This is totally new!"

In her book *Eating in the Raw*, Carol Alt says that as a cooked food eater and model under pressure to stay thin, she constantly felt deprived. It was only after switching to a raw diet that she was able to indulge in foods formerly forbidden without fear of excess weight gain, foods like raw cheeses, cookies, pies and other desserts. Indeed, a raw diet is anything but boring.

## If we've been eating cooked food throughout history, what's the big deal?

You might wonder what the big deal is if we have been eating cooked food "forever," and most of us are still living to be more than 70 years old.

First, we have been brainwashed into believing that it is "normal" to live no more than 80-100 years. Longevity researchers have come to realize that the potential human lifespan is much longer than that. Researchers such as Dr. Roy Walford have found it to be a minimum of 120 years. Some feel it is longer still. Some intriguing human longevity records are presented in Hilton Hotema's *Man's Higher Consciousness.*

Second, we have been misled into believing that the absence of observable disease symptoms equates to health. This is because doctors study *pathology* rather than *health*. People who have devoted their lives to studying health have found that there is almost no limit to the potential of "super" or "ultra" health to be achieved. One can keep improving by, for example, finding and harnessing more and more of one's innate body/mind potential.

Sometimes people would tell Zephyr, author of *Instinctive Eating: The Lost Knowledge of Optimum Nutrition*, that they felt they were adequately nourished already. The proof was that they were still alive, after all. He would respond that years ago, before his raw instinctive diet, he had a pitifully more limited view of what it is to experience "being alive." In retrospect, virtually all raw fooders characterize their former levels of consciousness as "semi-comatose" or "barely awake." They feel they have left "the living dead" or "sleepwalkers" for a much more awake, aware, alive existence.

We have been brainwashed into believing it is "normal" to get sick periodically and even to have minor health impairments that we can live functional lives with, such as constipation, allergies, acne, headaches, premenstrual syndrome, aches and pains, indigestion and more. We are constantly reminded that half of those who live beyond age 85 will suffer Alzheimer's, and nearly half will have cancer in their lifetimes.

Nearly all of us take for granted that it is our destiny to eventually succumb to a fatal illness before actually dying. We assume that to spend the last 10-20 or even more years of our lives in low-grade or horrible suffering, using up our children's inheritance for health care, is "normal."

*Consider that illness may not be natural.* Consider that it is not what nature intended for us at all, that radiant health is instead the norm and our birthright. Consider that we can live our lives nearly free of exogenous toxins while keeping endogenous toxins to the essential minimum. Certainly the primary sources of toxins we encounter come from that which we put directly into our bodies daily through our mouths and noses.

Third, since the onset of electric cooking gadgets, as well as all the processed, packaged foods we buy, we are eating more cooked foods than ever. Whenever food is canned, packaged, boxed or bottled, it has nearly always been pasteurized, irradiated or heated in some way and then vacuum-sealed in order to preserve its shelf life.

I remember, as a cooked fooder, that I was often too busy to prepare dishes from fresh produce. To save preparation and shopping time, I would fill a cupboard with canned vegetables. Then I would make stir-fry, heating it up with tofu. The next day, I would reheat some leftovers in the microwave. By that time, the food had been cooked *three times*!

We are also cooking at much higher temperatures than in the recent past, which produces a lot of acrylamides and AGEs. (See Chapter 9.) While the techniques of cooking at high temperatures (grilling, frying and baking) have been around a long time, in most societies they were not used so frequently as now. They were reserved for special occasions, such as for entertaining guests and hosting gatherings. Daily cooking, even just a few generations ago, consisted mainly of boiling, steaming and lightly frying. Sixty years ago potato chips were uncommon, as were fast-food restaurants with their french fries.

The current generation eats an estimated 80-95% of its diet cooked. For some, the only raw food consists of the lettuce and tomato on the burger at the fast-food restaurant! When my grandmother was on her deathbed, she craved strawberries. I wonder what this generation of Americans will crave: Pop•Tarts? Twinkies? Big Macs?

Recently gathered statistics reveal that the current generation is horrendously unhealthy. Obesity has escalated to a point that according to statistics from the National Institute of Diabetes and Digestive and Kidney Diseases, as of 2001, 58 million Americans were classified as overweight; 40 million were obese (30% or more over target weights). The Centers for Disease Control and Prevention (CDC) reports that the average American was 24 pounds heavier in 2002 than he was as recently as the 1960s.

Overweight is a major precursor to 80% of Type II diabetes, 70% of heart disease, as well as a major contributing factor in cancer. According to the CDC, obesity is about to surpass tobacco as the leading cause of preventable death.

Furthermore, younger and younger Americans are becoming overweight. Currently 9 million children over the age of six in the USA are obese, while another 15% are borderline and at risk, according to the National Center for Health Statistics. Sixty percent of children ages 5-10 had at least one risk factor for cardiovascular disease according to 2004 data from the Institute of Medicine report "Childhood Obesity, Health in the Balance, 2004." In children as young as eight years old, the increase in Type II diabetes is so high that it can no longer rightfully be called "adult" onset diabetes.

People are getting cancer and even heart disease at younger and younger ages. Sometimes athletes even drop dead in their teens.

Furthermore, the alarming increase in the percentage of adults of childbearing age who are sterile, as high as 30% by some estimates, has some people thinking we may be on our way to extinction. Incidentally, Hallelujah Acres (see Chapter 12) has had great success in reversing sterility conditions with the living food diet in combination with other healthful living practices.

It is well known that wild animals thrive on exclusively raw diets. Yet if you captured a wild animal and fed it a cooked meal, it would not die immediately. It would take years of cooked meals, during which time it would suffer progressive degenerative disease long before actually dying.

This is also the way it happens with humans. The deadly effects of cooked food are insidious, slow to build up, yet cumulative. This means the toxins build up gradually as the body's digestive enzyme-making capacity is depleted slowly over the course of decades. This unnatural, premature, disease-building aging process proceeds so imperceptibly that the cause/effect relationship remains virtually unnoticed.

People tell me, "Oh, I don't care how old I live to be, so I may as well eat what I want." I then reply that this diet is not just about living a long, healthy life, but about adding energy and zest to the present years. It is about avoiding a future of living in a nursing home completely incapacitated, of staying out of a hospital with tubes hooked up to every orifice, of not having crippling arthritis or being a "shut-in" in old-age victim, of not spending one's last years with Alzheimer's. It is about *life*!

According to an article in *The Wall Street Journal* (February 21, 2001), more than half of all women and a third of all men who survive to age 65 are expected to spend time in nursing homes for the remainder of their lives.

The Health Insurance Portability and Accountability Act of 1996 makes it clear that the people, not Medicare or Medicaid, will have to foot the bill for their own nursing homes. How many Americans from the Baby Boom generation will be walking around homeless as a result?

One could die at middle age from a car accident, yet have no regrets about eating properly nonetheless, as her life will have been much richer while it lasted on a raw food diet. People who eat living foods are full of life, vitality, imagination and creativity.

Though it may at first appear so, this diet is not one of great sacrifice; it is one of *abundant life*. It is not a diet of deprivation! For most new raw fooders, cravings for cooked and unnatural foods greatly diminish within a few weeks, returning perhaps for a matter of a few seconds or minutes every day or week the first year. You quickly get to the point where you simply don't want to eat the old way. There is no sacrifice here once you adjust to the new, healthful way of eating. There is only an improved quality of life.

## Can't I just eat cooked foods with vitamin, mineral and enzyme supplements?

Countless people, myself included once, have thought, "Well, I will just supplement with a multivitamin/mineral tablet to compensate for any lost nutrients." But it is not so simple.

For one thing, nutrients from food are much better assimilated and utilized than those from pills. As pointed out in Chapter 10, new vitamins and nutrients continue to be discovered, so the pill may not contain all of them. Supplements are generally dead, lacking the life force of raw food. Micronutrients ingested in supplement form also arrive in unbalanced combinations our biology doesn't handle well. The questions with supplements are always Which ones? and What doses? Nobody knows. In fresh, raw foods, nature has provided nutrients in the proper balance needed for us to digest and utilize.

I personally do not feel that all supplements are worthless, however. As an acupuncturist and herbalist, I have found a number of herbal remedies that provide some nutrients the body uses to heal. However, they would be even more useful if they could be available in fresh, raw form rather than the processed pill form commonly found in jars or the brewed herbal teas used in traditional Oriental medicine.

While a cooked fooder may be better off adding certain supplements, a raw fooder taking no supplements gets much better results than a cooked fooder taking hundreds of dollars of supplements each month.

My husband and I used to be supplement junkies. We should have joined Supplements Anonymous if it had existed. Yet both of us agree that we feel much better now that we are eating raw without about 75% of the supplements we used to take. Raw food simply provides better nutrition than any number of supplements you could ever buy!

Our soils are nonetheless extremely mineral deficient, as discussed in Chapter 17. A steady diet of foods grown in mineral-depleted soils throws everything off, including our enzyme balance. Because of this, even some prominent raw fooders take supplemental enzymes, minerals and mineral-rich super foods.

Recall from Chapter 8 that Dr. Kollath found only raw foods, not vitamin and mineral supplements alone, to provide the complete nourishment his animals needed to be restored to full health.

Furthermore, researchers from the Linus Pauling Institute reported that a raw diet fed to mice had the same anticancer properties as high doses of Vitamin C, indicating that supplementation was not necessary when eating raw. (See Chapter 8.)

Dr. Campbell relates in *The China Study* that his work in the 1982 report (and now book) *Diet, Nutrition and Cancer* led to a huge boom in the supplement industry. He attributes this to the fact that the committee organized the scientific information on diet and cancer by nutrients, with separate chapters for each nutrient.

He now feels this was a mistake. They did not emphasize that the nutrients should be obtained from *whole foods*. He theorizes that all nutritive and nonnutritive elements in a whole food provide nutrients in synergistic combination, that it is misguided scientific reductionism to think that we can obtain proper nutrition merely by adding supplements to our diets.

Of course if you are on a cooked diet, taking enzyme supplements is better than eating cooked food without them, as their active catalytic properties help digest the cooked food. But they do not fully compensate for all of the enzymes, biophotons, phytochemicals and other ingredients of live food, many of which, undoubtedly, have yet to be discovered. I have taken cooked food with literally dozens of enzyme supplements at one meal and still suffered that sluggish, "cooked-food" feeling.

Several raw food authorities, including Aajonus Vonderplanitz, claim that unheated honey is so rich in enzymes that it may assist in the digestion of cooked food. David Wolfe found that raw honey might even be better than enzyme supplements. The problem with taking extra honey instead of enzyme supplements is that if it is overconsumed, it can result in hypoglycemic reactions. Of course unprocessed, unheated honey is less damaging than what you normally find in the store. Truly raw honey is the only kind that retains its active enzymes.

Additionally, consider that supplementation may compensate for some lost food value, but it does not negate the fact that the cooked food contains toxins. So even if you supplement with enzymes to compensate for enzymes lost in cooking, you are still ingesting cooked food toxins. (See Chapter 9.)

Many supplements are inorganic and therefore are poorly utilized by the body, but they can help in cases of severe deficiency. For example, inorganic iodine added to salt helped give thyroids a boost in areas of the country where iodine levels were low. But in order to obtain the ideal amount of iodine, one would have to take doses from *inorganic* sources that would be seriously toxic, or at best, inferior to natural iodine in plant foods.

Jan Dries says, "Only natural food supplements contain substances that are accepted by the cells. All other substances are rejected or lead to pollution of the body" (*The Dries Cancer Diet*, p. 103). He shows that supplements, though correcting one area, may wreak havoc on another area. For example, frequent use of carotene stimulates lung cancer in smokers. Megadoses of Vitamin C in supplement form can negate the positive effects of selenium.

Most supplements also contain binders (glues), fillers (so-called inert ingredients that have no business being in the human body) and sometimes toxic "preservatives" or "natural" flavorings. Great liberty can be taken with the word "natural."

Even the vitamin "nutrients" themselves are often chemically created and don't have the correct geometric configurations of naturally occurring vitamins. Some of these *isomers* are toxic. Nor do they contain all the natural cofactors that occur in whole foods that enable these vitamins and minerals to be optimally utilized by the body. These artificial chemicals may thus be poorly assimilated as well. An additional concern for vegans is that supplements usually contain animal or insect extracts among their unlisted ingredients. For example, gelatin capsules, unless designated as vegetarian, are made from horse hooves.

If you use supplements, try to get them in their active, "living" forms. Take dehydrated, living grasses if you don't have time to grow wheatgrass. If you use hormonal therapy, take bioidentical hormones from plant extracts that your body can recognize, as recommended by Suzanne Somers in her book *The Sexy Years*. But never fool yourself into believing that what you are doing by taking supplements, even in their most natural forms, is as good as obtaining your micronutrients from whole, fresh, raw foods.

## What if I lose too much weight or muscle strength?

People who are naturally thin may fear getting too skinny eating raw diets. What happens with many of them is that they actually reach their ideal weight, putting on some pounds. If this does not happen automatically, they can always eat more fat (avocado, nuts, olives, seeds) or sprouted grains and legumes to reach desired weights while undertaking an exercise program.

Victoria Boutenko found that when people who had become too emaciated on raw food diets began drinking her green smoothies (see Appendix C), their increased hydrochloric acid secretions improved nutrient absorption so much that they reached and maintained healthy weights.

Typically, if someone who does not need to lose weight goes raw, he may lose a few pounds initially but eventually regain it.

As for one's musculature, the fatty tissues marbling its fibers lose fat, leaving leaner, stronger muscles. My husband certainly noticed that. Lou Corona has described this as an increase in "core strength." Although he has not worked out in years, he can do a yogic posture which many heavyweights and athletes cannot: that of sitting down, legs extended in front, hands by the sides, followed by raising the body and legs using only arm strength.

## I've been on the diet awhile, but still haven't lost as much weight as I would like. What can I do?

To lose more weight on a raw diet, you first need to reduce your intake of fatty raw foods: nuts, seeds, avocados, olives, durians and oils.

Second, detoxify more deeply! One of the body's uses of fat is to store toxins to protect the organs from those poisons. If we can release those toxins, the body no longer needs that fat. Many of us have toxins stored since childhood or even birth, such as fluoride from water, toothpaste and antidepressants, as well as mercury from fish, dental fillings and vaccinations. The body adapts to the presence of such toxins by holding onto more fat in which to store them.

I knew a woman who had been eating about 80-100% raw for thirty years, yet she still had an obvious pear shape. I figured it was because she hadn't been 100% raw. Well, one day I saw her, and she had lost 40 pounds. She said she had gotten chelation treatments, and the weight came off in just two weeks without any dietary change!

Since I couldn't afford $9,000 for those treatments, I intensified my detoxification program by taking in more wheatgrass, the sea vegetable chlorella and cilantro, reputed to be a good heavy metal chelator. Fasting is also effective at reducing the body's toxic burden.

Third, make sure you get enough sleep. Studies show that people who don't sleep enough have intensified appetites due to a lack of the hormone *leptin.*

I have also found coconut oil or butter to be extremely helpful in burning fat. Coconut oil contains medium chain fatty acids, or triglycerides (MCTs). Most vegetable oils are composed of long chain triglycerides (LCTs). LCTs are usually stored as fat, while MCTs are burned for energy and increase metabolic rates, leading to weight loss.

One study showing that MCTs help keep weight down is "Overfeeding with medium-chain triglycerides in the rat" (*Metabolism,* 1987). The study points out that the body is less inclined to store fat with MCTs and that eating them is *even better than a low fat diet at decreasing stored fat.*

Farmers have known for years to feed animals LCTs, such as soybean and corn oil, to fatten them up, and to feed them MCTs to trim them down. Now that people are demanding leaner meats, some farmers feed their animals coconut oil to get them trimmer. I try to eat about two or three tablespoons a day.

A minority of raw fooders, especially women, find that there are *pockets of fat* on the hips or waist that remain despite years of eating 100% raw. These stubborn areas can disappear using the protocol outlined in *The Weight Loss Cure "They" Don't Want You to Know About* by consumer advocate Kevin Trudeau.

Finally, in *The Health Seekers' YearBook*, Victoria BidWell offers "The Natural Weight-Loss System in a Nutshell." These 17 points have been edited by Dr. Vetrano. *The Natural Weight-Loss System* first appeared in a 500-page book/course published by T. C. Fry in 1984.

▶ Eat raw food properly combined. (See page 555.)

▶ Eat modest amounts. Do not stuff to abdominal distension and pain. Do not self-medicate with excess raw food. Do not use raw food as an antidepressant or as an escape drug. Ideal foods, being raw and without protoplasmic poisons laced into them, will not give you the "SAD fix" that cooked, salted, condimented and otherwise addictive foods do. Overeating on pure, raw foods can be very disappointing if you are looking to get that "fix" satisfied. Your tastebuds must make a paradigm shift from cooked-SAD to raw-glad!

It should be noted that the term *ideal foods* herein refers to raw foods that are *not* toxic, not protoplasmic poisons. It refers to nontoxic foods in their natural state that have neither been seasoned and condimented nor dressed with poisons. All seasonings, condiments and dressings, therefore, must be raw and natural, neither fermented, salted, heated nor turned into poisons in any way. If mild herbs and spices are used, such as basil and dill, they must not burn to the taste.

Purists are concerned, not just with taste, but with energy conservation to build health. T. C. Fry and Dr. Shelton taught that if a food cannot be touched to the eye or to an open body wound without resulting in a burning sensation, the food item in question should not be taken into the body. This rule of thumb does not hold true for acid fruits, however.

Also, remember that the stomach comfortably holds approximately one quart. Stop at one quart or sooner if your natural sense of satiety is not yet established.

▶ Minimize the more caloric sweet fruits and dried fruits.

▶ Minimize nuts and seeds, 3-4 ounces a day being totally sufficient for most health seekers with mild-to-moderate activity and stress levels. Eat nuts and seeds early in the day. Do not completely eliminate them however!

▶ Emphasize the less caloric vegetables, especially leafy greens and nonstarchy vegetables.

▶ If eating three meals a day, make your breakfast of fruit; and take vegetable plates or salads for lunch and dinner. More fruit means more calories and slower weight loss.

▶ Avoid all snacking whatsoever between meals to establish a habit of self-discipline and to give the digestive system resting periods between meals. If snack you must, do it on nonstarchy vegetables. Dr. Tilden recommended cucumbers, celery and lettuce. T. C. Fry called eating the nonstarchy vegetables "The Zero Calorie Diet," which is made up of foods that require more calories to process them than are in them.

▶ Take the evening meal no later than 6 or 7 PM so that the entire gastrointestinal tract can have a long break from its work and take a rest, revitalize and then use that restored energy for cleansing.

▶ Eat monomeals by selecting one kind of a favorite ideal food for an entire meal. This will help you develop a sense of self-control. A feeling of genuine satiety and emotional satisfaction is readily recognized when monomeals are taken because the health seeker is not tempted to overeat since there is not a displayed variety of delectable foods.

▶ Fast and rest completely for one full 24-hour period a week.

▶ Once a month when complete rest can be taken, fast for one full three-day period.

▶ Instead of whole-food meals, go on a juice diet. For one to ten days, take five cups of fruit and vegetable juices made from lower calorie, ideal foods. Spread the juices throughout the day in eight-ounce servings.

▶ Keep hydrated by drinking pure water as needed. Avoid dehydration.

▶ Dine only if you are in emotional balance. This will avoid stress-related eating and overeating, and it will help develop self-control.

▶ Practice slowing down your eating behaviors. (See "How to Slow Down Your Eating" as described on page 244.)

▶ Exercise regularly. Include stretching, aerobics and weight training to the extent that you are comfortably capable without overstressing yourself and/or causing injury. Emphasize aerobics to increase calorie output. Mini-trampoline exercise can be done aerobically. Aerobic or not, mini-trampoline workouts are especially useful for stimulating the lymphatic system to move out bodily waste.

▶ Become especially familiar with the number of calories in raw foods: a cup of diced celery has far fewer calories than a cup of diced dates! For this purpose, I have prepared a palm-sized calorie reference just for raw fooders, including hygienic purists: *The Fruit and Vegetable Lovers' Calorie Guide.*

Keep in mind that a *calorie* is the amount of heat needed to raise one kilogram of water by one degree centigrade. An excess of 3,500 calories taken in beyond the body's needs lays on one pound of fat. *The Calorie Guide* also has a table of calories burned per minute engaging in everyday activities.

## Can't I just go on a diet of 50-95% raw food?

Sure you can, but studies show that seriously sick people may require 100% raw food diets to fully recover. A number of experts have found that chronic illness calls for nothing less, as this is what best promotes healing. If you are seriously ill, I recommend you obtain guidance from a naturopathic or other holistic doctor, a Natural Hygiene specialist or a healing-center specialist. (See the Resource Guide.)

Most likely your diet will consist exclusively of raw fruits and vegetables during your initial revitalization, detoxification and healing stages, omitting even nuts and seeds in order to build up energy reserves.

On the other hand, some hold that while a serious illness calls for great diligence, discrimination and direction with every morsel of food entering the body, it should not be 100% raw initially. Nutritionist Natalia Rose feels that "cleansing foods can release too much waste matter into the bloodstream and eliminative organs" and that those organs may not be strong enough to keep up with the increased load. A condition of severe autointoxication could result as the toxins cycle through the bloodstream (*The Raw Food Detox Diet*, p. 46). These symptoms could become too uncomfortable for some people to tolerate.

Frankly, my strong suggestion for *relatively* healthy people would be to go 100% raw because that is the surest way for cooked food temptations to disappear. It is also the fastest way to rid the body of toxins accumulated over a lifetime. Once you eat cooked food, your body stops eliminating old debris in order to work on the incoming arrival of the new toxins.

Or you could do as I do at times and go 95% raw, allowing that 5% for special occasions when a loved one makes you a treat that you will politely nibble at or for that favorite food on a special occasion. Just be sure that the definition of "special occasion" doesn't become diluted until it's every day! One woman I know stays 100% raw except for Christmas, her husband's and daughter's birthdays. Because she has set these limits, she is not tempted to let her mind trick her into eating cooked food on other days.

It will be much easier for you not to have to battle the urge to eat favorite cooked and processed "goodies" if you commit to going *radically raw*. Knowing this, I was tempted to leave out advice on how to manage a less than 100% uncooked diet.

However, I also know that many people simply won't go for the 100% raw diet, at least not from the start. People already relatively healthy may not have the necessary motivation to commit to a 100% raw diet. Obviously, it is far better to eat 50% raw than only 5%.

I have counseled people willing to commit only to 50% raw. Even then they delighted in their improved health and newfound energy. The greater your percentage of raw food, the more you are avoiding toxic cooked foods, and the more you are nourishing your body with nutrients found only in raw food.

So, the greater the percentage raw, the better your health will be. You will benefit accordingly — the more raw, the better. Researchers and raw food advocates have found that a diet of 75-85% raw foods calorically is sufficient for reasonable health maintenance. Dr. Gabriel Cousens has found that he cannot get results with anything less than 80% raw food. Rev. George Malkmus, who attributes his cancer recovery to the raw food diet, found that once he became cancer free, he could maintain his health on an 85% raw food diet.

A friend of mine suggested I write a section about "how to cheat" on the raw food diet. I would say that if you are only committed to being say, 90% raw, just don't keep any cooked food items in your house. Save them for special occasions: a baked potato when dining out, steamed vegetables when visiting a friend or other occasional indulgences at parties and potlucks. If you keep "cheat food" in your cupboard, you will easily slip back into a greater percentage of cooked foods.

If you decide to eat only partially raw, it is best to decide beforehand exactly which cooked foods you will allow yourself to eat. For example, if your goal is 90% raw, you could calculate the number of calories you need and pick something each day that you eat cooked. For example, one item could either be steamed vegetables, a baked potato or some stir-fry. But under no circumstances would you consume dairy, junk food, sugary desserts, candy bars, potato chips, baked bread, cooked meat or other very unhealthful foods.

If you select a more ambitious goal, such as 95% raw, you might want to be very precise and only allow for a few of your favorite cooked foods and only seldom when eating or dining out. For example, the first year I went raw, I was committed to staying 95% raw. I figured this way I could have my occasional baked potato, a favorite food, despite its 450 novel chemical byproducts.

I also wanted to have popcorn when going to the movie theater a couple of times a month. I knew that the popcorn at theaters had hidden MSG. So I smuggled in my own dry air popcorn. But I prevented myself from falling back into an all-out cooked food addiction by limiting myself to those two cooked foods: dry air popcorn and potatoes fixed any way, with each consumed but once a week.

The reason I chose those two was that they were my favorite foods, and I could not find any raw counterpart. I was not tempted to eat a baked cake, for example, because I knew I could have my raw cake. It tasted even better. I almost never allowed myself to eat cooked food even while at a party.

Once I ate some cream-cheese icing off a piece of carrot cake and, on a few occasions, croutons or turkey dressing. But the price, with my newly awakened sensitivity, was heavy for eating wheat: a sluggish mind and extremely slowed digestion that included being constipated for a day. In addition, I acquired an intense craving for wheat for several days thereafter due to its physiologically addictive nature. (See Appendix A.)

If you aspire to 99% raw, that does not give you much leeway. In that case, the 1% might consist of occasional irradiated spices showing up in otherwise completely raw dishes at raw food potlucks. Or it could be for when the salad bar looks bleak except for the coleslaw with its pasteurized mayonnaise. It might even be comprised of food you eat that you think is raw, but isn't. So you should never consciously eat anything cooked in that scenario, but don't get fanatically upset if you do so inadvertently.

Also, remember that *even at raw potlucks*, you will invariably end up eating a small percentage of cooked food. You can only avoid this if you become a "raw food cop," drilling every contributor over whether he had checked with his supplier to verify the oil was unpasteurized, the was tahini not heated (which many labeled "raw" are), the fruit was not irradiated, and so on.

There is a big health difference between a 90-95% raw food diet and a 100% raw food diet, so the goal is worthwhile. The difference is much more than 5-10%. This is because on a 100% raw food diet, your body is continually detoxifying old toxins stored in your body for years or decades, and you are continually rejuvenating. The moment you eat cooked food, the detoxification of the old stuff stops because your body will be busy detoxifying the incoming toxins. You may still detoxify some of the old toxins at night to a certain degree, depending on just how energy-conserving your other health habits are. Still, revitalization and detoxification will proceed much more slowly overall than for a 100% raw fooder.

There are many people nonetheless who say that they feel just as good while eating 90% raw as they did when eating 100%, providing the 10% cooked is not processed foods, but rather something much less toxic, such as steamed vegetables.

Another concern is that the 90-95% raw fooder still has one foot in both worlds. This makes it much easier to backslide, especially during holiday seasons. For one thing, unless you border on obsession with calculations, you won't really know exactly what your percentage of cooked foods is. It may become easy to deceive yourself.

Eventually, the partial cooked fooder may encounter the frustrations of "yo-yoing" back and forth between a healthful diet and a cooked food one. Whereas a 100% raw fooder eventually completely loses all desire for dead food, one who is less than 100% will be continually battling cooked food addiction.

Victoria Boutenko has found through years of research that many people who are not 100% raw slide back into cooked food much more easily because cooked food is addictive. For people who use comfort foods as a way to de-stress or suppress their emotions, surely 100% raw is the easiest way to stay on this diet. (See "Is Cooked Food Addictive?" on page 183.)

Raw fooders who remain 100% or very close can go to cooked parties, potlucks and restaurants and have no temptation to eat those foods. They may enjoy some of the aromas, but they don't salivate and don't feel deprived.

# How do you get enough protein?

Initially, obtaining sufficient protein is a great concern for many approaching the raw food diet, especially those embarking on a vegetarian or vegan raw diet. However, it has been shown that the body does not need as much protein as formerly thought. As Dr. T. Colin Campbell says, "The story of protein is part science, part culture and a good dose of mythology" (*The China Study*).

In the late 1800s, the dairy and meat industries in Europe popularized the idea that we needed lots of protein. The average American eats about 60-120 grams of protein per day. It has been proven that we need only 25-45 grams a day and maybe even as little as 15 grams.

Certainly dietary protein is essential, but that does not mean we need excessive amounts of it. The truth is that most Americans eat far too much protein, which leaves them with toxic acidic residues that stress the body, often resulting in numerous diseases.

In an excellent Internet article entitled "Protein — How Much is Right for You?" Dr. Robert Sniadach explains that the heavy amount of protein that Americans eat is hazardous to their health. "The metabolism of proteins consumed in excess of the actual need leaves toxic residues of metabolic waste in tissues, causes autotoxemia, overacidity and nutritional deficiencies, accumulation of uric acid and purines in the tissues, intestinal putrefaction, and contributes to the development of many of our most common and serious diseases, such as arthritis, kidney damage, pyorrhea, schizophrenia, osteoporosis, arteriosclerosis, heart disease and cancer. A high protein diet also causes premature aging and lowers life expectancy."

Dr. Sniadach estimates that we need but 20-40 grams of protein a day. He also points out an article in a 1978 issue of the *Journal of American Medicine* that states that athletes do not need any more protein than nonathletes. It is a myth that protein increases strength. In fact excess protein takes greater energy to digest and metabolize. In his Natural Hygiene course, he explains in detail that the body is actually able to recycle proteins.

Dr. Gabriel Cousens also notes that research on people fasting on water indicates that their serum albumin levels (the amount of protein in their blood) remained constant during fasting despite no protein intake.

The body maintains a pool of amino acids, continually sending some free amino acids or protein complexes to wherever they are needed for tissue repair. This is explained in the classic physiology textbook authored by Dr. Arthur Guyton.

Also, keep in mind that cooked protein is only about 50% assimilated, so you only need on a raw diet half of what you needed on a cooked diet. Not only is the cooked protein less assimilated, but much of it is also denatured or lost in cooking. When you cook protein, you lose half of it in its true, assimilable form, according to research at the Max Planck Institute in Germany.

In his Great Experiment (see page 150), Dr. Szekely invariably found that less food facilitates speedy healing and that 30-40 grams of protein from uncooked and unadulterated foods was as efficient as 60-80 grams from cooked food.

If you are a vegan, you will get enough protein from leafy green vegetables, nuts and seeds. Even fruit is about 1% protein by volume — it has much more, up to 30%, if you go by caloric content. Denser sources of protein include sprouted grains and beans, although those are more energy expensive to digest and should be used only in small amounts, such as a few ounces in one day.

Human mother's milk is only about 5% protein by calories. Keep in mind that this is consumed during the time when the baby is growing most rapidly! I am not saying that 5% is the optimal percentage of protein, but only that one could survive on 5%, if necessary, providing that the digestive tract and trillions of body cells have been cleaned out for optimal absorption and assimilation.

In *Errors in Hygiene?!!?* Dr. Vetrano points out that we should never neglect getting sufficient protein. She has ascertained that one of the chief factors resulting in the early demise of Natural Hygiene leader T. C. Fry, who died prematurely at age 70, lay in his insistence that his diet of nearly all fruit and vegetables would contain sufficient protein. The version of Natural Hygiene that he adopted, which he dedicated 20 years of his life to promoting, was similar to that of hygienic doctor Doug Graham, one that precludes more than minimal consumption of nuts and seeds.

Dr. Vetrano asks all to take heed of "the early symptoms of a low protein diet: listlessness, apathy, slow healing of wounds, edema, skin and hair changes" (*Errors in Hygiene?!!?* p. 253). When people with these symptoms consult her, she advises them to eat nuts and seeds in addition to fruit. The symptoms then disappear, sometimes almost overnight. (See her article "Genuine Fruitarianism" beginning on page 346.)

She also notes that increased stress in one's life increases the amount of protein necessary. Stress also contributed to T. C. Fry's early demise. At a time when his protein needs were increased, he still refused to eat much of it.

In *The China Study*, Dr. Campbell points out that the most efficient (i.e., fastest) way to provide building blocks for our replacement proteins would be to eat not only animal flesh, but *human flesh*. Of course *he is not suggesting that anyone eat actually human flesh but making this absurd comparison simply to prove a point*: the greatest efficiency doesn't always lead to the greatest health. In the case of protein, plant protein shows that "slow and steady wins the race."

In his exhaustive research, he found those depending on plant foods for protein were able to achieve their height and weight potentials, even if it took a bit longer. Yet they remained free of degenerative diseases like cancer and heart disease, which eventually manifest in those who eat cooked meat heavily.

In her book *Green for Life,* Victoria Boutenko mentions that dieticians have lumped greens in with other vegetables in their food charts, so the high protein content of greens has been largely hidden from us. A diet emphasizing raw greens, combined with a regular weight-training routine over a period of weeks and months, is a way to put on quality muscle, since they contain high-quality amino acids freshly photosynthesized by plants as opposed to eating secondhand proteins obtained from meat.

I would like to add here that my husband's biggest fear of eating raw was getting insufficient protein. He is a bodybuilder. He has been nearly 100% raw for close to six years now and realizes that his fear was unfounded. He lost weight initially and then gained most of it back. Although he does not weigh as much as he used to, he is stronger and can actually lift more weight than when he ate cooked food. (See Chapter 2.)

## Won't I miss my comfort foods?

Because we often eat for emotional reasons, you may initially miss some of your favorite "comfort foods." However, as you learn to prepare some of the popular raw food recipes, including rich desserts and gourmet dishes, you will soon realize that raw foods can be equally comforting. Although they may not be what your mother fed you, you will soon find that eating things like delicious, raw, creamy carob mousse will taste just as decadent as chocolate. Even a few medjool dates will usually hit the sweet tooth spot.

Whenever you feel you need a special treat, you can buy a large-size juice from a juice bar. Just make sure they don't add anything like sugar, protein powder or yogurt. Buy that instead of the white chocolate mocha latté from Starbucks. Or treat yourself to an organic melon, which might be too expensive to buy on a daily basis.

Since I became raw over six years ago, the movement has caught on to such a degree that there are now tremendous numbers of raw, gourmet, packaged treats that can be purchased at health food stores or online. These are usually dehydrated and high in fat. They therefore should not be eaten as a dietary staple that replaces fresh, whole produce. But they do make wonderful comfort foods or treats.

Victoria Boutenko nonetheless warns us in her second edition of *12 Steps to Raw Foods* that many of the effects of standard comfort foods are actually from their addictive properties: "Raw foods don't have addictive substances in them and thus cannot 'provide freedom from worry.' "

In other words, we are finding "comfort" from the mind-altering addictive effects of many cooked comfort foods! For example, meat, poultry and fish contain opioid peptides. Dairy and wheat have addictive opioids too. Salt is also very addictive. Even sweet receptors in the mouth are hooked to brain areas that release endogenous opiates. See Appendix A for more information.

The conclusion is that we need to start finding comfort from our internal compass instead of from outside pleasures.

## What about my family? How can I ever get my family to eat my raw food dishes?

At first, when I told my husband I intended to become a raw fooder, he was very much opposed to it. "I will not eat a diet of rabbit food!" he complained. But he had to, by default, because I was the only one willing to do any food preparation.

I made sure the dinners were elaborate and tasty so that I would not be tempted to return to cooked food myself. So of course he also relished the raw gourmet "stir-fry," raw "meatloaf" made of nuts and seeds, raw avocado salad dressing, raw carrot cake and all the other dishes I delighted in experimenting with.

After a few weeks, he grew very excited. "I have so much energy! I am never tired! I feel younger! We need to go all the way with this raw food thing!" Now he is sometimes even more fanatical than I am about staying 100% raw. So, I am convinced it is sometimes easier to inspire people to switch with the taste of the food than with the logic behind the diet.

For those who have teenagers or kids, I recommend the recipe book *Eating without Heating*, written by two teens, Sergei and Valya Boutenko. Of course written by kids, many of the recipes are for cakes, cookies, candies and raw burgers. But these use high quality ingredients: nutritious dates, honey, nuts, seeds and such. More delicious than any junk food, they are also quite valuable to the body.

For preadolescent children, involving them in the process of preparing raw food recipes will engage their interest. This is what Victoria Boutenko did, as her kids were only eight and nine years old when the whole family went raw. She purchased for them their own blender, for example, so that they could make their own smoothies. When their friends visited them, they loved to "play" at making raw food dishes.

Make food a game for the kids. Make it look especially pretty, playful and inviting, such as making a flower out of a tomato. Be creative and decorative, just as you would be with cooked food on special occasions. For example, make a face on an orange, using toothpicks to attach olives as eyes and berries to form a mouth.

If your kids get teased for being "different" because of their diet, invite their friends over for a party, lunch or picnic. They will love the raw goodies too, and your kids will earn new respect. You might even have to watch out for other kids wanting to trade lunches with yours!

Remember to be gentle with your family. Pushing them will not convince them. Think of all the times someone preached to you about something. Did it make you want to do what they insisted you needed to do? Chances are you felt they were trying to control you. Your knowledge and wisdom about raw foods may impress your loved ones, but your living example of superior health and the superior food will especially inspire them. Your partner is an adult and has to make his/her own decision.

As for your children, *you were the one who got them addicted to cooked food*. So, you can also condition them to eat healthfully. But don't expect them to change overnight. Instead, prepare scrumptious goodies that will win them over and gradually substitute "treats" and cooked dishes with raw ones, slowly increasing the number of raw snacks and main dishes.

In her book *I Live on Fruit*, Essie Honiball tells how she maneuvered her husband into fruitarianism without being at all pushy or preachy. She started by serving him fruit with every meal, gradually replacing cooked food with more fruit. When one morning as a test she fed him a former favorite meal of eggs and ham without any fruit, his reaction was, "Do I have to eat this slop? Can't I just have fruit?"

Rhio explains in *Hooked on Raw* that she did the same thing with her boy-friend, serving him his cooked food and also some of her raw gourmet dishes until all he wanted was the raw food.

Tanya Zavasta cautions newly raw women, "Don't give up a good man just because he won't eat grass with you!"

If your family refuses to switch, stick with your own resolve to stay raw. Sooner or later they will catch on. Of course it will not be easy at first if you have to prepare your own food plus the cooked dishes. But it has been done. If you stay 100% raw, the cooked food temptations will gradually dissipate. You might also strike a deal with your family: if they choose cooked food, they must contribute to most, or all, of its preparation, providing they are able.

A word of caution: If you decide to put your children on a 100% raw diet, I would advise against telling others. We live in a society in which miseducated "authorities" tend to interpret this practice as "child abuse." They have a way of believing that veganism is somehow bad, which it can be if kids are not getting sufficient protein, Vitamin $B_{12}$, sunshine (Vitamin D) or other essential nutrients.

If your children are old enough, teach them to be discreet. When the "authorities" came knocking on the Boutenkos' door after hearing reports that the family was on a "weird" diet, the kids, who were home alone at the time, answered the caseworker's query with, "We just got back from Burger King!" After she left, satisfied that they were eating "nutritious" fast food like everyone else, the kids would jokingly refer to drive-in as "Murder King."

As for your extended family and friends, unless they are health seekers, don't overwhelm them. When I first went raw, I was sure that if everyone simply tasted the raw gourmet food, they would switch. I went to visit a friend and spent four days making her delicious raw pizza, soup, "meatloaf," cakes and other goodies. Her remark at the end of my visit? "I could simply never do this. It is too *labor intensive!*"

Years later, however, she did switch to a 90% raw diet on her own, making salads, smoothies and other quick meals.

# Does my pet need to eat raw? If so, how can I get my pet to eat raw food?

Animals in the wild do not suffer degenerative diseases, but those eating table scraps or processed foods — bagged, canned or boxed — do. Such foods have been heated and had inorganic mineral supplements and preservatives added to them. Another reason is that owners wouldn't be able to stomach feeding their beloved pets such perverted food if it weren't disguised by processing.

If your pet is young, it will naturally prefer raw food. If, however, you have gotten the poor creature addicted to cooked food, you will have to transition it back to raw. You cannot reason with it the way you can a human.

There are two possible methods to do this: the gradual way and the fasting method. With the first way, you will gradually mix raw food into its customary chow. For example, you might try 10% raw one week, then 20-30% the next week. Eventually, your pet will be eating 100% raw. You will observe that its energy and vitality will increase. Pustules, avenues for elimination of cooked food toxins, will no longer form. Its excrement will no longer stink! The animal itself will smell healthy and fresh. Indeed, it will experience the superlative health its raw-eating owner does.

Pets need live enzymes too, which is why they eat grass and even the excrement of other animals, which contains digestive enzymes. Often an animal will eat so much grass that it vomits. This may be because it is detoxing too quickly. The same happens to people who drink excessive wheatgrass juice during transition to raw diets.

A quicker way to transition your pet would be to fast it on water for a few days. This is something to consider, especially if it is sick. Even if it is seemingly healthy, fasting will speed up the detoxification from all the cooked food. You will not know how many days the creature needs to fast, and so it is best to put out fresh pieces of raw food for it after a couple days and let the pet decide when to break its fast.

I have a long-time raw food friend who once "cat-sat" for two obese cats. He decided to give them "tough love" and put them on a fast (water only)! They lost weight, and one of them was converted to eating raw meat within three days.

However, when the owner returned from vacation, despite their admittedly healthier appearance, he decided it would be too much trouble to keep buying fresh, raw meat. So, the poor felines were forced to resume their former kibbles diet that had resulted in worms, indigestion and numerous vet visits for one of them. No doubt, they went back to being lazy and fat.

Whenever people or animals revert to cooked food, the change they undergo reminds me of the movie *Awakenings*. Catatonic people were given a brief chance to live again and awaken to the wonders of life with immense awe and delight, but they eventually regressed to their previous, catatonic state.

Bruno Comby points out that animals in the wild, eating natural diets, can remain very healthy despite harboring a virus that would greatly sicken the same animal living on processed foods designed for pets. He explains, "*The animal whose diet has not been changed fares better every time.* Again and again, one finds a kind of peaceful coexistence between the virus and the animal that eats a natural diet" (*Maximize Immunity*, p. 27). He also cites the case of a veterinarian who fed a natural diet to two cats. After four months, there was a complete remission of "feline AIDS" in both cats.

If you are not convinced your pet needs to eat a raw diet, read the animal studies referenced in Chapter 8, especially the one on the cats. I showed this study to a good friend of mine about a year ago. She said it couldn't be true because her cats all ate processed food (which was organic, but still heat treated), and her three cats were all very healthy. A year later when she complained about how sick they were and how much her vet bills were, I reminded her of the study. Now she wants to try the raw diet on her cats!

Another friend of mine spent a great deal of money to get orthodox drug treatment for her cat that came down with leukemia. The cat recovered, and my friend asked, "Now, how can you be so strongly opposed to drug treatment? Look at her! She is playing like a kitten!"

Six months later the cat died of another form of cancer. This happens to humans all the time. Give them chemo or radiation, and one cancer goes away. Then due to the resulting weakened condition of their bodies, another cancer kills them a few months or years later. This doesn't happen on raw food. The body strengthens and regenerates on a raw food diet. People and animals alike, once cured by the body's innate healing mechanisms empowered by natural, raw food, may live out their normal lifespans even after recovering from full-blown cancer.

Tawana Jurek, a woman I met at the 2004 Raw Food Festival in Portland, Oregon, told this touching story of love and recovery after adopting a very sick dog, Pepper, which had also suffered severe burns and injuries from deliberate abuse. Veterinarians said he had a fatal disease. Tawana fasted Pepper and then fed him a 100% raw diet. He recovered completely. Pepper is still very healthy today. His story may be found on www.healthyhealing.org. Unlike most people I have come across who feed their pets raw food, this dog owner was smart enough to get onto a raw diet herself!

One note of caution: Some of the meat you buy at the grocer's has been irradiated. If it comes in hermetically sealed plastic, your suspicions should be aroused. The only way to tell for sure, since its appearance is often unchanged, is to talk with the store manager. You may have to go directly to a butcher to make sure the meat has not been irradiated. If it has been irradiated, it won't have intact enzymes or some of the other important nutrients of raw meat and will contain a new class of toxic compounds called *radiolytic byproducts*.

## Aren't you hungry all the time?

First of all, you need to learn the difference between *genuine hunger* and the *jaded appetite.* (See *The Health Seekers' YearBook*, p. 163.) Genuine hunger is a tingly, insistent mouth/throat sensation, often accompanied by salivation. It is a genuine demand for food, based on physiological need, which most Americans rarely experience. Those with jaded appetites experience "hunger" as one or more pathological symptoms: stomachache, gastric rumblings, fatigue, weakness, trembling, headache and/or "food" cravings, often stimulated by external cues.

Actually, I get hungry less often on a raw diet because my body is being better nourished. On SAD foods, which are designed for stimulation and overeating, I always felt hungry for something, usually sweet or salty, not even knowing what.

Initially after switching to a raw diet, I often needed fat in my diet — nuts, avocados, olives, seeds, coconut butter — because fat stays in the stomach longer than carbohydrates. Now I can have nothing but juice all day and not feel hunger.

When we were cooked fooders, my husband would always crave two big platefuls of whatever we were eating. After we switched to raw, I marveled that one plate was usually enough for him. I figured it would be the opposite, that he would want more of the raw food. But his body was being fully nourished, and so he came to be satisfied with less.

We have been eating raw for six years at the time of this writing and notice that our grocery bills have diminished, despite the use of more organic food and the rising cost of food. Our natural, unperverted, genuine appetites are serving us so well that our need for food has diminished.

This may sound unappealing because we Americans love to eat. But when eating a primarily raw, nonaddictive diet, the desire for food diminishes naturally, leaving no feeling of deprivation.

Famous model Carol Alt explains, "When I was eating cooked food and starving myself to stay thin as a model, I was very literally hungry almost all of the time. I am never hungry now. I eat all the time. I feel great. I have lots of energy. I'm thin now, but not hungry at all" (*Eating in the Raw*, p. 102).

## If this diet is so great and healing, why doesn't my doctor know about it? Why isn't it all over the news?

Medical schools are funded primarily by pharmaceutical companies, which have little interest in teaching future doctors about unprofitable healing methods. (See Appendix B.) Most doctors take only a few (if any) course hours of instruction in nutrition during the entire four years (or more) of medical school. They are taught that diet is not important to health and that drugs and surgeries must be their main tools.

A few doctors have heard about healing on raw food but have been trained by their instructors to think of it as quackery. They ask if there is any research to prove that the raw diet promotes such radical healing.

This is really a catch-22 situation because no one wants to fund the expensive research that would irrefutably prove the advantages of a raw diet. Even organic farming is not a highly profitable industry unless done in high volume. *No one profits from this diet except the person who employs it.*

Physicians have invested their whole adult lives in their methods of pharma-cology and surgery. It can be a radical ego blow to learn they have been on the wrong track, or at least, not on the highest track.

Guy-Claude Burger worked with a medical doctor who had lost his hearing in his left ear and couldn't move or feel anything in two of his fingers. The car-diac nerve that controlled his heartbeat was also seriously affected. After six months on the instinctive raw diet, he was back to normal. Yet Burger felt the doctor was *annoyed* at his recovery because it proved to him that food was more important than medicine!

What most people don't realize is the tremendous pressure medical doctors are under to maintain their status quo protocols. As Rev. George Malkmus says, "They find themselves in a very difficult dilemma because the laws protect them from the adverse side-effects and deaths that occur from the dispensing of drugs and the other accepted medical treatments. But if they prescribe God's Natural Laws and simple health principles to their patients, they can, in some states, lose their license to practice medicine, go to jail and be fined" (*God's Way to Ulti-mate Health*, p. 48).

One friend of mine was lamenting that the people in the raw food movement who get publicity are portrayed as "weird" and "nonmainstream." I told her that even if there were a "Martha Stewart of the raw food movement," she would take time to get widespread, complimentary publicity from the media. Trillions of dol-lars are at stake to keep the masses misinformed. It's really too bad that these major corporations don't channel their energies and money into the highest road for healing the planet. Yet that's the way it is, at least right now.

The raw food movement has always been a grassroots movement and al-ways will be until huge numbers of people around the world go raw. Until then it will never be promoted by mainstream government agencies or the corporate-controlled media. There are too many political and industrial interests involved in keeping people on the SAD that makes all too many people *feel* sad!

As Dr. David Darbro wrote in the foreword to Rev. Malkmus' book *God's Way to Ultimate Health*, "Powerful political and economic forces exist through-out the land which thrive upon the public's health misfortunes. These vested in-terest groups, because of financial reasons, do not wish to see these people freed from disease and pain. They hire expensive lawyers, influence the media, and bitterly oppose those who say there is a better way."

Dieticians and nutritionists also receive their fair share of brainwashing. Food companies, such as the sugar industry, often subsidize university nutrition departments the way drug companies support medical schools. (See Appendices A and B.) Look at the food served to hospital patients! One friend of mine who considered becoming a nutritionist remarked, "I don't want to go to school only to prescribe Jell-O to hospital patients."

As for the news media, newspapers and television have mostly treated the raw food movement as an eccentric fad or oddity rather than the real solution to many of our physical, mental and societal problems that it actually is. This is un-derstandable when you ask who funds the advertisements that ultimately fund the media. TV, newspapers and magazines are largely funded by pharmaceutical corporations, restaurants and processed-food companies through their advertising.

These companies also prepare press releases with "news stories" by "experts" touting the latest drug or processed-food product. Such releases are often shown on the news, actually becoming free commercials for the sponsoring company! This is done mainly because people will believe a seemingly "objective" news story more readily than a paid advertisement.

The most powerful force at present that is helping people find out the truth about how drugs and foods affect our health is the Internet since people can erect web sites at little cost. Big money is not necessary. Before the Net, the only people who really had freedom of speech were those who owned or controlled the mass media and the printing presses. Now the big corporations are even trying to buy out the Internet, our last vestige of free speech. The government is threatening to use "terrorism" as an excuse to censor it!

Personal-care product companies are also major players in the media industry, and of course they would be none too happy if the healing power of the raw diet ever caught on. Who would need drugs? Who would buy Coca-Cola? Who would even need deodorant or mouthwash after a few years of detoxifying?

And because a raw food diet makes one ever more health conscious, many other products would also lose their markets: toxic cleaning products, shampoo or toothpaste with toxic ingredients and so on.

Moreover, after a year or two of eating raw diets, many people no longer care to watch much TV, preferring instead to use that time tending to their gardens, growing their own food, spending quality time with their families, taking hikes in the wilderness, indulging in creative projects or writing books to tell others about the miracles of eating raw food.

The enchantment of cooking is deeply imprinted upon the psyches of everyone everywhere. People don't want to give up their favorite foods. Addiction can be blinding to even the most sincere seekers of health and the fountain of youth. Most people will scoff at the idea of the raw diet's role in healing, even relegate it to quackery rather than give up their potatoes, hamburgers, steaks, pasta, convenience foods, popcorn and the rest.

Finally, the idea that one can heal oneself with natural food sounds rather simplistic. Most people think life is cruel. *We are meant to suffer and fall ill.* Scientists believe they must create the elixir of health in a chemical lab, and the public think they must pay huge sums of money for health care. In her book on her own raw food recovery from cancer, Dr. Nolfi quotes Goethe, "Mankind is annoyed because the truth is so simple."

Don't wait for scientific research to confirm these truths! What good will it do you if scientists' findings finally concur with the research in this book and become mainstream knowledge 15 years from now, but you are six feet under by then?

# Don't you miss eating something warm?

I missed hot food at first. I would eat things straight from the dehydrator just to get the warmth, but I stopped eventually. I was about 95% raw my first year. Sometimes I would eat a baked potato while dining out. Often after a few months, the heat annoyed me, and I would wait for it to cool down to room temperature to eat it.

High heat actually harms the gastric mucus membranes of the mouth, esophagus and stomach. After a few months of eating raw, I found the heat annoying to my tender lips and the tissues of my mouth lining.

We associate warmth of food with comfort, but this association can easily be broken. Just get good and genuinely hungry, and then eat something good and genuinely raw.

# Shouldn't I wait until the summer, or at least spring, to begin eating raw? Won't I be too cold eating raw in the winter?

For psychological reasons, people think they need hot foods to keep them warm in the winter. They think it would be too difficult to eat only raw foods. By such logic, however, one would never eat *hot* foods in the *summer*!

In all fairness, people in transition often do feel chilled. However, these same people may feel that same chilliness even in the summer if they decide to transition during that season.

This feeling of chilliness is part of the healing process, as the body directs the blood, warmth, oxygen and nutrients inward to heal the most vital organs and tissues first, cleansing and rebuilding the body from the inside out. The feeling disappears in time, the length depending on the individual's state of health going in. In my case, it only lasted about a month. It is definitely profound, however, when I fast.

Jan Dries writes, "What is important about the thermodynamic aspect is that it stabilizes the central temperature by activating the capillaries. Both the organs and the tissues receive more blood, larger quantities of oxygen, warmth and nutrition, while the discharge of homotoxins improves. In the beginning, switching over to the diet can lead to chills, but only until the thermoregulation has adjusted itself" (*The Dries Cancer Diet*, p. 184).

Dr. Gabriel Cousens writes that he felt somewhat colder on raw foods until the second or third year, after which he grew comfortably warm and could even go out barefoot in the frost. He also met some raw fooders in Alaska who reported feeling warmer in the cold Alaskan winters after being on a raw diet for some time.

Victoria Boutenko wrote about this topic and explained that a hot meal, cup of coffee or even a shot of ice-cold vodka "warms up the body" a bit via the same mechanism as cooked food does. They all contain toxins that the body tries to violently expel, if it has the reserve capacity to do so, by enlisting the adrenals to pump out epinephrine, norepinephrine and a variety of steroid hormones. Boutenko explains this:

> These hormones stimulate our sympathetic nervous system, which is why we feel awake at first. They also force our heart to beat faster and to pump larger amounts of blood through our body, which makes us feel warm. This feeling doesn't last long, and we pay a high price for it. After 10-15 minutes, our body gets exhausted from performing extra work.

She further explains that over the long haul, the weakened adrenals leave you feeling colder, which is why older people have to wear sweaters even in the summer. By allowing the body to heal itself via raw diet, you gradually regain the extreme cold tolerance of your youth. *You should actually eat raw to feel warm!*

Eighty percent of all blood in the body is moving through the capillaries, only 20% through the arteries. If the arteries are clogged by cooked food remnants, the blood doesn't circulate efficiently. If the blood is cleansed by means of a 100% raw diet, circulation increases, along with tolerance to cold weather. Boutenko writes further that her raw family jumps into ice-cold mountain rivers year round, sleeps outside under a gazebo in the rain or snow. Her son even goes snowboarding wearing only shorts.

In *Fruit: The Food and Medicine for Man*, the author Morris Krok quoted one Dr. Barbara Moore as follows, "I have found that neither energy nor heat of the body comes from food."

She went on to relate that she spent three months in the mountains of Switzerland and Italy, eating nothing but snow and water, yet walking 15 miles to the foot of the mountain and climbing to at least seven or eight thousand feet. Then she would come down and walk another 20 miles to her hotel. She did this year after year, but found that she could not do this in civilization because the air was not pure enough.

Additionally, Iranian American Arshavir Ter Hovannessian, author of *Raw Eating*, regularly slept outdoors without feeling too cold.

People eating all-raw also report being able to tolerate heat and humidity better. In general, a raw diet enables one to better tolerate both temperature extremes. This is why we never see wild animals needing additional blankets or air conditioners.

Acupuncturists I know will think I am a heretic for preaching a raw food diet since Chinese medicine advocates the macrobiotic diet, a diet of whole foods, most of which are cooked, especially when a patient has what is termed a "cold" condition.

My former partner in an acupuncture business asked me in fact how I could promote a diet that went against the ancient Chinese tradition. I pointed out what one of our teachers once said. He had asked a Chinese acupuncturist master why they had the liver pulse on the left hand when the liver organ is located on the right side of the body. "We were wrong," was the humble reply of the Chinese master.

If they were wrong about that, then they could also be wrong about their diet. It is not just the Chinese; virtually every culture has been entrenched in cooked food culinary arts for tens of thousands of years.

Nutritionist, author and raw food chef Brigitte Mars has a lot to say on the topic. She studied Chinese herbalism under Michael Tierra and Bob Flaws, two of the American masters in the field. When she went raw several decades ago, they warned her about eating cold food in a cold climate, and so she switched back to cooked food.

Decades later her daughter went raw. At first, Brigitte felt a need to rescue her daughter from this "error." Then she began to wonder, "If the diet in the health food stores is so great, why are there so many supplements for sale there? And if the Chinese diet is so great, why do they need so many herbs?"

So she again took up the raw diet and noticed that she actually began to feel *less cold* than usual because her circulation had improved. She now declares, "Raw food is the perfect marriage between yin and yang." She explains this is because *yin* represents (among other things) the fluids, and *yang* represents (among other things) the life force and energy. Cooking destroys both of these in the food.

Joe Alexander has some interesting comments about people who use climate to delay their journey to raw diets (*Blatant Raw Foodist Propaganda!* pp. 116–117):

I have met many people who say that they would like to live on raw food if they lived in a warm climate, but it is too cold where they live. When I lived in Canada, I met such people. Then in Northern California, where there is hardly any winter at all, compared to Canada, I met people who said it was too cold there to be a raw fooder. Now here in Arkansas, which, to me, coming from Canada, is like a tropical jungle, I still meet people who say it is too cold here to be a raw fooder. And when I have visited the area around Austin, Texas, which is so far south that I was able to stand outside all day painting a landscape between Christmas and New Years, I still met people who said it was too cold there to be a raw fooder, which makes me wonder where these people think it is warm enough to be a raw fooder — the center of the sun maybe?

I have never had problems being a raw food eater in cold weather. In fact it helps me stand cold weather better. As a cooked food eater, my hands and lips used to crack and bleed when it got cold. That doesn't happen when I stay on raw food. And I have more energy to run around and be active to generate body heat. There are millions of wild animals living in Canada. Every one of them is a 100% raw food eater. So what makes people think they are special and need cooked food? Eating raw food doesn't mean you have to eat it ice cold from the refrigerator. You can warm it up to room temperature or body temperature. Anthropologists have apparently discovered that cooking began in northern Europe, where people would put frozen foods over a fire to thaw them out. Fine. Then they got careless and left them over the fire too long, and that's when our troubles began.

Conversely, raw food diet helps me to stand extremely hot weather better, too.

All that having been said, I can suggest ways to cope with the winter cold better during and after transition to raw eating. When indoors, add more clothing layers or blankets, turn up the thermostat, take your food out of the refrigerator a couple hours before you eat it to let it warm up to room temperature, and exercise until you sweat whenever you still feel cold.

If you are already in good health and not deep into pathology, spend some time daily outdoors running, jogging, or walking briskly. The heat generated during exercise will warm your body. Prepare for the cold season by exercising outside in the fall long enough each day to work up a sweat, wearing as little as possible to permit your bare skin to adjust to colder temperatures. You will be surprised at the difference this makes.

Finally, try ending your day with a relaxing, warm bath. Your body will accommodate you by becoming hardy!

## Why does cooked food seem to taste better?

The short answer is addiction. Cooked food does *not* taste as good as raw food once you have successfully transitioned to a 100% raw diet. However, at first, during the first few months or even the first year, there may be some cooked foods you miss or even give in to the temptation to eat. But if you allow your tastebuds time to adjust, you will eventually come to prefer raw food over cooked.

For example, I used to love a spicy, baked carrot cake. But once I tried the raw carrot cake recipe in Juliano's *Raw: The Uncook Book*, I was delighted with it. People get so excited when they find a baked cake that is moist. Baking dehydrates nearly all of the moisture from a cake. But a raw cake is always very moist. There is no comparison!

Cooked food is caramelized from the interaction of heated sugars and amino acids. Even though these are toxic, mutagenic substances, they taste good to jaded appetites.

Cooking also releases very strong aromas, making the food smell stronger. Much of what we think is taste is actually smell. As we have observed with instinctive eaters, our instincts associate an alluring smell with the desire to eat. Instinctively, we associate strong-smelling food with its nutritional value. Cooked foods have much stronger aromas because the heat disperses food molecules into the air. So the smell of cooked food deceives us. However, I suspect that as the heat disperses aromas into the air, much of the flavor is also being dispersed. Arnold Ehret expressed the opinion that cooking sends the most vital nutrients out of the food and into the atmosphere!

Cooked, processed foods nearly always contain additives and flavor enhancers, many being unsafe excitotoxins like MSG and aspartame, as explained in Appendix A. Food companies add these to their foods to make them addictive and thus more profitable.

Dairy, wheat and sugar are put into nearly all processed foods for their subtle, sometimes not so subtle, addictive qualities. Unfortunately, after decades of eating food strongly overwhelmed with condiments, spices, additives and artificial flavorings, our overstimulated tastebuds can barely discern the delicate natural flavors of raw foods.

The main reasons cooked food tastes good are that we have been physiologically addicted and psychologically conditioned to prefer it. If you take a baby and wean her from mother's milk with cooked, processed, commercialized baby food as most mothers do, chances are she will instinctively spit out the food repeatedly. If forced to eat dead food, she will likely cry. Only after repeated attempts at rejection will she give in.

Instinctively, she knows it is not good, doesn't taste good and isn't good for her. She may cry, get rashes and fall ill, but eventually her body gives up struggling against the forced feeding and attempts to adjust to it. It's "eat this awful stuff my mother is forcing on me or starve."

Those feeding their babies a 100% raw food diet have observed that they go through none of these stages and in fact avoid all the childhood illnesses thought to be "normal," such as rashes, earaches, fevers, frequent colds and the like, even named textbook diseases like mumps, chicken pox and measles. Vaccinations are also not needed.

Cooked food is addictive and disturbs our normal instincts. As Guy-Claude Burger says, after one has been eating "initial foods" and then eats a bit of cooked food, one is soon "completely taken over by cooking. Cooked foods jam the instincts, overload the body and make initial foods quickly lose their appeal; one compensates by adding more cooked foods, and it soon turns into a vicious cycle." He reports that the pleasure of raw, whole foods is much more complete and intense than that of cooked foods, but not at first. It takes time and occurs only after not having eaten cooked food for some time.

Finally, eating hot foods literally burns the tissue surfaces that house the microscopic tastebuds! When you stop destroying these tissues, they will regenerate. The tastebuds will then be able to sense a wider variety of natural flavors. In time, cooked food will not taste better than raw or even as good.

## Doesn't cooking result in better digestion and allow for better absorption of certain nutrients?

Once you are accustomed to the raw diet, you will find uncooked food is easiest to digest. After all, raw, living food has food enzymes within it to assist in its own digestion, whereas cooked food pulls much more from your body's limited ability to produce these enzymes. This is why you feel fatigued after a cooked meal, but light after a raw one.

People mistakenly think that raw food is hard to digest because they may have some initial difficulty. The truth is that their "digestive fire" has been weakened by so many decades of eating cooked food. Thus novice raw fooders may experience some gas or stomachache. Or they may experience diarrhea. This is a sign that their bodies are detoxifying — which is good!

People who begin raw diets in their forties or older often would do well to eat their vegetables in raw, blended soups or juiced, making them easier to digest. With time, their digestive systems will strengthen, and they can eat more raw vegetables. (See the Roseburg Study on page 167.)

Even experienced raw fooders may have to limit their intake of raw vegetables that are difficult to digest, such as broccoli or cabbage. Some people do not consider raw vegetables an "original food" but believe we started eating them only since 10,000-20,000 years ago when agriculture began. Vegetables contain a lot of humanly indigestible cellulose fiber, which is not always easy to pass through your digestive system, unless you are a cow. Processing high amounts fiber may initially cause stomach bloating, especially for people who have digestive problems.

Yes, cooking will make it easier to absorb certain nutrients from broccoli and cabbage, but it also destroys most of the other nutrients and creates toxic byproducts. It is better to avoid certain vegetables entirely, getting nutrients from fruit and other raw foods, than to eat them cooked! Better yet, just juice them!

Media reporters always have to show a downside in order to display their "objectivity." In nearly every newspaper or magazine article I have read about the raw food movement, the authors use as an example that cooked tomatoes allow for more lycopene absorption. But what about the Vitamin C and other nutrients destroyed in the cooked tomato? What about the toxins that go along with the cooked tomato? What about the toxins that are created while cooking the tomato and turning it into a salted, spicy paste used to flavor other toxic foods like cooked meat and french fries?

The reduced lycopene concentration in raw tomatoes does not warrant cooking, especially since there are many ways to get sufficient lycopene, such as eating watermelon or strawberries. According to Dr. Atkins, *blending* the raw tomatoes releases the lycopene just as well as *heating* them anyhow.

Another example sometimes cited to indicate the superiority of cooked food is that cooking a carrot softens the tough cellulose cell wall, thus enabling more absorption of beta-carotene. Yet cooking the carrot denatures or destroys other nutrients, such as Vitamin C, and completely kills all the enzymes.

One solution to this pseudo-problem is to liquefy the carrot in a heavy-duty blender, which breaks down the bulk of the cellulose cell walls without destroying nutrients.

Another criticism of raw food is that cooking starches converts them to sugars that are easier to digest. While this is true, vitamins, minerals and enzymes are destroyed and toxic byproducts produced, as discussed in Chapter 9. Besides, given the obesity rampant in many "civilized" countries, maybe some of the calories in these starchy foods are best left undigested and unassimilated. Many raw fooders believe that starchy foods, such as beans, rice and many grains, are simply not our genetically ideal foods to begin with and better left to the birds!

George Meinig writes, "There is a common misconception that cooking makes food more digestible. While this is true in a few isolated instances, on the whole it is utterly false. Cooking or heating often makes a bad food safe to eat, but it never makes it a better food."

He goes on to suggest taking the following test: Eat some cooked corn and notice the undigested corn kernels in your stools. Then eat the corn fresh from the cob without cooking it. This time you will not see as much undigested corn. Go to www.price-pottenger.org/articles/rawfoods.htm for his article.

## I have bowel problems. Can I do this diet?

People who have irritable bowel syndrome should be very careful to eat monomeals or very carefully combined foods. (See Chapter 17.) Blending foods is very helpful: raw smoothies or soups. According to nutritionist Natalia Rose, steamed vegetables, raw vegetable soups, avocados, young coconuts and fish are easiest to digest initially. Fruit may inspire the body to detox at an uncomfortable rate initially.

With Crohn's disease or diverticulosis, food — especially nuts and seeds — should also be well powdered or blended, making it easier to digest. Avoid whole nuts or seeds. Fruit in moderation is usually well tolerated.

Recommended books on this topic are *Healing Inflammatory Bowel Disease* by Paul Nison and *Self Healing Colitis & Crohn's* by David Klein, both of whom healed themselves of bowel disease on the live food diet.

## What if I just *have to* eat some cooked foods? Which ones are the least bad?

If you find yourself in a situation in which you must eat cooked food, then quick wok cooking in water, not oil, and brief steaming are preferred. Much of the insides of those foods will still contain active enzymes and other intact nutrients. Boiling would be acceptable too, but some of the nutrients would end up in the cooking water. Drinking this water is not recommended. By the time nutrients have left the food and have been boiled into the water, much of their nutritional value is lost, with toxic compounds created.

Food cooked at very high temperatures, prepared by deep-frying, barbecuing, pressure cooking, grilling and baking, is best avoided. The resulting advanced glycation end products are very toxic.

Probably the worst form of cooking is microwaving, which severely deranges food molecules, creating a toxic mess! Dr. Hans Hertel of Switzerland carried out a small, but well-controlled, study on the effects of eating microwaved food and was fired from his job as a food scientist because of it.

He learned from his experiment that microwaved food causes abnormal changes in human blood and the defense mechanisms. Additionally, microwave appliance leakage, which often goes undetected, can lead to skin cancer, birth defects, cataracts, dizziness, headaches and blood disorders.

If you must eat cooked foods, try to eliminate the very worst ones, such as dairy, wheat, processed foods, cooked meat and table salt. (See Appendix A.)

Try to eat only one cooked food per meal. That would mean, for example, cooked eggs but no cooked cheese mixed in. Eating simply like this will aid digestion. Always have a salad with the meal, along with enzyme supplements or unheated honey, which is rich in enzymes. If you choose to have only one cooked item per day, eat it in the evening so you can still feel light and energetic throughout the day.

Finally, carry enzyme supplements with you so you can take a dozen or so before eating any cooked food. Honey may be even richer in useful enzymes, so carry a small container of unheated honey to restaurants or parties.

## If raw food isn't available, isn't it better to eat cooked food than to eat no food?

Guy-Claude Burger ran an experiment with some field mice. One group was fattened up with cooked food. The other was lean, having been fed only raw food. Then he enforced a "famine," fasting them on water for some time. One might think that the cooked food eaters, having more body fat to live on, would have withstood the famine better.

However, when eating was resumed, the cooked eaters didn't fare as well. Some even died, whereas none of the raw eaters died. His conclusion was that the stored fats from cooked food are toxic, which make the cooked eaters lose any advantage those fats may provide during a famine.

Of course in a prolonged famine in which one is faced with death from months of starvation, it might be wise to compromise on a 100% raw diet if given the chance to eat cooked food. Hopefully, few of us will ever face such drastic situations.

From a raw food chat room, I did hear of a 100% raw woman imprisoned unjustly for being a whistleblower. She chose to fast (water only) rather than eat the prison food! She managed to get released on bail before having to eat anything cooked.

I also know of long-term raw fooders who find it much more appealing to fast a few days when there is no raw food around.

## Isn't there a danger of bacteria in raw food?

Raw food is not dangerous. Bacteria, such as salmonella, are present in small quantities in all foods. As explained in Chapter 5, bacteria and other microscopic "critters" are only dangerous to a body with weakened defenses — a toxic body ecology. If bacteria were so dangerous as we have been brainwashed to believe, why aren't all the wild animals dropping dead from bacterial infections? They have no stoves and no means of sterilizing their food.

Humans, on the other hand, eat very little raw food and have lost much of their natural resistance to bacteria. Their defense systems are weakened. The whole obsession with the "war on germs" has led to a very weakened population. We actually need to replenish ourselves with good bacteria by eating raw food!

You may become temporarily ill from raw food bacteria if you have compromised defenses from having eaten too few raw foods or having destroyed too many friendly bacteria with excessive antibiotics.

You can also be harmed by consuming foods containing far too many bacteria of the wrong types. Such food would smell rancid and might even look spoiled and partially decomposed.

Bacteria are in you and all around you. Physiologists tell us that every square inch of our bodies are homes for about 100,000 tiny living critters! There is no way to get rid of bacteria unless, as Aajonus Vonderplanitz says, you cook yourself to death!

All the evidence to date points to the fact that humans and other animals have adapted to bacteria and other microorganisms through millions of years of cohabitation with them. But we have not adapted to the thousands of years of cooked food. The foreign molecules created in heating food are dangerous to us.

However, raw animal foods — such as meat, dairy and eggs — have the potential to contain *much* more pathogenic bacteria than raw plant food. (See Appendix C.)

## Does this diet cost more money?

Initially, after you switch to organic produce, you may become alarmed at the amount of money you are spending. (Review Chapter 17 for a list of reasons to eat only organic.) Yet you will spend far less eating *in* organically than eating *out*. You will save a lot by not buying meat. You will also save the cost of buying processed, prepared foods. After a few years of eating a raw diet, you will need to eat far less. Review "Economy" on page 17 for more information. But in general, good, raw, organic food *is* more expensive than junky, processed, dead food made mostly out of grains, processed fats, refined sugars and artificial chemicals.

Rev. Malkmus offers us this test to determine if it's cost-effective to buy organic: Calculate the money you spend and the quantity of food you eat. Then switch to an organic raw vegan diet and make the same calculations for the same time period. Log how much you spend, how much you eat and how you feel before, during and especially *after* eating. See if it is worth it in terms, not only of money, but also of health to eat a raw organic diet (*The Hallelujah Diet*, p. 158).

Victoria Boutenko offers tips that her family has used to cut corners on produce expenses: arrive at farmers' markets just before closing to get the best deals; offer help to organic farmers in exchange for produce; learn from local experts which wild plants can be safely foraged; offer farmers $20 for a large box of edible weeds they would normally throw out.

Victoria BidWell offers these additional ideas that she constantly uses to save money on raw foods:

- Grow your own sprouts. They very least expensive, most nutritious food you can possibly find.
- Ask owners of fruit-bearing trees if you can glean their unharvested fruit.

- Pick berries and other foods in the wild.
- Befriend local fruit-stand owners, and take home free boxes of perfectly good food but rejected because of cosmetic imperfections.

Even if you find yourself spending more than you did before, your body is worth it. You wouldn't put junk in your gas tank. Your body is the only vehicle your consciousness or soul has in this lifetime.

# Can I drink alcohol?

Of course alcohol is a protoplasmic poison, toxic to every cell in the body, but with an affinity for killing brain and liver cells. If you must "enjoy" an occasional drink, choose organic wine. Wine is fermented and has enzymes to help digest at least the nonalcoholic part of it. Nonorganic wine is full of toxic sulfites, which may disturb your sleep and give you a hangover.

Be aware that you will not be able to handle as much alcohol as you used to. It will go through you faster since your body is more efficient at detoxifying. It also may interfere with your sleep, especially if you eat food along with it.

Guy-Claude Burger says, "There are better things than that [wine]. Fermented coconut milk, for instance — it's light, sweet, pungent and pleasantly alcoholic. It tastes better than champagne when instincts like it."

I also have found that a bit of kombucha tea, a raw drink of fermented mushrooms, satisfies my desire for a drink. There is just a tiny bit of alcohol in it.

One thing to consider about drinking alcohol: If you drink enough of it to impair your judgment, you may lose your will to resist cooked food.

Victoria Boutenko reminded us in a lecture that no matter how much money we pay for that organic wine, alcohol is the one "food" item highest in acidity!

# Can I drink tea or coffee?

Some raw fooders are not ready to give up other addictions, such as cigarettes or coffee. Joe Alexander said that even as a raw fooder, he was addicted to coffee until he got an ulcer from it. He defends the use of hot drinks, including vegetable broth from boiled vegetables, saying, "My experience is that drinks consisting almost entirely of boiled water don't spoil the raw food high" (*Blatant Raw Foodist Propaganda!* p. 117).

Many report that these desires for coffee and tea fade away on their own. As your body becomes more pure, even one cup of coffee a day can feel very toxic and acidic. Some raw fooders enjoy a cup of green tea, although drinking caffeine is less than ideal. Others enjoy herbal tea. Some wean themselves from coffee and tea but drink warm water with lemon, which is quite pleasing.

According to Frédéric Patenaude, "Anything liquid is better than anything solid, as far as cooked food is concerned, and with few exceptions. Solid food has to be turned into a liquid for your body to absorb it. . . . Tea, while not viewed as a 'living' food, is nothing more than herbal flavoring steeped in warm water" (*The Sunfood Cuisine*, p. 220).

Personally, I have found the psychological addiction to a hot drink (especially containing caffeine) much harder to give up than cooked food. When I went raw, I gave up coffee and switched to the milder organic green tea for my morning brew. Later I had to wean myself off green tea after learning that both green and black teas contain high concentrations of fluoride, which has been linked to osteoarthritis and hypothyroidism, along with other maladies. Since making this discovery, I sometimes have yerba maté. I also occasionally indulge in a cup of coffee, half decaf.

I enjoy occasional herbal tea as well but find that I can no longer tolerate those with "spices" or "natural flavorings" in them. I get a reaction like the one I get after accidentally ingesting MSG, which is often hidden in the most innocuous-sounding ingredients.

Be sure to drink your hot brew plain or sweetened with unheated honey — after the drink cools a bit — or stevia. If available, use raw milk or cream instead of pasteurized. Better yet, use nut milk.

The goal for the purist should nonetheless be to eventually wean oneself off hot drinks. According to a study in the British medical journal *Lancet*, hot beverages and food irritate the throat and tongue and are associated with increased throat and tongue cancers (*Lancet*, Dec 1973, p. 1503). According to the author, Dr. McCluskey, we should dip our little finger in the hot drink for ten seconds and drink only if the finger is not scalded. Another *Lancet* study, cited in *Life in the 21st Century*, associates drinking hot beverages with gastric enzymatic abnormalities.

Be aware that coffee, even decaffeinated, and tea are also very acidic, stimulating the body to produce mucus as the vehicle for expelling these poisons. This is the biggest price to pay. If I indulge in an occasional cup of brew, I feel the adverse effects within an hour and sometimes immediately.

Another big price to pay by drinking hot drinks is that your tastebuds may suffer burn damage in addition to the desensitization they suffer with other cooked foods, so you never really get to experience the full flavor of food that a strict raw fooder does.

A final word about hot drinks that contain caffeine: Caffeine is a potent addictive substance. Most people are unaware of just how bad it is. Stephen Cherniske explains in his book *Caffeine Blues* that this seemingly innocent drink contributes to a very unhealthy condition within the body.

The body resists the presence of caffeine by producing one or more of the following symptoms: energy swings, fatigue, depression, headaches, diarrhea, tension in the neck, PMS, fibrocystic breast disease, insomnia, anxiety, tooth grinding, irritability, irregular and accelerated heartbeat, ulcers, memory loss, ringing in the ears, panic attacks, osteoporosis and anemia.

Caffeine ingestion also results in high blood pressure. In fact I know someone who used a lot of coffee to pump up his blood pressure so he would fail the medical test after being drafted to Viet Nam: it worked!

Caffeine addiction can even lead to heart attacks. Blood levels of cortisol increase, which lowers levels of the hormone DHEA, thereby accelerating aging. Because the body reacts with increased cortisol production, the progression of AIDS becomes accelerated.

Caffeine ingestion causes the body to expend precious energy either to expel the poison or to store it. Either way, caffeine ingestion "robs energy." It is a huge factor in caffeine users' complaints of fatigue, poor sleep patterns, exhausted adrenals and blood sugar abnormalities. Thus it is perhaps the main cause of chronic fatigue rampant in America.

Think about that the next time you pass by a Starbucks!

## Can I eat frozen foods?

Freezing destroys 30-60% of the enzymes in fruits, so eating them frozen is not really ideal. However, during the transition period, a frozen banana can satisfy the urge for ice cream. It tastes wonderful in a smoothie.

The enzymes in frozen foods low in water content, such as nuts and seeds, are more resistant to destruction. Thus it is not so bad to freeze them as it is fruit. Nuts and seeds contain almost no water.

Unlike most other chemical compounds that contract when they freeze, water expands as it forms ice. The tiny ice crystals in all cells that contain water are like little bombs going off inside the food. These destroy enzymes, vitamins and all sorts of other molecules. That's why nuts, seeds and dehydrated foods are not much damaged by freezing. Their enzymes remain largely intact. If you freeze a sunflower seed, it will still sprout later. Try it!

If you want to maximize the nutrients in frozen fruit, dehydrate it first. Of course doing so will cause it to lose that creamy texture reminiscent of ice cream.

## What do *you* eat?

It always seems so funny when, after I tell someone I am a raw fooder, her face scrunches up in bewilderment and she asks, *"What do you eat?!"*

This makes me laugh because we have gotten so far from natural food that most people cannot even imagine going without processed, refined or cooked food.

So I answer with whatever happens to be my routine at the time. But in the years spent researching and writing this book, I have had to revise this section three or four times because I keep changing my eating habits, fine tuning them.

This is what I wrote a few years ago:

> Usually I have fruit with nuts for breakfast. Later I had heard that this was "bad food combining," so decided to just have fruit. But then I found I got very hungry soon after. So I went back to the raw trail mix idea of fruit and nuts.
>
> In proper food combination, fruit should be eaten alone or 20-30 minutes before another food, but if the fruit is dehydrated, it seems to work okay. The nuts slow down the fruit's digestion so that I don't get hypoglycemic reactions. The fat

in the nuts stays in my stomach for hours, and so I don't get hungry. It works out fine. Just be sure to floss after eating dehydrated fruit, as it can get stuck in the teeth, feeding the bacteria that build plaque.

For a snack I have 10-20 raw olives or maybe more fruit.

For lunch I have a salad. At first, I used to make elaborate raw salad dressings. After a few months, I got tired of that and simplified things by just having a mixed green salad with a cucumber and avocado. The fat in the avocado kept me full until I got home for my mid-afternoon snack.

For my late snack I may have a smoothie. Or I may have flaxseed crackers with nut butter. Sometimes I put honey on them, and it tastes like the peanut-butter-and-honey sandwich that my mother used to make.

For dinner I will have a raw food recipe dish. Often I will make a simple dish or eat leftovers from the day before. Sometimes, however, I will not be in the mood to plan or prepare a meal for days or even weeks. In that case, I will just munch on more olives, nuts, fruits or vegetables.

Now for my updated version: Like so many raw fooders, I have found that I require and crave much less fat than when I initially switched to raw. I have found that I can get through a stressful workday with relative ease if I eat almost no fat until dinner.

For breakfast, I usually have a green smoothie with dehydrated wheat grass (available at www.livefoodfactor.com), fresh-squeezed orange juice, a table-spoon of raw coconut butter and a tablespoon of unhulled sesame seeds (for calcium).

For lunch, I will have a salad with minimal or no dressing or other fat. Sometimes I will put a few olives or soaked and dehydrated sunflower seeds in it to spark up the taste.

For dinner, I will have raw soup or whatever leftover gourmet dishes I have around from the weekend. I sometimes go out to eat, now that more places serve raw entrées.

I used to eat popcorn at movies. My first year of raw food, I was only 90-95% raw. I smuggled in some dry air popcorn, as the theaters sell only popcorn loaded with MSG, heated oils and salt. Later it seemed too bland. I realized it was just the habit of eating little bits of food while in a movie that mattered to me. So now I smuggle in cherry tomatoes, olives, flax crackers, sprouts, baby carrots or even a bag of raw, organic greens!

My diet is slowly becoming more simplified. It is always evolving. Currently, I prepare or eat the fancy gourmet dishes only when I have guests or attend a potluck. I enjoy the time saved by not fixing food and therefore have time for other activities, such as writing this book!

A lot of times, I just relish an avocado or a couple of pieces of produce. This might not sound exciting to you if you are at all new to the raw diet, but this snack combination tastes great. Furthermore, as I become healthier, less and less of my excitement in life depends on food.

Shortly before going to press with the first edition of this book, I read Victoria Boutenko's *Green for Life* and began experimenting with green smoothies every day. By the time I drink one, there isn't much room for anything else. I have enjoyed much more alkalinity, weight loss and a feeling of well-being. I plan to make this a mainstay of my diet.

## Why should I go on a raw diet if I am young and healthy?

Many people think they are quite healthy already and thus do not need a raw food diet. Some people I counsel say that they will wait until they are older. This is especially true with young people, whose energy is already high and not drained from decades of toxic living and whose enzyme-producing capacity is also high. The young still produce so many hormones and enzymes that even though they eat a diet of 90% cooked food, they maintain a surplus of energy.

But I always tell them, *"If you feel great now, just think of how much better you would feel on a raw diet!"* and, "You are only 20-something now. What if you could look and feel the same, or only slightly older, when you are in your 50s?" And, "Just think of the edge you'll have at work!"

Indeed, I marvel at what I might have accomplished in life had I learned about this diet several decades ago!

One's life goals on a raw diet typically change for the better. One gets in closer touch with her true nature. Mental or emotional problems get solved that otherwise wouldn't. This is an especially important factor for young people who are struggling to find meaning in their lives and who deserve to live out their grandest dreams and fulfill their greatest callings.

If you want to *remain* young and healthy, this is the secret. I surely wish I had discovered this secret when I was in my twenties or even younger! This diet is not only a factor in preventing disease, but also in slowing down the aging process and facilitating rejuvenation. I have *seen* people who are in their 50s who started this diet in their 20s, so I *know* this fountain of youth secret is for real.

Moreover, there are higher levels of health to be attained, as mentioned in Chapter 1. It is truly an adventure to see how much you can improve your health. Your vision can improve, you can lessen your need for sleep, and you can heighten your senses. Your athletic abilities can be further enhanced. Perhaps best of all, you can experience a deeper spiritual awakening.

It is exciting to be on the cutting edge of health! We have been poisoned and held back by cooked food for so many generations that we raw fooders are all pioneers in this arena. Indeed, we have barely tapped into our *health potential.*

# 20
# Raising Live Food Children

*Now children, eat up your raw fruit and vegetables! Just think of all the nutritionally starved children in America who have nothing raw to eat.*                    —Susan Schenck (1956–)

Some frequently asked questions are so dear to us that they warrant a separate chapter. If we can only start our children off with a live food diet, they might never have to suffer cooked food addiction. People who have done so say that their children, once old enough to make their own food selections, rarely stray from an at least 85% raw diet and usually remain 100% vegan or vegetarian.

## Can I start this diet while pregnant?

One school of thought claims that while the raw diet is an excellent way to facilitate the body's cleansing and prepare for pregnancy, as well as a superior way to eat while pregnant once you have already cleansed, pregnancy is not the best time to start.

The argument is that while you are heavily detoxifying, you may stir up toxins that will cross the placenta and adversely affect the fetus. The more toxic accumulation you have stored in your body, the greater the danger. But even those who conservatively take this stance will agree that you may begin a *60% raw* diet while pregnant since such a diet will benefit you and your unborn child while not stirring up as many toxins for elimination.

On the other hand, there are those who say it is safer for the baby, as well as the mother, to begin a 100% raw diet while pregnant than to continue eating cooked food. Indeed, there are women who began nearly all-raw diets while pregnant and delivered very healthy babies. (See Chapter 2.) The reasoning here is that toxins from the daily incoming cooked food would otherwise cross the placenta and injure the fetus.

In fact a recent study of the umbilical cord blood of ten American newborns commissioned by the Environmental Working Group proved that pesticides and other chemicals are found in the blood of newborns. The analysis found 287 foreign, toxic chemicals in total, while the babies averaged 200 contaminants each!

Ideally, one should come to pregnancy having already been cleansed and raw for years. But that is not always possible, as in the case of unplanned pregnancy. In such a case, there are those who feel pregnancy is nonetheless *a great time* for a woman to go raw. Food instincts become sharpened and clear-cut as the mother's body tries to build the best possible nest for the incubating fetus. If the well-known food cravings that occur during pregnancy are satisfied in the context of whole, fresh, raw food choices only, a woman would be most likely to succeed as a follower of the instinctive nutrition branch of raw foodism. (See Appendix C.)

For example, a pregnant woman may crave pickles or potato chips because her body knows that more sodium is needed during pregnancy, and her mind is suggesting foods that it "remembers" as being high in what's needed. But if raw foods that are naturally high in sodium, such as celery, spinach or seaweed, are presented for smell/taste testing, the mother's body will likely choose one of those instead.

The morning sickness problem has a ready-made solution in Natural Hygiene — fasting! The nausea is the body's only way of communicating its need to stop the feeding process while it proceeds to clean house. Any form of eating while a major cleanup operation is in progress would just interfere with it, and the body often responds by immediately ejecting these intrusions via vomiting.

While the body is thus loudly proclaiming the need for a fast, the rational mind, the one that often gets us into trouble, is fearful that she would be starving the fetus by fasting. Wrong! There is a reason that morning sickness is primarily limited to the first trimester of pregnancy when the size of the embryo/fetus is smaller than a marble. Sure, it's growing, but the fasting mother's stored up nutritional reserves are more than adequate to meet the challenge of feeding such a tiny being.

The reason this nausea occurs in the morning is because the body had already entered fasting mode overnight during sleep. It has found projects to work on that it wants to complete. Ideally, the woman would go back to bed and stay there until this feeling of nausea passed, however long it took, until a clear-cut call for food came from her body. Dr. Tosca Haag clearly states, "A pregnant woman in reasonably good health can safely fast for three to five days without any harm to the fetus."

Some people fear that episodic detox reactions induced by a sudden switch to raw foods might poison the fetus and cause a miscarriage. These people do not understand the nature of detox reactions, which are merely symptoms of the healing process in action. The real danger lies in continuing to eat in the old, habitual, toxic way, which continues to poison the fetus throughout the entire pregnancy period.

The bloodstream detoxifies very rapidly once energy reserves are revitalized by following an energy conservative lifestyle, especially on raw foods. It is this revitalization that permits gradual autolysis of excess fat tissue and movement of other sequestered toxic matter slowly into the bloodstream. Once in the blood, the autolyzed tissues are broken down and viable nutrients recycled. Toxic matter is excreted via the primary avenues of excretion: the liver, kidneys, lungs, bowels and skin. Thus impediments to the proper functioning of all the body's tissues and organs are eventually removed.

Deeper levels of detoxification may take months or years to complete, but even a short fast will help the mother's bloodstream and tissues to achieve a healthier condition than they would have had she done nothing to reform her diet.

# Is it advisable for a lactating mother to go raw?

It is true that infants have been known to refuse the nipple in rare instances when the raw-eating mother is going through an acute detoxification crisis. This is because some of those toxins are being released into the milk, souring its taste. These episodes are only temporary while the quality of the milk that follows is raised to a higher, more healthful level of purity. The persistent mother and patient infant win out in the long run. See "The Prisoner of War Diet" on page 154 for a case of breastfeeding on a raw diet.

# Is this diet healthful for my kid?

It cracks me up when someone asks me this. Do you really think, after all the research you have seen so far, that it could possibly be healthful for your kids to eat *cooked* food? Furthermore, if this diet were not healthful, how do you think children survived over the eons on raw food diets prior to the invention of cooking?

I saw a CBS news segment on the raw diet in which someone said it was "unsafe" for children to eat this way. Someone who knows the facts would say that the odds of a child on a raw, plant-based diet getting sick from bacteria are insignificant. The odds of the child getting slowly poisoned from a diet of cooked food are 100% however.

Gabriel Cousens, MD, saw the need for a study on this subject because too many parents are being harassed by the government when they put their kids on a living foods diet. He therefore has begun one of the few studies being done on raw vegan children. Preliminary results of his study were given to those who attended his lecture at the 2004 Raw Food Festival in Oregon and are summarized in Chapter 8.

Dr. Cousens also informs the parents of the need to be sure their children get enough Vitamin $B_{12}$, which is often lacking in vegan diets. (See Chapter 17.)

I have seen kids who were raised eating 100% raw food diets, and they never got sick. No earaches, no fevers, no colds! None of the usual childhood diseases! Most amazingly, they do not crave or want cooked or junk foods. Even given the choice between a raw gourmet pizza dish, or something fancy like that, and nature's cuisine of plain, simple produce, they prefer the latter!

Victoria Boutenko relates that the raw diet radically improved not only her kids' physical health, but also their mental abilities and behavior. Once, she invited 18 raw teens over to her house, kids that her children had been corresponding with on the Internet. Although she was apprehensive about having so many American teenagers at her house at one time, she said they all behaved "like angels."

Addiction to cooked food begins shortly after weaning from mother's milk. For those not breastfed, it begins even sooner with pasteurized milk or formula. This is why babies get colicky, suffer from rashes and so on. It explains the phenomenon that when you try to feed them their first cooked food, they spit it out. This is why they cry. For some, this may be why all they want to do is sleep.

Rev. George Malkmus warns, "One of the most cruel injustices we commit as parents is when we place cooked (pasteurized) milk, cooked cereal and cooked baby foods into the beautiful living body of little children designed by God to be nourished _only_ with raw, living foods!" (*God's Way to Ultimate Health*, p. 83).

Natalia Rose explains that it is important not to be obsessively strict with kids, however. There will be times that they will go to parties in which others are consuming cakes, pizzas and sodas. She explains that it is important psychologically to let them make their own decisions. If they eat right at home, chances are they won't even like the cooked, chemicalized stuff anyway. The amount they eat on such occasions will be minimal. Once they are home, it's back to the good food (*The Raw Food Detox Diet*, p. 87).

There is even a book on helping your kids make the switch to the most healthful diet on the planet: *Raw Kids: Transitioning Children to a Raw Food Diet* by Cheryl Stoycoff.

Now let's see what Dr. Vetrano, Dr. Tosca Haag and Victoria BidWell have to share on raising raw kids.

# The ABCDs of Feeding Mothers, Infants and Children Hygienically

Drs. Tosca Haag and Vivian Virginia Vetrano have joined forces with Victoria BidWell to prepare a manuscript that will replace Dr. Shelton's now out-of-print book *The Hygienic Care of Children*. Only Victoria offers Dr. Shelton's classic, now in photocopy form, presented at www.getwellstaywellamerica.com. List A below should supersede Dr. Shelton's directives on feeding when using his text where new information from these three women calls for doing so.

Dr. Vetrano raised Tosca on strict hygienic practices. In turn, Tosca raised four healthy, happy children on the same. While Victoria never wanted children, she did teach high school students for ten years and managed to trick them into enjoying, if not loving, what has been found to be the most detested subject on the curriculum, English!

Now Tosca, with her hygienic child raising, and Victoria, with her trickery in getting high school kids to enjoy the unenjoyable, combine their life experiences with Dr. Vetrano's Natural Hygiene parenting and teaching skills to bring us the "ABCDs" from their upcoming book *The New, Natural, Hygienic Care of Children*.

List A is taken from the chapter entitled "For Mothers and Other Adults Who Feed Kids!" by Dr. Tosca and endorsed by Dr. Vetrano.

# A: Feeding Mothers, Infants and Children Hygienically

**1.** The mother's care of herself and her prenatal care of the child must follow the ten energy enhancers strictly if she is to thrive and if the fetus is to develop in a normal, healthy fashion. The mother-to-be should not eat more just because she is pregnant: she should eat only when genuinely hungry, according to the dictates of nature. The amount of nuts and seeds needed is different for each woman, depending upon her emotional habit patterns, wellness and body weight. Usually 1-2 ounces more than she would usually eat when not pregnant will be adequate.

**2.** The mother must eat the Natural Hygiene diet, especially plenty of raw fruits, raw greens and raw vegetables. While most women do well on 3-4 ounces of nuts/seeds a day, the nursing mother should take 4-6 ounces of raw, unheated nuts/seeds a day, but not all at one sitting.

**3.** If a nursing mother becomes pregnant, she can continue nursing without harm through the pregnancy and then nurse both newborn and baby after the second birth. But the mother must take care to be well nourished and to secure plenty of rest and sleep and all the other needs of physiology represented by the ten energy enhancers.

**4.** From birth to three months, the baby should be nursed exclusively. Newborns to approximately two weeks need more frequent nursing because their tummies are small and hold very little at a time. A newborn will probably want to nurse every two hours. This helps to regulate the milk production of the mother as well. Actually, newborns should be fed *on demand*, a little here and a little there, even up to ten times a day, mostly during the day and possibly once or twice during the night.

**5.** To maintain a good, on-going supply of mother's milk, the woman must nurse from both the breasts at each feeding, although a complete emptying of both is not needed.

**6.** Commercial, heated milk formulas and baby foods are typically laced with table salt, refined sugar and other protoplasmic poisons and should be absolutely and completely avoided. Formulas and baby foods from supermarket shelves are toxic, cooked, counterfeit quasi-foods. All wonderful, wholesome baby foods and even nut milks can be made at home with a good juicer or a Vita-Mix machine.

**7.** Once the newborn is 2-4 weeks old and up to two months, milk feedings should be 2-4 fluid ounces. At two months and until solid foods are taken at about 18 months, 6-8 fluid ounces is best. Separate feedings at two months and on should not exceed 8-9 fluid ounces.

**8.** Breast-fed babies have a far, far better start in life! They are more vigorous and healthy and more resistant to the disease process, and they grow into stronger children than formula-fed babies. Mother's milk is the perfect food for a newborn through to 18 months, more or less, depending on the appearance of baby's teeth.

Mother's milk should be supplemented with fresh, raw fruit juices and occasionally nonstarchy vegetable juices. The general rule of mouth is that a baby without teeth requires milk only. The exception of feeding fruit juices is done to supplement the mother's milk, just in case it is inadequate.

**9.** If the mother's milk is lacking or contaminated for some reason, the next best source is a wet nurse's raw milk, then raw goat's milk, then raw cow's milk as the least desirable and the last resort.

**10.** From 3-6 months old, introduce fresh fruit juices, such as fresh-squeezed orange juice or watermelon juice, the two mildest juices that cause the least amount of digestive disturbance. Juices should not be served with milk feedings.

At this point, you will need to start scheduling feedings more regularly. As the infant wakes in the morning, he will tend to have the most energy and be most active. Give first a fruit juice. Then wait approximately an hour and a half before the next feeding, which should be nursed milk. After the larger milk feeding, the baby will probably doze off for a nap. He should not be fed again for at least three hours. By this time, the baby may be hungry again and can have another juice feeding. Again, wait for an hour and a half before the next milk feeding. Waiting another three hours, you can give the baby another milk nursing before he goes to bed.

This is a total of two juice and three milk feedings for the day. The baby might need another milk feeding sometime during the night. This is plenty of food.

**11.** From 2-3 months onward, the infant is not necessarily hungry every time he or she cries and need not be fed every time on demand. The human body, whether infant or adult, thrives on healthful routines. Develop a schedule early on for the baby and other people around the baby. Follow this feeding schedule in union with naps and a regular bedtime and rising schedule. Do not feed between scheduled times, even when the baby cries or fits.

Here is a follow-up suggested feeding schedule: 6 AM milk, 10 AM fruit juice, 12 PM milk, 3–4 PM fruit juice, 6 PM milk. The younger child may do well with a feeding before bedtime and once during the night if called for. Ultimately, you will develop your own schedule. Just be sure to allow adequate time for digestion and rest between feedings. Ideally, the baby will tell you when he is hungry.

**12.** Overfeeding is more damaging than slightly underfeeding. Constant feeding results in building disease with this sequence of events: (1) continual stimulation, (2) enervation (the first stage of disease) by overworking the child's entire being, but especially the digestive organs, (3) accumulation of endogenous and exogenous toxins, (4) impairment of digestive system function and finally (5) descent into acute and then chronic disease. Digestion will be good as long as a healthy newborn baby is not overfed and is getting the proper amount of sleep.

If the baby is getting too much to eat, he may become both enervated and toxic and start an elimination, what we used to call a *cold* before we knew about Natural Hygiene. Cut back the number of feedings or the amount at each feeding if this happens. Know that most so-called colds, the flu and other childhood diseases begin with this sequence of events, made far, far worse by feeding commercial milk formulas and cooked baby foods, as well as other SAD foods.

**13.** No starchy foods should be taken under age two. Starch digestion requires both thorough and complete mastication with insalivation and the presence of ptyalin, the salivary starch-splitting enzyme. For proper digestion of starches into assimilable sugar form, no starchy foods should be fed to infants before they have their teeth and before ptyalin secretion develops.

If fed starches before these two events, the baby will be poisoned by the alcohols of indigestible starches and their fermentation malmetabolites. Mother's milk and fruits are ideal and perfect baby foods since milk sugar and fruit sugar are easily digested, absorbed and assimilated, as are nonstarchy vegetables in juice and whole form.

**14.** A fat baby is not a healthy baby. Neither overfeed nor force-feed your infants and children. Let them develop a genuine hunger for ripe, natural, raw fruits, vegetables, nuts, seeds and sprouts. No seasoned, condimented and/or complicated recipe preparations as enticements to eat whatsoever should be used, especially during the first two years of hygienic life. Mother's milk and fruit juices should be fed prior to teething. Mashed or otherwise processed, puréed, pulverized fruits, vegetables, nuts and seeds are fed during teething to assist the child's limited chewing capabilities.

**15.** Although mildly painful at times for the baby, teething is a perfectly normal, natural process. Practically all young from six months to two and a half years are continually cutting. Babies can teethe on a wide variety of natural whole foods: for example, celery ribs, carrots and corn on the cob.

**16.** From 6-12 months, the teeth come in. When the baby feels inclined to sit at the table with the adults to eat, you can begin to replace a juice feeding with a blended vegetable salad or mashed and spoon-fed fruits, such as banana and avocado. Fresh, puréed apple and avocado are good, as are puréed tomato and avocado.

At about 18 months or when the teeth are fully developed enough to enable the child to mash soft fruits up well, fruit may be fed at one meal of the day. If four or five feedings have been allowed up to this time, three should now be taken. Continue introducing all fresh fruits and vegetables as baby grows and more teeth develop.

Infants can also begin having fresh, raw nut or seed butters (concentrated proteins) along with tomatoes as a meal by 18 months. Remember that any protein meal needs to have a space of about 3-4 hours before the next meal. The number of feedings per day needs to be adjusted according to how much the baby eats at one meal and how satisfied he is from that meal.

**17.** Early in life, the child should be taught to thoroughly chew all solid foods, however soft, and to eat slowly without bolting down foods. These two habits are the beginnings of developing emotional balance, a healthy relationship with food and avoidance of compulsive overeating and other eating disorders.

**18.** The best way to feed nuts to a two-year-old is to grind them into a meal and then show him how to form the meal into little balls which he can pick up and eat. When feeding ground up nuts, always give the child a few whole nuts and teach him how to chew.

**19.** Nut milks are fine to feed, but they tend to teach the child that he does not have to chew. Nut milks should therefore be used only occasionally, not daily. The recipe used should be totally liquefied into a smooth and silky milk for ideal digestion. This is most easily and best accomplished with the Vita-Mix machine. If only a cheap blender is used, the nut milk should be squeezed through a cheesecloth. The child may have 3-4 ounces of nuts/seeds daily.

**20.** Teach your children to enjoy lettuces, as many important minerals, vitamins and proteins are found in abundance in the different types of lettuce leaves: romaine, red leaf, green leaf and buttercrunch. Search for the mildly sweet, not bitter, lettuces. Many ways to serve lettuce can be used:

• Lettuce with sweet fruit is delicious. You can teach the child to eat a bite of lettuce with a bite of fruit.

• Lettuce dipped into any of the simple, nut-based sauces or fruit-based sauces Victoria has prepared in *The Health Seekers' YearBook* is wonderful! However, you will have to watch the lettuce dipping with these tasty recipes as children have a tendency to eat too much dip or sauce and too little lettuce!

• A child usually wants to eat what mommy eats by age two. He will want to try vegetable salads, lettuce and all. Encourage the child to eat vegetables with you, even if he cannot chew them well.

• At about 18 months, it is good to start feeding the child tasty blended salads with a wide variety of vegetables, including lettuce. By feeding blended vegetables early in life, children will develop a taste for all vegetables and will learn to like foods that are not so sweet as fruits always are.

**21.** The mother must maintain emotional balance while nursing. Drugs must not be taken. The mother's continuous and intense fight-or-flight response (fear and all fear spin-offs: anxiety, anger, depression and so on) and/or drug use can poison her milk and greatly harm, addict or, in the very most rare and extreme situation, even kill the nursing infant.

**22.** Any acute or chronic disease that deranges her milk and renders it toxic should cause the mother to wean her child.

**23.** If the child is upset, overly excited, overtired, overheated, overchilled, in pain, in distress, sick, fevered or feels bad, do not feed him until emotional balance and/or wellness is regained.

**24.** Once the child has a full set of baby teeth, he or she can best be fed and nourished on the adult hygienic diet as detailed in *The Health Seekers' YearBook* *with The Best of Common Health Sense.* We have perfectly prepared breakfast, lunch and dinner for every day of the year, without repetition, for all health seekers: mothers, infants and children included!

Dr. Vetrano notes, "See Victoria BidWell's *Common Health Sense,* Volumes I and II, for many more of our detailed eating specifics for parents, infants and children. Our 26-point list here is just bare bones."

**25.** Feeding babies hygienically is not something completely new. It is just new to some people, to new health seekers. Remember, you are always on the safe side with nature. Many more children are born today with enzymatic deficiencies, weakened digestive systems and other problems than were formerly born with these defects. Often the only thing which saves these children from much suffering, childhood diseases and sometimes death is to follow the Natural Hygiene way of feeding infants and babies as closely as possible.

**26.** Serve only properly combined foods and foods completely free of protoplasmic poisons. Avoid all SAD foods. Avoid all cooked foods. Feed infants and children live foods!

Lists B, C and D are taken from Victoria BidWell's chapter "For ALL Grownups Who Love Kids!"

# B: How to Make the Live Food Diet Fun for Kids!

The live food diet is energy enhancer number five. You can make this all-important enhancer fun in creative ways. Here are ten for starters:

**1.** Teach your kids to love animals every opportunity you find! Get creative! From short nursery rhymes, fairy tales and songs when infants to longer poems, stories and movies as kids get older, immerse them in the wonderful wide world of critters of all kinds! Keep a home pet the child learns to care for daily and to love. Visit farms, zoos and friends' animals. Encourage learning about animals wherever possible. Take adventures into the natural habitats of animals to appreciate their lifestyles.

Continually explain that all creatures have a right to live out their lives in health and happiness, as do all we humans, and that most animals have intense feelings and preferences, as well as sharp instincts. This will build an empathy between child and animals. Get your kids to clearly understand how animals become meat and why. Ultimately, encourage your kids not to eat anything that looks back at them and/or that has parents!

**2.** Read aloud from *Dr. GetWell's Book of Nursery Rhymes* to your children. I have rewritten Mother Goose and added more of my own rhymes, all with an engaging hygienic spin. Two Dr. GetWell CDs teach Natural Hygiene to children and children-at-heart. I tell my favorites with delightful dramatic interpretation! Too fun!

Challenge your children to make up some of their own rhymes and fairy tales. Memorize some of these rhymes, and act them out while telling them. Put them to song and enjoy songfests! Other specifically vegetarian literature in book and film form will enrich your children's vegetarian lifestyle: *Black Beauty*, *Gordy*, *Victor the Vegetarian* and many, many others can become family favorites forever.

**3.** Color in *The Fruit & Vegetable Lovers' Coloring Book* and *Dr. GetWell's Apples to Zucchini Coloring Book*. I offer these two delightful, oversized, 32-page coloring books for raw food kids. You can color with your kids. You and your kids can even create your own drawings, photocopy them on stiff paper and find family fun in coloring and admiring each other's artwork!

**4.** As soon as your child is old enough, intimately involve him or her in grocery list making; in selecting, checking out and loading up the raw foods where you shop; and in unpacking the groceries, preparing raw meals and cleaning up at home! Sing and dance, laugh and hug, play and delight in all these stages so that your child and you bond in utter happiness and high joy with every aspect of the live food lifestyle!

**5.** With regularity, make recipes and food arrangements that are works of fun and primitive art or even works of sophisticated gourmet art! Take pictures of this art, and keep a photo album you frequently open to share and enjoy with friends and family for fun!

These raw artworks can be as simple and quick as birthing little critters made of raisin-eyed bananas sitting on beds of lettuce for every day or as time consuming and elaborate as carving out a big watermelon basket filled with many kinds of little melon balls studded with American flags for the Fourth of July.

*The Health Seekers' YearBook with The Best of Common Health Sense* is full of such gourmet, display, live food preparations, mostly simple and some elaborate. So much fun can be had with little cookie cutters and slices of jicama, beet, apple and so on, as well as with gourmet tools, such as crinklers, spiralizers, fluters, zesters and so on.

**6.** Family and friends who have fun together have won forever! Every time a meal, snack or beverage is enjoyed together is another moment for bonding forever! Such moments are times to make faces of satisfaction and yummy sound effects and to celebrate out loud how good the raw food is and how blessed everyone is to be dining on and drinking up such natural, colorful, healthful, joyful lusciousness!

It's a simple fact of human psychology that children copycat those they love. If adults will be in the moment and totally appreciate the raw foods being shared with their beloved children, the children will just naturally emulate their esteemed adults. That's the easiest way to turn fun-loving, copycatting, raw kids into gratitude-expressing, fun-loving, raw adults!

**7.** Specialize in sweet temptations for kids to taste and revel over in place of refined sugar and high fat, chemicalized, SAD, counterfeit quasi-foods and junk foods. Again, *The Health Seekers' YearBook with The Best of Common Health Sense* is loaded with such treat recipes: especially simple formulas of few ingredients for making endless variations in cookies, pies, sauces, puddings, nut milks, smoothies, frozen blitzes and so much more!

While food combining rules may not be strictly followed in some of these sweet temptation recipes, none have protoplasmic poisons and are otherwise hygienically correct.

**8.**   Encourage your school age kids to take part in the planning and preparation of their lunches so that they will look forward to making them, eating them and taking pride in them! My *Brown BagWell & StayWell!* book is a wonderful lunch place to start for raw ideas.

**9.**   Encourage your young ones to share raw delights with their visiting friends and even to share your raw food stories, rhymes, coloring books and lifestyle! When especially yummy foods are offered, your little ones will have the positive experiences of turning others on to the live food adventure. Likewise, encourage your young ones to share when they go abroad with teachers at school and with friends at church and at other social shindigs.

**10.**   As soon as your children are capable of abstract thought and when the right occasions present themselves, begin your relentless and systematic counterculture education on the health hazards of the SAD, counterfeit quasi-foods while, in the next breath, point out the endless benefits of live foods. Do this in fun ways! Ask them questions, and express delight when they have the right answers! Children thrive on attention and positive reinforcement! They love to get enthusiastic! Most are just longing for the chance to get happy! Make *Health by Healthful Living* your family motto and extreme adventure!

Many more items have been added to this list in our new book in the making. Basically, the important thing to remember here is to get creative in promoting the live food family lifestyle at home and on outings to friends' places. *Make it fun so it can get done!*

# C: How to Make the Other Nine Energy Enhancers Fun for Kids!

•   Energy Enhancer #1: Cleanliness. Children understand the concept of keeping clean on the outside with soap and water. Now you must extend that understanding to keeping clean on the inside, explaining that what goes into the body must be natural, clean and pure too. Very early in their lives, introduce the word *toxic* and the concept that *it's all about energy*. Then help them see their daily choices through these two lenses.

Dr. Tosca adds, "Observe bowel and urinary function. Breast-fed infants tend to have egg yolk-colored stain on the diaper rather than a formed bowel movement. With the healthy baby, stool odor is mild, not overly odorous. Bathe the baby in warm water once a day with a mild natural soap to remove cradle cap, urine and bowel residue."

•   Energy enhancers #2 and #3: Pure air and pure water. Teaching even very young children that *pure equals good* is very easy. Reinforce these two purities with regularity. Teach them about their lungs and the big role water plays in their bodies. Very young children can be taught about their circulation and their cells, organs and systems and how all need pure air and pure water. Also, don't encumber the infant 24/7 with bulky clothes. Give the baby *air baths*. Let the little body breathe and move around without any clothes or diapers for a short period, at least once or twice a day.

• Energy enhancer #4: Adequate rest and sleep. The body loves regular schedules. Reinforce #5 with naps, regular bedtime schedules and time-out periods to rest and relax. Speak in "childese," and teach your young the lessons from "Dr. Vetrano with Victoria on the Priceless Benefits of Adequate Rest and Sleep" on page 545.

Dr. Tosca adds, "Securing sleep is more important than keeping to a feeding schedule. Don't wake the baby up for a meal. The baby should sleep approximately 18 hours total in a 24-hour period, day and night. Handling and cuddling are very important, but don't wake an infant just to show him off. Put the baby to sleep in a comfortable, well-ventilated room with fresh air, leaving a window open a crack even in winter to let in fresh air. This helps the infant sleep better. Finally, securing quietness and darkness is not so very important. A baby can get used to sleeping where the activity is. This prevents light and noise neuroses and sensitivities as adults. It also helps a child to be able to sleep in noisy situations without everything having to be drop-dead quiet and dark."

• Energy enhancer #6: Right temperatures. Use *Goldilocks and the Three Bears* to teach about "not too hot and not too cold" for starters. Then take it from there to expand the concept to other practical temperature lifestyle choices.

• Energy enhancer #7: Regular sunshine. Teach the importance of sunlight. Make sure your children get plenty of it and preferably daily! Sunshine is a nutrient like food, air and water. Enjoy gentle sunshine every day when possible for 5-10 minutes on the entire body. This is helpful for growth and development, as well as for nutrition. No sun blocks are needed for such short exposures.

• Energy enhancer #8: Regular exercise. Teach your children about their skeletons and muscles and their nervous systems. Help them count the ways regular exercise makes them healthier and happier, stronger and smarter. Make sure your children get regular exercise in fun, challenging, delightful and even exciting, self-motivating, intrinsically rewarding ways! Encourage stretching, aerobics and even a little weightlifting fun. *Make it fun, and it will get done!* Ideally, find fabulous ways to exercise with your children that involve the great outdoors and even animals!

Absolutely do limit the number of hours spent in front of video screens and plugged into various electronics to a sensible two or so a day. This will free up time for more physical activities.

• Energy enhancer #9: Emotional balance, which includes freedom from addiction, high self-esteem, a purposeful life and meaningful goals. Although these are grown-up terms, even a five-year-old or a precocious, even younger child, can appreciate these concepts if the right questions are asked.

Pulling answers or concepts out of an individual's mind by asking the right, highly simplified questions is called the *Socratic method*, named after the genius philosopher Socrates who lived during the Golden Age of Greece. "Dr. GetWell Teaches Natural Hygiene to Children & Children-at-Heart" on CD is geared to helping adults get this idea.

Even very young children are aware of adults having very bad habits (addictions), feeling bad about themselves (low self-esteem), leading bad (undirected and unhappy) lives because they have bad ideas (goals). You can teach your children this energy enhancer in so many ways and then reinforce for them the idea of having good lives (fascinating, challenging lifestyle and career choices) they thoroughly enjoy — trademarked with emotional balance!

- Energy enhancer #10: Nurturing relationships. This is not rocket science. Even this can and must be taught to a very young child so that he or she can give and receive love and live happily ever after! Never shake the baby or perform any rough, harsh or nonnurturing act. Read, talk, coo and sing to your baby and cuddle, touching throughout the day, and introduce him or her to other people who do the same. Babies and children need to live with cheerful, loving family members and friends. And they need to have fun!

# D: How to De-brand and De-drug Your Kids!

- Realize that Corporate America and her big brother, Corporate Globe, are both geared to capture the very minds, hearts and souls of our children in order to make them loyal consumers of corporate commercial brands — for life! Motivational advertisers are skilled pied pipers, designing media campaigns to put our children into fantasy worlds of materialistic glory that promise them the world and all of its excitement and thrills if our children will just — in a thoroughly programmed, relentless and hypnotic mode — happily obey the ads and follow all dictates: "Consume! Consume! Consume!"

When such goods and services are clearly products of the disease industrialists, our only hope to keep our kids is to fight this brand-washing, brain-claiming makeover at the hands of the powers-that-be with our very minds, hearts and souls! We need to educate our offspring and the children in our lives, from birth until they leave the nest, to think for themselves, to identify truth from lies, to understand the economic interpretation of history, to appreciate both the pitfalls and the beauties of the capitalist system, to understand that the SAD food supply is toxic and to realize that many corporations deliberately tell out-and-out lies to sell their disease-promoting products. We need to help our children see what those lies are, especially concerning poisoned food and drink and toxic drugs. This means educating our children as early as possible about the medical mentality at its very worst versus Natural Hygiene at its very best.

- In simple "childese," teach your children about "The Natural, Physiological Laws of Life" presented on page 549. We must help our children develop minds that declare humanitarian values, make distinctions on the basis of those values and then discern physiology's truths from advertisers' lies.

We need to spend time in as entertaining a way as possible, perhaps in game formats or by using the Socratic method, to help our children analyze advertisements and identify the natural laws that have been violated and the corporate lies that have been perpetrated in commercials, in print and on radio, television and the Internet. We must teach our children what the liars have to gain if they successfully hypnotize the people into becoming brand-buyers for life. Even a very young child can understand that the body heals itself and that live food is lively! But we must point these realities out before our kids get kidnapped!

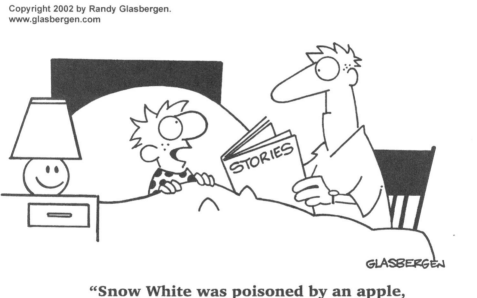

"Snow White was poisoned by an apple,
Jack found a giant in his beanstalk, and look
what happened to Alice when she ate the mushroom!
And you wonder why I won't eat fruits and vegetables!?"

# 21
# Raw Pleasure

There is no love sincerer than the love for food.
—George Bernard Shaw (1856–1950)

What we eat is more than nutrients or even the particular energy of the food. We also eat the mental state of those who grew the food, picked the food, prepared the food, and of the one who is eating the food. Food that is grown with love, picked with love, prepared with love, and eaten with love has a different quality than food that goes through those stages with a different consciousness relating to it. —Dr. Gabriel Cousens, MD (1943–), *Spiritual Nutrition and the Rainbow Diet*

Now that we have learned all about the benefits of eating raw, the raw food and Natural Hygiene movements, the scientific explanation for the health benefits of eating raw and how to go about changing one's lifestyle to eat raw, *let's eat*!

If someone had told me four or five years ago that I would become a quasi-chef, I would have had a good laugh. My life was always too active to get excited over a recipe. In fact as a cooked fooder, I don't recall ever inventing a recipe in my life. I don't even recall exchanging recipes with anybody. Let others do the cooking. My life was too full to be messing around in the kitchen. Yet here are my now-favorite recipes that I have fine tuned over the years and are always popular with guests.

At first I dreaded the idea of preparing my own food. My idea of preparing my own food before was sticking a TV dinner into a microwave. For special occasions I might have made some stir-fry or baked potatoes. Often I just ate out.

How and why did I get over my aversion to food prep and even go so far as to make my own mustard, salad dressings and even soup from scratch? *Only the desire to attain new levels of health motivated me.*

But I knew I had to change my attitude and make it _fun_. *Music was the key in my case.* I went out and bought some CDs that I knew would put me into a high, yet energetic, state of consciousness: Enya, Basia, Al Jarreau, Ronnie Jordan's "smooth jazz," as well as the ethnic music by Strunz and Farah worked great for me. More recently I enjoy fixing food to Joan Kurland's awesome CD "Looking Up."

But everyone has her own taste in music. The more you can sing and dance around while fixing food, the more fun it will be, the more you will actually enjoy it, and most importantly, *the more love you will transmit to the food.* Although there hasn't been a lot of research in that area, I am sure that food prepared with love is much more healthful to eat than food prepared by someone stressed out.

At first going raw may seem like a lot of work since you have to make so many things from scratch that you would normally buy prepared, such as crackers and salad dressing. But to quote Tonya Zavasta, "The day will come when you will no longer care for recipes. At first you cannot stand the lightness that consumption of the raw foods produces, but after several years on this lifestyle it is the fullness that becomes insufferable" (*Beautiful on Raw*, p. 13).

Note: Some of these recipes use nama shoyu, which is unpasteurized soy sauce made from cooked soybeans. If you are extremely sensitive to MSG, I would leave this out, as it does contain a little MSG, just as soy sauce does. If you are unable to get unpasteurized miso, you may use a pinch or so of powdered sea vegetables. Any time you are unable to use lemon, lime or grapefruit juice, use raw apple cider vinegar.

Typically, raw food recipes use unpasteurized miso, Himalayan or Celtic sea salt or nama shoyu for a salty flavor. But if you are trying to heal, do not use salt in any form as it is a protoplasmic poison. It also increases food addiction! If you feel a strong desire for a bit of salty flavor, use celery or powdered sea vegetables, such as dulse. It will taste much saltier after you detox the salt from your system.

If you are a strict vegan, there are numerous things you can substitute for the honey. You can use agave, which comes from cacti. Or you could use dates or raisins or other sweet fruit, but dried fruit is more concentrated than fresh fruit.

Stevia extract is especially good as a sweet substitute if you are sensitive to sweets and don't want any excess insulin output from your pancreas. Stevia is a plant. Though it is probably not raw when you get it from the store, stevia extract is used in such minute quantities that it won't matter too much. Since it is 200 times sweeter than sugar, $1/8$ teaspoon per serving is often all you need. It is also very easy to grow your own stevia plant. However, many find that it leaves a bitter aftertaste.

As you can see from the following recipes, I adore cilantro! It is said to be a good heavy metal chelator to aid in detoxification. I put an entire bunch of it in almost anything that is not a dessert. Feel free to reduce the amount. You could also use parsley or your own favorite herb as a substitute.

When I first started preparing raw dishes, I omitted many of the fresh herbs because I didn't want to pay two dollars for some fresh organic herbs when the recipes called for so little of them. Then I started buying my own pots of herbs, such as oregano, thyme, basil and parsley, and plucking a few leaves as needed.

I found that herbs make all the difference! They are truly the spice of raw food. Once I made nut and seed cheese with a handful of thyme and basil and discovered it had an overwhelmingly familiar taste. I closed my eyes and tried to remember where it came from. It was the bologna I ate as a kid! To think, all that time it was not the pork or beef that was tasty, but the hint of herbs mixed into it.

I highly recommend that you purchase herbs in pots so that you can keep growing your own. Fresh herbs cost several dollars at a grocery, and that is a needless expense when so many recipes call for such small amounts. Grow your own, and you can pluck a few leaves for extra flavor in whatever dish you are making.

Eventually you will want to alter these recipes or experiment with creating your own. The rule used by successful chefs is to attempt to excite all the taste-buds. To get an exciting taste, it is often fun, though not necessary, to have a bit from each of the five flavors: spicy, sweet, salty, sour and bitter. Many herbs are spicy, and you can also use organic spices. Use agave, honey, stevia, fresh or dried fruit for a sweet taste. Use celery or powdered sea vegetables, such as kelp or dulse, for a salty taste. Lemon, lime or grapefruit juice or raw apple cider vinegar hits the sour spot. Add green leafy vegetables for the bitter taste.

When dehydrating, keep the temperature at 100°-105° F since the enzymes start to die off at about 105° F. You may even want to tape down the thermostat so it won't accidentally be bumped.

Note: Unless otherwise stated, *store all the leftovers in the refrigerator*. Try to use them up within the next few days for best flavor and health benefits. Generally, most raw dishes will keep three to six days, but the fresher, the more nutritious and better tasting.

Now let's take a look at how we can make a raw food recipe fit the standards of Natural Hygiene. (See Controversial Foods and Seasonings on page 336 for the subtle differences from the simply raw food framework.)

# Victoria BidWell's Secret Touches for Perfectly Prepared, Hygienic, All-Raw Recipes!

The raw food movement's recipe books are wonderful. Susan and I both urge you to build a library of them and turn to yummy dishes and drinks instead of counterfeit, SAD foods while going for 100% raw.

The Natural Hygiene movement's teachings take recipe preparation a step further, however, so as to avoid the nerve energy drain of having to detoxify from the exogenous toxins in certain raw foods and from the endogenous toxins created by the body when poor food combinations are taken. The following simple, secret steps you can take to conserve your nerve energy while hygienizing the raw food movement's recipes were taken from *The Best of Common Health Sense*:

- Be selective: completely throw out hopelessly toxic raw recipes.
- Serve your salads with true transition, hygienic salad dressings.
  Remember, the nontoxic salad dressing recipe uses only fruits, vegetables, nuts and seeds. No stimulating, toxic salt of any kind, no hot spices, no onion, no garlic. And also remember, a dressing can be as simple as just lemon juice or or-

ange juice or carrot juice — or any juice! And of course fruit salads don't really need a dressing at all.

Arnold Shircliffe, in *The Edgewater Beach Hotel Salad Book*, warned us of the "powerful irritating effects" of toxic salad dressing ingredients. He reminded us that most seldom experience these effects for the first many years of their lives because the delicate mucous membranes of the gastrointestinal tract are supplied with comparatively few nerves of sensation. One does not experience the toxic effects and consequent pathology of the gastrointestinal tract until usually, years into a jazzed-up, condimented lifestyle. But in time these effects add up to a significant remote source of toxemia.

Shircliffe further reminded us that toxic salad dressings also "create an artificial appetite similar to the incessant craving of the chronic dyspeptic whose irritable stomach is seldom satisfied. Drinking alcoholic drinks and the excessive use of condiments are two of the greatest causes of overeating since they remove the sense of satiety by which the stomach naturally should call out with 'enough!' "

See Chapter 10 of *The Health Seekers' YearBook* and the extensive recipe section of *The Best of Common Health Sense* for many dressing recipes.

• Most raw recipes from the raw food movement already use all-raw ingredients. But many on the market also have cooked foods. Do substitute all-raw ingredients for cooked, canned or otherwise processed whenever possible.

And note that it is almost always possible! Except for those very few vegetables that absolutely must be eaten cooked, you can always substitute raw. But certainly whenever the recipe specifies, for instance, canned pears, you can use fresh!

• If you are presently committed to eating all-raw, please, never compromise yourself for the sake of a recipe!

Throw the salad out if it is built completely around cooked food and if you cannot come up with a pleasing substitution. Do not compromise yourself, and do not ruin your all-raw record! And never let a *recipe* be an *excuse* for getting you off the right track!

• Use nut milks for cow or goat dairy.

When raw milk, raw cream, raw sherbet, raw ice cream and so on are called for in the recipes, use nut milk recipes instead. And you do have banana ice cream instead of raw cow's milk ice cream. Most of the time, nut milks and their derivatives will substitute deliciously!

• Follow proper food combining rules.

• Visualize and "imaginate" as you read the raw recipe; see if you can make each dish or drink a work of art!

• This is a fun and creative challenge! *VISUALIZE.* Turn your dishes and drinks into Garden of Eden masterpieces!

• Enjoy your dishes or drinks slowly and in peacefulness and gratitude.

• Bring in foods the author of the recipes never thought of using to add even more high life to the adventure!

You can use such simple, common, inexpensive foods! Or you can use the expensive and the exotic! Get out your list of hygienic foods available in "Classification of Foods." Do not forget the whimsical sprouts and the many dried fruits!

## Garnish! Garnish! Garnish!

- Fruits and vegetables are natural garnishes! What fun you can have making a "nest" with sprouts and "boats" with cucumbers! The hygienic garnishes are endless — and all edible!

- In most raw food movement recipe books with fruit and vegetables as the centerpieces, most of the recipes are hygienizable. But some just are not: ignore these few recipes, and focus on the many salvageable dishes and drinks!

Now let's get on with the raw food recipes! They are presented here with better hygienic alternatives in parentheses.

# Soups

## Everybody's Favorite Celery-Cilantro Soup

1 bunch celery (about 8 stalks)
1 bunch cilantro
1 bunch fresh dill
1 cup unpasteurized olive oil (or substitute ½ cup water and ½ cup nut or seed butter for greater hygienic purity)
½ cup raw almond butter or raw tahini
3 cloves garlic
2-4 T unpasteurized miso (optional — substitute dulse)
2 T nama shoyu (optional — substitute dulse)
¼ cup lemon juice (if not available, raw apple cider vinegar)
8 cups water

Blend in a Blend-Tec or Vita-Mix, adding a little of the ingredients at a time until creamy. This is a big hit everywhere I have taken it. I always get requests for the recipe! If you want to make it creamier, simply add more celery stalks and a little more almond butter or olive oil.

Serves about 10.

# Creamy Carrot Soup

3 cups carrot juice
8-10 T raw almond butter
1½ avocados
4 T nama shoyu
2-3 garlic cloves
2 T honey or agave
1 bunch celery (about 8 stalks)
6-8 cups water

Blend in a Blend-Tec or Vita-Mix, adding a little at a time until creamy. Use the leftover carrot pulp from the juice to make almond carrot cookies (see "Desserts").

Makes about 10 servings.

# Cream of Tomato Soup

3 tomatoes
2-3 celery stalks
½ red bell pepper
Small handful of sun-dried tomatoes
1 t powdered sea vegetables
Juice of 1 lemon
6 dates, pitted
5 oz raw cashews
¼-½ cup unpasteurized olive oil (or substitute half nut butter, half water for the
    whole food alternative)
Enough pure water to make it as thick or thin as you like

Blend in Blend-Tec or Vita-Mix, adding a little at a time until creamy.

Makes about 5 servings.

# Cream of Celery Soup

1 bunch celery
1 bunch parsley
2 cups water — use sesame milk for creamier taste (see "Beverages")
¼ cup olive oil (or substitute $^1/_8$ cup nut butter $^1/_8$ cup water)
1 tomato
1 T honey (or agave)
Juice of 1 lemon
1 t powdered sea vegetables

Blend in Blend-Tec or Vita-Mix, adding a little at a time until creamy.

Serves about 4-6.

# Vegetable Chowder

Everybody's Favorite Celery-Cilantro Soup (see above)
2 zucchinis, grated
2 carrots, grated
2 avocados, cut up into chunks
Corn kernels from 3 ears of corn
1 bell pepper, chopped

Put the vegetables into the celery/cilantro base. Gently stir. This is a big hit at potlucks, even cooked ones! People like this one for winter and the celery/cilantro base alone for summer.

Serves 10-12.

# Cream of Spinach Soup

1 avocado
1 cup water
2 cucumbers, skin and all
2 cups spinach
2 cloves garlic
1 bell pepper
1 bunch cilantro

Blend in Blend-Tec or Vita-Mix, adding a little at a time until creamy. You may need to add more water.

Serves 4.

# Corn Chowder

4 cups corn kernels
1 avocado
1 cucumber
¾ cup almonds, soaked 6-12 hours, rinsed and drained
1 bunch cilantro
3 T dulse flakes
4 cloves garlic
Enough pure water to make it as thick or thin as you like

Blend in Blend-Tec or Vita-Mix with water, adding ingredients a little at a time, using only enough water to blend. Add more water until it is the right consistency, thick and creamy.

Serves 5-8.

# Creamy Cauliflower Soup

5 cups sesame or almond milk (see "Beverages")
1 medium or small cauliflower, chopped up
1 bell pepper, any color
½-1 avocado
Juice from 1 lemon or lime
3 T raw tahini or nut butter
3 T unpasteurized miso (or substitute dulse)
½ jalapeño pepper (optional — omit for hygienic purity)
3 cloves garlic

Blend in Blend-Tec or Vita-Mix until creamy.

Serves 5-8.

# Lorenzo's Tomato-Avocado Soup

A friend of mine serves this soup every time we go to his house, and my husband and I can't get enough! He says he has experimented with it a lot and found that the only crucial ingredients that cannot be omitted or substituted are the avocado and tomato, which is why I gave it this name.

2 cups water
1 large tomato
1 ripe avocado
2 cloves garlic
Juice from a small lime
¼ onion
½-¾ cup broccoli
1 big red kale leaf
4 small chilies or 1 jalapeño (optional — omit for hygienic purity)
4-5 stalks bok choy
1 inch fresh turmeric
1 red bell pepper
¼ cup flaxseeds
1 t powdered sea vegetables
2 T raw apple cider vinegar (or substitute lemon juice)
2 T nama shoyu (optional)

Blend ingredients in Blend-Tec or Vita-Mix until very creamy.

Serves 2-4.

# Entrées

## Spaghetti

Squash, zucchinis or daikon radishes (about 8-12 inches of any of these for each
    serving)
Tomato Sauce (see "Sauces, Salad Dressings, Condiments")
Tahini Sauce or Pesto Sauce (see "Sauces, Salad Dressings, Condiments")
Parmesan Cheese (see recipe under "Salads and Salad Trimmings")
Bits of vegetables, such as bell pepper or broccoli, chopped into small bits, or
    cherry tomatoes sliced into two (optional)

Using the Saladacco spiralizer, make spaghetti out of the vegetables. This wonderful gadget will make long, stringy strands just like spaghetti! If you have a large group to feed, this can be quite tiresome, as the spiralizer is a hand-crank gadget. Perhaps as this diet catches on, someone will invent an electric one or at least a spiralizer attachment to the food processor. If you do not have a spiralizer, or if you simply don't have the time or energy to crank out the spaghetti strands, you can use the grating attachment of the food processor to get mini-strips. Next, add tomato sauce and top with tahini sauce. Sprinkle with Parmesan cheese. Top with vegetable bits.

## Nori Rolls

This is the "fast food" of the raw diet. It is like making a sandwich.

1 Nori sheet (Note: The green ones found at Oriental groceries are much
    cheaper, but heated. Black ones are truly raw.)
Sprouts of any kind, a small handful
Tahini sauce (see "Sauces, Dressings, Condiments") *or*
Sunflower Seed Pâté (see "Appetizers and Dips"), about ½ cup
Grated or thinly chopped carrots, bell peppers, zucchini or beets
Small handful chopped green onions (or red onions), 1 T per serving
Chopped avocado (optional), ¼ avocado per serving

Put the Nori sheet on a plate. Put a tablespoon or two of sauce in the middle, followed by some sprouts, onions and chopped vegetables.

Note: This recipe cannot be made ahead of time, as the sheet will get very damp from the sauce and break. Therefore, you must make them just before serving. This recipe makes great appetizers as well as a snack or lunch entrée.

# Chinese Stir "Fry"

1 foot-long daikon radish
4 carrots
1 bunch green onions
5-6 stalks celery
½ head small cabbage
2 zucchinis
1 red bell pepper
1 cup mung bean sprouts
¾ cup watercress
3 stalks broccoli
1½ cups snow peas
Slivered raw almonds or raw cashews
Sesame seeds
Tahini sauce (see "Sauces, Salad Dressings, Condiments")
Tempeh (optional)

With the food processor, grate the daikon radish, and slice the carrots, celery, green onions, cabbage, zucchinis and bell pepper. (This is one time you will be especially thankful for your food processor: a job that could otherwise take an hour will be finished in minutes!) Put into a large bowl. Cut off florets from broccoli and toss into the mixture. Chop off tips of watercress and toss in, along with mung bean sprouts. Cut off stringy ends of snow peas and toss in. Fold in about a cup of tahini sauce. Top off with almond slivers (or truly raw cashews, sliced) and sesame seeds. Chop up tempeh and fold into mixture.

Serves 8-10.

# Tomato Raviolis

Tomatoes
Hummus (see "Appetizers and Dips")

Slice tomatoes about ½ inch thick. Put hummus between two slices of tomato, like a sandwich. Dehydrate at about 105° F for several hours.

# Buddy and Cherrie's Barbecue "Chicken" Nuggets

This recipe was contributed by my friends Buddy and Cherrie. They used it in one of their workshops on how to have a "raw picnic in the park." It is so delicious, you'll swear it's chicken! I personally prefer to double the amount of curry and poultry seasoning given in their recipe below.

2 cups carrots
2 cups almonds, soaked and drained
¼ cup orange juice
¼ cup onion
¼ cup olive oil (or substitute $^{1}/_{8}$ cup nut butter $^{1}/_{8}$ cup water)
2 T agave
1 T poultry seasoning
2 t powdered sea vegetables
¼ t black pepper
½ t curry powder
1 recipe Barbecue Sauce

In a food processor, process carrots until diced. Add remaining ingredients and blend until well mixed. Mold into nugget-size shapes and place on Teflex sheets. Brush with Barbecue Sauce. Dehydrate at 105° F for about 5 hours, flip onto a mesh screen, spread with more sauce and dehydrate about 5 more hours until dry but not crisp. Serve with additional sauce as dip, if desired.

For a plain nugget, leave the Barbecue Sauce off and dehydrate the plain nugget.

Yield: 37 nuggets, using a 2 T-size scoop

**Barbecue Sauce for Nuggets:**
1½ cups sun-dried tomatoes, soaked
1 cup chopped tomatoes
1 clove garlic
¼ cup dark agave
1 powdered sea vegetables
3 T lemon juice
¼ t dry mustard powder
1 t Chili Powder
1 T liquid smoke (optional — not a raw product)

Combine all ingredients in a blender and blend until smooth.

Yield: 1 cup sauce

# Burritos

Tortillas: To make the burrito tortillas, mix the following ingredients and dehydrate at 105° F for 12-24 hours until completely dry. Cut with scissors into squares for wraps. Store the remainder in a sealed container.

3 cups pure water
4 carrots, chopped
4 T unheated honey or raw agave
4 tomatoes
1 cup sun-dried tomatoes, soaked for at least 30 minutes and cut into pieces with
    scissors
2 celery stalks
¼ cup nama shoyu (or substitute 1 T dulse)
1½ cups flaxseeds, soaked overnight and rinsed
1 t cayenne powder (optional — purists omit)
½ bunch cilantro (optional)

Filling: "Sunflower Seed Pâté" or any of the other dips listed under "Appetizers and Dips."

Top off with alfalfa sprouts (or shredded lettuce) and roll into a burrito shape. These are always a big hit at potlucks!

Note: When you don't have time to make the burrito tortillas, you can use raw nori sheets instead.

Serves 10-12. You can make them smaller and have a great deal more if this is served as an appetizer instead of a main course.

# Beet Burgers

This recipe has been adapted from a recipe in *The Raw Gourmet* by Nomi Shannon.

1 cup pulp left over from beet juice
1 cup ground sunflower seeds (soaked, rinsed, dried, then ground in coffee
    grinder)
½ cup finely chopped celery
¼ cup finely chopped green onion
½ bunch cilantro
3 T flaxseeds, ground in coffee grinder
½ cup water
¼ cup finely chopped bell pepper
1 T unpasteurized miso or powdered sea vegetables

Mix everything in a food processor using the "S" blade. Form patties on a dehydrator and dehydrate about eight hours.

Serves about 10.

# Raw Pizza

1-2 medium, ripe eggplants (Note: Skin should be wrinkly; if green inside, they
    are not ripe and may be harder to digest)
Tomato sauce (see "Sauces, Salad Dressings, Condiments")
Deluxe macadamia nut cheese (see "Appetizers and Dips")
1 bunch green onions, chopped

½ cup fresh olives (more likely to be raw if from a jar, as canned olives are usually heated)
1 bell pepper, grated and chopped into small pieces

Remove the skin from the eggplants, and slice about ½ inch thick. Cover little
mini-pizza circles with tomato sauce. Next, add a thin layer of deluxe macadamia
nut cheese. Top with chopped green onions, bell peppers and olives. Dehydrate
for about 4 hours at 105° F. What's really amazing is that the eggplant shrivels
up and tastes almost like wheat! These can be refrigerated and taste really great
even if you don't heat them up again in the dehydrator. These are a big hit, especially for pizza lovers. They can also be used as appetizers. The following is an
optional crust that actually looks and tastes remarkably like cooked pizza:

**Optional crust:**
2½ cups buckwheat groats, soaked 6 hours, rinsed, drained and sprouted 24
hours
½ cup unpasteurized olive oil (or substitute ¼ cup nut butter ¼ cup water)
1 bunch cilantro

Blend all ingredients until creamy. Dehydrate 2 hours, and then add the toppings.
Dehydrate 2 more hours or until dry. The only caveat about this kind of crust is
that grains are much harder to digest than eggplant, even when sprouted. Digestion will probably get easier the longer you are eating a diet close to 100% raw.

Serves about 8-10 people, or use the little pizzas as an appetizer.

# Desserts

## Raw Cake

**Crust:** Blend until creamy 2 cups almonds (soaked overnight, rinsed, drained), 1
cup finely ground almonds (ground in coffee grinder or Blend-Tec or Vita-Mix), 4-
5 T unheated honey, 1 t cinnamon.

**Icing:** Carob Cream (see next).

Serves 10.

## Raw Candy

Nuts, soaked 6-12 hours, rinsed and drained
Dates
Raw carob powder, to taste (optional)
Raw shredded coconut or unhulled sesame seeds

Mix nuts, dates and carob in food processor. Mix in a food processor with the "S"
blade until the mixture forms a ball that bounces around inside that machine.
Remove and form little balls. Roll the balls in sesame seeds and/or raw shredded
coconut. These keep a long time in the freezer. Experiment with ingredient proportions and quantities to suit your own taste.

# Carob Cream

This tastes and looks like chocolate mousse. You won't be tempted to eat chocolate with this dessert! It can be eaten alone or used as an icing for a cake or a dip for strawberries, bananas and so on.

1 avocado
½ cup raw carob
¼ cup raw coconut butter
½ cup unheated honey or agave

Blend in food processor with the "S" blade until mixture is creamy and it looks like Hershey's chocolate. If it doesn't taste sweet enough, add another tablespoon of honey. Alternatively, you can thicken this with coconut butter or sweeten it with agave.

Serves 6-8.

# Peanut Butter & Carob Cups

This is the raw version of Reese's peanut butter cups. Take paper cupcake or confection holders such as the ones that cupcakes come in or the smaller ones that chocolates come in. Fill the bottom half with raw almond butter. Then fill the top part with the carob cream recipe in this section. Freeze and keep frozen until you serve them.

# Ice Cream

1½ cups nut or seed milk (see "Beverages")
2 cups pulp left over from nut or seed milk (use half as much if you want a less "pulpy" texture)
2 T coconut butter or oil
½ cup unheated honey or agave
1 T organic vanilla extract

Blend in food processor with the "S" blade until creamy. Then pour into ice-cream maker. In a Cuisinart, it will take about ½-¾ hour for it to become ice cream. If you want chocolate flavor, add about ½ cup raw carob powder. Store any leftovers in the freezer, but it will get very hard and be difficult to eat, so best to use it up now.

Serves 6-8.

# Frozen Fruit Ice Cream

Handful frozen strawberries (or blueberries)
1 frozen banana
Juice from 1 orange
8-10 grapes, frozen or fresh

Blend in food processor with the "S" blade until creamy. Or, if you have a centrifugal type juicer, push ingredients through, using the blank screen. The consistency will be like soft-serve ice cream. Store any leftovers in the freezer, but it will get very hard and difficult to use, so best to use it up now.

Serves 2-3.

# "Pumpkin Pie" Pudding

5 figs
10 pitted dates
1 cup walnuts, soaked 6-8 hours, rinsed and drained
¾ cup grated carrots
¾ t each of cloves, nutmeg, cinnamon (or just use "pumpkin pie spice")

Blend in food processor with the "S" blade, adding ingredients a little at a time. Blend until creamy.

Serves 4.

# Carrot Almond Cookies

4 cups grated carrots
4 cups almonds, soaked overnight and rinsed, drained
3 inches fresh ginger, chopped
¾-1 cup unheated honey
¾-1 cup sun-dried raisins
4 T unpasteurized white miso (optional — purists omit)

Slowly blend the mixture in a food processor, using the "S" blade. Take heaping tablespoons and put on the dehydrator sheets. Flatten them with the back end of spoon so that they are about half an inch thick. Dehydrate them 4-8 hours at 105° F. They will be nice and crunchy if dehydrated enough. Store in the refrigerator and eat within three or four days. Makes about 4 dozen. For fewer, simply halve the recipe.

# Peppermint Patties

For the "chocolate" layer, make recipe for carob cream. Make 6-7 times the amount, possibly even a bit more.

For the white-colored peppermint layer, blend in a food processor using the "S" blade:

3 cups shredded dehydrated coconut (call the company to be sure it is truly raw)
$1/_3$ cup raw honey or agave nectar
1 t peppermint or mint extract

Spread thin the layer of coconut mixture for the peppermint part on the bottom of a container, topping it with a thin layer of carob cream." Freeze for several hours. This tastes better than the peppermint candies you buy in wrappers, yet it is *much* more healthful!

Serves 10.

# Buddy and Cherrie's Carob Nut Taffy

This recipe was graciously contributed by my friends Buddy and Cherrie.

1 cup walnuts, soaked, dehydrated and chopped into large pieces
1 cup almonds, soaked, dehydrated and chopped into large pieces
1 cup brazil nuts, soaked, dehydrated and chopped into large pieces
½ cup agave or unheated honey
2 T raw carob powder
2 T cacao nibs, crushed or ground

Chop the nuts coarsely. I do it by hand so that the chunks are in large pieces. Place in a bowl and mix well with remaining ingredients. Place on Teflex sheet and dehydrate for 8 hours. Remove from sheets and place on mesh screens and dehydrate for 24 hours. They will be soft but will harden up as they cool. Store in an airtight container. They will be a little sticky. If you are looking for a crunchy, chocolate type of treat, this is wonderful.

# Sandy's Apple Pie in Ten Minutes

This was contributed by Sandra Schrift from Chapter 2:

**Crust:** Soak 1 cup of pecans and 1 cup of walnuts for a few hours. Drain and mix with four coconut-covered dates in food processor. (I buy mine in bulk at Whole Foods Market.) Place mixture in a glass pie plate (use your hands) and refrigerate overnight if possible.

**Filling:** 3 apples chopped (with their peels) in food processor. (In summer time use peaches.)

½ t cinnamon
¼ t nutmeg
1-1½ t lemon juice

Spread the filling over the crust.

**Toppings:** Sliced strawberries, blueberries, kiwis or any fruit you wish. This makes it look pretty — and taste good.

## Buddy and Cherrie's Cashew Ice Cream

Here we go again with another fantastic recipe from Buddy and Cherrie. This is their favorite raw ice cream.

3 cups raw cashews, soaked overnight and drained
3 T raw carob powder
3 T raw cacao powder (buy it that way or grind the cacao nibs in a coffee grinder until powdery)
4 cups coconut milk
1¾ cups raw agave nectar
½ t vanilla extract

Blend ingredients in food processor with the "S" blade or in a Blend-Tec or Vita-Mix until creamy. Put into an ice-cream machine.

Here is Buddy's updated version for the ice cream:

4 cups raw cashews
1¾ cups raw agave nectar
3 cups coconut milk
2 t vanilla extract
9 T cacao or 8 tsp. vanilla extract

Directions are the same.

## Frozen Persimmon Pudding

This recipe is contributed by Victoria BidWell.

5 fully ripened, "soft-style" persimmons
5 very ripe bananas
2 cups sweet, seedless grapes

Prepare and freeze all these fruits. Thaw them slightly. Then smash the persimmons and bananas together. Sprinkle the whole grapes on top. Serve.

Serves 4.

# Beverages

## Seed Milk

1 cup seeds (sesame seeds are especially good)
6 cups water

If you are using sesame seeds, be sure to get the unhulled kind, as they are richer in calcium. Mix seeds with water in Blend-Tec or Vita-Mix or use the non-heating option of the Soyajoy machine. If you use the Blend-Tec or Vita-Mix, liquefy the seeds. Then strain the liquid with a cheesecloth if you prefer a thinner consistency. (A Soyajoy has a built-in strainer.) Use the pulp to make ice cream (see "Desserts"), or use the pulp to make spinach dip (see "Appetizers & Dips"). The milk keeps for three days.

Makes about 6 servings.

## Nut Milk

1 cup nuts of choice
6 cups water

Liquefy the nuts and water completely as for seed milk. No cheesecloth straining is necessary when nuts are used. Of course if nut butters are on hand, they may be used to make nut milks, in which case, less liquefying time is required. The milk keeps for three days.

Makes about 6 servings.

## Banana Milk Shake

1 frozen banana
1 cup nut or seed milk
2 dates or 1 T unheated honey or 1 T agave

Blend in Blend-Tec or Vita-Mix or food processor (using the "S" blade) or blender.

Serves 1.

## Smoothie

2 frozen bananas
Juice from 2-3 oranges
2 T bee pollen or spirulina flakes

Blend in Blend-Tec or Vita-Mix or food processor (using the "S" blade) or blender.

Serves 2.

436

# Carob Mint Soda

1 cup nut or seed milk (see recipe above)
1 T unheated honey or ½ T stevia extract (liquid)
2 T raw carob powder
½ capful peppermint extract

Blend in Blend-Tec or Vita-Mix until it is foamy like a soda.

Serves 1.

# Super Smoothie

This is the best breakfast ever! It really gets you going. Who needs a latté? This will get you through the most stressful job ever. If you live alone, save half for lunch or to get a second wind when you get home. Upon taking this drink, I have experienced being able to clean my condo or do the laundry after working 11 hours straight at a stressful job!

½ bunch kale
2 cups fresh juice from sweet-tasting fruit (e.g., orange juice)
1 banana
2 T bee pollen
1 pinch cayenne (purists omit)

Blend in a Vita-Mix or Blend-Tec machine, adding water as needed to achieve your preferred consistency.

Serves 2-4.

# Pineapple Spinach Drink

1 bunch spinach
1 cup or more fresh pineapple
1 cup or more pure water

Put all ingredients into a Vita-Mix or Blend-Tec machine. Fill close to the top with pure water. Blend until creamy.

Serves 2-4.

# Strawberry Shake

1 batch almond milk (see "Nut Milk" recipe above)
2 qt baskets strawberries
1 T vanilla extract
$^2/_3$ cup agave
2 T coconut oil or butter (optional)

Blend in blender or Vita-mix or Blend-Tec machine.

## Green Drink

½ bunch kale
2 cups freshly squeezed fruit juice or carrot juice
1 dash cayenne (purists omit)

Put all ingredients into a Vita-Mix or Blend-Tec machine. Fill close to the top with pure water. Blend until creamy.

Serves 2-4.

# Beverages from *The Health Seekers' BeverageBook* Manuscript (Upcoming Book)

Victoria BidWell shares, "I am presently working on a 300-page book designed for health seekers who want drinks without protoplasmic poisons; that is, drinks made exclusively from the five food groups of the nontoxic Natural Hygiene diet: fruits, vegetables, nuts, seeds and sprouts. However, a few optional ingredients are allowed, defined as *true transition* ingredients by Dr. Vetrano and myself. Only two machines are used, the Champion juicer and the Vita-Mix blender. Following is a *tasting party* for your drinking pleasure from this upcoming protest against SAD drinks, *The Health Seekers' BeverageBook — A Happy Hour Guide of 20 Freedom Formulas for Bartending Endless, Yummy, Hygienic Drinks!*"

**General directions:** Clean, core, pit, peel, husk, shell and otherwise; likewise, prepare all the fruits, vegetables, nuts and seeds for pleasurable consumption! Always use distilled water when the recipe calls for ice cubes or water.

Health seekers' beverages calling for the Vita-Mix are to be blended to smoothness or according to directions, usually only 1-2 minutes, sometimes even less.

## The Waldorf Classic

The old Waldorf Astoria Hotel in New York City first served this salad: apples, celery and walnuts. Now you may enjoy this salad for the rich and famous as a health seekers' beverage!

3 cups celery juice
3 cups apple juice
2 big handfuls walnuts

## The Sweet Waldorf Classic

1 cup celery juice
5 cups apple juice
2 big handfuls of walnuts

# The Barely Sweet Waldorf Classic

4 cups celery juice
2 cups apple juice
2 big handfuls of walnuts

# The Pear Waldorf

Substitute pear juice for apple juice in any of the three versions of the Waldorf Classics above. Crispy pears make a smooth, clearer, thinner juice. Soft pears tend to come out of the juicer as a purée, yielding a thicker, grainier health seekers' beverage.

# The Nutty Waldorf Variations

Substitute any choice of your favored nuts in the any of the four versions of the Waldorf Classics above.

# The Pineapple Slushy

3 parts frozen pineapple chunks
1 part frozen strawberries
1" of very cold water

Blend just seconds to a coarse-grain slush. Add a few ice cubes for a finer-grain, sloshier health seekers' slushy.

# The Sweetest Tomato Beverage

This is one of my favorites and a great health seekers' beverage choice when left with an abundance of tomatoes, whether on sale or in the garden! Tomato juice by itself is often flat to the tastebuds. Just a little grape juice stirred in or whole grapes blended into the tomato juice tastes like the Sweetest Tomato Beverage was made from the sweetest tomatoes in the world!

8 parts tomato juice
2 parts grape juice or whole grapes

# The Mellowed-Out Grape — Choice 1

Straight grape juice is just too cloyingly sweet for some tastebuds! Mellow out grape sweetness with just a little tomato juice. Stir well.

# The Mellowed-Out Grape — Choice 2

The simplest, easiest, least costly way is to mellow out the too sweet grape juice is by adding plain, pure water or ice cubes. Stir well.

## The Mellowed-Out Grape — Choice 3

The all-time stand-in for mellowing out too sweet grape juice, and creating a salty taste as well, is by adding celery juice. Stir well.

## Dr. Scott's Refreshment

Dr. D. J. Scott is now in his mid-80s and runs a chiropractic clinic full-time and Scott's Natural Health Institute full-time too! I once saw him enjoy a tall glass of light green, frothy, sweet straight cabbage juice in one quaff! Amazing!

## The Hygienic Retreat Traditional Trio

Equal parts of apple, carrot and celery juice. To make less sweet and more salty, add more celery juice.

## Mango, Go! Go! Go!

Fill the Vita-Mix half full of sweet orange juice. (The small, thin-skinned oranges are often the very sweetest and also have the very best price when purchased by the case.) Add the slippery mango flesh. Use very little for just a hint of mango taste. Use much more for a thick health seekers' smoothie in which a straw can stand up. Blend the two ingredients until smooth. The Mango, Go! Go! Go! is a heavenly taste treat.

## Nutty Mango, Go! Go! Go!

Prepare the Mango, Go! Go! Go! above, adding just enough mango to the orange juice to make this health seekers' smoothie on the thin side. Add a big fistful of your favorite nut meats: cashews are divine! Blend the ingredients until the nuts are completely assimilated into the mango and orange juice. Remember, you have a whole new recipe and taste treat, depending on which nut you use. And you have a whole new consistency treat, depending on whether you make the smoothie thick with more mango and nuts — or thin with less mango and nuts.

## Ginger Mango, Go! Go! Go!

Prepare the Mango, Go! Go! Go! above, with the desired thinness or thickness. Before blending, however, add an inch of fresh, raw ginger root. Peel the ginger first. Cut it into a few small pieces. Try starting with 1" of ginger. Add more if you want more "kick"! Blend until the ginger is completely assimilated. The kick of the ginger makes a wonderful, real-food substitute for the SAD counterfeit of carbonation.

# Ginger Nutty Mango, Go! Go! Go!

Prepare the Nutty Mango, Go! Go! Go! Then add the ginger as described in Ginger Mango, Go! Go! Go!

# Chunky Mexican Salsa — In a Glass!

Add to your Vita-Mix the following typical Mexican salsa ingredients:

6 quartered tomatoes
2 stalks celery cut into 1" chunks
1 small onion in large dices (optional)
Juice of 2 lemons or 2 limes (or 1 of each)
2 tomatillos in large dices
Fresh cilantro and parsley to taste, slightly chopped

Blend these Mexican salsa ingredients very slowly, using the tamper, until they are thoroughly mixed into a chunky, but still drinkable, salsa. A few seconds will usually do it. Pour your Chunky Mexican Salsa into a glass. Garnish with a tall stalk of celery as a swizzle stick.

# Mexican Salsa In a Glass — Variation 1

Use 6 quartered, small, sweet oranges instead of the tomatoes for a sweet salsa.

# Mexican Salsa In a Glass — Variation 2

Use 4 quartered, sweet oranges and 2 quartered lemons for an unusually refreshing flavor.

# Mexican Salsa In a Glass — Variation 3

Add more liquid for a thinner drink, either citrus juices, tomato juice or water. Blend until silky smooth.

# Banana Cream Pie In a Glass

3 frozen bananas
¼ cup shredded coconut
½ cup pitted dates
1 cup very cold coconut milk
½ cup walnuts
1 cup ice water

Blend on high speed the coconut milk, walnuts, dates and water to make a creamy nut milk. Add the bananas, breaking into chunks as you go, and the shredded coconut. If using dried coconut, turn it into a fine meal in a nut grinder first. If using the fresh, moist coconut meat, turn it into the blender with the other nut milk ingredients first. As always, reach the smoothie smoothness you most enjoy by adding more liquid or more frozen bananas.

# Veggie Smoothie

4 cups chilled tomato juice, made with the Champion's large-hole screen
1 cup sweet corn kernels
15 spinach leaves
A few salad greens, such as lettuce and parsley
4 ice cubes, more or less

Blend until a health seeker's Veggie Smoothie! Use more of the sweet corn for a thicker, sweeter smoothie.

# Plumb Yummy Smoothie

8 very ripe, sweet plums
3 frozen bananas
1 cup apple juice
1 pinch cinnamon (optional)

Some beverage bartenders prefer to peel the plum skins, but their tart taste is part of what gives plums their sharp flavor. (Don't forget that just under the skin is where the highest concentration of nutrients burrow!) Blend all ingredients until a health seeker's Plumb Yummy Smoothie!

# The Ginger-Mint Pear Smoothie

3 ripe, soft to the touch pears
1 T fresh-grated ginger
6 fresh mint leaves
1 cup apple juice

Most health seekers prefer to peel the pears, as the skins — even blended — leave a grit. You decide. Blend into a smoothie! Add more ginger to flavor it more!

# Golden Delicious Smoothie

3 cold, quartered golden delicious apples
¼ cup pecans
½ cup golden raisins
1 cup very cold water
8 large ice cubes

Blend to a health seeker's Golden Delicious Smoothie!

# Banana Nutnog

3 large bananas at room temperature
3 rounded T almond butter
$\frac{1}{8}$ t nutmeg (optional)
½ t fresh vanilla bean paste scrapings
$\frac{1}{8}$ t cinnamon (optional)
2 cups boiling water

Blend until smooth and warm. Experiment with amount of liquid and number of bananas used to get the thickness you most enjoy. Stir in a handful of chopped almonds. Serve with a spoon, sit by an open fire, and enjoy. Instead of a counterfeit eggnog with booze, have a health seeker's Banana Nutnog without compunction!

# Sauces, Dressings, Condiments

## Tahini Sauce

1 cup raw tahini
¾ cup unpasteurized olive oil (or substitute $\frac{3}{8}$ cup nut butter $\frac{3}{8}$ cup water)
$\frac{2}{3}$ cup orange juice (about 2 medium-sized oranges)
3 cloves garlic
1½ inches fresh ginger
1 T nama shoyu (optional)
1-2 t powdered sea vegetables
¼ cup fresh cilantro (optional)

Mix in food processor with the "S" blade, adding ingredients a little at a time. Mix until creamy. This is great on raw Oriental vegetables for a stir-fry or on Nori Rolls.

## "Thousand Island" Salad Dressing

2 oranges, pulp, seeds and all
4 T unpasteurized olive oil (or substitute 2 T nut butter 2 T water)
2 T unheated honey
2 T nama shoyu (or 1 T dulse)
¼ cup raw almond butter
2 T raw apple cider vinegar or lemon juice
4 cloves garlic

Blend in food processor with the "S" blade, adding ingredients a little at a time. Mix until creamy. Add a bit of water if needed to thin, or add more oil.

# Honey Mustard Dressing

½ cup raw mustard (see recipe below)
½ cup unpasteurized olive oil (or substitute ¼ cup nut butter ¼ cup water)
½ cup unheated honey or agave
½ cup water (less makes it creamier)

Blend in food processor with the "S" blade until creamy.

# Oil and Vinegar

1 cup unpasteurized olive oil (or substitute ½ cup nut butter ½ cup water)
1 cup raw apple cider vinegar or lemon juice
1 T finely chopped fresh basil (optional)

Mix the ingredients and shake or blend in blender or food processor.

# Curry Spinach Dressing

2 cups spinach
1 cup cilantro
1 T curry powder
2 T unpasteurized miso (or dulse)
2 T raw almond butter
½ t powdered sea vegetables
½ t cayenne (optional)
¼ cup water
¼ cup unpasteurized olive oil (or substitute $1/8$ cup nut butter $1/8$ cup water)
¼ cup raw apple cider vinegar or lemon juice
¼ cup agave nectar
¼ cup water (if you want to make it thinner)
1 avocado (if you want to make it thicker)

Blend in a food processor with the "S" blade. This is great to pour over a tossed salad and mix thoroughly.

# Raw Mustard

8 T whole yellow mustard seeds
4 oz mineral water
3 oz lemon juice
2 T unheated honey or agave

Soak mustard seeds in water and lemon juice overnight. Add honey and blend in food processor with "S" blade until creamy. Keeps for months in the refrigerator.

# Tomato Sauce

1 cup fresh tomatoes
½ cup sun-dried tomatoes
½ cup pitted dates
½ bunch cilantro
3-4 cloves garlic
¼ cup chopped red onion
4 leaves basil
1 t powdered sea vegetables
3 T unpasteurized olive oil or nut butter

Blend in Blend-Tec or Vita-Mix until creamy. Liquefy all ingredients until smooth and you attain the desire consistency. For a thicker and sweeter sauce, use more dates and sun-dried tomatoes. You could blend it in a food processor with the "S" blade, but the dates and sun-dried tomatoes will be very hard to blend, causing the machine to vibrate, and the ingredients may even splatter! But this splattering can be avoided if you soak both the dates and sun-dried tomatoes for at least two hours first.

# Parmesan Cheese

½ cup ground flaxseeds
1 T dehydrated cilantro or parsley flakes
½ t garlic powder

Mix the ingredients evenly. Sprinkle on vegetable spaghetti, salads or other main dishes.

# Natural Hygiene Salad
# Dressings, Sauces and Dips

These recipes are excerpted from Victoria BidWell's *The Health Seekers' YearBook with The Best of Common Health Sense*. She explains:

I have been helping health seekers toward superlative nutrition using strict Natural Hygiene recipes since 1986. I remember a rough time when only one good hygienic recipe book was available, put out by T. C. Fry. Over the years, I have learned that the single biggest problem for those starting on, and staying on, the nontoxic raw food diet was getting down the dry salads, especially the vegetable salads. I know this situation has not changed. Therefore, I am thrilled to share some of the simple salad dressings from my *Health Seekers' YearBook with The Best of Common Health Sense* collection of 60 with the hope that they will get you past any of those tough SAD salad dressing, sauce and dip addictions and ever further into the live food lifestyle.

## Cashew Tang

Blend until smooth, 2 cups tangelo juice, the juice of 1 lemon and 8 ounces cashew butter or cashews.

## Tart Cashew Crème

Blend until smooth 2 cups grapefruit-tangelo juice with 8 ounces cashew butter or cashews.

## Cashew V-4 Crème

Blend until smooth 2 cups tomato-carrot-celery-beet juice with 8 ounces cashew butter or cashews.

## Apple-Sweet Cashew Crème

Blend until smooth 2 cups apple-celery juice with 8 ounces cashew butter or cashews.

## Almond Tang

Blend until smooth 2 cups pineapple-orange juice with 8 ounces almond butter or almonds.

## Almond V-2

Blend until smooth 2 cups carrot-cucumber juice with 8 ounces almond butter.

## GetWell's Waldorf Special Sauce

Blend until smooth 1¾ cups tangelo juice and ¼ cup lemon juice with 8 ounces walnut butter.

## Tomato-Pecan Dip

Coarse chop 2 large, quartered tomatoes in the blender. Juice 2 stalks celery. Then mix the tomatoes and celery juice in a bowl by hand with 8 ounces pecan butter.

## Sunny Tomato Topping

Blend until smooth 2 large tomatoes with 8 ounces sunflower seeds or sunflower seed meal.

## Piña-Tahini

Blend until smooth 2 cups pineapple-celery juice with 8 ounces sesame butter.

## Taste of Brazil

Blend until smooth 2 cups tomato-cucumber juice with 8 ounces brazil nuts or brazil nut butter.

## Hawaiian Dream

Blend until smooth 2 cups pineapple juice with 8 ounces macadamia nuts or macadamia nut butter.

## Tomacado

Blend until smooth 2 tomatoes, 1 large stalk celery and 1 large avocado.

## Applecado

Blend until smooth 2 cups apple juice with 2 medium avocados.

## Avocado Special

Blend until smooth 2 cups very sweet soak juice from any soaked dried fruits with 2 avocados. Especially sweet and tasty are raisins, figs and apricots.

## Avobutter

Mix 2 avocados and lemon juice together until a buttery consistency is reached. Avobutter will be stiff and spreadable like the soft, SAD counterfeit. Enjoy Avobutter with the many recipes and dishes with which you used to take butter.

## GetWell Guacamole

Coarse chop 3 tomatoes, blend and pour them into a mixing bowl. Dice into very small pieces yet another tomato. Mince 2 tomatillos, 1 celery stalk and 1 red bell pepper. Mash 2 large avocados. Juice 1 lime and 1 lemon. By hand, turn all these ingredients into each other thoroughly.

## Dieter's Delight Sauce

Coarse chop 3 tomatoes and blend. Juice 1 grapefruit. Cut into quarters 12 cherry tomatoes. By hand, mix all the ingredients thoroughly.

## Fig Ambrosia

Place 8 dried figs in a little over 1 cup water and soak overnight. Blend with 1 cup soak water until smooth.

# Fruit Fixin's Sauce

Blend until smooth 1 cup apple juice with the flesh of 2 small papayas.

# Old-fashioned Apple Sauce

Take 3 golden delicious and 3 red delicious chopped apples, ½ cup tart apple juice and ½ cup soaked raisins. Blend these ingredients until smooth.

# Mexican Salsa

Juice 2 lemons and 2 limes, chop 2 red bell peppers, dice 4 celery stalks, and mince 4 tomatillos. Mix these ingredients with 4 cups of coarse-chopped tomatoes.

# GetWell's Fruit Jam Formula

Any variety of dried fruit can be made into a tasty fruit jam, with all the advantages of live food and none of the poisons of counterfeit, SAD food. Simply soak the chosen fruit in an equal amount of water for 8-12 hours. Then cut the fruit into small pieces. Put it into the Vita-Mix. Next, run it in spurts. Stop between to stir GetWell's Fruit Jam Formula. To reach the desired consistency, add more or less soak juice. Also, you may try combining two or more fruits for a *merry taste medley*!

Serve the Jam Formula a variety of ways: spread on lettuce or celery as a filling, scooped onto a sliced fruit as a garnish, poured over a fruit salad as a dressing, set into a dish as a dip, piled onto a banana ice cream sundae as a topping, blended into a fruit smoothie as a sweetener and so on!

# Victoria BidWell's Nut and Seed Butter Secrets

Nut butters can be used in an endless array of recipes, but especially as thickeners in juices, soups, dressings, dips and sauces. Nut butters are delicious served with a raw vegetable finger food plate as well.

**Butter prepared with a juicer using the blank screen (homogenizing plate):** Some juicers, such as the Champion, have a homogenizing plate that slides in and replaces the juicing screen. Any nut can go through to make nut butter without adding oil, although adding a few teaspoons of liquid allows homogenizing the nuts more quickly and with less effort.

**Butter prepared with a Vita-Mix:** A slight amount of liquid must be added to the nuts when making Vita-Mix nut butters. Water or fruit or vegetable juice is more healthful than any oils for this purpose.

**Butter prepared with a grinder:** The various kinds of grinders will pulverize nuts into a powder, light and fluffy with a small amount of liquid and stirred into a nut butter.

448

## Victoria BidWell's Favorite Recipe: Traditional Cranberry Relish

1½ lbs fresh cranberries
1½ cups raisins
3 oranges, cut in sections
3 diced pears

Run all the above foods through the food grinder or through the food processor set for purée. Mix the foods thoroughly, cover with a tight seal, and let chill. This recipe is best when chilled overnight to let the flavors mingle one with the other. It's delicious!

# Appetizers and Dips

## Raw Hummus

2 zucchinis
¾ cup unhulled sesame seeds, soaked 6-12 hours, rinsed and drained
¾ cup raw tahini
¼-½ t cayenne (optional)
½ t celery salt or dulse
3-4 garlic cloves
1 t powdered sea vegetables
¼ cup lemon juice

Blend in a food processor with the "S" blade, adding ingredients a little at a time until creamy. Serve on flax crackers or use as a vegetable dip with sliced zucchini, baby carrots, sliced bell peppers and fresh broccoli.

## Nori Rolls

See "Entrées."

## Creamy Spinach Dip

½ lb spinach (about 5-6 cups)
½ red onion
3 cloves garlic
¾ cup raw tahini or leftover pulp from nut or seed milk
½ bunch cilantro
3-4 T lemon juice
½ t powdered sea vegetables

Blend in food processor with the "S" blade, adding spinach a little at a time. Mix until creamy. Serve on flax crackers, or use as a vegetable dip for sliced zucchini, baby carrots, sliced bell peppers or fresh broccoli.

## Deluxe Macadamia Nut Cheese

12 oz (3 cups) macadamia nuts, soaked 6-12 hours, rinsed and drained
1 t powdered sea vegetables
2 cloves garlic
1 T fresh cilantro
¼ cup lemon juice
$^3/_8$-½ cup unpasteurized olive oil (or substitute equal amount of half nut butter half water)

Blend in food processor with the "S" blade, adding the nuts a little at a time. Mix until creamy, the texture of cream cheese.

Note: For a creamier mixture, you could put the nuts through a juicer with the blank screen before putting them into the food processor. In that case, you will need about half the olive oil! You might have to add one or two tablespoons more of oil.

Blend until it has the creamy texture of cream cheese. Serve on flax crackers, or use as a vegetable dip with zucchini, baby carrots, sliced bell peppers, fresh broccoli and so on.

## Pecan Pesto

2 cups pecans, soaked 4-8 hours, rinsed and drained
1 bunch cilantro
1 medium red onion
4 cloves garlic
4 T ginger
Juice of 1 small lemon or lime

Mix in food processor using the "S" blade. Use just as you would pesto sauce. It is great over zucchini or squash noodles.

## Pumpkin Seed and Macadamia Nut Cheese

1½ cups macadamia nuts, soaked 4-8 hours, rinsed and drained
1½ cups pumpkin seeds, soaked 4-8 hours, rinsed and drained
Juice from small lemon
3 T unpasteurized olive oil (or substitute nut butter)
3-4 fresh basil leaves
3-4 any other fresh herbs (tarragon, mint, thyme)

For best results, put nuts and seeds through the blank screen of a juicer (e.g., Omega or Champion). Then mix everything until very creamy (with a texture like cream cheese) in a food processor using the "S" blade. If you do not have a juicer, simply put the nuts and seeds into the food processor right away with the other ingredients. You may have to add more olive oil, though, to help it get creamier.

# Guacamole

2 Roma tomatoes or ½ cup other tomatoes
2 large avocados
½ bunch cilantro
Juice from ½ small lemon
1 t jalapeño, chopped (optional — omit for hygienic purity)
2 cloves garlic
1 t powdered sea vegetables
½ red bell pepper

Blend in food processor using the "S" blade. For a chunky texture, cut the pieces first into small chunks; then blend for only about 3 seconds to get slightly smaller chunks. For a creamy texture, blend longer.

# Sunflower Seed Pâté

1 cup sunflower seeds, soaked overnight, rinsed
1 cup pumpkin seeds, soaked overnight, rinsed
½ cup pitted olives
2 red bell peppers
½ bunch cilantro or favorite fresh herb
1 t powdered sea vegetables
½-1 cup sun-dried tomatoes, soaked for 30 minutes and cut into small pieces with scissors

Combine the seeds and make butter according to "Victoria BidWell's Nut and Seed Butter Secrets." If using a food processor with the "S" blade to make the seed butter, it will not be as creamy with the true pâté consistency. Combine the seed butter with all the other ingredients, and blend in either the Blend-Tec or Vita-Mix, or process in a food processor.

# Salads and Salad Trimmings

## Arabian Salad

2 tomatoes
1 bell pepper, green or red
1 cucumber
¼ bunch cilantro
1 bunch green onions
Unpasteurized olive oil (or substitute half nut butter half water)
½ t powdered sea vegetables
1 lemon

Chop cilantro finely. Chop other vegetables into bite-size chunks. Add salt. Sprinkle on olive oil, but don't let it be so much that vegetables get soggy. Squeeze lemon juice over salad. Gently stir. This is a tasty, cool salad enjoyed in Middle Eastern dinners.

Serves 2-3.

# Cheesy Spinach Salad

½-¾ cup unpasteurized olive oil (or substitute half nut butter half water)
Juice of 1 lemon
1 cup pumpkin seeds, soaked 6-8 hours, soaked and rinsed
1 T mustard (see recipe in "Sauces, Salad Dressings, Condiments")
4 garlic cloves
½ t powdered raw sea vegetables
1 lb chopped and cleaned spinach
1 red onion

Mix all ingredients except the spinach and onion in food processor with the "S" blade or in a Blend-Tec or Vita-Mix. If the dressing is too thick, you may have to add more oil or a tiny bit of water. Chop the red onion, and put it with the spinach into a big bowl. Pour the dressing over it and toss.

Serves 6.

# Waldorf Salad

1-2 apples, grated
1-2 sprigs asparagus, grated or sliced in small pieces
½ cup sun-dried raisins
½ cup walnuts
3-4 cups lettuce and/or spinach

Toss salad ingredients. Top with honey mustard dressing (see "Sauces, Dressings, Condiments").

# Coleslaw

1 cabbage (green or purple)
½ red onion
1 red bell pepper
1 green bell pepper
3 carrots

**Dressing:**
$^1/_3$ cup raw apple cider vinegar (or $^1/_3$ cup lemon juice)
$^1/_3$ cup unpasteurized olive oil (or $^1/_6$ cup nut butter $^1/_6$ cup water)
$^1/_3$ cup unheated honey
1 T mustard or mustard seeds
1 t powdered sea vegetables

Grate the carrots with the food processor using the grating blade. Slice the other vegetables using the slicing blade. Next, blend the dressing using the "S" blade and pour over the salad.

Serves 8-10.

# Holiday Salad

5-6 cups spinach (about ½ lb)
1 cup pecan croutons (see recipe below)
½ cup raw olives
½ red onion, sliced into halved ringlets

Toss pecans, olives and onion ringlets into spinach. Top with oil and vinegar or dressing of your choice.

Serves 5-6.

# T. C. Fry's Super Salad

This favorite of T. C. Fry comes from Victoria BidWell's *The Health Seekers' YearBook*:

6 large tomatoes
4 stalks celery
4 red bell peppers
1 head bok choy
1 head cauliflower
4 medium avocados

Dice the tomatoes. Chop the cauliflower: stalks, leaves and all. Dice the avocados. U-cut the celery. Mince the red peppers. And chop the bok choy: stalks, greens and all. Combine the ingredients into a large bowl, and mix them thoroughly.

Serves 4.

# Marinated Kale

1 bunch kale (stems removed and saved to put later into a juice)
1 small red onion
2 carrots
1 red bell pepper
2 zucchinis
1 bunch cilantro or mint
½ cup red cabbage or 2-3 stalks celery

Chop in a food processor using the slicing blade. Then the dressing (below) over it and let it marinate overnight. Sprinkle with raw sesame seeds before serving.

**Dressing for Kale:**
½ cup coconut oil or unpasteurized olive oil (or ¼ cup nut butter ¼ cup water)
Note: If you plan to store this in the refrigerator, I would avoid using coconut oil, as it congeals.

2 cloves garlic
2 inches ginger
½ cup lemon or lime juice
2 T nama shoyu (or powdered sea vegetables)
1 dash cayenne (optional)

Chop the garlic and ginger, then blend with the other ingredients using a food processor with the "S" blade.

Serves 6-8.

# Arame Salad

This makes a very large salad. You may want to cut the recipe in half.

1 head green cabbage
1 head red cabbage
2 beets
5 carrots
3-4 bell peppers (red and green)
1 red onion
½-¾ cup arame seaweed (sun-dried)
½-¾ cups sesame seeds (soaked overnight and rinsed)
½ cup each of agave or unheated honey, raw apple cider vinegar and unpasteur-
    ized olive oil

With a food processor, slice the cabbages, bell peppers and onions. Grate the carrots and beets. Sprinkle in the arame and sesame seeds. For the dressing, mix the agave or unheated honey, raw apple cider vinegar and olive oil. Pour over the salad.

Serves 15-20.

# Dill Coleslaw

½ head red cabbage
½ head green cabbage
4 bell peppers
1 bunch parsley
1 bunch dill
1 cup sunflower seeds
4 carrots
¾ cup olive oil (or $^3/_8$ cup water $^3/_8$ cup nut butter)
½ cup unpasteurized miso or powdered sea vegetables
4 T mustard
3 T agave

Slice cabbage, carrots and peppers in food processor with the slicing blade. Use the shredding blade for the dill and parsley. Blend the rest of the ingredients to make a dressing to pour over vegetable mix.

# Greek Salad

3 tomatoes
2 cucumbers
2 red bell peppers
1 red onion
1 t oregano
¼ cup lemon juice
½ tsp basil
½ cup pitted greek olives
½ cup olive oil (or ¼ cup nut butter ¼ cup water)

Dice the vegetables. Blend the lemon juice, oil or nut butter with water, and spices to make a dressing to pour over the vegetables. Sprinkle with pitted olives.

# Pecan Croutons

1-3 cups pecans
Cinnamon
Unheated honey

Soak the pecans overnight, rinse and drain. Roll them in a mixture of honey and cinnamon. Dehydrate them for four hours or so until they are dry. Toss them in a salad.

# Salad Sprinkles

Soak overnight a few cups of flaxseeds, sesame seeds or sunflower seeds. If you like, you can soak them in Celtic sea salt or Himalayan rock salt. Rinse and thoroughly dehydrate. Sprinkle onto your salad for extra flavor and crunch.

# Buddy and Cherrie's Mock Potato Salad

8-10 cups jicama, peeled and diced
$^1/_3$ cup diced bell pepper (core and seeds removed)
2 cups chopped celery
2 ears of corn kernels
½ cup chopped onion
1 diced avocado
1 recipe of the following dressing

Put all ingredients in a large bowl and mix well.

Dressing for Mock Potato Salad
2 cups cashews
½ cup pure water
2 t powdered sea vegetables
½ cup agave
¼ cup lemon juice
¼ cup raw apple cider vinegar
½ cup olive oil
½ t paprika
½ t cumin
½ cup fresh dill

Add all ingredients and blend until smooth. This recipe makes 11 cups of salad. Enjoy!

Serves 11.

# Snacks

## Cauliflower Pâté ("Mashed Potatoes")

3 cups cauliflower, cut up
1 cup macadamia or pine nuts, soaked 4-8 hours, rinsed and drained
¼ cup lemon juice
¼ cup water
¾ T powdered sea vegetables
½ T garlic

Put into food processor, using the "S" blade, adding cauliflower a little at a time. Blend until the mixture looks light and fluffy like mashed potatoes. The mixture will not only look like mashed potatoes, but the taste will also be reminiscent of mashed potatoes!

Serves 8.

# Garlic Cilantro Flax Crackers

2-3 cups of flaxseeds, soaked overnight (Note: Seeds will expand with water, so it will become 4-6 cups the next day.)
1 bunch cilantro, chopped
1 T powdered sea vegetables
5-6 cloves garlic
5-6 T nama shoyu (optional)

Blend cilantro, salt, garlic and shoyu in the food processor, using the "S" blade. Put the seeds into a big mixing bowl and fold into the mixture, mixing until it is spread throughout the seeds. Put onto dehydrator sheets, and dehydrate until it is completely dry on both sides. (Some people like to turn the cracker over after 6 hours or so, but it is not absolutely necessary.) It may take up to 24 hours to dry completely. Store in a closed, airtight container with some moisture absorption packets. (These are often found in supplement or vitamin bottles.) The crackers can keep a month or so if dry.

# Barbecue Flax Chips

$^1/_3$ cup flaxseeds (soaked overnight)
$^1/_3$-$^2/_3$ cup pulp from carrot or orange juice (if not available, use another $^1/_3$ cup flaxseeds)
3 dates or ¼ cup agave nectar or unheated honey
1 celery stalk
2 tomatoes
1½ cups water
$^1/_2$-$^2/_3$ cups sun-dried tomatoes (if a heavy-duty blender is not available, such as a Vita-Mix or Blend-Tec machine, be sure to soak them for an hour before blending to soften them)
1 dash cayenne powder (optional)
1 t powdered sea vegetables
2 carrots

Blend all ingredients except seeds. Then add seeds, blending mixture until it is smooth. Dehydrate in the shape of small crackers or large ones that can be broken later. Dehydrate at about 105° F for about 24 hours until very dry. Store in an airtight container with moisture absorption packets such as found in vitamin and other nutritional supplement containers. This will enable them to keep much longer.

# Breakfast Dishes

Any of the drinks listed in the "beverage" section are also a great way to start out the morning. But if you need something to munch on…

## Al's Cereal

1 banana
2 heaping T sun-dried raisins
1 heaping T bee pollen
1 heaping t almond butter
1 heaping T hemp seeds

Mash the banana with a fork until it is creamy. Stir in other ingredients.

Serves 1.

## Trail Mix

1 cup almonds, soaked, drained, rinsed and dehydrated or left out until dry
½ cup sun-dried raisins
½ cup shredded coconut
½ cup sunflower seeds, sprouted and dried

Mix together. This is also great as a snack or travel food.

Serves 6.

# Sample Menus for One Week

The following menus are suggestions that may be modified according to taste. Portion sizes will vary and hence were generally not specified since people have differing caloric needs according to their sizes, ages and activity levels. Many of the suggested menu items are described in the recipe section of this chapter.

These sample menus contain a wide variety of dishes. *In reality, however, your own menus will more likely consist partly of leftovers from the previous day* since it is so much easier to prepare a single dish that will last for several days.

If you are pressed for time, you might make a few raw gourmet dishes on the weekends with plenty of salad and just live on that for the week, along with raw fruit, raw trail mix and flax crackers. Every two weeks or so, make some flax crackers with your favorite spices and vegetables. If they are dehydrated enough they can last several weeks, even longer.

Believe it or not, it does not get boring to eat the same raw dishes a few days in a row. Most people already do that with cooked food.

I was encouraged by many people to make this section available for those of you who may need some guidelines to get started, but I encourage you to experiment and find the foods that resonate with you. For example, you may find that you want to drink the "Super Smoothie" every morning as I do.

One thing to remember is that after six months to a year, you will no longer crave complex recipes. You will be satisfied more and more with eating foods just as Mother Nature gives them to us in their simplest, most perfect, whole raw forms.

## Day 1

**Breakfast:** ½ cantaloupe

**Snack:**     1 handful of olives

**Lunch:**     Cream of Spinach Soup (see recipe)

**Dinner:**    Raw Pizza (see recipe)

**Snack:**     Garlic Cilantro Flax Crackers (see recipe) with raw almond butter or Deluxe Macadamia Nut Cheese (see recipe)

# Day 2

**Breakfast:** Banana Milk Shake (see recipe) or Super Smoothie (see recipe)

**Snack:** Fruit of your choice, one piece

**Lunch:** Arabian Salad (see recipe)

**Dinner:** Chinese Stir "Fry" (see recipe)

**Snack:** Frozen Fruit Ice Cream (see recipe)

# Day 3

**Breakfast:** 3 T raw, dehydrated, green vegetable juice with a pinch of cayenne

**Snack:** Fruit of your choice, 1 or 2 pieces

**Lunch:** Coleslaw (see recipe)

**Dinner:** Nori Rolls (see recipe)

**Snack:** Garlic Cilantro Flax Crackers (see recipe) or other flax crackers of your choice with Guacamole (see recipe)

# Day 4

**Breakfast:** Smoothie (see recipes)

**Snack:** Fruit of your choice, 1 or 2 pieces

**Lunch:** Fresh green leafy vegetable mix with Honey Mustard Dressing (see recipe), sprinkled with soaked and dried walnuts

**Dinner:** Vegetable Chowder (see recipe)

**Snack:** Raw Cake (see recipe)

# Day 5

**Breakfast:** Fruit of your choice, 1 or 2 pieces

**Snack:** Trail Mix (see recipe)

**Lunch:** Holiday Salad (see recipe)

**Dinner:** Tomato Raviolis (see recipe)

**Snack:** Carob Mint Soda (see recipe)

# Day 6

**Breakfast:** Trail Mix (see recipe)

**Snack:** Fruit of your choice, 1 or 2 pieces

**Lunch:** Everybody's Favorite Celery-Cilantro Soup (see recipe)

**Dinner:** Spaghetti (see recipe)

**Snack:** Cauliflower Pâté ("Mashed Potatoes") (see recipe)

# Day 7

**Breakfast:** Al's Cereal (see recipe)

**Snack:** Raw Candy (see recipe)

**Lunch:** Raw Hummus (see recipe) with fresh cucumber slices

**Dinner:** Creamy Carrot Soup (see recipe)

**Snack:** Freshly cut cucumbers, tomatoes, carrots and celery dipped in Creamy Spinach Dip (see recipe)

# Sample Seasonal Hygienic Menus

On the next page, Victoria BidWell shares some menus from *The Health Seekers' YearBook*, Chapter 9, "The Year in Live-Food Menus":

The meals are all-raw and properly combined for ideal digestion, with exact amounts specified to serve one person. These whole food menus are completely wholesome with neither protoplasmic poisons nor transition compromises. They are stunning to the eye when attractively arranged. They are satisfying and filling when genuine hunger is brought to the table. They take just two minutes to prepare and even less time to clean up after. They are neither fragmented nor compromised in nutrition due to processing. And of course when a health seeker cannot chew effectively, these menus must be Vita-Mixed or otherwise processed.

Enjoy!

### Spring Breakfast

½ head butter lettuce
¼ pineapple
1 grapefruit
2 oranges
2 oz almonds

### Spring Lunch

3 leaves green cabbage
1 beefsteak tomato
1 cup mung bean
    sprouts
1 stalk broccoli
1 red bell pepper
2 stalks celery
1 avocado

### Spring Dinner

½ head butter lettuce
$^1/_8$ head savoy cabbage
10 cherry tomatoes
1 cup peas from the pod
12 snow peas
2 oz sunflower seeds

### Summer Breakfast

3 romaine lettuce leaves
6 apricots
1 peach
1 nectarine
3 fresh figs
3 huge strawberries
1 celery heart
1 avocado

### Summer Lunch

1 baby bok choy
3 tomatoes on the vine
3 pickling cucumbers
1 red bell pepper
1 young zucchini
12 sugar snap peas
2 oz cashews

### Summer Dinner

3 leaves red leaf lettuce
10 large strawberries
1 cup raspberries
1 cup blackberries
2 stalks celery
2 oz walnuts

### Fall Breakfast

mixed lettuce leaves
3 oranges
3 kiwis
1 grapefruit
2-3 oz almonds

### Fall Lunch

1 heart buttercrunch
    lettuce
3 ears sweet corn on the
    cob
½ cup each sprouts:
mung, lentil, alfalfa
1 avocado

### Fall Dinner

bed of mixed lettuce
    leaves
1 tart apple
1 sweet apple
1 persimmon
1 pear
3 fresh prunes
2 stalks celery

### Winter Breakfast

3 romaine lettuce leaves
2 tangelos
2 tangerines
1 pomegranate
2 stalks celery
1 oz each: pecans,
    filberts, brazils

### Winter Lunch

3 leaves green leaf
    lettuce
2 bananas
2 persimmon
1 cup red flame grapes
5 dates
2 stalks celery

### Winter Dinner

6 leaves purple cabbage
6 leaves spinach
10 cherry tomatoes
3 florets broccoli
3 florets cauliflower
1 kohlrabi
1 cucumber
2 stalks celery
1 avocado

# Veggie Volt! Tomato Bolt! Ginger Jolt! Instead of Coffee!

Victoria BidWell and I want to give you a final, best kept food preparation secret: how to stay raw with dried, live food seasonings that contain no SAD, protoplasmic poisons whatsoever and that add flavor beyond description! The small amount of onion used in the four formulas is considered a natural "true transition seasoning" by Dr. Vetrano and is allowed by the purists in small amounts as an item that will not compromise health. Victoria just turned me on to all four flavors, and I am hooked! She serves them up, packed tight, in traditional glass quart canning jars. But you can be sure that they have not been canned with heat. The glass jars and their rubber seals do keep the moisture out, the flavors in and the eyes attracted when the "uncanning" jars sit on my kitchen counter.

Victoria shares the following:

Dear Health Seekers! Fruit-based recipes are so yummy, you never need to season them up! But the raw veggie, sprout and nut-based recipes for appetizers, beverages, salads, slaws, patés, mock meats, "handwiches," pizzas, burgers, burritos, spaghettis, croutons, crackers, breads, soups, chowders, stews, dressings, dips, sauces and so on can sometimes be so bland and boring that all they do is inspire some of us to head for greener SAD pastures and get our kicks from the protoplasmic poisons in processed foods. By contrast, in my special raw seasoning formulas, the flavors of the ingredients are all kicked up several notches from their fresh versions because the water has been dehydrated out, and the natural aromas and tastes have been concentrated within. You get an electrifying high-voltage kick in Veggie Volt! You get a lightninglike deliverance in Tomato Bolt! You get the highest kick of all four in Ginger Jolt! And you get something warm, calming, soothing, delicious and good for you to sip on with Instead of Coffee! Following are the descriptions and ingredients of my four flavors.

• **Veggie Volt!** is the mildest in flavor and the most favored of the four by most of my GetWell friends: raw and dried carrot, tomato, spinach, parsley and onion powder; parsley and celery flakes, and celery seeds and sweet basil.

• **Tomato Bolt!** is my most favorite: raw and dried tomato, beet, parsley and onion powders; parsley and celery flakes, and celery seeds, dill weed and sweet basil.

• **Ginger Jolt!** is preferred by those who want a bigger kick than any of the others give, as the ginger root jolts the tastebuds and brings otherwise flat recipes to life: raw and dried tomato, parsley, onion and a tiny amount of ginger powder; celery seeds, and dill weed and sweet basil.

• **Instead of Coffee!** is made of raw, dried and powdered tomato, parsley and onion. With no added crunchy ingredients, the powders dissolve completely and instantly in warm water, and the brew is an amazingly comforting drink to have — instead of coffee!

# Appendix A
## Killer "Foods" to Avoid

If people let the government decide what foods they eat and what medicines they take, their bodies will soon be in as sorry a state as are the souls who live under tyranny.
—Thomas Jefferson (1743–1826)

If you're going to America, bring your own food.
—Fran Lebowitz (1950–), US journalist

Some "foods" are simply not natural foods for humans. They slowly poison us and are therefore deadly. "But aren't we omnivores?" you might ask. Most of us are omnivores in practice, but that doesn't mean our bodies are omnivorous by nature.

You might decide to call your car an "omnifueler" and mix some other ingredients into your tank along with the gasoline, but how long would it take before the engine would be messed up? How much mileage would you get for the gallon? How long would your car last?

Most people would never imagine doing that to their vehicles yet think nothing of doing it to their bodies. They worry about the financial cost of repairing or replacing their ruined cars, rarely pondering that their bodies are irreplaceable regardless of the amount of money they have.

Nutritionists point out that we have expanded our range of foods throughout history. Chefs are proud of their culinary creativity. Food engineers tempt us with their sweet and salty inventions. Yet few have realized the correlation between our degenerating health and all the new food variations.

"Well, I have to die someday," is a common response when someone is invited to consider that just maybe these innovative food novelties contribute to bad health. It is true that we are all destined to die, but how many of us want to spend our final years with crippling arthritis, diabetes, Alzheimer's and the numerous other pathologies of old age? Wouldn't it be prudent to find out what some of the dietary blunders of modern man are so that you could remain in great health right up to the end?

There is an old saying, "The history of disease is the history of agriculture." Humans did not begin eating grains until the dawn of agriculture, which was only 10,000-20,000 years ago, not much time compared to our millions of years of evolution. The development of grain consumption, along with its processing and preparation techniques, led to the use of refined sugar, salt, fats and alcohol. It also led to the refining away of most of whatever nutrition these grains once contained.

Adherents to the paleolithic diet are quick to point out that heart disease, cancer, obesity, diabetes, osteoporosis, rheumatoid arthritis and other diseases of affluence were very rare or nonexistent among recent hunters and gatherers, such as the Bushmen, Amazonian Indians and Australian Aborigines, until they started to eat Western foods and adopt our lifestyles.

Around the same time that agriculture began, people started domesticating cattle and consuming their milk. They made vessels to store it in. Various experts have concluded from both anthropological and nutritional research that very few people can properly digest the milks of other species. Cow's milk is excellent for a baby calf but can be quite detrimental to a baby, child or adult human.

In addition, few of us can adequately digest grains, in particular gluten grains, especially wheat, one of the most common foods we eat. Grains are for the birds: birds are graminivores. Severen Schaeffer (*Instinctive Nutrition*) believed that the two classes of foods that contribute most severely to stress are cereals and dairy.

You might think, "Wait a minute! But I learned about the four basic food groups in school, two of which were dairy and bread!" (And cooked meat, don't forget, was another.) Internationally known nutritionist Dr. Mary Ruth Swope, among others, says that the "four basic food groups" were nothing but the result of a clever advertising ploy designed primarily to benefit the dairy and meat industries. I would add that this advertising campaign benefited the grain industries too, although they probably didn't invest as much money in its publicity.

In fact the dairy industrialists use the public school system as their primary advertising target. They give free "educational" (marketing) materials to teachers, who are often overwhelmed with curriculum development and welcome ready-made materials. They have a web site containing over 70,000 lesson plans for teachers to use! Dairy marketing is so effective that even the most health-conscious people, even the author of this book, cannot easily erase the implanted idea that "milk does a body good."

As David Klein says, "Our commercial masters, who endow our educational institutions and pay for most advertising, control the American dietary profession and almost totally determine the pathogenic American diet" (*Your Natural Diet*, p. 13).

The replacement for the four basic food groups, the original food "pyramid," is not much, if any, better. The revised food pyramid (dubbed "My Pyramid") is more of the same. *It actually includes salt, sugar, condiments, candies, syrups and other man-made atrocities as a food group!*

The biggest change from the old pyramid is that the food groups are no longer presented horizontally. Rainbow-colored, vertical stripes now represent much the same disastrous diet, all with official government approval.

Through studies, such as those done by the Food and Nutrition Board, the government tells us that a diet high in refined sugar, fat, animal protein and dairy is good for us. Most people don't realize the power wielded by the food industries over the conclusions reached in these studies. They are nearly always funded by food corporations, and the "independent" researchers involved know that their future grant money depends on their coming up with industry-favorable results.

Food conglomerate lobbyists court politicians to set government dietary standards in the industry's favor. Executives of these food giants buy influence by contributing to politicians' election campaign funds and offering countless other forms of gratuities. As the documentary *Eating* points out, "There's a politician in your kitchen, and he's already decided what you'll be eating tonight!"

Because so many unsuspecting people trust government to look out for their health and believe in these studies, *they affect the health of most Americans by influencing the food served in schools, hospitals, orphanages, prisons, mental institutions, day-care centers, nursing homes and the diets recommended by trained nutritionists and dieticians.*

Dr. T. Colin Campbell served on the committee that wrote the report (and later book) *Diet, Nutrition and Cancer*, one of the first investigations into the relationship between diet and cancer. He quickly learned that scientists in the world of health and nutrition were not free to pursue their research wherever it might lead.

"Coming to the 'wrong' conclusions, even through first-rate science, can damage your career," Campbell wrote in *The China Study* (p. 265). He learned that the career of a sincere scientist, trying to get the truth out for the sake of people's health, would be damaged due to the powerful forces of the food and drug industries that would lose huge profits if people actually ate more natural foods.

We are living in a world in which people subsist on what can barely be called "food." Some foodstuffs have been so transformed by technology, such as sugar beets/cane and wheat, that the final products made from these foods bear no resemblance to their original forms.

To top it off, nonfood chemicals have been refined or manufactured and added to nearly all processed foods and many restaurant foods. Most prominent and dangerous among them are salt, MSG, aspartame, various "preservatives," corn syrup, hydrogenated oils and "natural flavors."

As a teacher in the public school system, I always knew it would be much harder to teach after lunch. The easiest day I ever had teaching in the public school system was when I was substituting at a Los Angeles school in which the children ate lunch one hour before going home. More usual is two or three hours.

Teachers everywhere try to save the least important material for after lunch. The children become extremely hyperactive from having ingested all of these foreign molecules that interfere with their brains' functioning.

Teaching children is particularly difficult at the high school level where the kids can buy chips and sodas instead of the less harmful sandwich option. Some of them become hyperactive, while others fall asleep from hypoglycemia. School systems earn sales commissions by vending these junk foods. School officials rationalize that the kids would buy them anyway, so the schools may as well share in the profits from these sales.

However, there was one alternative school in Wisconsin where administrators were smart enough to change this practice by offering only whole foods, albeit cooked. (Search the Internet for "Miracle in Wisconsin.") The school was also filmed in the documentary *Super Size Me*. The kids in this school shaped up, focused on their schoolwork, and achieved better grades. The school ended up saving so much money from lack of vandalism that they still came out ahead despite paying more for the wholesome food and losing out on junk food kickback money.

Even if you decide not to pursue paradisiacal health with a 100% raw food diet, you would do well to avoid these "*killer foods*":

# The Four White Evils:
# Wheat, Dairy, Sugar and Salt

Even if you don't go the entirely raw route, you can gain tremendous health benefits by omitting the "four white evils" from your diet: dairy products, refined salt, sugar and wheat — as well as other processed gluten grains. *Many times, it is not just what we eat that keeps us healthy, but also what we omit from our diet.*

These four "foods" have been so highly refined and processed that they can no longer be considered real foods. Before the food pyramid, schools taught that we needed to get a certain number of daily servings of (1) dairy, (2) bread and cereals, (3) meat and (4) fruits and vegetables.

Decades later there was an attempt to update the recommendations with the development of the food "pyramid." But the food industry didn't approve release of its initial version — it was *too healthful*, which would have lost business for them! — so we ended up with a much watered-down, revised version, which has recently been revised again.

Mental and emotional health is very negatively impacted by eating these "foods." A chief probation officer, Barbara Reed Stitt, was able to get the criminals she worked with to turn their entire lives around simply by omitting these four unnatural foods! She proved that the delinquent mind could be healed by diet change alone and that the biochemistry of the criminal mind is created in part by the insane American diet. She wrote all about her work with criminals in her book *Food & Behavior*.

## Grains, but Especially Wheat!

Some people find that they can handle some grains in moderation, at least in sprouted form. Quinoa seems to be one of the easier ones. Many authorities on nutrition — including my own digestive system! — feel nonetheless that grains should not be one of the main staples of our diet. Though they can make great transition foods for raw fooders, most eventually choose to bypass grains, as they enjoy the lightness in their digestive system that comes from eating the foods that require less energy to digest.

Dr. Joseph Mercola points out in *The No-Grain Diet: Conquer Carbohydrate Addiction and Stay Slim for Life* that nutritional anthropologists have compiled data from fossil records and other sources that indicate humans are designed to fare better on a hunter/gatherer's diet than on an agricultural one. Since we began eating grains 10,000-20,000 years ago, there have been increases in infectious diseases, tooth decay, osteoporosis and diabetes. Even the organic, unhybridized grains of ancient times led to these negative health consequences.

Our genetic makeup is still that of the paleolithic hunter/gatherer, according to Dr. Loren Cordain, PhD, author of *Paleo Diet: Lose Weight and Get Healthy by Eating the Food You Were Designed to Eat*. In other words, we are meant to eat wild meats, fruits and vegetables, but not cereal grains.

Dr. Mercola concurs with Cordain and maintains that one of the most critical problems with grain consumption is the ensuing blood glucose elevation. This triggers cravings for sweets, the consumption of which further exacerbates the problem.

During the last few decades, doctors have recommended cutting back on fat. The result has been disastrous. Americans have consumed cooked grains and other highly glycemic carbohydrates more than ever, thus contributing to diabetes and obesity. "Fat-free" packaged foods are notoriously high in sugars and refined starches, which stimulate insulin release, causing fat storage and leading to diabetes.

High levels of blood insulin also suppress the secretion of human growth hormone and increase hunger. These levels are believed by longevity experts to be a key factor in aging. Chronic excess insulin released into the bloodstream contributes to a number of pathological developments: sustained food cravings, blood pressure and cholesterol elevation, cancer cell proliferation, osteoporosis, adult onset diabetes and a shortened lifespan.

Another problem presented by grain consumption is that grains are high in yeast/fungus/mold. Commercially stored grains ferment in 90 days, during which time mycotoxins are produced. Grains that are not stored for long periods in grain elevators — spelt, amaranth, quinoa, millet, buckwheat and wild rice — do not present such a mycotoxin hazard.

Yet another serious problem with grains is that most of them also leave an acid ash when digested, which can be very bad for health when overindulged. Amaranth, millet, buckwheat and quinoa are among the few grains that are alkaline forming upon digestion.

Most people are more or less "gluten intolerant" and should not eat the following grains: wheat, rye, barley, oats, spelt, triticale, kamut and farina.

Severe gluten intolerance without a proper diet leads to celiac disease or dermatitis herpetiformis. Celiac disease is characterized by diarrhea, weight loss, irritable bowel syndrome and/or other signs of indigestion. Milder forms of gluten insensitivity include allergies and asthma.

Many holistic doctors believe that grains are also implicated in autoimmune diseases, such as rheumatoid arthritis, MS, underactive thyroid and skin rashes.

In *The 80/10/10 Diet* (p. 92), Dr. Doug Graham claims that exposure to the insoluble fibers of grains, even raw and sprouted grains, is very harsh on our delicate digestive tracts. The sharp edges and points of these fibers scrape at the delicate digestive tract walls, thus irritating and cutting them as if we had eaten ground glass!

When wheat is referred to as the "staff of life," remember that a *staff* is a crutch, and a crutch is not something one needs for support when times are good. Grains have long shelf lives, thus proving vital in times of famine, thereby offering crutchlike support in the face of starvation.

While wheat may contain many nutrients, this does not necessarily mean it is good for us or easy to digest. In fact wheat is second only to dairy in the number of illnesses, both physical and mental, which its consumption has precipitated in unsuspecting consumers.

According to Carlton Fredericks, author of *Psycho-Nutrition*, "In Europe during World War II, when wheat imports were reduced by 50%, schizophrenic admissions to the mental wards fell by nearly the same percentage. In Formosa, the natives eating very little grain are reported to have a schizophrenic rate nearly two-thirds less than that of northern Europe."

Wheat contains morphinelike opioid peptides, which are addictive and stimulate the appetite. This explains why food manufacturers put wheat in everything. It is even hidden in items like ketchup under names like "modified starch." Gluten was found to contain fifteen different opioid sequences which, when ingested and assimilated, interfere with normal brain chemistry and result in learning disabilities.

In an article entitled "Schizophrenia and dietary neuroactive peptides," T. C. Dohan discusses how wheat and other glutens create endorphic activity, which is probably what makes them addictive, and also induce schizophrenia in people who are particularly sensitive. Whole wheat contains more fiber and nutrients than refined wheat, but whole wheat also has more gluten, which wreaks havoc on our nervous systems.

In a lecture, Dr. Gabriel Cousens described watching a normal, healthy woman being injected with a wheat extract. Within three minutes, the woman became schizophrenic, complete with hallucinations!

Grains are not considered an initial food by instinctive eaters (see Appendix C) since, as mentioned previously, humans have been eating them for such a brief time period historically. If you find a raw grain, it will probably taste bitter. Even if you sprout it, it won't taste that wonderful. Grains need a lot of processing to become tasty and edible. Because of this, the wheat we use today is so highly processed and genetically manipulated that the body does not even recognize wheat as a real food. It has become a toxin.

According to Severen Schaeffer, the wheat eaten today is so hybridized that it will not produce a taste change among instinctive eaters. Even chickens, which eat instinctively, will gorge themselves upon it.

The processing of grains employs many toxic chemicals, including mercury, cyanide, salt, chlorine, alum, aspartame, ammonium, mineral oil and fluorine.

Wheat is found in nearly every American meal in the form of bread, pasta, pizza, cereal, cake, cookies, doughnuts and more. Wheat can also be constipating because much of the fiber has been refined out.

I say, "Bread makes you dead." My mother was a big bread eater, and its toxic byproducts clogged her colon. Naturopathic doctors say that "death begins in the colon" because the large intestine is a primary excretory organ, second only to the liver. If the colon is compromised, toxins accumulate in the body. My mother died of kidney cancer, and I believe her high wheat diet had a lot to do with it. My suspicion was confirmed when the *International Journal of Cancer* (October 2006) published an Italian study linking bread consumption with kidney cancer!

Grains also contain phytic acid, which leaves a potentially unbalancing acidic residue when metabolized. Grains are therefore potentially disease producing. Excess acidity means the body will draw upon important alkaline minerals, like calcium and magnesium, from bones and teeth to maintain blood pH balance, thus leading to osteoporosis and dental problems.

Grains also may ferment in one's intestines, producing alcohol and gas. Many a classic case of liver cirrhosis has been recorded in people who have never touched alcohol.

David Wolfe, in *Eating for Beauty*, writes that products with wheat seeds can make the face puffy and the skin pale and pasty.

In *Grain Damage*, Dr. Douglas Graham explains why governments convince us that grains are good for us. It is because all government leaders know that they must feed their people in order to stay in power, and grains are cheap foods with long shelf lives. If people were told that they needed fresh produce for optimal health and didn't have the money to feed their families accordingly, there might be a revolution. Therefore, generations upon generations have been convinced that wheat is healthful. Now even government officials have been fooled into believing their own propaganda.

On an ecological note, before the agricultural revolution's advent, the world's human population remained almost stable for about 200,000 years, doubling about every 20,000 years. Today, partly because grains are such cheap sources of food for the masses, world population is skyrocketing. It went from three billion in 1960 to six billion in 1999. It is projected to double again by 2050.

Thom Hartman, author of *The Last Hours of Ancient Sunlight*, predicts that when we run out of oil to run the agricultural machinery, billions could starve. Perhaps this could be averted if we focused on growing fruit trees, which feed many more people per acre than grains do and which don't rely as much on heavy farm machinery that depends on oil.

# Dairy

Americans have been conditioned since preschool with intense propagandizing by the powerful dairy lobbyists to think that milk is healthful. Probably no other food has been associated with health as much as milk! Yet according to *The China Study,* casein, the protein that makes up 87% of cow's milk protein, is one of the most dangerous foods you can eat. The author says that dairy is probably *the most relevant cancer-causing substance that we eat* (p. 104).

In a study conducted in India, mice were divided into two groups, one eating a diet of 20% protein and the other consuming only 5% protein. The protein used was casein. Both groups were exposed to equal amounts of the cancer-causing agent aflatoxin. One hundred percent of the group eating a diet of 20% casein got liver cancer, whereas none of the ones eating a diet low in this protein got cancer (*The China Study*, p. 47).

Casein adversely affects the way cells, especially their DNA, interact with carcinogens and the way that cancer cells grow. A diet high in casein allows more carcinogens to enter into the body's cells. This allows more carcinogens to bind to the DNA, fostering more mutagenic reactions that turn the cells cancerous, which in turn allow faster growth of tumors once they have been formed.

By adjusting the amount of dairy that we eat, we have the power to turn cancer growth off or on and to override the cancer-causing properties of aflatoxin and possibly other carcinogens!

*The China Study* also implicates dairy in Type I diabetes, MS, osteoporosis, prostate cancer, breast cancer and other diseases.

The web site www.notmilk.com lists numerous diseases and ailments that have been eliminated by people who merely stopped consuming dairy. What more evidence is needed that dairy is not a natural food for humans?

According to the documentary *Eating*, 70% of the population is lactose intolerant, especially non-Caucasians. Yet due to the powerful dairy lobby in the USA, milk is required drinking for all kids enrolled in federal lunch programs, "which amounts to nutritional persecution of non-Caucasians due to their high rates of lactose intolerance."

When babies are given cow's milk to drink, they often become colicky. *Yet something is thought to be wrong with the baby rather than with the drink!*

Dairy is not only almost always pasteurized, but with the recent rise of agribusiness techniques designed solely for profit in the dairy industry, milk comes from sick cows that are pumped up with antibiotics and hormones. In fact milk is filled with pus cells from these sick cows' udders! This situation was exacerbated when Monsanto's artificial growth hormone began to be fed to dairy cattle to boost milk production. Their milk began to routinely exceed FDA guidelines for pus cell content. Rather than ban the growth hormone, the FDA simply increased the allowable pus cell content to match what the dairy industry was producing.

Dr. Cousens cites studies that show a correlation between an increased incidence of leukemia in cows and in children who drank these cows' milk. He also cites a study in which 100% of the chimpanzees drinking milk from leukemic cows for one year also developed leukemia themselves (*Spiritual Nutrition*, pp. 261–262).

A woman wrote this about her children's experience with dairy:

My two children are now in their 20s, but when they were little, every kid I knew was having tubes put in their ears because they all kept getting ear infections, and the parents got tired of giving them so many rounds of antibiotics for years and years.

Mine would get the same ear infections; so with my son, I made an appointment to have the tubes put in (a surgical procedure in which they create a drain in the ears). A friend asked me why I would have tubes put in when all I had to do was take my son off dairy.

I'd never heard this before. I canceled the appointment, took my son off dairy, and he never had another ear infection. I did the same for my daughter: no more dairy, and she stopped getting ear infections and strep throat.

Dairy and soy just breed infection; it's as simple as that.

It is ridiculous to believe we need dairy to get enough calcium. Tall hominid skeletons have been found dating back millions of years, while man has been raising cattle and drinking their milk for a mere 10,000-20,000 years. By eating nuts, seeds and greens, we can receive adequate calcium that is actually much better absorbed and assimilated than that from cow's milk.

The documentary *Eating* points out that *there has not been a single case of calcium deficiency of dietary origin in the entire history of the human race*. The milk industry created this myth. Osteoporosis is caused largely by lack of weight-bearing exercise, insufficient Vitamin D and bone demineralization due to excessive consumption of acidic ash foods: meats, milk products, refined sugar and wheat, along with all the thousands of supermarket foods made from these four foods, including all junk foods.

If milk were so good for our bones, you would think that we would have one of the lowest rates of osteoporosis in the world. In fact those countries and regions that consume the most dairy have the *highest* rates of osteoporosis: the USA, England and Scandinavia.

Dairy, like meat, is high in protein, which leaves an acid ash residue upon metabolism. In its homeostatic efforts to neutralize the deadly acidic ash, the body removes alkaline minerals from the bones and teeth in order to neutralize this acidity. Furthermore, dairy is low in magnesium and high in phosphorus, which makes its calcium less bioavailable. Twenty-five to thirty million Americans have been diagnosed with osteoporosis. Of that figure, a quarter will end up in nursing homes, a quarter will never walk again unassisted, and a quarter will die of conditions related to bone fracture.

Osteoporosis is extremely rare in cultures that eat traditional plant-based diets. The best sources of bioavailable calcium are green vegetables like lettuce, broccoli, spinach, kale, dandelion and Swiss chard, as well as nuts and seeds. Greens can be juiced or blended to make them quick and easy to consume.

Sergei Boutenko broke his clavicle in a snowboarding accident. Subsequently, he constantly craved sesame milk, which is rich in calcium if unhulled seeds are used. The doctors said it would take eight to twelve weeks for him to heal. However, his body made speedy use of his high consumption of sesame seeds to expedite his healing. After two weeks, he actually grew a calcified ball over the injury that isolated the bones so they could knit properly (*12 Steps to Raw Food*, p. 14).

In the book *Biological Transmutation*, Louis Kervran describes using the herb horsetail grass, which is high in silica, to recalcify broken bones. This worked much better and faster than calcium supplementation. In a lecture, David Wolfe talked about a woman who used this method with amazing results to reverse her osteoporosis, astonishing her doctors, who said she would never recalcify to that extent.

Dairy has been found to influence mental as well as physical health. "When I investigated hyperactive children, I found that many of them were 'wild and crazy' because they were sensitive to dairy products," wrote Lendon Smith, MD, in *Dr. Lendon Smith's Low-Stress Diet Book*. Alexander Schauss, author of *Diet, Crime and Delinquency*, worked with juvenile offenders and found that 90% had milk intolerance or allergy. Many of these also drank twice the amount of milk as their peers.

Interestingly, Severen Schaeffer reported that all cancer patients examined under instinctive eating conditions carried very unpleasant odors, often reminiscent of putrefied milk. When the tumors shrank, the odors faded. The same odor of putrid dairy products was observed among autoimmune-compromised patients.

It appears there *may* be some people, however, who are genetically adapted to *raw* dairy, at least to some extent. These are mainly people of Northern European ancestry, especially from Scandinavian countries. However, to be considered healthful, the milk should be raw and from animals that have not been given steroid hormones, antibiotics or unnatural feed.

For more information on the perils of dairy, see Appendix C.

# Table Salt

Table salt, the primary constituent of which is sodium chloride, is an inorganic substance that is toxic. Supplementing your diet with this compound is in no way essential to human metabolism, contrary to what you may have been taught, even though sodium and chlorine as separate molecules each play important roles as electrolytes within our bodily fluids. In fact any use of table salt contributes to bodily toxicity. Table salt is rendered even more toxic by the refining process that strips away all of its other inorganic trace minerals and by the addition of harmful stabilizers and anticaking agents that may contain aluminum. These unnatural additives amount to 5% of table salt's bulk.

In her book *The Salt Conspiracy*, Victoria BidWell states that table salt "is responsible for upsetting fluid homeostasis, debilitating circulatory system function and precipitating and/or aggravating a number of salt pathologies: edema, obesity, hypertension, coronary heart disease, myocardial infarction [heart attack], angina pectoris, stroke, congestive heart failure, kidney failure, PMS, manic depression and many more."

Table salt is a protoplasmic poison. In more than tiny amounts, it kills plants as well as animals, which explains its popularity as a preservative: bacteria are prevented from growing in meat or other foods that have been pickled in brine.

Sodium is nonetheless an essential nutrient. Victoria explains:

> Naturally occurring sodium is necessary to the body for optimal health. Its primary roles are responsibility for maintaining fluid homeostasis, regulation of circulatory system function and normalization of nerve impulses. . . .
>
> The human body needs an estimated 200-280 mg of sodium daily to carry on the aforementioned functions, an amount fully supplied in the raw, fresh food diet. The average American on the Standard American Diet consumes between 4,000 and 6,000 mg daily. The heavy-salt eater consumes 10,000 mg ($^1/_8$ of a fatal dose). While an estimated 15% of this daily ingested sodium chloride comes from a saltshaker, the other 85% comes through other sources — but primarily, processed foods.

While some of the sodium and chlorine atoms found in fresh produce do occur in free ionic form that could be considered inorganic, most of these atoms come to us chemically bound, or *chelated*, to organic molecules, the types of molecules to which animal life is biologically suited to assimilating.

Fresh produce, nuts, seeds, sprouts and especially seaweed all contain sufficient amounts of these nutrients to render additional supplementation not only unnecessary, but even dangerous. Vegetables high in sodium include celery, spinach, chard and especially sea vegetables. Flesh foods are also quite high in naturally occurring sodium. You can get organic iodine from sea vegetables, such as dulse or kelp. Table salt contains only inorganic iodine.

We should be looking to live foods as our nutrient sources, not rocks. If you feel you must use salt at all, substitute Celtic sea salt or Himalayan rock salt in all recipes demanding salt. These are less refined than common table salt and contain no toxic chemical additives. Much better is to use sea vegetables or make or buy your own organic "salt" from dehydrated, ground up celery. Victoria also offers Tomato Bolt! Ginger Jolt! and Veggie Volt! as salt substitutes. These raw seasonings are so full of flavor that table salt is never missed.

Be advised that the use of salt as a condiment reinforces cooked food addiction. Victoria adds, "Salt is an addiction within an addiction. Quit the salt addiction, and half the battle to quitting the cooked food addiction is won."

Nearly all processed foods contain huge amounts of added salt, listed as sodium on the labels. Salt extends shelf life, enhances flavor, creates addiction and thus increases profits. Salt adds flavor to bland, lifeless food. Remember, the body needs merely 200-280 milligrams of sodium daily, yet the average American takes in 4,000-6,000 milligrams.

In *The Salt Conspiracy*, Victoria further points that since salt in the body holds 96 times its weight in water, the average American carries about 10-15 pounds of edema, or excess water weight, due to salt accumulation. This disrupts fluid balance, increases blood pressure and causes dehydration of blood capillaries. Half of Americans have high blood pressure by the age of 65, and high blood pressure is called a "silent killer" since one in four doesn't even know he has it.

According to Aajonus Vonderplanitz, four grains of salt (and he includes sea salt) destroys approximately two million red blood cells. It takes three hours to replace them and 24 hours to clear out the dead cells. Because the body removes nutrients from its tissues during these processes, salt speeds the aging process.

Victoria further argues that for all practical purposes, there is a conspiracy to lace so many foods with high doses of salt. When health professionals petitioned in 1981 for a bill to limit and label the sodium content of processed foods, over 100 Representatives signed on as co-sponsors of the legislation, and numerous health organizations, including the American Medical Association, were in favor of it. But the bill was withdrawn after Congressmen were wined and dined by food producers.

# Refined Sugar

Since the early 1900s, sugar consumption in America has increased tremendously. The average American today consumes 130-150 pounds of refined sugar a year. When sugar was rationed during World War II, the rate of diabetes dropped sharply. Refined sugar is largely responsible for the rise in processed carbohydrates that Americans eat. Refined sugar consumption results in raised insulin levels as well as rising rates of obesity, heart disease and diabetes.

Author T. S. Wiley declares, *"We are as addicted to a low-fat, high-sugar diet as alcoholics are to alcohol* because high insulin levels create the same brain state that alcohol does."

Most experts view refined sugar, or table sugar, as a drug rather than a food. In 1973, a Senate committee declared it to be an antinutrient. An *antinutrient* is 'any substance or drug that is in some way antagonistic to nutrients, interfering with their use or metabolism'.

At least 78 ailments have been linked to sugar consumption, which has skyrocketed in America, especially during the last few decades. The body reacts to refined sugar consumption the same as it does to any ingested toxin — with increased energy expenditure accompanied by lowered function, especially of its defense mechanisms. Body chemistry and mineral balances are disrupted as well. Refined sugar is implicated in tooth decay, alcoholism, obesity, diabetes, arthritis, asthma, hyperactivity, kidney damage, cancer, hypoglycemia, varicose veins, osteoporosis, depression and other mental disorders, headaches and many other ailments and diseases.

Yet sugar continues to be one of the main "comfort" and pick-me-up foods of Americans. We crave it because the fungi in our bodies (see Chapter 5) love sugar and will push us to eat sweets so that they can multiply and thrive. Eliminating sugar and even sweet fruits spells death to the fungi!

Good books on the pitfalls of sugar are *Lick the Sugar Habit* by Nancy Appleton and *Sugar Blues* by William Dufty.

# Excitotoxins

"Excitotoxins" are toxic, addictive chemicals, such as aspartame and MSG, commonly added to foods to "excite" (unnaturally stimulate) the brain and nervous system. They trick the brain into thinking the food is delicious, deepening addiction while causing cumulative damage to the nervous system over many years. Thus we have advertisements for chips that taunt us, "I bet you can't eat just one." This slogan defied 1970s consumers to eat "just one" as these chips were infused with MSG to induce bingeing and addiction.

Most people have complete trust that if a food additive were harmful, the FDA would outlaw it. In actuality, this organization works for the food and drug companies. (See Appendix B.) As Howard Lyman puts it, "[The] American people have been raised to believe that someone is looking out for their food safety. The disturbing truth is that the protection of the quality of our food is the mandate of foot-dragging bureaucrats at the US Department of Agriculture and the Food and Drug Administration who can generally be counted upon to behave not like public servants, but like hired hands of the meat and dairy industries" (*Mad Cowboy*, p. 20). In fact there have been cases in which someone working for the food industry temporarily got a job at the FDA in order to get a chemical approved for consumer use and then went back to the more lucrative position with the food company!

In the book *Excitotoxins: The Taste That Kills*, Dr. Russell Blaylock, MD, documents the cover-up to keep these chemicals legal despite the evidence that they are toxic to the brain and nervous system. Some of the potentially severe forms of damage include Parkinson's disease, Amyotrophic Lateral Sclerosis (ALS) — also known as Lou Gehrig's Disease — Alzheimer's, Huntington disease, brain tumors, seizures and learning and emotional disabilities. A pregnant woman consuming excitotoxins risks damaging the brain of her unborn child. This is thought to be one of the major causes, along with mercury from vaccinations, of the increase in learning disabilities and autism among children.

MSG has been used by food companies for about 50 years. Reactions vary from person to person. They intensify when one has not been ingesting it for several weeks. Reactions may include headache, insomnia, itching, nausea, vomiting, diarrhea, asthma, anxiety, panic attack, mental confusion, brain fog, mood swings, neurological disorders — Parkinson's, MS, ALS, Alzheimer's — behavioral disorders (especially in children and teens), skin rashes, runny nose, depression, bags under the eyes and more.

You might read a food label and think the product is safe if it does not list MSG. However, this is absolutely not the case. The FDA does not require the labeling of MSG if it is blended in with a mixture of spices or food additives, so it is usually hidden. This is because, in the 1970s, consumers became aware of the damage it does.

MSG is definitely hidden in anything labeled with the following: hydrolyzed protein, sodium caseinate, calcium caseinate, autolyzed yeast, yeast extract or gelatin. It is quite possibly in anything labeled with these ingredients: textured vegetable protein, carrageenan, vegetable gum, seasonings, spices, flavoring, natural flavorings, chicken, beef, pork, smoke flavorings, bouillon, broth, stock, barley malt, malt extract, malt flavoring, whey protein, whey protein isolate or concentrate, soy protein, soy protein isolate or concentrate, soy sauce or soy extract. One of the most common forms is "hydrolyzed vegetable protein." In other words, MSG is in nearly all boxed, canned and bagged foods, often even when you buy them at a health food store.

MSG is commonly found in soups, Chinese food, chips, processed foods (anything premade and packaged), nearly all fast foods and nearly all chain sit-down restaurant dishes. It enhances the flavor of dead, bland food. It intensely stimulates the tastebuds and olfactory nerves, an event the brain perceives as salty, high flavor. Many restaurants also use it to give their food a burst of flavor. It's what gives foods such as the skin of Kentucky Fried Chicken, most potato chips and microwave popcorn that strong, addictive flavor.

A research assistant at the University of Waterloo, John Erb, was wondering what was causing the massive obesity epidemic. He went through scientific journals and was shocked to learn that hundreds of studies around the world have shown that MSG is both toxic and addictive.

He learned that MSG is injected into rats and mice to make them obese when overweight rodents are needed for experiments since these animals are not naturally obese. The presence of MSG *triples* the amount of insulin the pancreas secretes, and insulin is a hormone that causes *fat storage*. In his book *The Slow Poisoning of America*, John exposes the food industry for getting people addicted to their food by adding this known poison.

Two good web sites to further educate you on this very important matter are www.truthinlabeling.org and www.msgtruth.org.

Sadly, the FDA has no limits as to how much MSG may be added to food. As a result, more and more gets used over the years. MSG poisoning has doubtless added to behavioral and health problems among children. Think of all the pregnant women eating at fast-food restaurants, risking their babies' health!

Aspartame is another primary excitotoxin. It has been used for years as a sweetener in soft drinks and has lately been put into numerous other foods. It is hidden in canned juices, protein powders, protein bars and much more. Its use has been linked to MS symptoms, brain tumors, sudden death in athletes, Parkinson's disease, brain fog, learning disabilities, ADHD, birth defects, diabetes, emotional disorders, seizures, migraines and more. Diabetics and young women are at particular risk, as they drink a lot of diet soft drinks.

A good web site for information on aspartame is www.dorway.com. A good book on its perils is *Sweet Poison* by Dr. Janet Starr Hull. There are two documentaries about aspartame entitled *Sweet Misery* and *Sweet Remedy*.

A friend of mine performed an experiment in which she fed aspartame to mice. She wrote a report about it and showed me the photos of the poor mice with tumors half the size of their bodies!

After being about 95% raw and cleaned out for some time — and therefore acutely sensitive — I unknowingly drank something with a bit of aspartame in it.

I experienced, for a brief flash, a loss of muscle control, spilling a container of raw soup all over the floor! I knew it was not clumsiness on my part but rather a brief experience of what it was like to have MS. My husband reported similar nerve problems after taking the same beverage. This chemical is insidiously being sneaked into processed foods in America without even being labeled as such.

Not only is aspartame deadly, but also this "diet" product actually makes you *gain weight*! The body reacts to its ingestion with suppressed thyroid function. Aspartame is thought to make you store fat. Kevin Trudeau describes an experiment he conducted in which people replaced their diet sodas with regular sodas, and 80% of the people lost weight after two weeks (*Natural Cures "They" Don't Want You to Know About*, p. 160).

For those seeking low-calorie, low-carbohydrate substitutes, Splenda — the brand name for sucralose — is also very dangerous. Some of its side effects include: a shrunken thymus gland, enlarged kidneys and liver, atrophy of lymph follicles, decreased red blood cell count, aborted pregnancy, decreased fetal weight, diarrhea and more. "Splenda Is Not Splendid" is one of the web site articles that expose its toxic qualities, located at www.wnho.net/splenda.htm. Just plug "toxic reaction Splenda" into an Internet search engine to learn more.

The best low-calorie sweetener is stevia, a natural and nontoxic plant. Because it is 200 times sweeter than sugar, only tiny amounts are needed. Because stevia often has an unpleasant aftertaste, many people are replacing it with raw agave nectar. It is very sweet and does not induce low blood sugar since it does not stimulate the pancreas to produce or release insulin.

# Soy

It may come as a shock to many readers to learn that soy, having been cleverly marketed as a health food for many years, can actually be toxic! While it contains all the essential amino acids, omega-3 fatty acids and B Vitamins, its toxic properties make it an undesirable food choice except when fermented and used sparingly as a condiment, which is how the Asians consume it. They generally have only two teaspoons of soy a day.

The Gerson Institute puts soy on its forbidden food list. The Vitamin $B_{12}$ analogs in soy are not absorbed and actually increase the body's need for $B_{12}$. The high levels of phytic acid in soy reduce assimilation of calcium, magnesium, copper, iron and zinc. The high temperatures used to process soy make its protein largely indigestible and useless as a nutrient.

Children fed soy are especially at risk due to the high levels of phytoestrogens in soy. Girls fed ample soy products develop prematurely. Boys experience delayed or retarded sexual development, some even becoming sterile or developing breasts. *Some boys have sexual organs that don't mature!* Infants fed exclusively soy-based formulas have 13-22 *thousand* times more estrogen compounds in their blood than babies fed milk-based formula. This is the estrogenic equivalent of five birth control pills a day!

Soy consumption leads to many more problems. The excess of phytoestrogens is thought to lead to estrogen-dependent tumors as well. Soy foods are also bad for the thyroid and can cause fatigue, weight gain, depression and/or moodiness in people with an existing thyroid problem. Soy contains high levels of aluminum, toxic to the nervous system, kidneys and brain. Free glutamic acid (MSG) is formed during soy processing, and MSG is added to many soy foods. A Hawaiian study found a correlation between eating two or more servings of tofu a week and accelerated brain aging and even development of Alzheimer's disease. The vast majority of soy in the USA is genetically modified. Soy is found in an estimated 70% of processed foods in the USA.

# The Corruption of Our Food Supply through Processing, Refining and Preserving

Victoria BidWell describes how the food processing industry denatures our food:

> The food giants employ three artificial techniques to create the thousands of designer foods placed before us in today's supermarkets: heat processing, refining and preserving. These techniques render whole, fresh, raw foods unrecognizable when competing for shelf space against fresh produce, our natural diet:
>
> • Heat processing (cooking) destroys certain vitamins, minerals and all of the enzymes.
> • Refining breaks the food into various parts, resulting in fragmentation of the whole food into a fiberless material and/or an otherwise unbalanced source of nutrition.
> • Preserving employs the addition of chemicals, euphemistically called "nonnutritive substances," to basic foodstuffs. All of these substances are protoplasmic poisons. Chemical adulteration includes these toxic additives: preservatives, buffers, neutralizers, moisture controls, coloring agents, flavorings, physiologic activity controls, bleaches, maturing agents, stabilizers, processing aids and other supplements.
>
> Now consider what happens when you apply all three of these techniques at once to the food! Is it any wonder that this food is making us chronically unhealthy?

By contrast, raw fooders may employ minimal processing via chopping, dicing, shredding and so on. They employ minimal refining via juicing and use minimal preserving via dehydration and chilling/freezing, which slow down the enzymatic degradation of fresh foods.

Americans eat more processed foods than ever: foods from boxes, cans, bags, jars and the like. Most of these foods have the life force cooked out of them several times over and are loaded with salt and sugar to enhance their taste and preserve them. In addition, most contain excitotoxins, wheat, sugar, salt and other chemicals to enhance taste, create addiction for the consumer, and/or preserve the food. Processed foods have far less food value than natural foods apart from calories. They do not enhance life but only destroy health, slowly sucking out your life force. As Jack LaLanne says, "If man made it, don't eat it!"

America's processed, refined and adulterated foods are so altered and contaminated that many overweight people could eat the same exact food types living abroad and yet lose weight! This happened to me when I lived in Mexico. It also happened to Kevin Trudeau, as he explains in *Natural Cures "They" Don't Want You to Know About* (p.157). This is because the chemicals found in our domestic processed-food products wreak havoc on our digestive organs, preventing them from operating correctly.

According to Trudeau, who has talked to many food industry insiders, *there are over 15,000 toxic chemicals added to our food that do not require labeling*. Since our brains are 70% fatty tissue, a large percentage of those consumed chemicals are stored in the brain, leading to depression, stress, anxiety, learning disabilities and possibly Alzheimer's disease. He estimates that over 95% of all processed food purchased has up to 300 chemicals added to each product that are not even listed on the label. The power of the food lobbyists working for the food industry rivals that of the drug company lobbyists working for the medical/pharmaceutical complex. (See Appendix B.)

Most of the sugar Americans eat is concealed in processed foods. Of the 2½ pounds of sugar the average American eats per week, 1½ pounds comes from high fructose corn sweetener used in processed foods, and it is six times as sweet as sugar. Low-fat or zero-fat foods are especially high in this sweetener to compensate for the loss of flavor from omitting the fat.

Processed foods are also loaded with hydrogenated fats. During the process of hydrogenation, the shape of the fatty acid changes into a dangerous "trans" configuration, or *trans fat*. Hydrogenated soy or palm oil is in most packaged foods, as this extends their shelf lives. The body simply can't handle hydrogenated oils. Some symptoms of ill health that seem to come out of nowhere are actually caused by trans fat ingestion: examples are bloating, sore throat and acne.

Research shows conclusively that trans fats contribute to Type II diabetes. Their ingestion also increases the risk of heart disease, cancer and autoimmune disease. Over 100 studies have been ignored by the FDA and mainstream media because of the potential economic impact on processed food industries. Furthermore, as a person continues to eat fat in this form, he is getting even less of the essential fatty acids needed for mental and physical health. New York City has even banned trans fats from restaurants!

Processed foods may also contain Olestra (also known as Olean), a substance found in fat-free snack foods. Olestra is a fat substitute that goes through the body undigested but unfortunately takes fat-soluble vitamins with it. Because it is a fat substitute, it becomes a large percentage of the food item. As a result, large quantities of what T. S. Wiley calls a "nonfat, two-molecules-away-from-plastic solution" are consumed.

For example, one fat-free potato chip with Olestra is made up of one-third Olestra. When Olestra is allowed to be placed in nonsnack foods, Americans who fall for the fat-free gimmick will find themselves slowly dying of vitamin and essential fatty acid deficiencies — if they aren't already.

Those who consume Olestra are also denying themselves the health benefits of real, raw, healthful fat. Real fat is needed by the body to create hormones, feed the brain, and perform many other vital bodily functions. Real fat is also needed to control the glycemic response to food, slowing down the absorption of sugar so that hypoglycemia and, later, diabetes do not evolve.

Additional killer ingredients in processed foods are sucrose, fructose, maltose, dextrose, polydextrose, corn syrup, molasses, sorbitol, maltodextrin, high fructose corn syrup, margarine, BHA, BHT, sulfates, sulfites, dyes and colorings.

Here is the list of ingredients for the popular cake snack known as Twinkies:

> **Ingredients:** Enriched bleached wheat flour (flour, ferrous sulfate [iron], B vitamins [niacin, thiamine mononitrate {B$_1$}, riboflavin {B$_2$}, folic acid]), sugar, water, corn syrup, high fructose corn syrup, vegetable and/or animal shortening (contains one or more of: partially hydrogenated soybean, cottonseed or canola oil, beef fat), dextrose, whole eggs. Contains 2% or less of: modified cornstarch, cellulose gum, whey, leavenings (sodium acid pyrophosphate, baking soda, monocalcium phosphate), salt, cornstarch, corn flour, mono- and diglycerides, soy lecithin, polysorbate 60, sodium and calcium caseinate, soy protein isolate, sodium stearoyl lactylate, wheat gluten, calcium sulfate, natural and artificial flavors, sorbic acid (to retain freshness), color added (yellow #5 and #6, red #40).

The only ingredient that is really a natural, unadulterated food is the "whole eggs," which comprises only a minor part of the recipe and is no doubt also cooked.

Now compare that with this recipe, adapted from *Eating without Heating* by Sergei and Valya Boutenko, for a delicious raw cake:

> **Body of cake:** Mix in blender or food processor 2 cups raw almond butter, 3½ cups shredded coconut, ½ cup agave and ¼ cup sun-dried raisins or dates.
>
> **Icing:** Blend together 2 cups raw cashews, 4 T raw agave nectar, 2 t vanilla extract, ½ cup fresh coconut butter (use fresh dates if not available) and ½ cup water.
>
> This recipe takes 15 minutes to prepare.

Which one do you think would taste better, the raw cake or the processed cake? Which one do you think would be more health enhancing to your body? Of course the raw, natural cake does cost more. It won't keep for more than a week. Which one would be cheaper and more profitable to mass-produce?

Here is something Dr. Max Gerson said in a speech *in 1956*. If it was that bad in 1956 — the year I was born! — think how bad it must be now!

> But our modern food, the "normal" food people eat, is bottled, poisoned, canned, color added, powdered, frozen, dipped in acids, sprayed — no longer normal. We no longer have living, normal food. Our food and drink is a mass of

dead, poisoned material, and one cannot cure very sick people by adding poisons to their systems. We cannot detoxify our bodies when we add poisons through our food, which is one of the reasons why cancer is so much on the increase. Saving time in the kitchen is fine, but the consequences are terrible. Thirty or fifty years ago [and remember, this speech was written in 1956] cancer was a disease of old age. . . . Now one out of three dies of cancer.

This was published in *Physiological Chemistry and Physics*, 1978, Vol. 10, Issue 5, pp. 449–464.

Now because of the nightmarish consequences of processed foods, we are experiencing a nearly 50% rate of cancer in the USA. Soon, it will be much worse if people don't wake up and reclaim their health from the processed food industries!

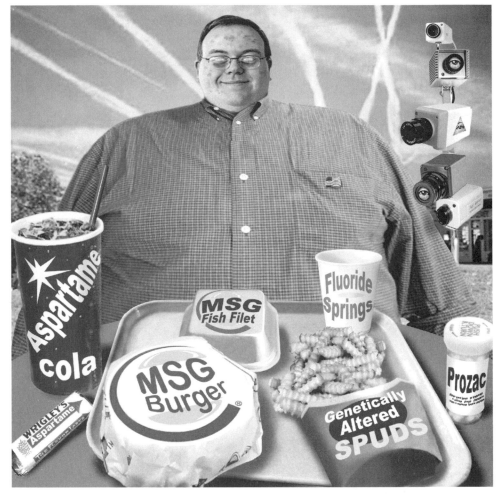

# Appendix B
## The Drug Story

The whole imposing edifice of modern medicine
is like the celebrated Tower of Pisa — slightly off balance.
—Charles, Prince of Wales (1948–), *Observer*

You might wonder why I am going into the "dirt" on the pharmaceutical industry. It is because of Claudia. Claudia was one of my first raw food students. She was enthusiastic about the diet but couldn't let go of her chemotherapy to treat her breast cancer so insisted on using both. I tried to warn her that even a raw food diet could not compensate for the toxicity that she would be exposed to. She died about a year later. I suspect it was *from the treatment*, not the cancer. You will understand when you read this appendix.

In writing this brief exposé of the pharmaceutical companies, *I do not wish to imply that no one has ever been helped by drug therapy, toxic as it may be.* Even if drugs don't *cure* disease, they can alleviate symptoms. Be aware, however, that symptoms are part of the body's natural healing processes. Symptoms may be acute and remedial, or they may be chronic and degenerative once illness reaches the point that disease reversal is no longer possible. They may also serve as cries for help from the body, warning signs for you to change your ways toward a more health-supportive lifestyle. Alternatively, if you don't want to give up your barbecued spareribs, you may choose to take drugs to relieve the symptoms that will eventually arise before you age and die prematurely.

In a society that professes to be free, there should be no tolerance for suppression of alternatives that are far more healthful that, unlike drugs, do in fact enable the body to recover from disease. Drugs should be a choice, not a forced option.

Drugs are flat out toxic. Just flip through the *Physician's Desk Reference* and see for yourself! Just as humans have not evolved to incorporate and benefit from the thousands of new chemicals produced by cooking, we have not evolved to be able to tolerate drugs. Drugs are just as unnatural to our bodies as cooked food but *much* more toxic. So how did this penchant for drug taking come about?

In the book *The Drug Story*, Morris A. Bealle explains how John D. Rockefeller built perhaps the most lucrative industry in the history of the world. Americans now spend about half a trillion dollars ($500,000,000,000) on pharmaceuticals every year.

Because Rockefeller interests owned, or controlled through lavish advertising, most of the mass media, Bealle had to self-publish his book. It was first published in 1949, and even though it received no media attention, it was already into its 33$^{rd}$ printing in the 1970s.

Rockefeller was once perhaps the wealthiest man in America, owning Chase National Bank and Standard Oil. He wanted to make even more profit from the waste products of petroleum refining; so in the 1860s, he patented bottled raw petroleum as a cure for cancer and the popular maladies of the day. This "miracle cure," called Nujol (from "new oil"), had a placebo effect for some users, meaning that the belief people had in it created a certain amount of results. His cost to produce it was $1/5$ of a cent, and it sold for $28^2/_3$ cents for eight fluid ounces.

Of course some of these petroleum-based drugs appeared to have a certain value, such as for poisoning insomniacs into unrestorative sleep. However, people would soon enough experience a huge price to pay in "side" effects.

Rockefeller nurtured his drug industry until there were 12,000 drugs in the early 1900s. His "charitable" Rockefeller Foundation became an instrument for "educating" medical students into his excessive — and exclusive — patented pharmaceutical therapy. With some of his drug profits, he granted scholarships to medical students, but not one penny did he give to any of the chiropractic or natural therapy schools, even though he himself used homeopathy, knowing full well that the drug empire he was erecting was a scam. One way he helped build his medical monopoly was funding, with millions of dollars, only those medical schools that made medical students memorize the uses of his thousands of patented drugs.

Knowing the power of the written word, Rockefeller then set out to control the media, making sure that only drug-friendly articles were printed and that anyone promoting an alternative natural therapy would be labeled a "quack." Newspapers and magazines dependent on him for his bountiful drug advertisements would not dare print antidrug articles. *He controlled about 80% of all advertising by 1948.*

Rockefeller put his men on the directorship of the Associated Press, thus controlling the "news" on health matters so that of all the healing modalities, only drug treatments were published in a favorable light. One of his puppets, Morris Fishbein, director of the American Medical Association, was made the official "science editor expert" of *The Journal of the American Medical Association, even though he never practiced medicine a day in his life* and in fact did not even complete medical school! Several mainstream magazines were purchased with Rockefeller money: *Time, Newsweek, Life* and *Fortune.* Thus began the pro-drug brainwashing of the public via the media.

Furthermore, the house of Rockefeller got its hooks into the FDA, using its political power and leverage to influence the agency to become one of the drug cartel's puppets. To this day, this government bureau covertly works for the food and drug companies, not the public. This agency strives to keep medical drugs and practices legal that should *not* be.

It tries to outlaw, persecute and/or otherwise suppress alternative, nondrugging practices proven to help people regain health. The FDA cracks down on those who impinge upon the Drug Trust's self-defined domain. Former FDA Commissioner Herbert Lay, MD, once said, "The thing that bugs me is that the people think the FDA is protecting them. It isn't. What the FDA is doing and what the public thinks it's doing are as different as night and day."

Bealle has this to say about the FDA in *The Drug Story* (pp. 39–40):

This Bureau — known as the Food and Drug Administration — is used primarily for the perversion of justice by "cracking down" on all who endanger the profits of the Drug Trust. The Bureau occasionally prosecutes, on its own initiative, small-time opportunists who should be prosecuted. Thus, in a few small cases, the Bureau does good work. Its principal activities, however, are as servants of the Drug Trust. Not only does the FDA wink at violations by the Drug Trust (such as the mass murders in the ginger Jake and sulfathiozole cases), but it is very assiduous in putting out of business any and all vendors of therapeutic devices which increase the health incidence of the public and thus decrease the profit incidence of the Drug Trust.

After a thorough investigation of the FDA, Elaine Feuer exposed the truth about it in *Innocent Casualties: The FDA's War Against Humanity*. She documents that the FDA goes after the companies that offer natural cures for those diseases most lucrative to the drug companies. An example of their hypocrisy is their making *herba ephedra* illegal after 153 deaths were linked to it; yet thousands of people die every year from taking *recommended amounts* of *aspirin*.

Bealle wrote and published another tell-all book, *The House of Rockefeller*. He documents how the Rockefeller power elite set up stooges and puppets not only in the FDA, but also in the US Public Health Service, the Federal Trade Commission, the Better Business Bureau, the Army Medical Corps, the Navy Bureau of Medicine, the Centers for Disease Control and Prevention and among thousands of health officials all over the country.

An updated version of the story that reveals more of this corruption is found in the writings of Dr. Leonard Horowitz, Harvard-educated public health researcher, who wrote *Death in the Air: Globalism, Terrorism & Toxic Warfare* and *Emerging Viruses: AIDS and Ebola*, among other titles.

With his enormous wealth, Rockefeller founded and lavishly endowed education boards, thus gaining control of federal government health policy and also the output of the intellectual and scientific community. In fact no Pulitzer, Nobel or any similar prize endowed with money and prestige has ever been awarded to a declared foe of the Rockefeller cartel.

Thus began the brainwashing of the American public and eventually the world, as Rockefeller's empire spread worldwide. It didn't matter that most of the drugs were not only worthless for healing, but were actually harmful and even dangerous.

Studies have shown that the poisons in vaccinations are a major cause of learning disabilities, autism and mental retardation in children. *Evidence of Harm: Mercury in Vaccines and the Autism Epidemic: A Medical Controversy* by David Kirby is one of several books exposing this danger. The drug companies even lobbied to get a rider attached to the Homeland Security Bill that prevents people from suing them for the damage done by vaccinations!

Furthermore, a number of antidepressant medications have actually been proven to arouse suicidal and homicidal tendencies in users, especially among children, teenagers and young adults. Hormone replacement therapy has been shown to increase cancer risk. If you still have doubts about the dangers inherent in drugs, I again urge you to scan the *Physician's Desk Reference* for all the "side" effects of whatever drug interests you.

The brainwashing continues to escalate. Today, approximately two-thirds of all advertising expenditures are for drugs. People are convinced by TV ads that they need to see their doctors and demand various advertised drugs. People's minds are so altered by these ads that viewers feel that parents who don't give their children drugs or vaccinations are guilty of child abuse. Yet these drugs are harmful, and many are physically and psychologically addicting.

Always remember that it was only half a century ago that medical doctors appeared in cigarette commercials and advertisements, advising which brand of cigarettes was good for digestion and stress and even advising pregnant women to smoke!

"One of the major reasons why there is so much sickness and disease is because of the poisons you are putting in your body. The number one poison you put in your body consists of prescription and nonprescription drugs!" says Kevin Trudeau. "That's right. The prescription and nonprescription drugs you are taking to eliminate your symptoms are in fact one of the major reasons that you get sick" (*Natural Cures "They" Don't Want You to Know About,* p. 33).

When Dr. T. Colin Campbell got on the committee to write the first report on the connection between diet and cancer (*Cancer, Diet and Nutrition*), he quickly discovered there existed a "Medical Establishment." He explains in *The China Study* that the hostility of Harvard Medical School and other medical universities surprised him. But when the American Cancer Society also joined in making the committee's life difficult, at that point he realized that a kind of medical mafia was in charge of things. Only after being in the system for many years did he learn that an honest search for truth in science is rare. Entrenched forces of money, ego, power and control take priority over the real quest for health.

Although more and more people are catching on to the importance of diet to good health, medical schools persist in failing to educate medical students about nutrition. Most doctors I have met took only two course hours of nutrition classes in their entire medical training.

Dr. Julian Whitaker, MD, President of the American Association for Health Freedom, points out, "Many people are aware that doctors are woefully ignorant in nutrition. Only about one-third of the nation's 125 medical schools require students to take courses in nutrition, and most of those courses are very brief. This is a shocking statistic, considering that six out of the ten leading causes of death are directly related to diet."

Dr. Campbell points out that not only do medical students receive only about 21 classroom hours of nutritional instruction, but also that this "instruction" is largely influenced by the food corporations themselves! Joining forces to provide the Nutrition in Medicine program and the Medical Nutrition Curriculum Initiative are no less than the Dannon Institute, the Egg Nutrition Board, the National Cattlemen's Beef Association, the National Dairy Council, Nestlé Clinical Nutrition, Wyeth-Ayerst Laboratories, Bristol-Myers Squibb Company and others.

The reason that medical schools fail to teach medical students the truth about health is that drug companies fund their scholarships and want to create doctors who function as professional and legal drug pushers. The indoctrination techniques used in medical schools resemble those used by certain religious and cult organizations to brainwash their followers into a narrow belief system: sleep deprivation from having to study hard and work 24-hour shifts while in training, isolation from the outside world from forced immersion in the doctrine, and fear of failure to conform to the almost unachievably high standards set by frequent and excruciating exams. A great eye-opening book on this topic is *Confessions of a Medical Heretic* by Dr. Robert Mendelsohn, MD.

Yet in prescribing drugs as primary treatment, medical doctors are breaking their Hippocratic oath, "First, do no harm." Since medical drugs are made up of molecules totally foreign to anything the body can absorb and metabolize to provide energy or to assimilate into fluids and tissues, they are by definition *protoplasmic poisons*. They cause definite harm. *Drugs are worse than cooked food.*

With every prescription, the MD is violating his Hippocratic oath. As T. C. Fry stated, "In studying organisms, biology lays down its first law: that while a plant can make use of inorganic elements and by means of solar energy build them up into its own substance, animal organisms do not have this power and are dependent for their sustenance on the plant kingdom. . . . Every inorganic material becomes a foreign element in the animal organism and consequently a poison to it" (*The Health Formula*, p. 122). Could this be where the raw food company Nature's First Law got its title?

Pharmaceutical companies cleverly use the term *side effects* instead of simply *effects* to explain the damage done by drugs. The use of the word *side* softens the impression, making this damage seem like a small, insignificant thing, like a small portion of salad dressing *on the side* or a *side dish*, as opposed to the main course. Sometimes these "side" effects include cancer, heart attacks or even death, *symptoms much worse than the ailment being treated.*

In fact a 2002 study published in *The Journal of the American Medical Association* (*JAMA*) indicates that one in five new drugs will either be withdrawn from the market or get a "black-box warning" indicating a previously unknown, serious, adverse reaction that may result in death or severe injury.

At the time of this writing, for example, Viagra has been implicated in causing blindness in some poor, unsuspecting men! Fosamax, a drug taken to reduce the risk of osteoporosis, actually causes the jawbone to dissolve in some women!

Ambien, a sleeping pill, was causing the "side" effects of sleepwalking, sleep eating and even sleep *driving*! Needless to say, numerous car accidents occurred as a result. My husband knows a woman with no history of thievery who was sentenced for shoplifting while under the influence of this drug!

Another *JAMA* article ("Incidence of adverse drug reactions in hospitalized patients," 1998, pp. 1200–1205) showed that 20% of all new drugs have serious unknown side effects (on top of all the *known* effects). More than 100,000 Americans die every year from *correctly* taking their *properly prescribed* medications! Remember, too, that this is a confession *from within the system*. Mightn't it be that the true situation is actually *even worse*?

Dr. Joseph Mercola, MD, who has one of the world's most widely read health Internet sites (www.mercola.com), writes in one of his Internet commentaries, "Unless we are able to break the connection to drug support of medicine, we are not likely to see much of a shift in the traditional paradigm. It is a very subtle, pernicious and persistent influence that is very difficult to break out of. In retrospect, I believe I was 'brainwashed' in medical school, and it took me nearly five years to break out of that mold, despite the fact that I was resistant to it going in."

In recent years, the drug push has gotten much stronger as billions are spent on TV advertising, as well as on lavish gifts and incentives to medical doctors.

Orthodox medicine is quick to yell quack when unproven alternative methods are used for healing. The irony is that most of the dangerous and deadly drugs used in traditional allopathic medicine have not been proven to be effective or safe. And of course those that *have* were proven using tunnel vision, looking only at the symptoms being treated and not at the overall resulting health consequences.

David Darbro, MD, wrote in the foreword to *God's Way to Ultimate Health*, "I learned that the Office of Technological Assessment of the United States Government had shown that 80-90% of the therapeutic approaches which were accepted by the medical profession as standard care *were actually unproven*! No wonder I wasn't seeing anyone cured! I suddenly realized that 80-90% of what I had been taught in medical school was UNPROVEN!"

Dr. Mercola points out there are "hundreds of articles published in top medical journals claimed to be written by academic researchers that are actually written by ghostwriters working for agencies which receive large amounts of money from pharmaceutical companies to market their products. These are the very journals medical professionals rely on when determining treatment options."

Most of the studies done to prove drug effectiveness are funded by the drug companies themselves, which is like letting the fox guard the chickens. Can you spell *conflict of interest*?

A man I once talked to told me that he quit working for a drug company because he noticed that *doctors were encouraged to drop from studies patients who were not responding to the drug being tested* to increase the percentage of good results!

According to the report "Death by Medicine," the number one cause of death today in the USA is *iatrogenic*, meaning caused by errors made by medical caregivers. This study was compiled by Gary Null, PhD; Carolyn Dean, MD, ND; Martin Feldman, MD; Dorothy Smith, PhD, and Debora Rasio, MD, from government health figures and medical peer-reviewed journal articles.

They tallied up deaths from adverse drug reactions, medical errors, bedsores, infections, unnecessary procedures and malnutrition that occurred in hospitals. They added in deaths of outpatients, which totaled 783,936 in 2001. The deaths in 2001 from heart disease were 699,697. Those from cancer numbered 553,251. These researchers also estimated that the number of deaths due to errors is actually 20 times greater since many go unreported or misreported due to fear of lawsuits and confusion about the actual cause of death. Often doctors mistakenly list the cause of death as the disease, when many times it is actually the toxicity of the drug treatment itself, as with the use of chemo-"therapy."

The study puts the blame for these needless deaths on the medical industry. Current medical practice actually exacerbates illness via drugs, excessive surgeries, toxic and invasive diagnostic testing procedures and even counterproductive, harmful dietary advice. The practitioners do this instead of teaching patients to minimize disease-causing factors like improper diet, pollution, inadequate sleep, excess emotional stress and insufficient exercise! The pharmaceutical juggernaut and its pocketbook are *holding the health care field hostage.*

The report concludes that drug companies control, via curriculum, the brainwashing of medical students as well as the outcomes of "scientific" studies. As the authors, three of whom are MDs themselves, are quick to point out, "It appears that money can't buy you love, but it can buy you any 'scientific' result you want."

Medical doctors are even complaining about this situation in medical journals, as in an article published in 1994 in *JAMA*, "Errors in Medicine." Author Dr. Lucian Leape calculated the 0.1% failure rate at intensive care units to be comparable to two unsafe planes landing at O'Hare Airport a day, 16,000 pieces of mail lost in the post office per hour or 32,000 checks deducted from the wrong bank account every hour! If six jumbo jets a day were crashing, wouldn't there be an outcry and a boycott of airlines until the situation was fixed?

The report by Null et al. points out that the equivalent is happening in modern medicine, yet the media will not give the issue any feature coverage because they depend upon drug company advertisements. The entire report can be found at various Internet sites, including here: www.mercola.com/2003/nov/26/death_by_medicine.htm.

This danger of death at the hands of those who are supposed to heal us never existed before widespread drug usage; doctors and hospitals once employed gentler treatments, including herbal potions and fasting.

Nowadays when hospitals or doctors go on strike, death rates drop in those localities. These strikes are always brief affairs lest people catch on to how dangerous allopathic treatments can be.

In 1973, a strike in an Israeli hospital lasted a month, and the death rate dropped by 50%. Similar results happened again in Israel in 1983 and 2000. In 1976, doctors refused to treat all cases except for emergencies in Bogotá, Colombia, for a period of 52 days. The death rate fell 35%. In 1976, a slowdown of Los Angeles doctors resulted in 18% fewer deaths.

Patients trapped in the medical matrix must wake up. We should not have to fear entering hospitals. *Healing sites should not be life threatening!* They should be places of *rest, relaxation, revitalization, detoxification*, and *recovery*.

I remember spending nights in hospitals with loved ones. When my mother was on her deathbed, I was allowed to sleep over but wasn't able to get any actual sleep due to lights, noise and regular interruptions by nurses barging in. Even a healthy person like me would get sick after a few such sleepless nights added to the abominable hospital food and toxic drugs! So how can a sick person be expected to *heal* in a place like that?

Cancer treatment is perhaps the biggest example of the complete insincerity at the medical pyramid's pinnacle. As discussed in Chapter 17, a major contributor to cancer, systemic acidity, was discovered by a Nobel Prize winner in 1931 decades before the "war on cancer" began! Its natural cure was also discovered — eliminating the cause by restoring the body's natural alkalinity.

There is simply too much money to be made in cancer treatment as practiced today. Since it is a $120 billion dollar a year industry, the medical monopoly will let it go about as readily as a hungry dog will release a juicy bone.

Yet Dr. Hardin B. Jones, PhD and professor of medical physics and physiology at U. C. Berkeley, found that people diagnosed with cancer who received *no allopathic treatment* (chemotherapy, radiation, surgery) actually lived longer than those who did! They lived an average of 12½ years longer. Those receiving no therapy lived, on the average, four times longer than those who paid huge sums of money for medical treatments (*Transactions of the N. Y. Academy of Medical Sciences*, 1956, Vol. 6).

Though this research was published decades ago, today's "gentler, softer" toxic treatments are not much better because they are still based on the false premise that poison ingestion will heal a sick body. The basic chemical used in chemotherapy is similar to mustard gas, a World War I weapon used to kill soldiers on the battlefield. It was so terrible that wartime treaties banned its future wartime use.

Radiation is nearly as bad. It is actually quite absurd to think that rays that would kill *healthy* people with strong defense mechanisms should heal very sick people with weak defense mechanisms!

Orthodox cancer treatment consisting of chemo or radiation very often kills people before their cancers do. This occurs because the effects of the drugs and/or radiation include malnutrition due to loss of appetite, vomiting and destruction of the digestive tract, as well as debilitation of the body's defensive army as the result of killing blood and bone marrow cells. Hence, the patient often dies of emaciation and consequent starvation or of infection before he can die of cancer.

Chemotherapy itself is carcinogenic, which is why the patient, even if pronounced "cured," will usually die of the same or a different form of cancer within a few weeks, months or years. In fact the arbitrary definition of "cured" is that the cancer patient is still alive five years after the onset of medical treatment, even if he dies five years and a day later!

This is the real reason why early detection leads to more "cures." If the patient is going to die within six years, whether he gets the treatment or not, then detection within the first year may result in a "cure" since he will have begun treatment prior to five years before his death!

Even surgery, the third quiver in the oncologist's bow after chemotherapy and radiation, yields less than optimal results due to the inherent limitations of surgical procedures. Surgeons can remove only self-contained tumors, not cancers that have spread systemically throughout the body. Even then surgeons remove much healthy tissue along with the sick tissue, even entire organs that could have been saved by natural healing, which operates at microscopic levels that the surgeon's scalpel can't match.

Author G. Edward Griffin writes, "Excluding skin cancer, the average cure rate of cancer by medical doctors is 17%" (*World without Cancer: The Story of Vitamin $B_{17}$*). So, not only is the cure rate low, but the definition of "cure" *hardly paints a healthy picture.*

We have been blinded by the big pharmaceutical companies to believe that there is significant merit in orthodox treatments for cancer when studies have in fact shown quite clearly the opposite to be true.

A German epidemiologist from the Heidelberg/Mannheim Tumor Clinic, Dr. Ulrich Abel, wrote up a comprehensive review and analysis of every major study on chemotherapy, even writing to 350 medical centers around the world to be sure he had everything published on the subject. After several years of study, he concluded that there was no scientific evidence anywhere that chemo could in any way appreciably extend the lives of cancer patients. He said it was like the story of "The Emperor's New Clothes."

Few mainstream journals published his data, naturally, since they are highly dependent upon pharmaceuticals for their funding. But by the time Dr. Abel published his report and subsequent book, *Chemotherapy of Advanced Epithelial Cancer: A Survey*, he knew more about chemotherapy than any person in existence. His report, published in *Lancet* in August 1991, described chemotherapy as a "scientific wasteland" that doctors were not willing to give up even though there was no scientific evidence that it worked.

T. S. Wiley points out, "A review article in the *Journal of Clinical Oncology* in October of 1998 compiled the results of a twenty-two year study following 31,510 women with breast cancer. Their overall conclusion was that over the course of twenty-two years of reviewing twelve different therapeutic regimens in various combinations, the cancer therapies only provided 'a modest improvement in survival rates' " (*Lights Out*, p. 144).

Dr. Ralph Moss, MD, has written several books exposing the horrors of cancer industry. Of course these books are given no media attention. There are also several interviews with him on the Internet in which he blasts the cancer industry.

In his video *How to Eliminate Sickness*, Rev. George Malkmus refutes the integrity of the alleged "war on cancer," which began when President Nixon was in office and has squandered to date over forty billion dollars in search of a cure.

"Research," he explains, "is nothing but a guise to keep the American people in ignorance." At Hallelujah Acres, Malkmus is able to boast that people heal completely at his healing center not only from cancer, but also from AIDS. "If the medical community were getting these results, it would be front page news."

At the end of the video, a medical doctor speaks about how he healed himself with the raw food diet and wished he had only known about this during his 30 years of medical practice.

When people used to ask me if acupuncture really worked, I answered, "Hey, it's been around for 5,000 years. Don't you think the Chinese would have figured it out by now if it didn't work?" Folks, the alleged war on cancer has been for over 30 years now. How many more people will have to die before we realize these methods are not working?

When Dr. Lorraine Day, MD, got cancer, she refused chemotherapy and radiation because she knew the statistics, and she wanted to live. For several years, her breast lump continued to grow. She became bedridden for six months as she tried 40-odd different alternative remedies, including the macrobiotic diet and supplements. She then discovered Natural Hygiene via Seventh Day Adventist books and used live fruit juices, vegetable juices and wheatgrass, along with other supportive lifestyle practices. The tumor disappeared in eight months. She regained full health after another ten months.

Dr. Day now promotes a living foods diet. She has made over a dozen videos, including *Cancer Doesn't Scare Me Anymore* and *Drugs Never Cure Disease*. She remarks that the medical industry keeps looking for answers in the wrong places because they are stuck in the wrong paradigm. How ironic it is, she points out, that the medical establishment admits that people can *prevent* cancer with diet and lifestyle but maintains that they cannot *recover from* cancer with diet and lifestyle!

When Dr. William Donald Kelley found an enzymatic cancer cure that had a 93% success rate, including patients whose natural defense mechanisms had been severely compromised by chemotherapy, what was his reward from orthodox medicine? *He was jailed!* In order to continue his practice, he was forced to go to Mexico. His book, *Cancer: Curing the Incurable without Surgery, Chemotherapy or Radiation*, tells of his treatment and its success rate.

To me, it seems very strange that when orthodox treatment fails to cure cancer 80-90% of the time, it is said, "The cancer killed them." *But when an alternative approach works 93% of the time, the doctor is persecuted, accused of killing the 7% he failed to save, and jailed because he did not give patients the orthodox, toxic medicine that would have greatly increased their mortality risk!* Clearly, as far as those behind the drug cartel are concerned, *the issue at stake is money and not lives.*

Some people wonder why insurance companies do not sponsor fasting retreats and other alternative methods that work so well, when these methods are infinitely less expensive than standard treatments. The reason is simple: if people knew the truth about the causes of disease and how to retrace their symptoms back into health, they would refuse to pay hundreds of dollars a month for health insurance. People might pay a bit for accident insurance, but the chances of a catastrophic accident are miniscule compared to the chances of developing a disease condition (nearly a 100% chance). Insurance rates and insurance company profits, which are typically a percentage of insurance rates, would thus logically have to be much lower.

At the disease industry pyramid's apex, those who control the insurance companies are no dummies. They know that fasting and proper diet provide ideal conditions for health recovery and maintenance. But they are financially invested in keeping the masses locked in the wrong paradigm. Keeping people in fear that they have no control over their own health justifies large health insurance premiums.

In her book *The Medical Mafia*, Guylaine Lanctôt, MD, explains that our health care system is controlled by a group of three: the American Medical Association, the health insurance industry and, most of all, the pharmaceutical companies.

She once practiced medicine in the USA, as well as in France and Canada where medicine is socialized. She urges Americans not to socialize medicine, explaining that the only ones who profit are the pharmaceutical companies. Allopathic medicine focuses only on treating illness, not on creating health. Taxpayers' money would go much, much further in creating real public health by funding natural therapies and preventive measures via health education. Not only would this be cost effective, but there would also be no adverse side effects. This is not happening because people have been brainwashed into believing that the men and women in white laboratory coats always know best.

Michael Moore's film *Sicko* has revived interest in socialized medicine. Surely, emergency and trauma care should in some way be made available to the masses. The documentary also makes the valid point that socialized medicine at least focuses more public attention on preventive measures in the name of cutting costs.

However, the film does not at all address the pattern of deterioration we have seen whenever government takes over an institution and runs it as a monopoly. An example is documented by Charlotte Thompson Iserbyt in her book *The Deliberate Dumbing Down of America*, which shows dozens of court documents proving that forces within the federal government have intentionally and gradually bestowed upon us an inferior educational system, perhaps for the purpose of population control.

Likewise, in socialized medicine, only the drug companies will profit from mass consumption of their poisons.

The pharmaceutical industry is a vast business, a cartel dangerous even to children. In fact wise and loving parents who wish to provide their children with safe and more effective cancer treatments than chemotherapy or radiation often have to fight in court and *risk losing custody of their own children*! I heard of a case from a raw food teacher of mine who knew of a couple whose child had brain cancer. They had to give up their jobs, leave their home, and go into hiding in order to be able to exercise their own health care choices for their child. The child was healed of cancer while on raw foods, but the parents lost everything in order to make that happen!

A case in which a young boy died because he was denied alternative treatment is presented on the web site www.ouralexander.org/war1.htm.

The medical mafia appears to own a patent on the word "cure." Their servant, the FDA, has issued a ruling that states that the only thing that can cure or prevent a disease is a drug! Just think, every time a body cures or heals itself, it is breaking this law!

Even though drugs do not cure, anyone who offers a real alternative, such as a raw food diet, is putting himself in serious legal jeopardy if he claims that his treatment cures. In acupuncture school, we were sternly warned never to use the word "cure." Doing so could cost us our licenses or even land us in jail.

The Federal Trade Commission (FTC) is another handmaiden of the medical mafia. Kevin Trudeau details how they harassed him when he was selling a natural remedy, coral calcium. He went to the FTC and asked if any of his ads would violate FTC or FDA regulations. They responded that the infomercial ads were acceptable.

Later, without warning, after profitable sales of this supplement, the FTC filed a lawsuit against him saying he was making unsubstantiated claims, *although they had approved these claims earlier*! They shut down his company and seized his assets.

He has since learned that this is their standard operating procedure. They wait until money is made so they can take it. And when the FTC files suit, it is not required to go to federal court. Instead, FTC suits are presented before an "administrative law judge" who is really an employee of the FTC. The "courtroom" is in the FTC building itself!

The media have relentlessly trashed Kevin for his best-selling consumer watchdog book *Natural Cures "They" Don't Want You to Know About*. Shows like *20/20* that usually attempt to give both sides of a story refused to interview any of the tens of thousands of people who had written to Kevin praising his book for helping them find true healing. Instead, show producers tried to distract their audiences from recognizing the validity of his message by focusing their efforts on assassinating the character of the messenger. He was, after all, attacking their drug sponsors.

The First Amendment to the US Constitution states, "Congress shall make no law prohibiting the free exercise of religion or abridging the freedom of speech or of the press."

Dr. Benjamin Rush, MD, who was a signatory to the Declaration of Independence and physician to George Washington, urged Congress to add the words, "or abridging the right of citizens to secure medical treatment from doctors of their own choice." He pleaded, "Unless we put medical freedom into the Constitution, the time will come when medicine will organize into an undercover dictatorship. . . . To restrict the art of healing to one class of men and deny equal privilege to others will constitute the Bastille of medical science."

There are undoubtedly countless cases in which people's lives are prolonged or even saved by allopathic interventions, but drugs are extremely inefficient and often futile tools for effecting the fullest possible recovery. Drug treatment becomes a case of shooting the messenger rather than addressing underlying causes.

First of all, if one is eating properly and practicing good preventive medicine via a healthful lifestyle, he will not contract infection or descend into disease.

Second, if he does become sick, fasting and eating properly gets much better results than drug therapy to restore health in nearly all cases. These methods are also gentler, kinder, safer and considerably less expensive.

Yet the medical mafia would have people, during their last few months of life, spend their last dimes and even go hundreds of thousands of dollars into debt in order to prolong the dying process a few months longer in sheer agony. These cases happen all the time. It has been estimated that the average American outlays 25% of his lifetime medical expenditures during the last year of his life. His children's potential inheritance is snatched up by the medical mafia so that he may endure a miserable existence, hooked up to machines and barely conscious or writhing in indescribable pain for another six months or so. The cost of this is bankrupting Medicare, Medicaid and countless individuals.

Painkillers are perhaps the most seductive of all drugs because pain is the most unbearable of all disease or injury symptoms. But even pain medications are not as necessary as one might think. On a raw diet, especially an instinctive one (see Appendix C), one experiences vastly less pain from injuries. Acupuncture is also remarkable in pain management.

For those who are extremely sick and hooked on morphine, coffee enemas are reported to reduce pain very effectively. Dr. Max Gerson weaned all of his cancer patients from pain medication with the use of coffee enemas, which he explains in "The cure of advanced cancer by diet therapy: a summary of 30 years of clinical experimentation" (*Physiological Chemistry and Physics*, 1978, Vol. 10, Issue 5, pp. 449–464). Medical monopolies don't like that kind of competition. Is it any wonder he was forced to move his clinic to Mexico?

Dr. J. W. Hodge, MD, of Niagara Falls, New York, has this to say of the medical monopoly:

> The medical monopoly, or medical trust, euphemistically called the American Medical Association, is not merely the meanest monopoly ever organized, but the most arrogant, dangerous and despotic organization which ever managed a free people in this or any other age. Any and all methods of healing the sick by means of safe, simple and natural remedies are sure to be assailed and denounced by the arrogant leaders of the AMA doctors' trust as fakes, frauds and humbugs. Every practitioner of the healing art who does not ally himself with the medical trust is denounced as a "dangerous quack" and imposter by the predatory trust doctors.
>
> Every sanitarium who attempts to restore the sick to a state of health by natural means without resort to the knife or poisonous drugs, disease-imparting se-

rums, deadly toxins or vaccines, is at once pounced upon by these medical tyrants and fanatics, bitterly denounced, vilified and persecuted to the fullest extent.

In her book *Dying to Get Well*, Shelly Keck-Borsits talks about her nightmarish experience with FDA-approved birth control injections of DepoProvera that were supposed to be "safe." She experienced migraines, fibromyalgia, loss of libido, chronic pain, muscle weakness and a huge list of other problems resulting in several years of hell until she discovered Natural Hygiene.

She documented this horrible nightmare of drug-induced symptoms, along with those of many other women, and sent it all to the FDA, thinking they would be concerned enough to do something about it. She never heard a word back from them.

Shelly laments that we are a drugged nation, constantly bombarded with brainwashing commercials to convince us that drugs are the answer to everything from A to Z.

We are taught not to deal with our emotions, but to pop a Prozac. We are taught not to eat right and exercise, but to run to the doctor for a quick-fix prescription drug. We are pressured, even by teachers, to drug our kids with Ritalin instead of finding the underlying causes of their hyperactivity, which are usually refined sugar, food additives and dyes (Appendix A) or pesticides (Chapter 17).

Take no responsibility for your health! Just pop a pill! And when you don't get well, it's the doctor's fault or the drug's fault or the hospital's fault. And when you have paid so much money for the treatments that didn't get you well, complain to the government that health care should be paid for by taxpayers, the health care that *didn't even cure you*. This all reflects the conventional medical paradigm thinking: it cannot get you well!

Researcher, medical school professor and author Bruce Lipton, PhD, believes that current medical theory is based on outdated Newtonian physics and needs to be updated with theories based on quantum physics and the impact of the mind. This shift has not happened because of drug industry financial interests. "Medical doctors are caught between an intellectual rock and a corporate hard place; they are pawns in the huge medical industrial complex," he laments (*Biology of Belief*, p. 108).

Lipton says that the placebo effect, which involves healing due to sheer belief, is brushed off as a fluke in medical school, glossed over quickly so students can get to the real "tools" of modern medicine.

"This is a giant mistake," he explains. "Doctors should not dismiss the power of the mind as something inferior to the power of chemicals and the scalpel. They should let go of their conviction that the body and its parts are essentially stupid and that we need outside intervention to maintain our health" (pp. 137–138). He claims this doesn't happen, however. Why would we need drugs if we learned to harness mental power to focus the body's healing energies?

Lipton was chagrined to learn that drug companies are now trying to decipher which kinds of patients respond to sugar pills so they can be eliminated from drug trials! "It inevitably disturbs pharmaceutical manufacturers that in most of their clinical trials, the placebos, the 'fake' drugs, prove to be as effective

498

as their engineered chemical cocktails." In fact he proceeds to point out that the history of medicine is largely the history of the placebo effect, with the use of bloodletting, treating wounds with arsenic and the use of rattlesnake oil.

The drug companies are worried because a growing percentage of the American health dollar is now being spent on alternative therapies: in fact half of all Americans have used alternative health care. Twenty-six drug companies have banded together to form an organization, now known as the "quackbusters," that tries to discredit true health care practitioners. They call them "quacks" and even stoop to the low level of sending false complaints to the FDA and other federal agencies. Visit www.quackpotwatch.org for more information.

On a positive note, many doctors and other health professionals are fighting back when the drug cartel hits them with accusations of quackery. The ongoing struggle between the "health freedom movement" and the "quackbusters" is covered by a newsletter entitled "Millions of Health Freedom-Fighters Newsletter." *Those who are persecuted for using nondrug treatments are now fighting for the right to treat patients as they see fit!*

Another problem we face is that the Codex Alimentarius Commission, an international regulatory body established under United Nations auspices in 1963 that has tried for over a decade to make dietary supplements available by prescription only. Codex is working to institute many other things to degrade our health. If you wanted anything more than a miniscule (ineffective) doses an herb or mineral supplement, you would have to get it from an MD.

Codex is already doing this in parts of Europe, and the World Trade Organization is trying to make sure it happens soon in the USA. They also plan to have all fresh food irradiated by December 31, 2009. Any food considered to have therapeutic effects would be considered a drug and be available by prescription only.

For more information, go to www.healthfreedomusa.org. That site also has petitions you can sign to help fight Codex.

Yet another pressure group is Operation Cure All, which has a plan to restrict health information, supplements and natural therapies. The World Health Organization, the United Nations, international banks and the multinational pharmaceutical companies are all working in concert to make this happen. This group has already conspired to outlaw all health claims for products sold on the Internet. Testimonials are not allowed either.

For more information, read the aforementioned *Medical Mafia* and any of Ralph Moss's books exposing the cancer industry, as well as *Racketeering in Medicine: The Suppression of Alternatives* by James P. Carter, MD, and *Politics in Healing: The Suppression and Manipulation of American Medicine* by Daniel Haley.

Dr. Marcia Angell resigned from her editorial position at *The New England Journal of Medicine*. She explained in an interview with the *LA Times* on August 9, 2004 that she had no choice after writing an exposé about how drug company leaders manipulate clinical trials and about their influence on medical journals, doctors and government agencies. Her book is called *The Truth about the Drug Companies: How They Deceive Us and What to Do About It.*

Drug companies are being sued so much for their toxic products that the FDA, their partner in drug proliferation for all practical purposes, enacted a "Final Rule." In an article on www.naturalnews.com, Mike Adams writes:

> June 30, 2006, is a day that will long be remembered as a dark milestone in the history of the FDA and its campaign against health consumers. On June 30, an FDA "Final Rule" goes into effect establishing a regulatory power grab of such scale and scope that it attempts to bypass all laws, the will of Congress and fundamental protections for consumers. This "Final Rule" . . . claims that consumers can no longer sue drug companies for the harm caused by any FDA-approved drug, even if the drug's manufacturer intentionally misled the FDA by hiding or fabricating clinical trial data.
>
> In one blatantly illegal act, the FDA is attempting to pull off the greatest Big Pharma coup of all: the outright elimination of any responsibility whatsoever for the suffering and death caused by deadly pharmaceuticals.

Clearly, the "war on drugs" needs to include pharmaceuticals. Perhaps Nancy Reagan should have said, "Just say no to *prescription* drugs!" Maybe, as I once told a friend, we should all join in partnership for a prescription-drug-free America.

In conclusion, let's consider these 17 quotations regarding the use of drugs in medicine, most of them made by MDs themselves:

- "The cause of most disease is in the poisonous drugs physicians superstitiously give in order to effect a cure."     —Charles E. Page, MD

- "Medicines are of subordinate importance; because of their very nature, they can only work symptomatically."     —Hans Kusche, MD

- "If all the *materia medica* in the world were thrown into the sea, it would be bad for the fish and good for humanity." — Oliver Wendell Holmes, Sr., Professor of Medicine, Harvard University (paraphrased)

- "Drug medication consists in employing, as remedies for disease, those things which produce disease in well persons. Its *materia medica* is simply a lot of drugs or chemicals or dyestuffs — in a word, poisons. All are incompatible with vital matter; all produce disease when brought in contact in any manner with the living; all are poisons."
  —Russell T. Trall, MD, in a 2½-hour lecture to members of Congress and the medical profession, delivered at the Smithsonian Institute in Washington, D.C. in 1862.

- "Every drug increases and complicates the patient's condition."
  —Robert Henderson, MD

- "Drugs never cure disease. They merely hush the voice of Nature's protest and pull down the danger signals she erects along the pathway of transgression. Any poison taken into the system has to be reckoned with later on, even though it palliates present symptoms. Pain may disappear, but the patient is left in a worse condition, though unconscious of it at the time."　　　　　　　　　　　　　　　　　　　—Daniel H. Kress, MD

- "The greatest part of all chronic disease is created by the suppression of acute disease by drug poisoning."　　　　　　　　　　—Henry Lindlahr, MD

- "Every educated physician knows that most diseases are not appreciably helped by medicine."

  —Richard C. Cabot, MD, Massachusetts General Hospital

- "Medicine is only palliative, for back of disease lies the cause, and this cause no drug can reach."　　　　　　　　　　　　　—Wier Mitchel, MD

- "The person who takes medicine must recover twice, once from the disease and once from the medicine."　　　　　　　—William Osler, MD

- "Medical practice has neither philosophy nor common sense to recommend it. In sickness the body is already loaded with impurities. By taking drug medicines, more impurities are added; thereby the case is further embarrassed and harder to cure."

  —Elmer Lee, MD, Vice President, Academy of Medicine

- "Our figures show approximately four and one half million hospital admissions annually due to the adverse reactions to drugs. Further, the average hospital patient has as much as a thirty percent chance, depending how long he is in, of doubling his stay due to adverse drug reactions."

  —Milton Silverman, MD, Professor of Pharmacology,
  University of California

- "Why would a patient swallow a poison because he is ill or take that which would make a well man sick?"　　　　　　　　—L. F. Kebler, MD

- "What hope is there for medical science to ever become a true science when the entire structure of medical knowledge is built around the idea that there is an entity called disease which can be expelled when the right drug is found?"　　　　　　　　　　　　　　　—John H. Tilden, MD

- "We are prone to thinking of drug abuse in terms of the male population and illicit drugs such as heroin, cocaine and marijuana. It may surprise you to learn that a greater problem exists with millions of women dependent on legal prescription drugs."　　　　　　　　—Robert Mendelsohn, MD

- "The necessity of teaching mankind not to take drugs and medicines is a duty incumbent upon all who know their uncertainty and injurious effects, and the time is not far distant when the drug system will be abandoned."

  —Charles Armbruster, MD

- "I have come to the conclusion that prescription drugs are causing a lot more harm in this country than the illegal drugs."

  —Ron Paul, MD, Texas Congressman and Presidential candidate

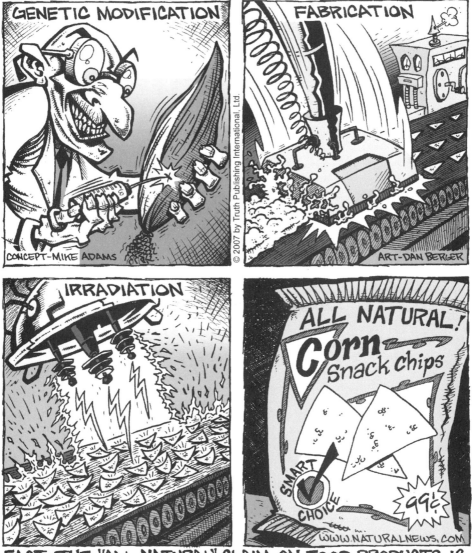

FACT: THE "ALL NATURAL" CLAIM ON FOOD PRODUCTS IS MEANINGLESS. GET THE FACTS:
www.HonestFoodGuide.org

# Appendix C

## Radical Branches of the Raw Food Movement

*Extreme measures are very appropriate for extreme disease.*
—Hippocrates (460–377 BC), *Aphorisms*

### The Green Smoothie Diet

Victoria Boutenko (see Chapters 2 and 12) is heralding a new "green revolution" with her diet consisting mainly of green smoothies, as detailed in her book *Green for Life*. Greens, also referred to as green leafy vegetables, include all lettuces and varieties of kale, collards, parsley, cilantro, spinach, carrot and beet tops, wild greens and the like. This is a pretty radical diet not just in content, but also since it involves becoming a "liquidarian" when taken to extremes.

The development of this diet began when Victoria was searching for answers as to why her family, having been 100% raw for over 11 years, nonetheless had minor health problems, such as fatigue, dental sensitivity and gray hair. In her quest for answers, she thoroughly researched our closest living relative, the chimpanzee, which shares 99.4% of our DNA sequences. In fact she found that chimps are so close to us, even intellectually (having their own sign language) and emotionally, that scientists at the Chimpanzee & Human Communication Institute at Washington Central University maintain that chimpanzees should be classified as "people"! Chimps even have the same A/B/O blood types and are used for studies on tissue transplants.

When studying their diet, Victoria learned that the diet of the average raw fooder was very different from that of the healthy wild chimpanzee. Typically, a raw fooder will eat a diet of about 45-50% fruit by volume, maybe 5-10% greens and 25-30% fats in the form of avocados, oils, nuts and seeds. The rest would be vegetables. On the other hand, chimps will eat a diet of 50% fruit, 40% greens and blossoms by volume and then about 10% pith, bark, seeds and insects or even — though rarely — small animals.

Victoria developed her green smoothies as a way for us to ingest a comparably vast quantity of greens and found that by mixing them with fruit, they became not only palatable, but also very tasty.

People writing to Victoria were concerned that mixing fruits with greens was bad food combining, but she concludes from her research that greens warrant being a food group by themselves since they differ so much from other vegetables.

For example, greens are much higher in protein. One pound of kale has more protein than the USDA recommendation for one day. Greens match human nutritional needs the most closely of all foods, making them "the most essential food for humans." They contain a high amount of chlorophyll, which is "liquefied sun energy."

Thus began her green smoothie diet, which is very close to the ratios of our chimpanzee relative, about 40% greens, 50% fruit and then some nuts and seeds.

The Boutenko family experienced dramatic health improvements after just a few weeks of consuming two bunches of greens daily. Warts and moles they'd had since childhood fell off. Her husband Igor's beard turned black. Wrinkles vanished, vision sharpened, and nails grew stronger. The children's tooth sensitivity stopped, and they needed less sleep. Furthermore, the family's cravings for fat and spices vanished.

You may wonder, why smoothies? For one thing, chimps spend about six hours a day chewing, something few humans have time for. It is necessary to chew greens intensely into a creamy consistency in order for the rigid cellulose walls to be ruptured, releasing their nutrients. Who has the time for that?

Secondly, as Dr. Weston Price, DDS, discovered (*Nutrition and Physical Degeneration*), we have damaged our jaws and chewing capacities through decades of eating soft processed foods. Most of us have had our wisdom teeth pulled due to this jaw deformation, and those teeth are also needed for such intense chewing.

Victoria's answer to these time and dental dilemmas is the Vita-Mix machine since a cheap blender's blades would go dull after just two weeks on this diet. The reason for using a Vita-Mix rather than a juicer is that we need the fiber that juicing eliminates. Chimps eat 300 grams of fiber a day, while the average American consumes only 10-20 grams. Though the usual recommendation for humans is about 30 grams a day, Victoria believes we need at least 70 grams.

Note: Most raw food diets also lack in fiber, although Dr. Vetrano's recommended Natural Hygiene diet offers 60-90 grams or more, depending on whether the person juices out much of the fiber.

Additionally, blending foods helps predigest them since most of us develop very low levels of hydrochloric acid production as we age. When the Vita-Mix processes the high-fiber greens in juice or water, cell walls are broken down and nutrients liberated. The net effect is a premastication of the nutrients. The green smoothie diet has been proven to supply the body with what it needs to regenerate stomach acid production. (See the Roseburg Study on page 167.)

Victoria found that the switch to a greens diet created much more alkalinity. Her family's urine used to test acidic despite their 100% raw diets. They had concluded there must be a glitch in the test since they were on the healthiest diet in the world. But since adding the large quantity of greens, they have tested consistently at the ideal alkalinity for human health!

She wondered why doctors don't routinely test for alkalinity. I think they do not learn its importance in medical school because the medical schools are funded by pharmaceutical companies that know how acidic drugs are. (See Appendix B.) Why promote alkaline foods when selling acidic drugs?

So many people have noted dramatic improvements so quickly on this diet that Victoria sees *the switch to green as more beneficial than even the switch to raw.*

One woman who had Stage IV pancreatic cancer tried a raw diet, but the cancer would not go away. She then tried the green smoothie diet, hoping to prolong her life a bit more. After her next tests, however, the doctor told her that not only was the cancer gone, but also her pancreatic juices were healthier than the average!

Other testimonials in her book describe no more cravings for coffee, meat, sweets and fats; freedom from need of a wheelchair; normalized $B_{12}$ levels, and healed eczema and cataracts.

Victoria notes that the jaw needs exercise. She sells a jaw exerciser that compensates for the lack of chewing. Most people would need this, even if not on her diet, since we no longer chew as much as we should. The body adapts to regular exercise using this jaw tool with improved bone density in the teeth, just as walking improves leg bone density. This tool also firms up sagging jowls.

I first met Victoria and Igor three years before this writing, and I must say that they look ten years younger now! I learned from her book that I had not been doing the diet correctly. For example, I was only taking about a fourth of the amount of greens I needed. I was also not getting nearly the optimal amount of fiber, which, as she details in her book, is crucial for eliminating toxins. Additionally, it is necessary to rotate the greens to get as much variety as possible. I am beginning to experiment with this diet the correct way with great results. The feeling of ecstatic well-being from normalized alkalinity is astonishing.

# Nonvegan Branches

Even though I am a vegetarian, I feel that no book on the raw food movement would be complete without mentioning these other two groups of raw fooders. However, since the version of the raw diet I practice, teach and promote is vegetarian, I decided that presentation of these somewhat radical schools of raw diet belonged in an appendix.

The purpose of writing this is not to convince anyone to eat meat. That is a personal decision people often agonize over. Meat lovers will only painfully forgo meat for better health. A small percentage of long-term vegans sometimes agonize over the decision whether to eat small amounts of meat after their health fails due to strict veganism. The purpose of this writing is not to persuade you, but simply to inform you of the issues involved and conclusions that some people have made.

Perhaps the majority of raw fooders transition to raw eating after first being vegetarian, or even vegan, for a number of years. Because of this, many of the raw vegan promoters prefer to think of themselves as entirely separate from the somewhat radical branches of the raw food movement described below.

Vegans are usually religiously adamant that people are meant to be frugivores, not consuming any animal products at all. Many feel that it was the animal products that made them sick in the first place before they discovered the health virtues inherent in the raw food diet. They cannot imagine that it may not have been the meat in itself that caused their cancers or other serious illnesses, but rather the fact that the meat was cooked.

Some researchers have concluded that although we as humans are all part of the same species, we vary somewhat in our genetic backgrounds and metabolic needs. It appears that at least a *few* people seem to do better with at least *some* raw animal protein. Others do much better on raw vegetarian or vegan diets. It does seem that even raw animal products are far superior to their cooked counterparts. As the authors of *Nature's First Law* are fond of saying, "Raw is law!"

Are there people who genetically require meat? If you research both sides of the issue, you may become humbled enough, as I am, to say that you don't really know. One thing I do believe: if we had a fraction of the billions in funding at our disposal that the drug companies have to devote to research, we would be able to get to the bottom of this matter.

# Beyond Raw Food: Guy-Claude Burger and Instinctive Eating

The instinctive diet is, in my opinion, possibly the *ultimate diet* in terms of getting back to the way we used to eat. It is the way we ate for millions of years, guided not by nutritional theory, but rather by sheer instinct. It is the lost art of trusting the nose and tongue to guide us to the exact food that produces optimal ecstasy and maximal health. But it is probably the hardest diet to adhere to now, as we are so far removed from natural settings and natural foods. We have to unlearn so much of our food conditioning. We have to learn so much to return to and trust our instincts.

Though the diet is practiced by animals in nature all over the world today, humans repopularized instinctive eating through a book, *Manger Vrai: Instinctothérapie* [Correct Eating: Instinctotherapy], written by the French author Guy-Claude Burger.

At age 26, Burger was told he had no hope of surviving cancer. Doctors said there was nothing they could do for him. So, with nothing to lose, he decided to look to nature, cancer being a disease of civilization. Possibly nature could heal him. He went back to his native Switzerland to live on a farm. After observing how animals use their instincts to select foods, he began eating only fresh food that he instinctively desired. *Within months*, his cancer diminished. Eventually he became completely free of it.

According to Burger, "Medicine is a few hundred years old. Instincts, on the other hand, have millions of years of experience behind them — all of which has accumulated in our genetic memory."

Eventually, Burger established a center for instinctive healing and teaching called the French National Anopsological Center. There, people healed themselves of nearly every kind of disease using the instinctive approach, which begins with sniffing the food as an animal does. One sniffs various foods from a smorgasbord and perhaps even tastes a bite or two until finding the one that smells and tastes the best.

Then one consumes this food exclusively until there is a distinct taste change, termed an *alliesthetic response*. If satisfied, one stops eating at this point. If hunger remains, one repeats the sniff/taste process with the remaining available foods until he finds another food that smells and tastes more attractive than the rest, continuing to repeat the procedure to repletion.

Herein lies the difficulty: with the instinctive diet, the food must be not only raw, but also totally unadulterated. It must be as found in nature: unheated, uncut, unseasoned, unfrozen, not chopped, not dehydrated, not mixed, not genetically modified and without pesticides, chemical fertilizers, fungicides, wax and so on.

Such foods are considered *initial*, or *original*, foods because they are in the state in which our ancient ancestors ate them. So a "walk on the wild side" for an instinctive eater (sometimes referred to as an *instincto*) would be to eat a mixed lettuce, tomato and cucumber salad! An instinctive eater, upon backsliding, might eat something that is everyday fare for a typical raw fooder, such as a nut and date trail mix.

An instinctive eater must thrive by eating only one raw food at a time. It is important not to mix the foods, as humans have traditionally done since prehistoric times. This is because the taste change does not occur if the food is altered in any way. Mixing just two foods together will get the smells and tastes confused, causing instinctive signals to become unreliable.

Why is the taste change so crucial? While attractive smell and taste are the body's ways of telling the person he needs that particular food at that particular moment, the taste change is the body's instinctual way of telling him that he has had enough of that food. Eating more of it could result in too much for the body's biochemistry and neurophysiology to handle, thus resulting in enervation and toxemia. (See Appendix F.)

Zephyr, author of *Instinctive Eating*, describes it as an intimate communication between "the eater's DNA and the food by way of a biochemical, sensual message. This type of communication takes place between two living entities — a food and an animal."

One never has to be afraid of overeating on this diet. The taste change, which becomes very distinct with practice, will let one know when to stop. The taste change will make it unattractive or unpleasant to continue eating that food. The books *Instinctive Nutrition* by Severen L. Schaeffer and *Genefit Nutrition* by Roman Devivo and Antje Spors have lists of foods and what the taste change for each particular food is. For example, cherries become bland tasting when no longer needed. Dates become sour. Plums lose their flavor or taste acidic. Other changes include tastes that become boring, biting, sharp, burning or dry. One's lips may even bleed (pineapple).

In *Manger Vrai*, Guy-Claude Burger recounts how this taste change is so reliable that it saved his children's lives when they tried some poisonous wild berries. The taste became bitter just before a toxic dose could be ingested. Conventionally eating neighbor children who ate from the same plants were not so fortunate.

An interesting thing about instinctive eaters is that they include raw meat as an initial food. Some of them let the meat dry in dehydrators or in the open air to enhance the taste, as it becomes similar to beef jerky. Perhaps this is because our ancestors scavenged meat from carcasses that may have been lying around for a few days. Instinctive eaters do not believe early humans were hunters initially, but rather scavengers. Our diet thus included carrion.

Instinctive eaters consider it important to consume flesh only from animals that were raised instinctively themselves. In France, a company called Orkos even sells meat especially for instinctive eaters from animals which themselves are third generation instinctive eaters, making the animals much healthier.

Although excess *cooked* meat in the diet is often associated with cancer, Burger noted that he knew of patients recovering from what was diagnosed as terminal cancer who would instinctively crave large quantities of *raw* meat. Some people believe that the body does not metabolize raw meat to produce acidic ash residues. Thus raw meat neither creates nor promotes degenerative diseases, such as cancer, arthritis, heart disease and osteoporosis, as cooked meat is notorious for doing.

Since it permits not only the vegan nuts, seeds, fruits, vegetables and sprouts, but also the animal products meat, eggs, honey and even insects, the instinctive diet is one of the most all-inclusive of raw food diets.

However, most grains were found not to generate proper taste changes and were therefore relegated to the category of *nonoriginal* foods, especially wheat, which has been extensively manipulated genetically by agricultural interests over the centuries. Grains are therefore typically excluded from instinctive diets.

Dairy was also found to be a harmful *nonfood* unless one is a baby consuming the milk of his own species. Burger ran experiments with raw, organic milk, including goat's milk, which is easier for people to digest than cow's milk. He and his wife even milked the goats by hand themselves to assure its natural quality. Members of his family alternated monthly periods of drinking and abstaining from milk in order to avoid confusing possible causes of any symptoms in the body.

Without fail, the milk drinkers experienced faintness, sunken eyes, weakness, diarrhea, bad breath, coated tongues (indicating phlegm build-up), greasy hair, moodiness and infections appearing in minor cuts.

Burger implies that they were disappointed to discover that milk was not an initial food. As a Frenchman, he undoubtedly loved his cheese. While Northern Europeans may retain the enzyme lactase to help digest the lactose in dairy, its casein still presents a problem. (See Appendix A.)

The most amazing thing about the instinctive diet is that those practicing it report levels of health that people have never even imagined possible, even beyond that of mere raw fooders.

For example, while a raw fooder may experience minimal labor time and almost no pain during childbirth, an instinctive eater does not even experience a water breakage until the moment of birth. Then the breaking water propels the baby hydraulically through the birth canal so that no pain is experienced! Labor becomes a matter of minutes rather than hours. This is no doubt what nature intended for us before we were "cast out of the Garden of Eden."

On the instinctive diet, pain, inflammation and infected cuts are almost non-existent. After an injury, an instinctive eater will experience the initial pain, which is necessary so that the body can tell the person that such an injury needs attention, but the pain stops after a minute or so. Because there is no inflammation, the throbbing pain that most of us experience after an accident doesn't exist for one who eats this way.

For an instinctive eater, wounds no longer become infected. We tend to assume it is normal for germs to infect a wound if no disinfectant is used, but germs only thrive in the toxic internal environment of a malnourished body. They are nature's garbage collectors. (See Chapter 5.) If there is no garbage to be collected, they do not thrive and proliferate.

Burger claims that he and his family never used disinfectant for over 20 years, despite cuts from rusty barbed wire and nails contaminated with manure, including pig's manure, which could theoretically cause tetanus. Yet they never got tetanus shots (which could theoretically result in tetanus) and never got tetanus.

Burger tells how surprised he was when his daughter had an injury that became inflamed and infected. She confessed that she had been eating cooked food at school, but her temptation ceased after experiencing so much pain!

Temperature extremes are well tolerated by instinctive eaters. Severen Schaeffer reports a man who fell into an ice-cold lake and spent the night clinging to his capsized boat until a morning rescue. After fifteen minutes in the ice-cold lake, he began to feel "warm all over" and suffered no lasting aftereffects from being in the cold water all night. Animals in the wild, eating instinctively, tolerate cold temperatures well. Why shouldn't people too?

The body's ability to make use of foods eaten instinctively on this diet appears to be greater than on a random raw diet. Dr. Catherine Aimelet, a consulting physician at the experimental Instinctotherapy Center near Paris, documented the case of a mother who refused surgery on her son's third-degree-burned hand, which the doctors claimed needed amputation. By the 30th day of an instinctive diet, he had no visible trace of burn, no scars, no aftereffects at all. Within one year on the diet, he experienced complete recovery from a preautistic state and from hemophilia.

Rheumatoid arthritis in a 61-year-old woman regressed almost completely in nine months. Often a heavy smoker or alcoholic on this diet quits his vice completely within days. In some cases, hair even grows back on bald men's heads.

When other diets have failed, the instinctive diet works in taking off unwanted weight. Guy-Claude Burger tells of having known "300-pounders who had given up on everything — diets, fasting and drugs, all to no effect — lose up to 110 pounds within three months." He believes instinctotherapy enables the body to find the dietary substances it needs to release metabolic deadlock.

Chimpanzees, man's closest relative, eat about 50% by volume, 68% by calories, of their diet in fruit. It has been observed by Burger that instinctive eaters eat about the same percentage of fruit.

Burger noted that when someone has habitually overeaten a particular cooked food, he or she would be repulsed by that food in the raw state for some time. Perhaps the toxic residues and overload of the cooked food must be detoxified before the body craves it instinctively in its raw state.

In France, scientist Bruno Comby has spent many years experimenting and researching the instinctive diet. It is extremely rare that someone with full-blown AIDS will return to the state of symptom-free carrier, yet his work documents several such cases in his book *Maximize Immunity*. Comby even cites a case in which the person became a *noncarrier* of HIV! His research is respected by medical doctors in France.

Interestingly, Comby has concluded that humans, as well as chimpanzees, benefit from eating insects. He wrote a book about which insects are delicious, although it has not yet been published in English.

Perhaps best of all, this diet confers great pleasure and even euphoria. Eating denatured food to one's heart's content creates guilt and physical discomfort, whereas the opposite is true with original foods. A person gets to eat his fill of whichever food he finds most attractive in taste and smell at the time of eating. People have set the following records for these one-ingredient meals, consumed all at one meal: 52 egg yolks, 156 oysters, 48 bananas, 120 passion fruits, 16 melons. Yet no digestive upsets occurred because the food was fulfilling what the body needed in each case. No one ate beyond the point of pleasure; no one forced himself to eat more than that.

Zephyr insists that he feels most alive and healthy when he stops eating a food that's no longer totally pleasurable. He claims that if science were to suddenly prove that the standard cooked diet were the most healthful, he would plunge into depression because the pleasure from eating cooked foods pales in comparison to the pleasure found in instinctively eating natural foods. Although people on the outside may think so, this is not the diet of an ascetic!

Instinctive eaters, more than any other raw fooders, speak of euphoria. Burger says, "When one eats initial foods . . . one is in a constant state of well-being. One can very well describe it as a form of euphoria, ecstatic joy that constantly wells up within."

Severen Schaeffer describes his delight in eating instinctively, "Once the senses have reawakened, the delight to be found in a native food the body truly needs can literally border on ecstasy."

Zephyr writes in his book *Instinctive Eating*, "My ecstatic experience those first few days of instinctive foraging was the undeniable 'proof' I had been searching for, the missing element of my other food experiments. . . . The high I was experiencing had many of the qualities of psychedelics. I experienced playful lucidity, freedom from many cultural programs, a more visceral sense of my connection to source, a more natural slower rhythm and shift of focus towards timelessness. . . . It was an intense awakening!"

Eventually, Zephyr came to eat insects and fruit skins. It has often been said by vegetarians that we shouldn't eat an animal unless we are willing to kill it. So he even describes the primal experience of killing some of his chickens by hand in order to be in moral integrity with eating meat.

Because of his interest in living communally, he became an active member of an instinctive community in Hawaii called Pangaia. More information can be found at www.pangaia.cc.

Perhaps the most difficult aspect of the instinctive diet is the lack of food variety we as individuals typically have available to us. We would certainly attract a lot of attention to ourselves if we were to start picking up, sniffing and tasting produce at a grocery store in order to test whether or not it is what our bodies need.

A friend of mine saw someone doing this at an all-you-can-eat salad bar and thought the man was mentally challenged! Besides, the artificial chill of such foods weakens their odors.

Yet who can afford to buy large quantities of vast numbers of foods? If it turns out, for example, that a cucumber passes the test, you may need to eat quite a number of them before satiation or taste change. How would you know how many to buy?

Having a smorgasbord of raw, organic produce to select from while the rest of the food is left to rot is not economically feasible either. Therefore, it would help either to live down the street from the organic grocery or to live in a community that practiced this together, everyone pitching in some food.

Practitioners of this diet say nonetheless that once you have become trained to follow your instincts in a few workshops, you begin to notice what your body typically needs and develop a system so that this does not become a problem.

## Aajonus Vonderplanitz and the Raw Animal Food Diet

Aajonus Vonderplanitz's raw animal food (RAF) diet is in a category of its own. He is perhaps the most controversial of all raw food leaders. His story is one of going from *eating rabbit food* to *eating rabbits*!

Aajonus suffered cancer as a child. A vaccination also caused him to become dyslexic and autistic. Yet with great determination to restore his health, he recovered from all of these problems by means of a raw vegetarian diet, which he followed religiously. He nonetheless still retained some health challenges.

After being a raw vegetarian for quite a few years in California, Aajonus biked around North America for three years, living off the land, hoping to learn the truth about optimal health by living in the wild. Occasionally, he lived with Native American tribes for a month at a time.

He went on a vision quest for his health dilemma in the summer of 1975, meditating, praying and fasting alone for four days and nights, at which time an

Indian spirit named Elk of the Black Moon appeared to guide him. Conversing with Aajonus, the spirit advised that raw meat would make him strong.

Aajonus protested that he could not kill an animal for food. The Native American responded that there is a natural agreement among all species. "Death is quick in the hunt. Suffering is a lifetime in disease. You choose," he instructed. He explained that the American Indians had lived peacefully while eating raw meat under harsh conditions for thousands of years. But Aajonus was not yet ready to hear the message.

He eventually decided he preferred to starve to death rather than return to Los Angeles, with its pollution and the survival-of-the-fittest rat race. So he began to fast himself into starvation and then to death.

Coyotes kept waking him up. This happened night after night. One night, a coyote rubbed his cold nose on Aajonus's leg and motioned with his head for him to follow. The coyote led him to the pack, and they all killed a rabbit in front of him. A female coyote placed the dead rabbit at Aajonus's feet.

He felt that the coyotes were helping him end his life faster since at that time he believed that eating raw meat would be toxic. Although Aajonus had not eaten meat in six years, it began to taste delicious after only five bites.

Aajonus woke up the next morning after what he describes as the best sleep of his life. He felt strong. He had found the missing link to his health recovery! He peddled back to Los Angeles to spread word of his great discovery. Everyone thought he was crazy. That was in 1976.

People who have seen Aajonus at work no longer think he is crazy. He is respected by medical doctors who have worked with him. He has touched many lives.

In his book *We Want to Live*, Aajonus relates that his teenage son was once brought to a hospital unconscious after a car wreck. Several doctors claimed he would probably die, but if he survived, he would be brain dead.

Aajonus describes in mini-novel fashion how when no one was looking, he emptied the drug bottles of antiseizure medications and replaced them with nutritious raw animal foods: honey, eggs and butter. His son came out of his coma within several days. Aajonus went on to feed him raw meat.

Eventually, the son regained speech and the use of his muscles and brain. Due to the raw meat, the son's muscles did not atrophy as commonly occurs among brain-damaged accident victims.

He completely recovered and went on to study at a university. Eleven years after the accident, his son remained free of any seizures or other complications from an accident in which doctors had left him to live the life of a vegetable.

Aajonus has worked with people having all kinds of ailments. In his book, he claims he facilitated 236 cancer remissions out of 240 cases. He has educated people and assisted them in beating chronic fatigue syndrome, hepatitis C, heart disease and more.

He describes many case studies, including that of a teenage girl who reversed her leukemia by eating fresh, raw animal bones with organic, raw ground beef instead of getting a bone marrow transplant. He even helped a man avoid surgery for his knees by having him eat raw animal food.

Aajonus's diet is radical, perhaps because it is almost the opposite of the raw *vegan* diet. The raw animal food diet, also known as the primal diet, consists largely of raw meat, raw eggs, unheated honey and raw dairy. Fruits and salads are kept to a minimum, as these result in an alkaline environment in the stomach when a strongly acidic one is required to digest meat.

He notes that since we are not herbivores with several stomachs, many raw vegetables are difficult for us to digest and thus best taken as juice. Nuts and seeds are also considered difficult to digest and are to be taken sparingly.

Aajonus proved that a raw plant diet can facilitate self-healing from serious disease. He also discovered that raw animal protein not only helps the body heal, but also provides the body with what it needs to reverse aging and regenerate its cells and tissues.

He claims not to have worked out or performed any other strenuous exercise in nearly twenty years while still maintaining a muscular physique. He also claimed in an interview with *Whole Life Times* that only about four percent out of 1,800 vegetarians he had known since 1969 did well on such diets, and only about 0.01% excelled.

I have met Aajonus on several occasions, as he attends potlucks and gives question and answer sessions in San Diego every few months. He had the muscles of a man who exercises and a very healthy, robust, youthful appearance for someone his age — about 56 when I last saw him. His hair was brown, and he had a youthful complexion.

However, as many have noted, most remarkable are his clear, radiant eyes. Iridologists have commented that his eyes indicate perfect health! But one need not be an iridologist to be dazzled by his eyes.

At the potlucks, I was amazed to meet a woman I had known from years earlier. She showed me photos of herself when she'd had cancer. After a few sessions of chemo, she had found it too invasive and tried the raw animal food diet instead. Within months, she was completely healed! She has been cancer free for many years now. I have run into her from time to time, and she continues to radiate health.

I met another woman who had been saying her goodbyes to everyone while dying of hepatitis C. She was in remarkable health when I last talked to her, thanks to her recovery on this diet.

Although raw dairy was impossible for me, as I explain in the next section, I couldn't question that it worked for Aajonus. He is very much in touch with his body. So, I cannot deny the facts: dairy is compatible with at least a small minority of people, so long as it is raw and from organically fed animals not polluted with antibiotics and steroids.

On the other hand, who knows whether consumers of raw dairy will not encounter health problems down the road? It is questionable as to whether we are truly able to fully digest casein. The instinctive eaters are adamant that this creates health problems.

Even if you are a militant vegan, I encourage you to read the book *We Want to Live*. It is a true testament to the powerful role played by raw food nutrition in recovering from both disease and trauma — trauma so horrific that one may otherwise be forced to live out his life as a "vegetable"!

Before reading his book, I thought orthodox medicine was at least superior to alternative health systems for accidents and trauma. Now I am not so sure. The first half is written in the form of a true mini-novel that *you will not be able to put down*. I just *had* to read the whole thing in one day, which is rare for me. The second half consists of frequently asked questions and answers, as well as dietary remedies for particular ailments. Recipes are in a separate book, *The Recipe for Living without Disease*.

Anecdotal reports on the Internet chat groups have nonetheless stressed that some people have suffered heart disease and even liver problems on a diet of so much animal fat. There is probably only a small minority who can thrive on this diet.

# Issues with Raw Meat, Dairy and Eggs

When the subject of eating raw meat comes up, the first fear that arises is that of bacteria. According to Aajonus, if one eats raw meat that is highly contaminated, the smell will be so putrid that no one would want to eat it. This instinctual warning signal of a strong, repugnant odor given to us by nature is destroyed by cooking. Cooked food will accumulate 50-60 times the bacterial count that raw food gets before it gives off this putrid odor. Therefore, the risk of getting harmful bacterial infection from *cooked* meat is much greater, as the taste and smell of contamination are so much harder to detect.

If bacteria from raw meat were so dangerous, why aren't all of the wild carnivorous animals dropping dead from salmonella and other infections? You don't see too many of them sterilizing their food.

Raw meat, especially pork, is not advised for the beginner or part-timer. However, when one has healthy intestines, having been cleaned out on a raw diet for some time, intestinal parasites will, theoretically, neither homestead nor thrive in the intestines. If one is still full of toxic debris from cooked or unnatural foods, then worms and other parasites can homestead, multiply and flourish. A parasitic infestation actually assists in cleaning up this debris by consuming the weak, dead and mutated cells of the intestinal lining. The parasites break these damaged cells down into substances the body can eliminate.

Bruno Comby gives an account of a person with a tapeworm that couldn't be poisoned away with medication, but it was completely passed in the stools after the individual switched to an instinctive raw diet.

Guy-Claude Burger even ate raw pork without getting trichinosis. He maintains that on an instinctive diet, the parasites simply don't thrive. He gives an example of a man who had been suffering pinworms and couldn't get rid of them until he tried the diet. *Within days* of eating raw foods exclusively and instinctively, his body expelled the worms. He has been free of them since. Remember, however, that Burger and the people he worked with were eating only very healthy animals: third generation instinctive eaters themselves.

Aajonus Vonderplanitz said in a 1998 interview with *Whole Life Times*, "Once, I ate pinworm-infested salmon and ten weeks afterward did not prove positive for any kind of intestinal parasite. I have eaten raw meat since 1976 and have never suffered parasites." If one is clean inside, the parasites don't have an environment in which they can survive.

On the other hand, I received word that a noted instinctive eater and author of a book on instinctive eating nearly died of trichinosis from eating a raw wild mongoose. These creatures have been known to eat cooked food scraps from human trash. Carnivore, beware!

Another point I wish to stress is that while in theory it may seem healthful to eat raw meat, things have changed with our modern animal farming and distribution methods. As Dr. Lorraine Day, MD, points out in her video *Drugs Never Cure Disease!* meat inspectors tell us that all hamburger meat in this country is made from what they call "4-D meat," which means the animals from which hamburgers are produced were dead, dying, diseased or disabled.

In this video, Dr. Day explains that the chickens we buy at the supermarket have had their intestines pulled out in the slaughterhouse. The excrement pours all over the chickens, and the chickens are actually soaked together in a vat filled with the excrement until they absorb 10% additional weight from this fecal soup!

Government regulators allow this practice because if they didn't, it would cost the chicken companies a lot of money. The Tyson company, for example, would lose an estimated 40 million dollars a year. You may be wondering why the government doesn't also consider the medical costs to the people eating this fecal-marinated chicken. Perhaps it is because the people don't have the lobbying power of Tyson Foods.

Finally, for those who still think fish is a healthful alternative, think again. The flesh of fish that are high on the food chain, i.e., tuna, shark, swordfish and other large ones, can concentrate up to a million times the pollution of the water they swim in! This is because a predator fish concentrates the poisons of the water in which it swims and the toxins of the smaller fish which it eats into its own tissues and fluids throughout its lifetime. These include not only mercury, but also dioxins, pesticides, cadmium, petroleum hydrocarbons and virtually all other poisons present in salt or fresh water. Bon appétit!

Perhaps one of the most toxic of all raw animal products is dairy. Humans stop making rennin, the enzyme needed to digest casein, at about age three, by which time they are weaned from their mothers' milk. *I remain unconvinced that there are very many, if any, people who can truly digest the casein in even raw dairy.*

After being on the raw vegan diet for nine months, I read Aajonus Vonderplanitz's books and decided to try the raw animal food diet as an experiment. I was thrilled to be able to eat dairy again, for I had been a real cheese lover, especially of feta cheese. I placed an order with some Amish for raw cottage cheese, kefir, yogurt and several flavors of cheeses. I was in dairy heaven!

I had just gotten off a two-week juice-only diet, so I was very clean inside. My sensitivity was thus heightened. If something was bad for me, my body was going to reject it immediately. There would be no time for me to be in denial!

To my chagrin, I got asthma attacks as bad as when I was a teenager. Since the phlegm layers had already been cleaned out, the toxins got to me more intensely. It felt like there was a tight band all around my chest, as if my lungs had been glued so that they could not expand! I couldn't sleep because if I lay down, I couldn't breathe. I could barely breathe at all, even when upright.

I wish I had the mutated gene (if such exists) that accepts dairy from another species, but I don't. And breathing is really important to me. If you have ever suffered from asthma, you know how horrible it can be and how little sleep you get in the night when there is an attack.

I can still digest raw cream and raw butter because those are pure fat. It is the protein in dairy that contains casein, *which is what glue is made of.* Casein sticks to the digestive tract, causing the body to produce abnormal mucus to serve as the fluid vehicle by which the body eliminates the dairy toxins in most people who eat dairy.

In *The China Study*, casein is implicated as one of the major cancer-causing substances humans consume! For more on the negative effects of dairy, see Appendix A.

While I was in great pain from the asthma attacks, I kept thinking, "So, the main reason I got such bad asthma when I was young was simply due to the dairy!"

I was told that I "outgrew" the childhood asthma, but what had really happened was that some of my internal tissues had formed such a thick mucoid layer that the dairy was no longer absorbed so quickly as to give me such acute reactions. Instead, it was slowly poisoning me into chronic degeneration as I was building up a tolerance to the dairy products.

If only doctors were educated in nutrition! It would have spared me decades of pain and addiction to stimulants (asthma pills and *herba ephedra*) had I known how simple it would have been to avoid the asthma altogether. I often wonder what my life would have been like if doctors were educated about nutrition. How much more would I have accomplished had I not taken that detour in my life?

Raw eggs are, in my opinion, the least harmful of raw animal foods. They have gotten a bad rap because of their link to salmonella infection. But salmonella, like other bacteria, is not the problem. A toxic body permits them to thrive in order to assist in detoxification. Only a sick, toxic chicken is going to be infected with it anyway, and you shouldn't be eating the eggs of such chickens.

If you are not up for a major cleansing, simply avoid eating eggs that smell or look bad or have yolk membranes that break easily. Eat eggs only from organic, vegan-fed, free-range chickens, as these are much healthier. As with meat, the uncooked egg will smell much worse than a cooked one when it is highly infected, contaminated and/or spoiling.

Osteopathic physician Joseph Mercola claims from his research that only one in 30,000 commercially produced eggs contains salmonella in high enough quantities to create illness. Check out his web site at www.mercola.com.

In *The No-Grain Diet*, he cites a study by the USDA in 2002 that found that 2.3 million eggs every year are contaminated with salmonella. But since *69 billion eggs* are produced annually, this means only one in 30,000 have salmonella. If you wish to minimize your chances of getting sick, buy eggs that come from healthy chickens. The carton should state "free range" and "vegan fed." These chickens are not fed other dead chickens or chicken excrement, so you don't have to worry about getting "mad chicken disease" in case that is later discovered to be a counterpart to mad cow disease, which reputedly arose from feeding infected, dead cows to live cattle.

Free-range and vegan-fed chickens, especially those whose diets include flaxseeds, always yield the best eggs. They are higher in beneficial omega-3 fatty acids, as opposed to the more common omega-6 fatty acids. Furthermore, such eggs taste much, much more delicious. The yolks are deep yellow and rich in flavor, whereas conventionally raised chickens lay eggs with pale yolks that are much blander in taste.

If you are avoiding eggs for ethical reasons, eggs from free-range chickens are not much better than from caged chickens. I have heard that at some factory farms, the poor "free-range" chickens only get to roam out of their cages for as little as five minutes a day!

The cholesterol in eggs has also given them an undeservedly bad reputation. Our society is suffering from heart disease because nearly all of the fat we eat, and certainly *all of the animal fat* we eat, is cooked. Harmful cholesterol accumulations result from fats that have been cooked or are rancid.

Arterial cholesterol accumulations actually *decrease* when eating *raw* fats. According to enzyme expert Dr. Edward Howell, raw fats belong in a category of their own. They contain the enzyme lipase, which is destroyed by cooking or processing. This enzyme helps the body properly digest the fat. Raw fats have no harmful effect on the arteries or heart. The Eskimos lived on a diet very, very high in raw animal fats, including raw eggs, and suffered no heart disease until introduced to cooking. Dr. Stanley Bass claims that the lecithin in egg yolks appears to counteract the development of cholesterol deposition in arteries.

According to Aajonus Vonderplanitz, raw fat is needed more than any other nutrient, even more than carbohydrates and protein. Raw fat not only functions as a fuel supply, but it also cleanses, lubricates and protects the body.

Some people caution against eating raw egg white because it contains avidin, an enzyme inhibitor that interferes with the absorption of biotin, a B vitamin. Dr. Mercola used to recommend eating the whole egg raw until Dr. Sharma, PhD, who is a biochemist with Bayer, investigated the matter. He concluded that there is not enough biotin in an egg yolk to bind to all the avidin present in the raw whites. He found that 5.7 grams of biotin are required to neutralize all of the avidin found in the raw white of an average-sized egg. There are only about 25 micrograms — or 25 millionths of a gram — of biotin in an average egg yolk.

Animals in the wild nonetheless consume the entire egg. Aajonus Vonderplanitz experimented with feeding people, as well as animals, yolks without the whites and found that eating both together was more conducive to metabolic and emotional balance. However, some people, including me, find egg white consumption to result in mucus formation.

One danger of raw animal foods is their high level of mycotoxins. Dr. Cousens is convinced that all animal products — no matter how raw, organic or home-reared — are high in mycotoxins. According to *The Fungal/Mycotoxin Etiology of Human Disease*, Vol. 2, 1994, a single egg contains 37 million pathogenic microorganisms. Even pasteurized milk has 5 million; beef, poultry, lamb and seafood contain 336 million per serving. While an average American meal of animal products has 750 million to a billion of these pathogenic microorganisms, the average vegan meal has less than 500! When you compare a billion to 500, this is a most convincing argument in favor of being at least primarily vegan.

On other hand, let us not fall into the trap of being too germ phobic, as so many have been brainwashed to be. A certain amount of bacteria is actually good for us, and there is a theory that our bodies' defense mechanisms have been weakened by our "war on germs" mentality.

# Meat: To Eat or Not to Eat

The human digestive tract is long, like that of a vegetarian animal. Man likely originated in a tropical area. As he migrated to colder climates, eating meat became necessary for survival because it was the only food around to eat in the winter. In practice, if not in theory, there seem to be a number of people who fare much better with *at least some occasional* meat.

After many years on a raw food diet, some people feel deficient in something, even weak, perhaps due to Vitamin $B_{12}$ deficiency. (See Chapter 17.) Aajonus Vonderplanitz claims that while initially his health improved on the raw vegan diet, he deteriorated despite following all the rules to get complete protein.

Some would have taken that as a signal that they should eat some cooked food, perhaps even cooked meat. But could it be that their bodies really need not cooked food, not cooked meat, but meat in its natural, raw state? Up to 85% of the nutrition in meat is deranged by cooking. The proteins are damaged, making them less assimilable and even toxic. Surely if meat is needed, it must be eaten from a healthy, organically fed animal and in its raw, natural form.

A dentist, Dr. Weston Price, DDS, lived with native peoples from all over the world before they were assimilated into modern society with its unnatural, refined diet. He found the healthiest people were not vegetarians, but meat eaters, especially the Eskimos, who were raw meat eaters. Their diet consisted of 90% raw animal food. Referring to the Eskimos, he wrote, "In his primitive state, he has provided an example of physical excellence and dental perfection such as has seldom been excelled by any race in the past or present."

On the other hand, it has been argued that Price studied only 14 groups of people, of which only a small minority were vegetarian. Perhaps those vegetarians did not have access to a wide enough variety of foods. Since his work did not really focus on the issue of vegetarianism, his remarks in that department do not carry as much weight as his main point that we need to go back to unprocessed, whole, natural foods. Additionally, the Eskimos maintained glowing health mostly because they were eating everything 100% raw. Price did not consider that a relevant factor, instead attributing their remarkable health to the meat.

Those on the path of instinctive nutrition eat raw meat very moderately. Severen Schaeffer claims that it is regularly observed in instinctive eating conditions that healthy infants, children and adults are spontaneously attracted to the smells and tastes of meat. Guy-Claude Burger talked about feeding meat prechewed by his wife to his newborn infant, who enjoyed it and slept peacefully that night.

Zephyr writes in his book *Instinctive Eating* that he once found his body craving something he hadn't been giving it. An inner voice told him to eat raw meat, and this turned out to be the missing link that liberated him from backsliding into cooked foods. He says that raw meat gave him power, drive and passion. He claims he has known only one person who has been able to remain consistently an instinctive eater for longer than a few years without eating raw meat and that certain states of consciousness are activated and nourished by eating and even killing animals.

Devivo and Spors point out in *Genefit Nutrition* that raw meat has tremendous therapeutic value under certain conditions but can also be the most dangerous of foods if overeaten. They even observed fast-growing tumors in people who ate excessively large amounts of raw meat over several years and attribute this to the accumulation of undigested foreign proteins that overload the body and poison its cells, resulting in mutations that stimulate the production of cancer cells. Devivo and Spors further claim that mammalian proteins are the worst "because they are closest to our own proteins; so the immune system might not always recognize them as foreign and might allow them to accumulate freely in the body" (p. 80).

Research indicates that some people fare better on vegetarian diets, while others appear to do better with some meat. This is thought to be related to the genes: those with tropical genes can live as vegetarians, while those with Northern European genes might need meat. If you find that you are what the authors of *The Metabolic Typing Diet* call a "protein type," who needs more protein, it may be difficult to get enough protein on a raw vegan diet, according to this theory.

However, you can still remain vegetarian, or even vegan, and still get totally sufficient, high quality protein by including in your diet greens, raw hemp seed powder, sprouted legumes and grains and soaked seeds and nuts. A few people may even handle raw dairy if they have the genetic ability to tolerate it.

As mentioned in Chapter 17, perhaps those who seem to require meat cannot assimilate sufficient Vitamin $B_{12}$ any other way. There is a lot of controversy as to whether we can get enough $B_{12}$ on a vegan diet.

Vegans even refuse any dietary supplements with gelatin capsules, which are made from animal protein. Some do it for health reasons, others because of their sheer love of animals. Still others do it because they believe it is immoral to eat animals or their products, possibly creating bad *karma*, the Eastern notion that what you do, good or bad, comes back to you later. This same notion is prevalent in virtually all spiritual belief systems. Christianity teaches, "As you sow, so shall you reap."

Personally, I do not believe there is bad karma from eating meat if one really needs it, or believes he does. But I do believe it is best to purchase only free-range animals; otherwise, you are eating an animal that has been treated harshly, like a slave. The animal should also have been fed organic food and be free of antibiotics, steroids and other drugs, for your health as well as for its, however cut short its existence on this earth.

If you do not eat organically fed or wild animals, remember you will be eating, by some estimates, ten times the toxic pesticides that you get from a like serving of produce. This is because high concentrations of toxins are stored in animal fat, and meat is about 50% fat. Most of the fat is in the flesh itself and cannot be trimmed off, but wild and properly exercised animals will be leaner, with higher proportions of omega-3 fats.

Many spiritual traditions claim that eating meat increases the "density" of one's consciousness and can even "lower one's vibration," which inhibits spiritual growth. (There is a theory that our molecules vibrate at a faster, or higher, level when our consciousness expands, thus accelerating spiritual growth.)

This may be true, and it may be truer for some people than others. It may also be that certain animals, such as cows, create more density when consumed by humans than others, such as fish. I once asked Aajonus Vonderplanitz what he thought about the spiritual side of eating meat. He answered that for him, he definitely became more centered and calm after incorporating raw meat, contrary to what he had been taught by his spiritual teachers! He said that the hypoglycemic effect of eating so much fruit created a lot of mood swings and even anger outbursts. Now even when confronted by angry vegetarians, he remains unperturbed.

It is also prudent to point out that raw animal foods are not the highest form of living foods in the same way that raw plant foods are. The theory is that by eating living food, we increase our life force. As Dr. Gabriel Cousens points out, "The sunlight energy, when transferred to us indirectly through our food, is almost completely lost to us if the transfer of the vegetarian nutrients is secondhand through animal foods" (*Conscious Eating*, p. 575).

Another factor to consider is that meat, whether cooked or raw, is generally considered acidic. (See "The Acid/Alkaline Balance" on page 331.) It is undoubtedly less acidic than cooked meat, but protein in general tends to leave acidic residues upon digestion. In my opinion, if one decides to eat raw meat, it should be only a small percentage of the diet, such as the less than 5% or so that the chimpanzees eat.

However, Dr. Ron Rosedale, MD, contends that raw meat contains sufficient ammonia, a highly alkaline compound which otherwise evaporates in cooking, for the body to utilize in neutralizing the acidity of the raw meat.

A huge factor in considering significant flesh consumption is that even raw meat has large amounts of saturated fat. If you have seen the video *Diet for a New America*, you will recall the scene in which Dr. Michael Klaper pulls a long, hardened tube of animal-derived, saturated fat from a man's artery. Saturated fat is solid at room temperature, and it is implicated in heart disease.

Not much research has been done with raw meat eaters. Still, it can be argued that the Eskimos ate a lot of raw blubber and remained healthy. Raw meat contains no trans fat, and perhaps this is the real culprit in heart disease. Cooked meat is definitely dangerous in this arena. Dr. Atkins, innovator of the infamous Atkins diet, which is tremendously high in cooked animal products, died indirectly as a result of his own heart disease!

My personal grand experiment with raw animal foods didn't last long. You already know the disaster that happened with raw dairy. While my encounters with meat were not as harsh, I quickly realized that it was not for me.

A few years ago, I decided to test the raw animal food diet for a month. I found that after eating raw meat, I maintained the light feeling that I had on a raw vegetarian diet. When I ate raw meat alone, it was actually easier for my body to digest than raw nuts, raw vegetables, raw sprouts or raw seeds. I even slept better, with no disturbances, on the days that I had meat instead of the usual raw vegan food.

I know a raw fooder who claims that eating raw fish soon after breaking a long fast enables him to recover his strength much more quickly than on plant foods alone. It seems hard for me to believe that we as humans are not capable of digesting raw meat when so many other people I know have reported the same.

On the other hand, when I mixed raw meat with raw vegetables, such as eating a salad and meat both in the same day, my intestines apparently became too alkaline to digest the meat properly. I became constipated, just as Aajonus Vonderplanitz warned.

On a diet rich in raw meat, one should have a salad only once in every two weeks or so, even though on a diet of *cooked* meat, salads help increase elimination. Just think of the people who, in times before cooking, migrated to the Northern Hemisphere. In the winter, they ate animals. In the seasons when plants grew, they ate plant food. Originally there may not have been much mixing of the two.

I found a diet of only animal products to be too limiting for me. I experimented with raw meat for a month and then gave it up with no desire for more. I just loved my salads too much. For me, it seems more natural to eat salads than meat. *Besides, raw vegan food tastes much better than raw meat.*

Another factor to consider in the decision whether or not to eat meat is its ecological impact. Forests and rainforests are being destroyed all over the world to raise farm animals, especially cattle. Our limited fresh water is being depleted. *Soon, our land may be covered in desert largely as a result of meat eating!*

While eating meat, at least raw meat, may be in the best health interest for some individuals, it is not in the best interest of an overpopulated planet. Within decades, eating meat will likely become a luxury only the wealthy can afford. For most of the world, *it already is.*

To most people, eating raw meat sounds thoroughly disgusting. However, if the body needs it, it may taste better than any cooked meat you have ever had. If you decide to eat meat, make it raw by all means, as cooked meat has been proven to contribute to the development of many diseases: heart disease, cancer, arthritis, kidney disease and gout, to name a few.

Even if you eat the best quality raw meat, be aware that it might be well to start off as a raw vegetarian for six to twelve months before adding raw meat. This is to ensure that you are cleansed enough so that any microscopic parasites in the meat will not have an environment in which to flourish within your body. Some people advise marinating meat in lemon juice overnight to kill parasites. This also makes raw meat look and taste more like cooked meat.

Keep in mind, too, that even the best meat is not usually very fresh. Some of it is imported from New Zealand, where cattle are grass fed and free range. Work carefully with a holistic doctor or health professional because eating raw animal products holds, perhaps, the only potential danger of the raw food diet.

Kosher meat is also advised for anyone eating meat, *cooked or raw.* This is because these animals have been slaughtered in a much more compassionate way. They are killed so quickly they don't even have time to realize it and there-fore do not have adrenaline and various fear molecules flooding their blood-streams and other tissues. We produce enough adrenaline in our stressful lives without adding still more stress by consuming an animal's adrenaline.

Another benefit to kosher animals is how they are fed: their usual vegetarian food replaces rendered feed, derived from dead chickens, cows, pigs, roadkill and euthanized pets. The practice of rendering is said to be responsible for mad cow disease. Who knows how many other mad animal diseases will be popping up? Also, kosher animals are guaranteed to have been healthy. As stated earlier, much of the meat we see at the grocery comes from very sick animals. If you can, get kosher meat from animals that have been fed organic plant food.

Kevin Trudeau claims to have a source of organic kosher meat. If you join his web site for a small monthly fee at www.naturalcures.com, you can learn where to buy it.

The web site www.eatwild.com provides a directory of numerous farms in the USA that sell eggs, meat and/or raw dairy products from naturally raised and/or organically fed animals.

If you live in Europe, it is best of all to get your meat from the third genera-tion instinctive-eating animals sold by Orkos distributors. Their web site is www.orkos.com/home_EN.php.

# Appendix D

## Studies from
## Scientific Journals

It is inexcusable for scientists to torture animals;
let them make their experiments on journalists and politicians.
—Henrik Ibsen (1828–1906)

In continuation from Chapter 8, various studies published in professional scientific journals are excerpted here, along with a few comments summarizing the findings. This list is by no means complete. Note that *mutagenic* means 'causing mutations', and *carcinogenic* means 'causing cancer'. Mutagens are typically carcinogenic.

### 48. "Advanced Maillard reaction end products are associated with Alzheimer's disease," *Proceedings of the National Academy of Science*, 7 June 1994, Vol. 91 (12), pp. 5710–5714.

As explained in Chapter 9, cooked food produces Maillard molecules, abnormal molecules that are usually toxic to the body. In 1916, French chemist Louis Camille Maillard proved that brown pigments and polymers that occur in pyrolysis (chemical breakdown caused by heat — in a word, cooking) are formed after the reaction of an amino acid group with the carbonyl group of sugars.

This study presents evidence that "the characteristic pathological structures associated with Alzheimer's disease contain modifications typical of advanced Maillard end products: pyrraline and pentosidine, immunocytochemically labile neurofibrillary tangles and senile plaques in brain tissue from patients with Alzheimer's disease." The study found, in contrast, little or no abnormal staining in healthy neurons of the same brain. It was concluded that the Maillard reaction-related changes could be the cause of the biochemical and insolubility properties of the lesions of Alzheimer's disease through the formation of protein cross-links.

### 49. "Analysis of cooked meat muscles for heterocyclic amine carcinogens," *Mutation Research*, 12 May 1997, Vol. 376 (1–2), pp. 129–134.

The study concluded that cooking meat makes it carcinogenic. The most carcinogenic method of cooking of those tested was shown to be flame grilling.

## 50. "Carcinogens in foods: heterocyclic amines and cancer and heart disease," *Adv Exp Med Biol*, 1995, Vol. 369, pp. 211–220.

Carcinogens occur naturally in the foods we commonly eat, including a number of heterocyclic amines (HCAs) identified in beef, pork, poultry and fish as a result of cooking. These compounds are formed during the normal cooking process by the reaction of creatine with various other amino acids.

HCAs were singled out because of their high mutagenic activity in the Ames test, which involves feeding the chemicals to rabbits to see how much it takes to kill half of them. The HCAs can be separated into two types, nonimidazole and imidazole, the latter being the predominant type present in Western foods.

Both types of HCAs have been found to be carcinogenic in rodent bioassays. A high proportion of the nonhuman primates tested also developed myocardial lesions.

The conclusions were that consumption of the HCAs formed by cooking meat may constitute a risk factor for both cancer and cardiovascular disease in humans.

## 51. "Characterization of mutagenic activity in cooked-grain-food products," *Food and Chemical Toxicity*, January 1994, Vol. 32 (1), pp. 15–21.

The study tested wheat gluten or flour from several plant sources heated at 410° F (210° C) for one hour, as well as baked or toasted grains and a heated grain beverage. The study found that heated grain products form aromatic amine chemicals during heating that are mutagenic in bacterial mutation tests.

## 52. "Cooking procedures and food mutagens: a literature review," *Food and Chemical Toxicity*, Sept 1993, Vol. 31 (9), pp. 655–675.

The abstract reads, "Commonly eaten meat products prepared from beef, pork, mutton and chicken show some level of mutagenic activity following normal frying. Food preparation methods have a significant influence on the formation of the mutagenic activity. The main food mutagens found in cooked meat products are heterocyclic amines. Several of them have been tested in long-term animal studies and shown to be carcinogenic in rodents. From a health point of view, it is desirable to reduce or prevent the formation of food mutagens. Therefore, a deeper understanding of the precursors and reaction conditions for mutagen formation during normal domestic cooking is very important."

The study goes on to show that several of the precursors in the formation of thermic mutagens are creatine or creatinine cross-linked with other amino acids and sugars.

**53. "Determination of heterocyclic aromatic amines in food products: automation of the sample preparation method prior to HPLC and PHLC-MS quantification."** *Mutation Research*, 12 May 1997, Vol. 376 (1–2), pp. 29–35.

The study found, "Heat-processing protein-rich foods may cause the formation of heterocyclic aromatic amines (HAAs), all of which are mutagenic, and some also have carcinogenic potential."

**54. "Effects of heating time and antioxidants on the formation of heterocyclic amines in marinated foods,"** *Journal of Chromatography B*, 25 March 2004, Vol. 802 (1), p. 2737.

Marinated food samples were cooked at 208° F (98° C) for 1, 2, 4, 8, 16 and 32 hours. Results showed that heterocyclic amines formed during heating increased in amount for each increase in heating time. Antioxidants (BHT and Vitamins C and E) helped inhibit HCAs, but the effect was minor.

**55. "Effects of temperature and time on mutagen formation in pan-fried hamburger,"** *A Cancer Journal of Clinicians Cancer Letters*, July 1979, Vol. 7 (2–3), pp. 63–69.

Mutagenic activity was found in hamburgers during pan-frying. It increased with temperature and time, but especially with temperature.

Uniformly frozen patties were fried at varied temperatures. Mutagenic activity was not detected in the uncooked hamburgers. In hamburgers fried at 289° F (143° C), mutagenic activity remained low for those fried from four to twenty minutes. However, when fried at 375-410° F (191-210° C) for up to ten minutes, mutagenic activity increased considerably. Mutagenic activity in fried hamburgers sold at selected restaurants ranged from very low to moderately high.

**56. "Food-derived mutagens and carcinogens,"** *Cancer Research*, 1 April 1992, Vol. 52 (7), pp. 2092s–2098s.

This study showed that cooked food contains a variety of heterocyclic amines (HCAs), byproducts of cooking found to cause cancer in animals. All the mutagenic HCAs tested were carcinogenic in rodents, most of these poor creatures ending up with cancer of the liver and other organs.

"Quantification of HCAs in cooked foods and in human urine indicated that humans are continuously exposed to low levels of them in the diet."

**57. "Formation of mutagens in cooked food. II. Foods with high starch content,"** *Cancer Letters*, March 1980, Vol. 9 (1), pp. 7–12.

Mutagens are formed when starchy foods are cooked. The study included fried potatoes, toasted bread, baked bread and fried bread to produce mutagenically active substances. Toasting white and dark bread produces mutagens at the same initial rate, but dark bread produces much higher levels of mutagenicity when toasted for long times.

The study concluded, "Significant mutagenic activity is produced when starchy foods are prepared by common cooking procedures."

## 58. "Health risks of heterocyclic amines," *Mutation Research*, 12 May 1997, Vol. 376 (1–2), pp. 37–41.

The study found, "Common cooking procedures, such as broiling, frying, barbequing (flame-grilling), heat processing — any pyrolysis of protein-rich foods — induce the formation of potent mutagenic and carcinogenic heterocyclic amines."

The cooked proteins produced organ tumors in mice and rats, as well as in nonhuman primates. The differences of risk from heterocyclic amines range greatly among humans, depending on exposure and genetic susceptibility.

## 59. "Lipid extracts isolated from heat processed food show a strong agglutinating activity against human red blood cells," *Food Research International*, 2002, Vol. 35 (6), pp. 535–540.

Agglutination of the blood cells refers to their stickiness, the cells sticking together as if glued together. (See Glossary.) In this study, the hemagglutinating (blood stickiness) activity of several mass market oils and several lipid mixtures isolated from different food items was evaluated against human red blood cells and against hamster red blood cells.

Unheated oils had a low agglutination effect, but when the same foods were heated at a common cooking temperature for 24 hours, the isolated mixture of lipids and oils showed strong hemagglutinating activity, which shows that heated oils have a toxic effect on humans. Agglutination of blood forms clots. Clots can block blood flow in arteries, leading to heart attacks and strokes.

## 60. "Metabolism of food-derived heterocyclic amines in nonhuman primates," *Mutation Research*, 12 May 1997, Vol. 376 (1–2), pp. 203–210.

The study found that the heterocyclic amines from cooked meat increased the risk of liver cancer in monkeys.

## 61. "Molecules heated in cooking generate compounds toxic for embryos," *Cahiers de nutrition et de diététique* [Journal of Nutrition and Dietetics], March 1982, pp. 36–37.

In this study, a mixture of glucose (the most common sugar) and lysine (an amino acid) was heated for two hours at 194° F (90° C). Fifty percent of both compounds reacted, forming Maillard molecules. Then the resulting mixture was blended with food and fed to rats, using only $1/6^{th}$ part of the compound mixture together with $5/6^{ths}$ part food. Results were that the number of embryos per litter decreased from 9.8 to 3.75. The weight of the embryos decreased, while placenta weight increased.

The researchers interpreted the weight decrease of the embryos as signifying food poisoning rather than lack of nutrition. Teratogenic (interfering with normal embryonic development), vascularized tumors of the navel were also observed.

## 62. "Occurrence of lipid oxidation products in foods," *Chemical and Food Toxicity*, Oct/Nov 1986, Vol. 24 (10–11), pp. 1021–1030.

Lipid oxidation products were found in food that is dehydrated (which is normally done at temperatures higher than 118° F), fried and cooked in other ways. These toxic chemicals contribute to coronary heart disease.

## 63. "Occurrence of mutagens in canned foods," *Mutation Research*, Nov/Dec 1984, Vol. 141 (3–4), pp. 131–134.

The study found mutagens in commercially heat-processed foods that are not present in the unheated raw material and appear to be produced during processing. Mutagens in these foods have been observed to display chemical behaviors and induce salmonella strains similar to those mutagens in grilled foods that have been shown to be mammalian carcinogens.

## 64. "Past, present and future of mutagens in cooked foods," *Environmental Health Perspective*, August 1986, Vol. 67, pp. 5–10.

Using a mutation assay with *Salmonella typhimurium*, the scientists who conducted this study detected various types of mutagens in cooked foods. Mutagenic heterocyclic amines were found in broiled fish meat and pyrolyzates of amino acids and proteins. Mutagenic nitropyrenes, some of which are carcinogenic, were found in grilled chicken. Roasted coffee beans contain mutagens, such as methylglyoxal. Mutagen precursors were found in food processing.

## 65. "Pyrolysis and risks of toxicity," *Cahiers de nutrition et de diététique* [Journal of Nutrition and Dietetics], 1982, Vol. 17, p. 39.

Cooking has been proven to produce millions of different Maillard molecules. The research in this paper verifies that the numerous substances generated are endless chains of novel molecules that are toxic, aromatic, peroxidizing, antioxidizing, mutagenic and carcinogenic.

## 66. "Toxicity of dietary lipid peroxidation products," *Trends in Food Science and Technology*, July 1990, Vol. 1, pp. 67–71.

This study concluded, "Humans are exposed to oxidized fats from fatty fish, fish oils, deep fat frying and powdered foods." The researchers found that even though primary hydroperoxides and lipid polymers produced from heated oils are not significantly toxic in themselves, toxic effects may be induced by secondary lipid peroxides. *Secondary* refers to products generated in the body when the initial substance is metabolized.

The study also points out that recent studies indicate that heated oils may play a role in the acceleration of atherosclerosis. "There is increasing evidence that cholesterol oxides found in deep fat fried and dehydrated foods can exert atherogenic effects."

## If You Want More Studies...

These are but a small sampling of the available evidence of the toxic effects of cooked food. Search PubMed on the Internet at www.ncbi.nlm.nih.gov/entrez/query.fcgi if you would like to do some research on your own. Plug in keyword searches like "cooked food," "cooked meat," "cooked starches" and "cooked fats." Then use the word "heated" instead of "cooked." Add some of the toxic byproducts that you have seen in this section of the book, such as "heterocyclic amines."

# Appendix E
## End Cooked Food Habits via Behavior Modification

Here is another tool in the fight to change old habits and over-come addictions: immediately remove your attention from the temptation; do not struggle; just keep your attention on another subject that interests you.    —Dr. Stanley Bass (1918–)

The following comes from Victoria BidWell's *GetWell ♥StayWell Affirmations for Americans* mind/body connection exercises, as well as from the behavior modification strategies presented in *The Natural Weight-Loss System.*

Behavior modification bypasses critical thinking and introspection and goes straight to work at changing one desirable habit for one undesirable habit. It must be practiced consistently. Each change should preferably come with a reward to reinforce the desired behavior. Exercises dealing with the mind/body connection operate at a nonmaterial, quantum level of thoughts and feelings. By deliberately and consciously changing your thoughts and feelings, your body constructs corresponding changes at the observable behavioral level.

Exercises that access the subconscious mind are superior for forming lasting behavioral changes. It is always more powerful to become aware of and release, or clear, the underlying emotional needs that motivate overeating or indulging in other unhealthful habits than to try to change those habits by conscious force of will, although the latter method will often suffice. It has been said that altering any habit for 21-28 days will leave it changed for good.

## The Addiction Syndrome at Its Very Worst

A descent into the miseries of addiction proceeds through these seven phases:

**1.** Ingestion of a toxic, addicting substance and/or indulgence in obsessive-compulsive thought patterns stimulate the body's biochemistry and neurophysiology into one of two opposite modes: (a) a sense of heightened fear or (b) a sense of great pleasure, superb well-being and/or euphoria. If the latter mode is activated, the addict feels he is in firm control of his life. And he has a strong sense of personal power with this new "ego food." The field of all possibilities opens up to him: the future looks encouraging.

**2.** The chronic stimulation demanded by the addict's habit eventually exhausts nerve energy reserves and leads to low energy levels, depression and malaise. Pathological symptoms invariably appear. Total enervation, toxemia and descent into disease are the dark destiny of the addict. The initially induced biochemical, neurophysiological drug high is no longer achieved.

**3.** When continued doses or thought/feeling indulgences do not induce the original drug high, stronger and more frequent doses are needed. The body must deal with the continual ingestion of the life-threatening substance and/or practice of the destructive thought/feeling habit.

As a lifesaving measure, therefore, the body develops a tolerance to the exogenous poisons in the substances and/or to the endogenous poisons resulting from toxic thought/feeling patterns. The body builds up this tolerance by making abnormal, retrograde, detrimental, disease-promoting changes in fluids, cells, tissues, organs and systems. All of these backward changes decrease the ability of the mind and body to function normally as they did before the addiction syndrome set in.

**4.** Painful withdrawal symptoms — both physical (material) and emotional/mental/spiritual (nonmaterial) — are experienced in periods of abstinence. Without counseling, the addict is likely to resent these periods of abstinence and spend his time listlessly, longing just to get back to his drug and/or obsessive-compulsive habit.

**5.** The addict becomes dependent on the substance or obsession/compulsion in order to "feel good" — or even function at all. Once the upper levels of tolerance are reached, the individual cannot achieve a sense of well-being or a drug high at all. The addict is now a full-blown addict who cannot manage his life without practicing the addiction daily. He socially isolates himself from those who care about him and prefers to keep company with other addicts or to be alone.

**6.** The addict continues his addictive habit. Often he will begin to experiment with other stimulating substances and mental/emotional, obsessive-compulsive modes in impossible, illusory attempts to recapture the original drug high.

**7.** The addict is finally "hooked." By now his social relationships are in tatters. His job is in danger. His socially appropriate grooming habits have been abandoned. He is controlled by the gamut of negative emotions — from hopelessness and self-pity to bitterness and anger. With no escape in sight, his lifestyle is a portrait of self-destruction. Indeed, psychological and social dysfunction, accompanied by acute and chronic diseases of various types and degrees, typify those caught in the addiction syndrome at its very worst. Misery remains until the addict can shatter his self-destructive bents of mind and emotions. The field of all possibilities has closed down for him: the future looks frightening.

Happily for the addict, a turn to Natural Hygiene's ten energy enhancers offers him an escape route to the health and happiness of mind and body. We bring nothing but good news for all members of society around the world and for all counselors who assist people with a history of addiction, deviancy and/or a criminal record! To heal ourselves and our planet, we simply get on the ten energy enhancers with an emphasis on the live food factor and get off all stimulants.

Doing so will bring about a normalization of physiology on the cellular level of every individual practicing health by healthful living. Mind, emotions and body will get well. Addictions will cease to control lives. Deviancy and criminality will cease to endanger society. New and healthy horizons will open up to everyone, including those labeled *addict* and *criminal.* The natural human inclination to do the right thing will kick in.

We will reach a critical mass, a hundredth monkey moment. We will all become less selfish and start exhibiting more concern for each other. In the best case scenario, health and compassion will override sickness and selfishness. Wars will end. We will become good stewards of our land, air and waters. Plants and animals will thrive. Our planet earth will heal. Until we, as global citizens, pay attention to and practice the live food factor and the other nine energy enhancers with a passion that passes all addictions and ignorance, we are missing this glorious get-well and stay-well boat!

# Self-Correction Strategies for Cooked Food Eating or Overeating

It has been said that the first spaceship to the moon was off course 93% of the time. The rocket only got there because of continual minor self-correction maneuvers. A health seeker can reach the goals of superlative health and a high joy through similar self-correction adjustments.

- **Enervation Avoidance:** Plan your 24 hours of each day deliberately, taking precautions to avoid getting too tired or exhausted. It is dangerously easy to eat food, especially cooked food, for its stimulating effects when just very tired but not genuinely hungry. It is also possible to overeat, even on raw food, when terribly tired. Strategically timed minutes of rest or catnaps can help you avoid enervation and its wrong-choice consequences.

- **Immediate Gratification List:** Writing down 10 a day for 10 days, make a list of 100 simple, mostly cost-free and readily available things that you *love* to do! In behavior modification psychology, this is called giving yourself *immediate gratification*. The goal is to practice pleasures not associated with food. The person who is addicted to cooked foods and/or spends too much time eating needs to shift his or her attention to nonfood activities and pastimes that bring peace, joy, pleasure and even excitement. If spiritual bankruptcy is the root cause of cooked food addiction and overeating, this strategy has amazing power to bring new pleasures and meanings into life.

- **Must Do List:** Writing down 10 a day for 10 days, itemize 100 large and small unfinished, or never begun, projects or chores, even unpleasant ones, that need attention. Use your immediate gratification activities as rewards for getting them done.

- **Short Fast:** Take a short fast of 24-36 hours to revitalize and detoxify. Use this *time-out* to get in touch with your innate sense of genuine hunger and to sharpen the tastebuds for appreciation of the natural flavors of raw foods upon breaking the fast.

- **Locking Up:** When finished with meals and evening snacks, clean up and close down the kitchen. Actually install a padlock on the door, or at least lock up the kitchen in your imagination. Turn your attention away from food whenever you get a message or a vision to eat beyond your needs or to prepare and eat cooked food.

THE LOCKED REFRIGERATOR: If so out of control with food that you cannot keep out of the refrigerator, wrap a rope around it — actually chain and padlock it shut, or imagine it locked. The act of having to untie or unlock the refrigerator door, physically or in your imagination, is a conscious reminder to open it and eat from it only when genuinely hungry. (This technique was used on the reality TV show *Honey, We're Killing the Kids*.)

- **Shock Therapy for the Overweight:** If the jaded appetite is roaring for more food when you have already eaten a sufficient amount, stand in front of a full-length mirror for 10 whole minutes with just a bathing suit on, studying front, back and sides. Ask yourself in all honesty, "Is this body underfed?"

- **Restaurant-Style Serving:** To avoid overeating, even on raw food, serve your meals restaurant-style, with the food already arranged and served on the plates and the table free of possibilities for second helpings.

- **The Food Carrier Blessing:** Keep with you wherever you go a small cooler or picnic basket filled with raw food so that an emergency situation does not throw you off into cooked food.

- **Dissociation:** Make a list of all *trigger places* that you associate with eating cooked foods or with eating beyond genuine hunger which you can realistically avoid completely in your daily schedule. Avoid these places until you are clear-headed and can enter them without eating cooked food and without overeating. Distance yourself until the neuroassociations are broken between the trigger places and eating cooked food or overeating. When you reenter them after this behavior modification process is complete, stay alert to keeping the dissociation going.

Make a list of the places and times when you typically want to eat cooked food or wrong amounts. Next to each entry, write an attitude or behavior you can substitute for the indulgence so as to break the automatic responses to these triggers. Keep totally conscious of replacing wrong eating habits with either eating correctly in these places or substituting new, nonfood habits.

- **The Blinders Association:** When entering a supermarket, put on imaginary blinders like those they used to put on workhorses to keep them focused on the furrow before them. Do not enter the aisles of cooked food products. Look away from checkout shelves and racks filled with impulse-purchase junk food. Do not give SAD food items your attention. Head straight for the produce section, shop, and get out.

- **The Produce Stand Solution:** Better yet, find the finest produce stands in town. Stay out of the supermarkets altogether.

- **The Eat before Shopping Safeguard:** Eat a satisfying meal. Take a brief rest. Then do the shopping. When tired and hungry, we are most vulnerable to feeding cooked food addiction and to overeating.

- **Social Events without Food:** Plan social get-togethers or personal activities that do not include any food: swimming, hiking, dancing, horseback riding. Learn to actively enjoy the company of others or yourself alone without food.

- **Social Events without Food at Their Cores:** Plan social get-togethers or personal activities that do not center solely around food. Bring out and enjoy raw foods for only a certain time during the event. Then put them away and clean up in order to further enjoy the people and the event without food as the core entertainment.

- **The Home Focal Point:** Plan for some other room to be the focal point of family life besides the kitchen. Let personal/family activities, goals and projects rule the mind and run your life rather than gatherings in the kitchen that entertain cooked or raw food obsessions and compulsions. Practice *out of sight, out of mind* except at meal times.

- **The Victory Kitchen:** Transform your cooking kitchen into a *victory* kitchen. Clean out the refrigerator, cupboards and pantry. Get rid of every cooked food item and gadget that cannot serve a transformed raw food purpose. Display raw food gadgetry instead.

- **The Recipe Reservoir:** Collect raw food recipe books. Prepare special occasion meals, snacks and/or beverages when the thought of just simple, whole, raw foods is giving way to cooked food yearnings and a desire to overeat.

- **The Babysitter:** If the urge to eat wrongly is upon you for a brief few hours or a day, ask a friend — or hire a helper — to be with you. Some health seekers may need this help momentarily and periodically to get through a really rough time.

- **The at Home Health Retreat:** If you realize that you cannot go it alone day after day, find a cohort who wants to live with you. Set up a Natural Hygiene health retreat in your own living space. Share the adventure of *The Natural Weight-Loss System* together. A few of the hard-core cooked food addicts and/or overeaters will need this support for speedy, successful progress.

- **The Coffee/Tea Substitutes:** Heat slightly the soak water from dried fruit, and nurse the warmed mug though your coffee/tea withdrawals. Or enjoy warm water with lemon juice.

- **Bedtime Routine without Food:** Some people go into bed with panic attack and self-medicate with a stomach full of cooked or raw food. Change this behavior by planning out a relaxing, rewarding, reassuring bedtime strategy that works for you. From mild stretching to a warm bath, from journalizing to visualizing, whatever routines bring a sense of peace without food.

- **The Gift Refusal:** If someone makes a gift of cooked food or invites you into a situation where overeating is a possibility, politely acknowledge the gift or invitation. Then refuse it.

- **BYOB:** At a conventional party where alcohol and bottled and canned juices, punches and sodas are served, bring your own bottle of distilled water. Prepare a glass with ice cubes and a twist of lime. Enjoy the party. Imbibers will not know the difference and will not feel threatened or annoyed by your abstinence.

- **Counting Crutches:** Lean on counting crutches, especially calorie and sodium counting booklets, to remind yourself of how bad SAD, cooked food is for you. Refer to these when standing before cooked food, reminding yourself of its punishments and the payoffs of raw food.

- **Count to 15:** Studies with the electroencephalogram show that a high-spiked and almost overpowering enough thought impulse, identified subjectively as a desire to eat that which we know we should not, lasts only a few seconds, after which the electrical impulse records as a weak, short spike, no longer overpowering in thought content to act on the previous desire. Therefore, it is suggested that if a person can get past those first few seconds by diverting attention or simply by counting to 15, the impulse will weaken sufficiently to successfully resist it. Count sheep to fall asleep, count pineapples to stay awake.

- **Buffet Table Sailing:** Turn your attention away from all cooked food at a feast. Focus on raw dishes only. Retreat from the smorgasbord, stand at a distance, and reaffirm your intention to eat only raw. Then consider the best choices, and identify the off-limit choices. Approach the table with resolve and delight. Enjoy your raw choices to their fullest.

- **Restaurant Insurance:** Take out these insurance policies:

  ✓ Seek out restaurants with the best raw food dishes and salad bars.

  ✓ Seat yourself as much as possible away from, or with your back to, the cooked food stimuli of dessert carts, barbecue pits and people loading up.

  ✓ Remove salt, pepper, sugar packets and the like from the table, as well as any colored pictures of desserts and drinks.

  ✓ Ask the waiter to bring the check with the meal to set up avoiding ordering a dessert at the last minute.

  ✓ Hand the waiter a *business card* to be presented to the chef requesting a raw fruit and vegetable plate that meets your special dietary/health needs. It could read something to this effect, "Dear chef, please prepare for me a plate of raw fruits and/or vegetables. I am unable to eat cooked foods. Your help will be much appreciated. Thank you so much. I am sure that I will be happy with what you bring me. Thank you again."

  ✓ Bring your own avocado or serving of nuts to eat with the raw plate.

- **The Painter's Mask:** If nonstop snacking, especially while around cooked food, has become an impossible habit to break, wear a painter's mask while around food to break yourself of this bad habit, much like wearing gloves to keep a person from biting one's nails.

- **One Day at a Time:** If so out of control with food, shop for each day so that the kitchen is not loaded with a week's worth of food that gets eaten in two days. Break this expensive habit one day at a time until you can trust yourself with excess raw food in your home.

# Mind/Body Connection Exercises for Ending Food Addictions

A much more powerful approach than eliciting a new conditioned response with proper application of behavior modification techniques exists: that is to spontaneously change into a new behavior pattern by making changes at the quantum level of thoughts and feelings.

A new science since the 1950s, alternatively named *psychoneuroimmunology*, *molecular biology* or *the mind/body connection,* it reveals that our thoughts and feelings (nonmaterial events) create neurotransmitters (material realities) that go out to communicate with our bodies. Happy thoughts and feelings create unique molecules that communicate with the cells of the body to make us feel happy. Fearful thoughts and feelings do the same, making us feel afraid. This new mind/body science teaches us how to take conscious control of our thoughts and feelings that directly impact our 75 trillion body cells in the direction of health — all this at the quantum level! How exciting is this?

If used with great enthusiasm, commitment and joy, quantum level changes can break addictions instantaneously and forever. All it takes is one sufficiently strong, highly charged, mental/emotional phenomenon sparked by a clear vision of infinitely better possibilities for the life one is presently living!

Following are mind/body connection level exercises to bring about freedom from cooked food addiction and desires to overeat on cooked or raw food. They are exercises that also have the potential to quantum leap you into freedom from all addictions and into much higher joy and deeper spirituality.

- **Get Clear about Your Great Purpose in Life:** Every person has a calling when brought into this life. Not all hear or see the calling. Not all who get the calling rise to it. But rising to your calling, doing that which you were born to do, doing what you love to do — that will bring happiness like nothing else. To know that you are doing what you were put on earth to do is deeply satisfying and a huge source of strength in times of trouble. If not yet clear on what your great purpose in life is, start journalizing, exploring that which would make you happiest. If clear already, log what challenges need to be faced and overcome to become a more powerful force for good as you fulfill your great purpose. Also make a list of lesser goals under this great purpose. Ask yourself what you can do to fully actualize your highest purpose in this lifetime.

- **Visualize Yourself at Your Very Best:** Psychologists have found in studies that the mind will believe what we give it and will strive, much like a computer, to bring the given "software" image into being. When you practice visualizing yourself at your best, your mind will rise to that image and strive to bring it into reality. The rules of visualization are as follows:

  ✓ In a quiet, peaceful spot, get comfortable, close your eyes, go through five minutes of relaxation and deep breathing, and let go of the day's concerns.

  ✓ Take five minutes to get a still life picture, like a snapshot, of how you look at your very best, of you interacting with others, of you in your private life and in various outside activities. Notice how wonderful you feel at your very best. Hold this picture in your mind's eye. Imagine this picture as a blueprint for your subconscious mind to build into reality.

  ✓ Be patient as visualization sessions progress: it may take weeks before you are good at creating visualizations from your linear left-brain commands. Making visions is a right-brain activity and takes some practice.

  ✓ After practicing the still life snapshot for a few days, start visualizing yourself in live, Technicolor scenarios in which you are thoroughly enjoying yourself doing the many things you would do if you were energized and in superlative health and high joy. Studies reveal that the finer the details of sight, sound, touch, taste and smell; then the more uplifting the emotions; the more positive the thoughts, the more powerful the resulting quantum leap into reality. The researchers actually tell us that the mind cannot tell the difference between a real experience and a vividly imagined experience. To the mind, these living scenes of you at your very best are really happening.

  ✓ Daily repetition of 5-10 minute sessions of these positive images interspersed throughout the day is absolutely paramount. Most people have several years of daylong negative self-talk and negative visualizations that must be replaced with visions of themselves at their very best. Time is needed. Thought/feelings that are carefully and consciously aimed, crystal clean in detail and supported with strong feelings of self-worth, self-love and positivity have the power to shatter cooked food addictions, end overeating, and move mountains.

- **Forgive Everybody for Everything:** Make a list of all the people throughout your lifetime, living or deceased, whom you need to forgive for any real, retrospective or possibly imagined wrongdoing on their part. If they are living and in whereabouts known, contact them to ask their forgiveness. If they are deceased, write and mail a letter with the forgiven's name but no address and no return address. Each person who carries unforgiveness in the heart also carries unforgiveness in his 75 trillion or so body cells, which eats away at the body and psyche, lowering the vital functioning of the immune defenses, inspiring wrong choices and otherwise adversely affecting body, mind and spirit.

- **Forgive Yourself:** In like spirit, make a list of unforgivenesses you hold against yourself. Work your way down the list over a period of time, checking off the now-forgiven as you go. Forgive yourself for every imperfect thing ever done, every bad choice ever made, every energy robber lived out, every everything. Give up fear and negativity in all its forms.

• **Self-Assurance:** Practice self-assurance when uneducated people want to persuade, coax, goad or intimidate you back to the basic four food groups or into overeating. Renew your mind with the *truth* and *proof* of the raw food diet's efficacy, and refuse to be moved by these uneducated people. They know not what they say.

• **Love Your "Fearfully and Wonderfully Made" Body:** Seventy-five trillion or so cells, all working in unison for your health and happiness, are an amazing ongoing drama! Here are 3 exercises to help you love your body:

✓ Lie down in quietude. Gently feel your body and all of its inner functionings. Send thoughts of unconditional acceptance and love for yourself as you are right now.

✓ Stand before a mirror and view your body for 10 minutes. Reject all negative thoughts and feelings as part of the old self that only contributes to wrong choices, addiction and disease. Embrace the new self with unconditional love and acceptance for yourself as you are right now.

✓ Throughout the day — wherever you are, whatever you are doing — practice sending your body thoughts of acceptance, love and appreciation for serving you as well as it does. Refuse to entertain thoughts from the old self that humiliate, blame, shame, hate, disgust, punish or lead to addiction. Give only love.

• **GetWell♥StayWell Affirmations:** My book and four compact disk course, *GetWell ♥StayWell Affirmations for Americans — How to Bust Up Old, Rigid, Fearful, Energy Robbing Patterns in Consciousness — and — How to Restructure a New, Flexible, Loving, Energy Enhancing Sense of Life*, provide 500 affirmations spread over the ten energy enhancers. In writing and using your own affirmations, here are guidelines:

✓ Affirmations should always be stated in the affirmative, the positive, without using words like *don't*, *not*, *never* and *won't*.

✓ Affirmations should always be stated in the present tense, as if they are happening right now, and never in the past or future.

✓ Affirmations should be one-sentence statements.

✓ Ideally, affirmations should have your name worded into the sentence.

✓ Affirmations should be spoken aloud with power, commitment, joy, exuberance, gratitude, amazement — any emotion from the gamut of the positive.

✓ Affirmations could also be written down and read with likewise powerful passion.

✓ The most significant affirmation should be written down in your journal 10 times a day.

✓ Affirmations can be written out on cards and placed about your home, taken with you to read for strength at crucial times, shared with friends, memorized and repeated as needed and so forth. Negative self-talk can be supplanted with such positive affirmations as these:

- My body right now automatically processes the raw foods which I, _____, eat to give me superlative health in mind, spirit and body.

- I, _____, enjoy only raw fruits and vegetables, nuts, seeds and sprouts. They turn to beauty and well-being in me.

- I, _____, deserve a fantastic, fit, fun body.

- My body knows raw food gives me the greatest health and pleasure. Such food is wholesome and pleasing to me.

- **The Attitude of Gratitude:** We ourselves cannot be completely healthy and happy in a world with even one sick person. It therefore behooves us to give away our knowledge of Natural Hygiene and the benefits of raw foods to open-minded health seekers and to those sick and suffering who do not even know health can be sought and built. We do this out of gratitude for what this knowledge has done for us and thereby do that '60s thing: make the world a better place. Begin by making a very long journal entry to which you add as time goes by: "Counting My Blessings." List and number all for which you are grateful. Think on these things. Then make another entry: "Sharing My Blessings." Practice the attitude of gratitude all the days of your life by reaching out in the endless ways you can to daily help people heal in mind, body and spirit.

- **Journalizing Out of Cooked Food Addiction and Overeating:** Keeping a journal is another technique for making changes at the quantum level of thoughts and feelings, which then inspire a person to spontaneously make behavioral changes to complement the new quantum level mindset. Studies show that when a person keeps a journal consistently to help make himself or herself more aware of daily thought/feeling/habit patterns that he or she wants to change, these patterns are changed more successfully than when a person keeps no journal. This finding only makes sense: where the attention goes, the energy flows. And journalizing is a way to flow attention to a situation needing change and to keep that attention focused.

*Insanity* has been jokingly defined as 'doing what you have always done and expecting different results from what you have always gotten'. Writing down new desired behaviors in specific terms and then keeping a record of how you are doing on a daily basis to achieve these new behaviors keeps a person awake, aware and alert to avoiding doing what he or she has always done. The following are journal topics:

✓ an evening layout of next day's schedule

✓ a Sunday night layout of highlights of the upcoming week's schedule

✓ a daily eating log — every meal and every snack

✓ a daily exercise log

✓ a weekly weight and measurement log if on a weight-loss program

✓ an evening journal of the day's activities and highlights

✓ a diary of anything new: thoughts, teachings, conversations, people, events, music and so on

✓ a list of what you would like to change in your life with periodic evaluations of how well you are progressing and what you can do to further speed your progress along.

# Appendix F

## Natural Hygiene and the Nondietary Health Factors

In addition to all your chores, you must make time in your daily schedule for adequate rest, sleep, exercise and sunshine.
—Dr. Virginia Vetrano (1927–)

I have carefully avoided, as far as possible, all extreme heat, cold, extraordinary fatigue, interruption of my usual hours of rest or staying long in bad air. I, likewise, did all that lay in my power to avoid those evils, which appear to have the greatest influence on our bodies. —Luigi Cornaro (1458–1560)

I am grateful to Victoria BidWell for sharing excerpts from *The Health Seekers' YearBook*. If you'd like to learn more about the crucial nondietary factors for attaining superior health status, read her book. It presents an easy-to-understand guide to Natural Hygiene, the comprehensive health system alternative to the conventional medical system. It makes a great complement to the book you are holding. Victoria's book is now sold as "two books in one," the second being excerpts from her Natural Hygiene periodical *Common Health Sense*.

People often buy her book just to get Chapter 9, which serves up menus for breakfast, lunch and dinner for every day of the year. They consist of 100% raw, nontoxic foods, with exact amounts specified and seasonal foods featured, all in proper combination for ideal digestion — with no repetition! Chapter 10 serves up 50 classic, all-raw, full-meal dishes in proper combination, as well as many wonderful salad dressings for both fruit and vegetable dishes.

Not only is there a menu for every day of the year, but Chapter 13 also presents a health quote for every day of the year! The January quotes are all by Dr. Shelton. The above two quotes were among the book's selections.

With the recent addition of *The Best of Common Health Sense*, hundreds more all-raw recipes are served up, as well as "Victoria's Secret Formula Recipes" for making an endless variety of appetizers, beverages, main dishes, nut milks and desserts.

*The Health Seekers' YearBook* covers such topics as exercise, emotional balance, in-depth discussion of the dangers of the SAD, as well as tidbits on topics like the advantages of monomeals, the distinction between true and false hunger and the value of fasting. It also includes writings by Dr. Vetrano, Dr. Shelton and other hygienic practitioners.

The book is very user friendly, with a lot of graphics. Best of all, it has been painstakingly edited for Natural Hygiene accuracy by none other than Dr. Vetrano, Dr. Shelton's protégée! It was also recommended and sold by T. C. Fry, whose review touted it as "better than my Life Science Health System!"

One of the things that Victoria emphasizes is that while many raw food books, including my first edition, claim that the raw food diet heals the body, it is not the diet that heals. It is only the body's trillions of cells that make up its many organ systems working together to take in food, water, air and sunlight to detoxify poisons and to eliminate bodily wastes that can achieve healing.

In Victoria's own words, "Raw foods supply the superlative nutrition the human body needs to conduct its ongoing metabolic processes in its 75 trillion cells that will result, over time, in a complete upgrading of the individual to ultimate heights of body, mind and spirit health. But keep in mind, it is the food that does the supplying. And it is the body that does the healing."

The remaining material presented below was written by Victoria BidWell and edited by Dr. Vetrano for hygienic accuracy. Victoria now takes the lead with Dr. Vetrano backing her up.

# The Medical Mentality at Its Very Worst

• The medical mentality holds that a person can appear "perfectly healthy" one day and then be mysteriously, inexplicably stricken with a dreaded disease virtually overnight. "Mysterious" is a favored word used.

• The medical mentality supports a belief in the germ theory as originally proposed by Louis Pasteur: disease is caused by microorganisms or viruses foreign to the body, which they invade and use as a host.

• The medical mentality holds that there are over 10,000 known and categorized and named diseases, each disease with its own cause or causes, known or unknown. Years of scientists' time and billions of Americans' dollars are spent annually, searching for the external, mysterious causes of various diseases and their antidotes.

• The medical mentality looks at the disease process as warfare, as an enemy which "invades or attacks the body" and therefore as something which can — and must — be stopped: the symptoms must be palliated or suppressed; the body must in some way be "treated" with some sort of doctor-prescribed drug, treatment, therapy or surgery to make the patient get well.

• The medical mentality teaches you that illness is to be expected as the years advance, as disease is an expected part of the aging process. Doctors hopelessly and coldheartedly state, "You will just have to learn to live with it!" ("it" meaning "the pain and degeneration") . . . if standard medical treatment cannot help you.

• The medical mentality is not interested in promoting dietary nutrition as an integral part of getting well or staying well, although it may make minor concessions such as recommending a reduction in dietary salt or the adoption of a weight-loss program. The prevailing pessimistic attitude, however, is that even if there were something to this "dietary nutrition," people would not change their eating habits, anyway. At its worst, the medical mentality does not have faith in the human being to change: a sense of hopelessness prevails.

• The medical mentality looks at the practice of fasting to be synonymous with starvation, and fasting is therefore viewed as a form of dangerous extremism.

• The medical mentality refuses to acknowledge the evidence that any of the many alternative health care systems have any validity whatsoever. It does this in the face of vast amounts of evidence and carefully kept records. Any improvement on the part of individuals under alternative health care systems is attributed to chance, to "spontaneous remission" or to other causes. Or the improvement is branded as "dangerous in the long run," regardless of how much the person has improved.

• The medical mentality encourages both a belief in and a dependence on the medical/pharmaceutical complex as the final authority on all health questions and the only real source of knowledge and power that leads to individual health. Conformity to establishment thinking and the medical mentality are systematically and relentlessly conditioned and brainwashed into the minds of the American people from birth to death, through both subtle cues and by means of open intimidation by those in power.

• Under the medical mentality, you subject yourself and your loved ones to continued medical treatment, disregarding the all-too-often reality: you will only get worse as the medical treatment continues. Furthermore, you have no hope or desire to search for a workable alternative health care system, no desire to learn how to take personal responsibility for your own health.

# Natural Hygiene at Its Very Best

• Natural Hygiene holds that health is the normal state of all living organisms and that health is maintained through natural, self-initiating, self-healing processes!

• Natural Hygiene holds that the one cause of all disease is the toxic saturation at the cellular level of the bodily tissues, bloodstream and fluids brought on by the depletion of nerve energy reserves through toxic living habits. This self-poisonous state is termed *toxemia*, *autointoxication*, or *toxicosis*.

• Natural Hygiene views disease as orderly backward degenerative changes at the cellular level as a result of toxemia. In order to prevent these retrograde changes and to forestall degenerative changes in the actual structure and consequent function of cells, tissues, organs and systems for as long as possible, the body isolates and/or eliminates abnormal accumulations of metabolic waste and ingested poisons. Such bodily conducted actions of elimination may be called "disease" (acute), but they actually serve to prevent further degenerative (chronic) changes.

- Because toxemia is "the one cause of all disease," Natural Hygiene refutes the concept that microorganisms — also called *germs* or *viruses* — are the sole causative factors of disease.
- Because only the body is capable of instituting renewing, cleansing, healing processes, Natural Hygiene rejects the ingestion of any substances which the body cannot metabolize and assimilate and which cannot be used in the normal metabolic processes for appropriation into bodily tissues and fluids. Such unnatural substances can only further enervate and poison the body and are not to be considered as *food* or *nutrition* in any way.
- Both medication and the *quasi-food* substances typical of the refined, chemicalized, processed Standard American Diet are included in this poisoning category. They are not only health threatening, but life threatening.
- Natural Hygiene recommends the following as the Ideal Diet and therefore as the only foods fit for the highest level of human health and well-being: whole, raw fruits, vegetables, nuts and seeds, prepared in proper combination and eaten in moderation and when one is in a state of emotional balance.
- Natural Hygiene advocates fasting for some health seekers. Fasting provides physical, physiological, sensory, mental, emotional rest. This deep and almost total rest provides the body with the ideal conditions which are necessary for the regeneration of nerve energy and mandatory for the elimination of toxins, cellular repairs and full restoration of health.
- Natural Hygiene maintains that health is the personal responsibility of each individual and that God-given health, happiness and Hygiene joy are achieved only by the most conscientious and daily application of the ten energy enhancers!

# *Nerve Energy* — A Formal Definition

*Nerve energy*, in Natural Hygiene, refers to the low-grade electricity generated by the brain that supplies current to and regenerates and repairs all tissues: brain, bone, blood, skin, muscles, nervous tissues, glands et al.

The health seeker best appreciates the human body as a wondrous electrochemical power system! It is nerve energy that runs the whole show, such that all bodily functions — and especially nutrition through diet, air, water, sunlight and the elimination of toxins from endogenous and exogenous sources — are performed within their normal parameters.

When a person lives in a state of high nerve energy, well nourished on the raw food diet, the body has the vital force it needs to keep itself well nourished and well cleansed, free of disease and full of vitality for the reasonable demands made upon it from a hygienic lifestyle of moderation in all things good and avoidance of all things toxic!

Joyful, superlative health results only when nerve energy is high and bodily toxicity is at healthful, homeostatic levels!

## How to Restore Your Nerve Energy!

The brain can also be likened to a high-powered battery that needs continual recharging on a daily and nightly basis. Its low-grade electricity can be recharged in one of four ways:

ADEQUATE SLEEP

REST AND CATNAPS during the day, as needed

COMPLETE REST — time spent in hygienic fasting

QUIET, STILL TIME — spent in meditation, biofeedback, prayer or some such calming inactivity proven to provide deep rest to the mind and body.

## Nerve Energy Is Not Plain, Old "Energy"!

Plain, old "energy" refers to …

anything the body consumes in the form of food and drink,

anything the body uses in the form of muscular output,

anything the body generates in the form of heat,

anything the body burns in the form of calories,

anything the body employs to secrete fluids,

anything the body experiences in the form of stimulation,

anything the body ingests to get "hyped up" or excited,

anything the body expends in the form of mental activity,

anything the body exudes in the form of charisma,

anything the body stores in the form of potential activity.

In other words, anything the mind and body consume from the outside, anything the mind and body generate in the form of creative thoughts or mental constructs or emotional output, anything the mind and body exert in the form of muscular output is not *nerve energy*. We may experience these activities, these "anythings" as stimulating and even feel fully energized by their undertaking. *But what we are engaging in with these "anythings" is the expenditure of nerve energy, not the generation of nerve energy!*

# Dr. Vetrano with Victoria on the Priceless Benefits of Adequate Rest and Sleep

Sleep is a period of complete unconsciousness of the individual and a function of the nervous system exclusively: with the advent of sleep, the body shuts down consciousness. Nonnervous tissues of the body, such as bone, muscle and blood, do not transmit nerve impulses; nevertheless, these nonnervous tissues too need the period of nightly sleep, as they too do have their own healthy functions and need revitalization for restoration.

Are adequate rest and sleep the missing energy enhancers in your life that are preventing you from reaching superlative health? Are you following the other nine energy enhancers but still suffering in ill health?

An estimated four out of six American adults report "daytime sleepiness." This makes them sluggish and irritable, unable to focus on tasks at hand. This much we hygienists have fully established: sleep is a part of the life of every animal and human in the world.

Sleep — and only sleep — is absolutely necessary for renovation and recharging of the nervous system and affords a period of revitalization for other structures so that the organism can continue to function normally and be *well*.

## The Two Primary Needs of Sleep

- A period of revitalization for the nervous system and renewing of nerve energy
- A time of decreased activity for the repair of organic damages and rebalancing of body chemistry

## Miseries of Sleep Deprivation

- Toxins which are eliminated more rapidly while sleeping accumulate to an abnormal, unhealthy degree if one does not take adequate sleep. These retained wastes damage tissues and organs throughout the body. If the nervous system is not recharged by nightly sleeping, it cannot send the proper number of nerve impulses to the various bodily organs for their proper functioning!
- Consequently these organs function poorly. The result is greater toxin accumulation; eventually the individual takes the relentless descent into disease.
- Enervation resulting from insufficient sleep results in a lowering of available vital nerve energy. This causes all organs to work less efficiently, resulting in poor digestion and in toxin accumulation from impaired liver, kidneys, lung and bowel.
- Drowsiness and inability to concentrate or actual impairment of memory and physical performance, particularly reduced ability to carry out mathematical calculations, cause endless everyday problems.
- Countless more miseries! Beware! This list could go on and on, adversely affecting every cell and organ of the body: hallucinations and mood swings, increased heart rate variability, irritation/inflammation of the digestive tract resulting in body messages causing insomnia, decrease in release of growth hormones, decrease in normal body temperature, significantly decreased metabolic activity of the brain after only 24 hours, decreased immune system function measured by decreased white blood cell count, abnormality in hormone production regulating hunger and appetite that causes a desire to eat well in excess of caloric demands to stimulate oneself into wakefulness and resulting in obesity and more.

## The Lifesaving Benefits of Sleep

- During sleep, the entire human body is permitted a priceless and profound rest. This deep rest cannot be bought for any amount of money!

- During sleep, sympathetic nervous activity decreases, and parasympathetic activity increases, reducing muscular tone to almost nil. This provides a much greater rest of the skeletal muscles compared to that of simple, wakeful resting.
- During sleep, arterial blood pressure falls; pulse rate decreases; skin vessels dilate. This deep sleep therefore affords deep rest for the heart and for the muscles of the arteries.
- During sleep, activity of the gastrointestinal tract increases, improving digestion and absorption of food to promote better nutrition.
- During sleep, skeletal muscles are completely relaxed; whereas, when in resting wakefulness — and especially when under stress — they are not.
- During sleep, the metabolic rate falls by 10-20%, thus permitting the bodily tissues, organs and systems a much-needed deep rest.
- During sleep, healing and repair wherever needed throughout the body increase. During sleep is when we get well! This healing and repair is especially profound while both sleeping and undertaking a fast, and especially while doing both!

## Recuperation and Recovery Come from Rest and Sleep!

Recuperation from temporary or partial exhaustion will take place with one or two days of extra rest and sleep. If, however, you persist in the excesses that waste nerve energy, then enervation will follow "as night follows day."

This leads to lowered functioning capacity of every tissue, organ and system in the body. At this point, it could take the enervated person many weeks or even many months (or years) of 12 hours a day or more of rest and sleep, along with strict, low-key, hygienic living to get well. Rearranging the lifestyle to align with Hygiene, relearning how to best deal with stress and taking time for adequate rest and sleep are your only antidotes. And happily, priceless as they are — they cost absolutely nothing!

**Note:** The hygienic raw diet does not "give" the body more energy. Eating raw does the very next best thing: consuming the hygienic raw food diet conserves precious nerve energy, as raw foods are so easy and efficient for the body to digest and do not contain all the exogenous toxins of the SAD, which must be expelled at the cost of even more nerve energy. Less energy used to process your raw foods equals more energy for detoxification, repair and the fun of your daily life!

## Dr. J. H. Tilden: The Seven Stages of Disease

To review, "the one cause of all disease" is termed *toxemia* and defined as 'the poisoning of bodily fluids and tissues'. We become sick because we became toxic in the first place. And we became toxic because, just prior to this event, we ran so low on nerve energy that the body could not keep the bodily tissues and fluids clean. The solution to the energy crisis in a toxic body, therefore, is to get the nerve energy back, to revitalize!

With restored reserves of nerve energy, the body can go about detoxification and repair.

Since disease is simply the body's adaptation to a toxic overload, the reversal of the disease process is simply a dedicated and disciplined, hygienic, energy-enhancing lifestyle!

This descent into sickness was first presented by Dr. J. H. Tilden in his landmark 1926 publication *Toxemia Explained* as the "seven stages of disease."

The role of the raw food diet in the ascent out of disease, regardless of the stage, early or advanced, is that (1) raw foods are free of exogenous toxins, (2) they provide the human body with the superlative nutrition the body needs to perform its basic metabolic tasks, and (3) they provide this nutrition in an energy-conservative package, being easy and energy efficient to digest. Less nerve energy used to process the food ingested means more nerve energy for detoxification and repair. Remember, it's all about nerve energy first and foremost! See Chapter 4 for the role of the raw food diet in getting well and staying well.

# The Seven Stages of Disease

**Stage 1 is enervation.** Nerve energy is so reduced or exhausted that all normal bodily functions are impaired, especially the elimination of endogenous and exogenous poisons. Stage 1 thus begins the progressive, chronic process of *toxemic toleration* of toxins that continues through all of the seven stages. The toxic sufferer does not feel his "normal self." He feels either stimulated or depressed.

**Stage 2 is toxemia.** Nerve energy is too low to eliminate metabolic wastes (endogenous) and ingested poisons (exogenous). These toxic substances begin to saturate first the bloodstream and lymphatic fluids and then the tissues themselves. The toxic sufferer feels inordinately tired, run-down and "out of it."

**Stage 3 is irritation.** Toxic buildup within the bodily fluids and tissues continues. The cells/tissues where buildup occurs are irritated by the toxic nature of the wastes, resulting in low-grade inflammation. The toxic sufferer often feels exhausted, irritable, itchy — even hostile or irrational. If the toxic sufferer goes to a standard medical doctor at this point, he can only guess at a name for the disease; or he cannot find enough disease symptoms present to pin a formal name to the complaints and declares, "There is nothing wrong with you! This is all in your head!" He may then recommend a psychiatrist.

**Stage 4 is inflammation.** The low-grade, chronic inflammation from stage 3 is leading to the death of cells. An area or organ where toxicants have amassed next becomes fully inflamed. The toxic sufferer experiences actual pain, along with pathological symptoms. The standard medical doctor now names the set of symptoms and begins his treatments.

**Stage 5 is ulceration.** Tissues are destroyed. The body ulcerates, forming an outlet for the poisonous buildup. The toxic sufferer experiences a multiplication and worsening of symptoms and pain. Standard medical doctors typically continue drugging and often commence with surgery and other forms of more radical and questionable treatment at this stage. The standard doctor easily names the disease and declares, "You're going to have to learn to live with pain!"

**Stage 6 is induration.** Induration is the result of long-standing, chronic inflammation, interspersed with bouts of acute inflammation. The chronic inflammation causes an impairment or sluggishness of circulation; because some cells may succumb, they are replaced with scar tissue. The toxic sufferer endures even more physical pain. In this 6th stage, standard medical doctors continue with both drugging and/or surgery and/or other modalities.

**Stage 7 is chronic, irreversible degeneration.** Cellular integrity is destroyed through cellular disorganization and/or cancerous proliferation. Tissues, organs and whole systems lose their ability to function normally. Biochemical and morphological changes from the deposition of endogenous and exogenous toxins bring about degeneration and death at the cellular level. The toxic sufferer is "a pathological mess" on his or her deathbed.

# The Natural, Physiological Laws of Life

**Life's Great Law:** Every living cell of the organized body is endowed with an instinct of self-preservation, sustained by an inherent force in the organism called *vital force* or *life force*. The success of each living organism — whether it be simple or complex — is directly proportional to the amount of its life force and inversely proportional to the degree of its activity.

The medical mentality at its very worst overrides Life's Great Law with propaganda to program the people into thinking that the 75 trillion cells of the body which make up *human life* must, without question and at all times, be subjugated to the dictates of the medical doctor and that lasting, reliable, dependable health and even *life* itself come only through such subjugation. In fact absolutely everyone in society is expected to "have" a medical doctor!

**The Law of Order:** The living organism is completely self-constructing, self-maintaining, self-directing, self-repairing, self-defending and self-healing.

Although most medical doctors do acknowledge that science has revealed much about how the body works, the medical mentality at its very worst overrides the Law of Order with propaganda to program the people into thinking that the presence of disease in the body is oftentimes a "mystery," with no known causes and no known cures, or that disease is an "enemy at war with the body," a war that can only be won by following the dictates of the medical doctor.

**The Law of Action:** Whenever action occurs in the living organism as the result of extraneous influences, the action must be ascribed to the living thing which has the power of action — and not to the lifeless, the leading characteristic of which is inertia.

The medical mentality at its very worst overrides the Law of Action with propaganda to program the people into thinking that the drugs pushed by those in control of the medical/pharmaceutical industry have the power not only to "act," but to "heal," as long as these drugs are introduced into the body exactly as doctors dictate. Likewise, dieticians are fond of promoting their foods by portraying them with powers of action which they absolutely do not, according to the Law of Action, possess!

**The Law of Power:** The bodily power employed, and consequently expended, in any vital or so-called medicinal action, is vital power used up (expended nerve energy) — in other words, "natural power from within and not from without."

The medical mentality at its very worst overrides the Law of Power with propaganda to program people into thinking that the bodily response to stimulation from ingestion of toxic medicines people experience comes from powers inherent in drugs. The hygienic truth is that the "power" experienced comes from the body's being stimulated by poison to rid itself of the drug.

**The Law of Distribution:** The power of the body, whether that power is great or little, is distributed in a manner proportionate to the importance and needs of the various organs and tissues of the body.

The medical mentality at its very worst makes no effort to attempt to override such an obviously common health sense affirmation of how the human body operates.

**The Law of Conservation, also termed the Law of Autolysis:** Whenever nutritive abstinence is effected to bring about improved health, the living organism's reserves are conserved and economized: living structures are autolyzed in the inverse order of their usefulness, while toxic substances are eliminated. This law refers to hygienic fasting, hygienic dieting for weight loss and hygienic detoxification while eating right.

The medical mentality at its very worst overrides the Law of Conservation with propaganda to program the people into thinking that any kind of fasting will ultimately lead to an unbalanced biochemistry ending in starvation and that fasting is a dangerous form of extremism.

Along these same lines, any dieting for weight loss that does not follow the basic four food groups, no matter how the foods are served, cooked or raw, condimented or plain, is termed "extreme and dangerous" by medical doctors.

**The Law of Limitation:** Whenever and wherever the expenditure of vital power has advanced so far that fatal exhaustion is imminent, a check is put upon the unnecessary expenditure of power; and the organism rebels against the further use of even an accustomed stimulant.

The medical mentality at its very worst overrides the Law of Limitation with propaganda to program the people into thinking that "extraordinary measures" must be used in hopes that science will kill the enemy disease. Limitations of the human body are absolutely not respected. This false paradigm employed *to cure* often translates in reality as *to kill*.

**The Law of Special Economy:** The vital organism — under favorable conditions — stores up all excess of vital funds above the current expenditures as a *reserve fund* to be employed in time of special need.

The medical mentality at its very worst overrides the Law of Special Economy with propaganda to program the people into thinking that no matter how deathbed weak a person becomes with the therapies and drugs prescribed by the medical doctors, war (against what hygienists correctly denote as "symptoms of toxic overload") should continue to be waged, that *reserve funds* (if this term were to even be recognized by the medical doctors) should bravely be deployed in hopes of winning victories over the dreaded enemy disease.

**The Law of Vital Accommodation:** The response of the vital organism to external stimuli is an instinctive one, based upon a self-preservative instinct which adapts or accommodates itself to whatever influence it cannot destroy or control.

The medical mentality at its very worst overrides the Law of Vital Accommodation with propaganda to program the people into thinking that the most effective way to train the body to accommodate so as to achieve self-preservation is to become dependent upon a chosen medical doctor's thinking and care and to follow the chosen medical doctor's dictates without question.

**The Law of Stimulation or Dual Effect:** Whenever a toxic or irritating agent is brought to bear upon the living organism, the body puts forth vital resistance — which manifests itself in an action at once accelerated, but also impaired. This resistance diminishes the bodily power precisely to the degree to which it accelerates action. The increased action is caused by the extra expenditure of vital power called out, not supplied, by the stimulatory process. In consequence, the available supply of power is diminished by this amount.

The medical mentality at its very worst overrides the Law of Stimulation with propaganda to program the people into thinking that the therapies and drug treatments prescribed by medical doctors should be followed without question, regardless of the fact that the people experience loss of energy, loss of mental clarity, loss of hope and finally, loss of life. In the medical doctor's paradigm, "to stimulate with drugs" is a good thing.

**The Law of Compensation, also termed the Law of Repose:** Whenever action in the body has expended the substance and available energy of the body, sleep and/or rest is induced in order to replenish the body's substance and nerve energy.

The medical mentality at its very worst does not negate the need for adequate rest and sleep. The medical mentality does, however, muddy the Law of Compensation with propaganda to program the people into thinking that to take sleeping pills, whenever falling asleep naturally becomes even slightly troublesome, is a perfectly harmless practice and a good thing.

**The Law of Selective Elimination:** All injurious substances which gain admittance by any means into the living organism are counteracted, neutralized and expelled as fully as the bodily nerve energy supplies allow by such means and through such channels as will produce the least amount of harm to living structure. It follows therefore that if nerve energy supplies are low, and a person has become very toxic, he will not have the nerve energy to expel endogenous and exogenous toxins and will take the descent into disease.

The medical mentality at its very worst overrides the Law of Selective Elimination with propaganda to program the people into thinking that the flesh and blood, nerve and brawn of the human body have a virtually unlimited ability to detoxify a virtually unlimited number of mild and even virulent toxins commonly served in the foods from the Standard American Diet, found in our polluted environment and omnipresent in prescription drugs.

**The Law of Utilization:** The normal elements and materials of life are all that the living organism is ever capable of constructively utilizing, whether it is well or sick. No substance or process that is not a normal factor element in physiology can be of any value in the structure of the living organism, and that which is unusable in a state of health is equally unusable in a state of illness.

The medical mentality at its very worst overrides the Law of Utilization with propaganda to program the people into thinking that virtually anything called a *food* by the SAD industrialists and anything called a *drug* by the medical/pharmaceutical industrialists can be consumed absolutely and positively without harm, with impunity, with benefit.

Pleasure-seeking people are therefore happy to be brainwashed into the "eat, drink and be merry, for tomorrow you surely will not die!" mentality.

**The Law of Quality Selection:** When the quality of nutriment being received by the living organism is higher than that of the existing, living tissue, the organism will discard lower-grade cells to make room for appropriating the superior materials into new and healthy tissue.

The medical mentality at its very worst makes no effort to attempt to override such an obviously common health sense affirmation of how the human body operates.

**The Law of the Minimum:** The development of living organisms is regulated by the supply of that element or factor which is least abundantly provided or utilized. The element or factor in shortest supply determines the amount of development. A chain is only as long as its weakest link.

The medical mentality at its very worst makes no effort to attempt to override such an obviously common health sense affirmation of how the human body operates.

**The Law of Development:** The development of any and all parts of the living organism is measured in direct proportion to the amount of vital forces and nutritive materials which are directed to it and brought to bear upon it.

As noted in Life's Great Law — the first law given — the medical mentality at its very worst does not acknowledge the *vital forces* (nerve energy) aspect of the Law of Development and overrides the *nutritive materials* aspect of this law with propaganda to program the people into thinking that the quality of the "nutritive materials" of the SAD are totally adequate to supply health and are certainly nothing to worry about.

# T. C. Fry's Twenty-Two Health Essentials

Formulated by T. C. Fry, these "22 Health Essentials" are synonymous to what Dr. Shelton called *the basic requisites of life* and what I distill down to the ten energy enhancers. We give tribute here to T. C. Fry and his mighty efforts while reminding our readers that there are what T. C. called 21 more *essentials of health* beyond diet to which we must attend if we want our healing to proceed speedily and mightily and our high energy to be on demand, bringing us the best nature has to offer from this new millennium: the *Natural Hygiene high*!

From T. C. Fry:

> If you want to enjoy happy well-being, you must take steps that build vigorous, sickness-free health. No one else can do it for you. Health is self-built, not conferred from without. For most, overcoming any disease can be easy. Discontinuing the causes of disease and establishing the conditions of health will eliminate the disease symptoms.
>
> The Life Science Motto is this: Exercise and a raw food diet build great health — try it!
>
> That really sums it up. These are the two areas in which we most sin against ourselves. The first commandment of eating is this: Thou shalt not poison thyself. Building health consists of meeting all of life's needs appropriately.

## Overcome Ailments and Achieve Health: Establishing the Essentials of Health

- **Good air:** Polluted air is destructive of health and well-being.

- **A comfortable body temperature:** Uncomfortable temperatures drain nerve energy.

- **Cleanliness:** Most of us are adequately clean externally but not internally, which contributes to our discomforts, pains and ailments.

- **Pure water:** Drink only distilled water.

- **Sleep:** Sleep is the condition under which the brain and nervous system regenerate a fund of nerve energy, heal tissues, make repairs and rebalance the body chemistry.

- **Raw fruits, vegetables, nuts and seeds:** Only foods consonant with our biological adaptation must be eaten. When we eat foods that our dietetic character decrees, we'll handle them efficiently and without problems. Most Americans are taught and most believe that the basic four food groups are required to furnish our needs. Of the basic four (meat/protein group, dairy group, grain group and fruit/vegetable group), three are contrary to our dietary character and precipitate or aggravate all kinds of diseases from which we suffer. Just giving up these three toxic food groups and eating fruits and vegetables alone, in the uncooked state, is enough to help many people regain much health!

- **Sunshine and indirect sunlight:** We should obtain at least an hour of sunshine on our bodies weekly.

- **Regular exercise:** At first, you may have to limit your exercise routines. But vigorous, high-exertion exercise is essential to high-level health. Activity is the foremost characteristic of life.

- **Rest and relaxation:** Like sleep, the body regenerates its nerve energy during rest and relaxation. They are essential after any kind of fatigue brought on by any kind of exertion: mental, emotional or physical.

- **Play and recreation:** Such activities rejuvenate the spirit: both combine well with exercise.

- **Mental and emotional poise, peace of mind and self-assurance:** These all derive from the foregoing "essentials" and the "requisites of life" cited hereafter. Stressful conditions will disturb you less as your health and equilibrium improve.

- **Pleasant environment:** An ugly, distressing environment drains our spirits and therefore our sense of well-being. Lovely and beautiful surroundings uplift us and contribute to health.

- **A sense of belonging to a group:** Humans are by nature social beings. We have a gregarious instinct. Being among pleasant, loving, joyful fellow beings or peers contributes to well-being.

- **Self-mastery:** This is a must if we are to competently cope with life's ups and downs, temptations and demands that face us.

- **Security of life and its means:** Insecurity leads to emotional stresses that rob us of well-being. We must have assurance that the necessities of life will be ours for reasonable efforts.

- **Creative, useful work:** No one wants to be a parasite or be unproductive. Everyone thrives when their needs of life are met by their efforts.

- **Inspiration, motivation, purpose and commitment in life:** Having realistic goals to achieve and working towards them is health promoting.

- **Instinct of reproduction.**

- **Satisfaction of the aesthetic senses:** We thrive on beauty, recoil from ugliness. We should stop to appreciate beauty when possible.

- **Love and appreciation:** We are exhilarated and exuberant when we are loved and appreciated. On the obverse side, we become depressed when others dislike and deprecate us, even if unjustifiably. These exalted feelings must be earned! To be appreciated most, you must genuinely appreciate others and make it known to them unmistakably by your words and actions.

- **Interaction with peers about feelings, matters of intellectual moment, life's affairs and life's problems:** While this is implicit in belonging to a social group, it needs to be highlighted.

• **Self-esteem, self-confidence, self-reliance and a sense of self-worth:** *Self-esteem* means 'you have a good self-image because you're equal to the demands life makes upon you'.

# The Food Combining Rules — Summarized

• Fruits are *best* eaten alone. Fruits are eaten according to acid, subacid and sweet compatibility. Acid fruits combine *fair* with subacid. Subacid combine *fair* with sweet. But acid and sweet make a *poor* combination.

• Eat melons with no other fruit or food.

• Acid fruit with nuts and seeds make a *fair* combination.

• Proteins are a *good* combination with nonstarchy vegetables.

• Eat only one type of protein at a meal. A variety of nuts is allowable.

• Starches are a *good* combination with nonstarchy vegetables.

• Proteins and starches are a *poor* combination. Proteins combine *best* with nonstarchy vegetables and combine *fair* with acid fruits.

• Lettuce and celery may be combined with all fruit — except melons.

• Dried fruit is *best* combined with lettuce and celery.

• The avocado combines *best* with nonstarchy vegetables. The avocado combines *fair* with starches and with acid and subacid fruit. The avocado is a *poor* combination with sweet fruits and with protein.

• The tomato is actually an acid fruit and combines accordingly. The tomato also is a *good* combination with nonstarchy vegetables. The tomato is a *poor* combination with starches or animal proteins. The tomato is a *good* combination with either nuts and seeds or avocados.

• Animal milk products combine *poor* with all foods and are inferior foods. All milk products should therefore not be taken at all or taken alone.

• All juices, or ideal food beverages, are best taken as an entire meal and are best not combined with whole fruits, vegetables, nuts or seeds.

• If thirsty, drink water 15-20 minutes before a meal, ½ hour after a fruit meal, 2 hours after a vegetable meal and 4 hours after a protein meal.

• Be particularly attentive to your own digestive system and what combinations work best for you! Dr. David Scott has advised that a person with a strong, uncompromised digestive system can eat outside the food combining rules with relative ease, but such compromises should be minimized for the sake of nerve energy conservation.

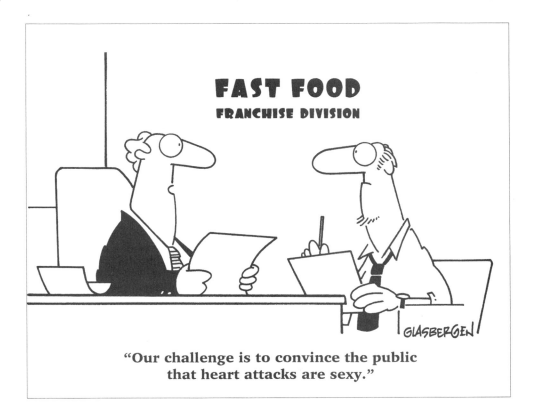

**FAST FOOD**
FRANCHISE DIVISION

GLASBERGEN

"Our challenge is to convince the public
that heart attacks are sexy."

## Classification of Foods for Food Combining Rules

Foods are classified according to which nutrients predominate. Nearly all foods have some proteins, fats and carbohydrates. But foods classified as *proteins* have the highest concentration of protein, likewise with *fats*.

*Carbohydrates* include the following: fruit (which is broken into four categories), starches, low-starch and nonstarchy vegetables, syrups and sugars. Because the classifications are somewhat arbitrary, some controversy among hygienic teachers as to which foods properly belong to which classes exists. Following is a revised *Health Seekers' YearBook* summary of five food combining experts' teachings.

**Note:** True transition and ideal foods are each preceded with a bullet (•) in this listing. Bulleted items are considered true transition or ideal foods only when consumed uncooked.

## ACID (SOUR) FRUITS

- cranberries
- grapefruits
- kiwis
- kumquats
- lemons
- limes
- oranges
- pineapples
- pomegranates
- pomelos
- strawberries
- tangelos
- tangerines
- tomatoes

## SUBACID FRUITS

- apples
- apricots
- berries (most varieties)
- mangoes
- papayas

- peaches
- pears
- plums
- nectarines

## SWEET FRUITS AND ALL DRIED FRUITS

- bananas
- cherimoyas
- cherries
- fresh and dried dates
- fresh and dried figs
- grapes and raisins
- persimmons
- sapotes
- melons (all ideal foods) of all varieties: canary, cantaloupe, casaba, crenshaw, Christmas, banana, honeyball, honeydew, muskmelon, persian, pie, nutmeg, watermelon and all varieties thereof

## STARCHES

- asparagus
- beets
- carrots
- chestnuts
- cereals — all varieties
- coconut (also high in protein and fat)
- corn, mature
- grains — all varieties, dried
- grains — most varieties, sprouted
- jerusalem artichokes
- lima beans
- peas, mature

- parsnips
- potatoes — all varieties and colors
- pumpkins
- rutabagas
- squashes — all winter varieties
  - acorn
  - banana
  - buttercup
  - hubbard
  - gold nugget
  - spaghetti
- sweet potatoes
- turnips
- yams

## LOW STARCH AND NONSTARCHY VEGETABLES: VIRTUALLY ALL GREENS

- alfalfa sprouts
- artichokes, globe
- bean sprouts, mung
- beans, all string varieties
- broccoli
- brussels sprouts
- bok choy
- cabbage
- cauliflower
- celery
- collard greens
- corn, sweet
- cucumbers
- eggplant
- garlic
- lettuces
- kale
- kohlrabi
- mushrooms
  - mustard greens
  - onions family — leeks, scallions
  - peas: sweet, sugar and snap
  - peppers, all bell colors
  peppers, hot
  - radishes
  - spinach
  - squash — all summer varieties
    - crookneck
    - patty pan
    - zucchini
- Swiss chard

## SYRUPS AND SUGARS — ALL SAD FOODS

sugar in all forms: white, brown, raw
syrups of all kinds
honey

## PROTEINS

eggs (a SAD food and also high in fat)
- grains, sprouted — most varieties (also high in starch)
meat — most flesh foods (a SAD food and also high in fats)
milk products — most types (SAD food and also high in fat)
- nuts and seeds — all varieties (also high in fat)
- legumes — all varieties (also high in starch)

## FATS

- avocados (also high in protein)
butter (a SAD food)
cream (a SAD food)
lard (a very SAD food)
margarine (a SAD food)
vegetable oils (a SAD food)

# Appendix G

## How to Get Strict with the Ten Energy Enhancers

> At some point you may begin to question why you are still eating the cooked foods at all. Sure, you love them; the question is, do they love you back? —Doug Graham, DC (1953–)

The following material was contributed by Victoria BidWell, who takes a stand throughout this book for Natural Hygiene and doing right by living the ten energy enhancers.

I cannot say it strongly enough. *It's all about energy!* We all know the word *strict* means 'disciplined and to the letter of the law'. Therefore, strict application of the ten energy enhancers is disciplined living to the letter of the natural, physiological laws of life. Only ten simple healthful living habits, practiced properly and consistently, day in and day out, provide the ideal conditions for health so that all the sick can hope to get well and stay well. This beautiful promise of hope is made to all health seekers willing to get educated, do right and get strict. Even those with advanced chronic, degenerative conditions can realistically hope for arrest or partial recovery, even near-complete recovery.

First, this "strict, do the right thing" approach means *stopping the energy robbers*. Stop the energy-draining habits. Stop burning the candle at both ends with energy-squandering pursuits. Minimize endogenous poisoning. Completely stop the exogenous poisoning whenever possible. Dr. Tilden's landmark book *Toxemia Explained* best teaches stopping all energy leaks and inspires health seekers to examine their lives with a microscope. Now out-of-print, you can get this foundational, lifesaving, inspiring book at www.getwellstaywellamerica. com. You can also order two extensive, powerfully useful, do-it-yourself questionnaire booklets at this web site to help you self-diagnose your own energy leaks: *Personal Health Profile* and *Cause and Consequence Survey.*

Second, this "strict, do the right thing" approach means *avoiding excesses of the ten energy enhancers*. It is possible to get too much of a good thing. Although you cannot get too much cleanliness, pure air and right temperatures, you can overdo the other seven energy enhancers. You can get too much water and over-tax energy reserves dealing with it. You can get too much sleep and get groggy with endogenous toxins. You can eat too much raw food at a meal or snack and get gastrointestinal poisoning, receive too much sun and get burned, get too much exercise and get fatigued and poisoned with lactic acid excess. You can get too emotionally involved in good pursuits and take on too many nurturing relationships and get poisoned with adrenaline and other endogenous toxins of emotional excess. Just as the ten energy robbers can drain energy and lead to autointoxication, so too can excesses of these ten good enhancers.

Now we can — Choose Life! Do Right! Eat Live! And Get High!

If you were to visit a hygienic or holistic health care professional, he or she would charge a fee, closely examine your daily living habits in great detail and recommend what to stop, what to continue and what to start. The few health seekers deep into chronic degeneration would need to seek this guidance and follow doctors' orders, all guaranteed to require strict discipline to get results. But by far the vast majority of health seekers not excessively tired and toxic can be their own doctors, applying self-initiated, strict, energy-enhancing choices while conserving their own healthier pocketbooks in the process!

Here is a concrete list, by no means complete, of what it means to "get strict":

✓ Do right by getting clean inside and out: get determined, get strict, get your energy reserves built up and get detoxified. Do not give up!

✓ Brush and floss your teeth everyday. Do yourself this huge favor while there is still time. As years pass for a person on cooked foods, and much less so for the person on raw foods, the gums recede. Little pockets around the teeth form in which food particles lodge. Bacterial interaction with these trapped particles builds a toxic plaque that poisons the tissues that feed the teeth. Then the teeth decay, only to go bad in time. Thorough chewing is essential for good digestion. It is a sad and terrible thing to let the teeth go.

✓ Use an electric toothbrush with a sonic (sound wave) technology: these waves have been proven to break up plaque and promote dental health like no other toothbrush.

✓ Take pride in your daily cleanliness and appearance. Virtually all who become sick and chronically fatigued experience emotional depression early in their disease evolution. Personal grooming is the very first thing to go when a person gives up. Love and pamper yourself to keep self-esteem high and your spirits up to encourage strict living of the ten energy enhancers.

✓ Live where the air is naturally fresh and pure to breathe.

✓ Let the fresh, pure air fill the house when outdoor temperatures allow. I crave the fresh mountain air where I live the same as I crave live foods! Fresh, pure air is every bit as much a nutrient as live food.

✓ Use air filters when indoors and in your vehicle if the air is not fresh and pure where you live, and moving is not possible.

✓ Go to lengths to secure and drink pure water; it too is a nutrient.

✓ Get adequate sleep and rest to allow the nervous system to revitalize itself. Both the simply tired and toxic in the earlier stages of disease and the seriously ill in the later stages may need ten to twelve hours, and even more, of sleep/bed rest a day for a period of weeks or months to sufficiently revitalize their nervous systems in order to successfully carry out needed detoxification and healing.

✓ Take one or more naps/rests during the day for energy boosting.

✓ Take a fast if your holistic doctor strongly recommends fasting.

✓ Get off all medications as your holistic doctor recommends.

✓ Chew foods slowly and thoroughly to greatly assist ideal digestion.

✓ Practice proper food combining for ideal digestion.

✓ Eat exclusively of unfired, sun-dried, raw, unheated, sun-ripened fruits, vegetables, nuts, seeds and sprouts.

✓ Drink raw juices rather than eat whole foods to conserve body energy for a period of days or a few weeks.

✓ Eat pure raw foods and true transition foods that are completely free of all known outright protoplasmic poisons: salt, condiments, hot peppers, hot spices, refined oils, fermented food and drink, garlic and more.

✓ Eat modest amounts so as not to overwork the digestive system.

✓ Do not snack, so as to give the digestive system brief periods of complete rest.

✓ Do not drink with meals. Diluting the normal concentration of the body's natural digestive juices prohibits ease and efficiency of digestion while wasting energy supplies. If a meal is high in dried fruit or nuts and seeds, always combine these water-deficient foods with lettuce and/or celery, which are high in water content.

✓ Do not use a machine that heats raw foods while processing them.

✓ Eat natural raw foods at room or near-body temperatures. The body has to warm up cold and freezing foods and drinks to body temperature, which results in an energy drain.

✓ Avoid extremes of temperature that leave you hot or chilled.

✓ Get natural sunlight on exposed skin on a regular basis, daily if possible; but avoid extreme heat and direct sunlight during the midday hours.

✓ Get natural sunlight through the eyes: it too is a nutrient.

✓ Get regular exercise: stretching, aerobics and weight training. But if the health seeker is severely enervated, strict bed rest and extra hours for sleep are absolutely essential until he or she is revitalized before an exercise regime should be undertaken.

✓ Use the antigravity BodySlant with regularity. This is a passive form of exercise for the lymphatic system. It is especially useful for the severely enervated and for the person with prolapsed organs and circulatory pains and problems, especially varicose veins and edema.

✓ Take an active role in creating your emotional balance. Overcome addictions. Pick rewarding goals. Create a career situation you enjoy or better yet, absolutely love! Living in negative emotions contributes to the disease process in a human body like nothing else! Not only do negative emotions result in endogenous poisons, but fear and all of its branching dark emotions can kill. Negative emotions play the leading role in all psychosomatically induced diseases.

✓ Get playful whenever appropriate and possible! Come to these moments as a loving child, with smiles, laughter, imagination and freedom! These moments engender a totally health-boosting biochemistry and physiology! They are wonderfully fun and bless us and others around us! They give us a natural, high joy alternative to drugs that promise emotional balance but give only momentary escapism.

A health seeker can be 100% raw and practice all other nine energy enhancers to the letter; but if the fearful fight-or-flight response is chronically activated, even at a low pitch of fear, the body inevitably adapts with malfunctions at the microscopic level that lead to diseased tissues, organs and systems at the macroscopic level. Stay with positive emotions. Count your blessings, starting with the reality that you are alive and have been blessed to find the superlative alternative health care system, complete with the ten energy enhancers, including the live food factor!

✓ Take an active role in creating your nurturing relationships with humans. But even if your primary nurturing relationship is with nature or an animal, these can be highly health promoting. Others find their very most nurturing relationship with God and derive a highly health-promoting strength from this spiritual relationship. Toxic relationships can result in so much misery that words cannot even do their descriptions justice. Toxic relationships are tremendously exhausting, as they are built on fear and generate endogenous toxins that can utterly poison a person into the disease process. Deal with all toxic relationships to turn them into at least neutral or better yet, nurturing ones.

It was Dr. Shelton who admonished all health seekers, "Forgive everybody everything!" Bible passages, as well as virtually all religions, likewise promote forgiveness. When love, joy and gratitude are the overriding emotional modes, peace reigns supreme in the body. And health flourishes.

# Bibliography
## General Bibliography

Abel, Ulrich. *Chemotherapy of Advanced Epithelial Cancer: A Critical Survey*, Hippokrates Verlag: Stuttgart, Germany, 1990.

Abramowski, Dr. O. L. M. *Fruitarian Diet and Physical Rejuvenation*, Essence of Health Publishing Co.: Westville, South Africa, 1911.

Airola, Paavo. *Are You Confused?* Health Plus: Phoenix, AZ, 1971.

Airola, Paavo. *How to Keep Slim, Healthy and Young with Juice Fasting*, the Age-old Way to a New You! Health Plus: Sherwood, OR, 1971.

Alexander, Joe. *Blatant Raw Foodist Propaganda!* Blue Dolphin Publishing: Nevada City, CA, 1990.

Alt, Carol. *Eating in the Raw: A Beginner's Guide to Getting Slimmer, Feeling Healthier and Living Longer the Raw-Food Way*, Clarkson Potter Publishers: New York, NY, 2004.

Angell, Marcia. *The Truth about the Drug Companies: How They Deceive Us and What to Do about It*, Random House: New York, NY, 2005.

Angler, Bradford. *Field Guide to Edible Wild Plants*, Stackpole Books: Harrisburg, PA, 1974.

Appleton, Nancy. *Lick the Sugar Habit: How to Break Your Sugar Addiction Naturally*, Avery Publishing Group, Inc: Wayne, NJ, 1988.

Arlin, Stephen. *Raw Power! Building Strength & Muscle Naturally*, Maul Brothers Publishing: San Diego, CA, 1998.

Arlin, Stephen, Dini, Fouad and Wolfe, David. *Nature's First Law: The Raw Food Diet*, Maul Brothers Publishing: San Diego, CA, 1996.

Baker, Arthur M. *Awakening Our Self-Healing Body: A Solution to the Health Care Crisis*, Self Health Care Systems: Los Angeles, CA, 1994.

Baker, Elizabeth. *Does the Bible Teach Nutrition?* WinePress Publications: Mukilteo, WA, 1997.

Baker, Elizabeth. *The Un-Diet Book: The All-Natural Lifestyle for Weight Loss and Eating, Good Health and Exercise by the Author of the Uncook Book*, Drelwood Communications: Indianola, WA, 1992.

Baker, Elizabeth. *The Unmedical Book: How to Conquer Disease, Lose Weight, Avoid Suffering & Save Money*, Drelwood Publications: Saguache, CO, 1987.

Baroody, Dr. Theodore A., ND, DC, PhD Nutrition, CNC. *Alkalize or Die: Superior Health through Proper Alkaline-Acid Balance*, Holographic Health Press: Waynesville, NC, 1991.

Bealle, Morris A. *House of Rockefeller: How a Shoestring Was Run into 200 Billion Dollars in Two Generations*, All America House: Washington, DC, 1959.

Bealle, Morris A. *The Drug Story*, Columbia Publishing Company: Washington, DC, 1949.

Bernays, Edward L. *Propaganda*, Ig Publishing: Brooklyn, NY, 2005.

BidWell, Victoria. *2 Books in 1: The Health Seekers' YearBook — A Revolutionist's Handbook for Getting Well & Staying Well without the Medicine Men — With The Best of Common Health Sense*, GetWell♥StayWell, America! Concrete, WA, 2005.

BidWell, Victoria. *GetWell ♥StayWell Affirmations for Americans!* GetWell♥ StayWell, America! Concrete, WA, 1993.

BidWell, Victoria. *Apples to Zucchini Coloring Book*, GetWell♥StayWell, America! Concrete, WA, 1989.

BidWell, Victoria. *Dr. GetWell's Book of Nursery Rhymes*, GetWell♥StayWell, America! Concrete, WA, 1989.

BidWell, Victoria. *The Fruit & Vegetable Lovers' Coloring Book*, GetWell♥Stay Well, America! Concrete, WA, 1987.

BidWell, Victoria. *The Fruit & Vegetable Lovers' Calorie Guide*, GetWell♥Stay Well, America! Concrete, WA, 1986.

BidWell, Victoria. *The Salt Conspiracy*, GetWell♥StayWell, America! Freemont, CA, 1986.

BidWell, Victoria. *The Natural Weight-Loss System,* Life Science: Austin, TX, 1984.

Bircher-Benner, Ralph. *Dr. Bircher-Benner's Way to Positive Health and Vitality, 1867–1967*, Bircher-Benner Verlag: Zurich, Switzerland, 1967.

Bland, Dr. Jeffrey S., PhD. *Genetic Nutritioneering: How You Can Modify Inherited Traits and Live a Longer, Healthier Life*, McGraw-Hill: New York, NY, 1999.

Blaylock, Dr. Russell L., MD. *Excitotoxins: The Taste that Kills*, Health Press: Santa Fe, NM, 1997.

Boutenko, Victoria. *12 Steps to Raw Foods: How to End Your Dependency on Cooked Food* (second edition), North Atlantic Books: Berkeley, CA, 2007.

Boutenko, Victoria. *Green for Life*, Raw Family Publishing: Ashland, OR, 2005.

Boutenko, Victoria. *12 Steps to Raw Foods: How to End Your Addiction to Cooked Food*, Raw Family Publishing: Ashland, OR, 2001.

Boutenko, Victoria, Igor, Sergei and Valya. *Raw Family: A True Story of Awakening*, Raw Family Publishing: Ashland, OR, 2000.

Bragg, Paul. *The Miracle of Fasting for Agelessness, Physical, Mental & Spiritual Rejuvenation: New Discoveries about an Old Miracle, the Fast Fasting Way to Health*, Health Science: Burbank, CA, 1966.

Brandt, Johanna. *The Grape Cure*, Benedict Lust Publications: New York, NY, 2001.

Bruce, Elaine. *Living Foods for Radiant Health*, Thorsons: London, England, 2003.

Bryson, Christopher. *The Fluoride Deception*, Seven Stories Press: New York, NY, 2004.

Bueno, Lee. *Fast Your Way to Health*, Whitaker House: New Kensington, PA, 1991.

Buhner, Stephen. *The Fasting Path: The Way to Spiritual, Physical and Emotional Enlightenment*, Penguin Group, Inc.: New York, NY, 2003.

Burger, Guy-Claude. *Manger Vrai: Instinctothérapie*, Editions du Rocher: Paris, France, 1980.

Campbell, Dr. T. Colin, PhD. *The China Study: Startling Implications for Diet, Weight Loss and Long-Term Health,* BenBella Books: Dallas, TX, 2004.

Carper, Jean. *The Food Pharmacy: Dramatic New Evidence that Food Is Your Best Medicine*, Bantam Books: New York, NY, 1988.

Carter, Dr. James P., MD. *Racketeering in Medicine: The Suppression of Alternatives*, Hampton Roads Publishing Company, Inc.: Charlottesville, VA, 1992.

Cherniske, Stephen, MS. *Caffeine Blues: Wake Up to the Hidden Dangers of America's #1 Drug*, Warner Books: New York, NY, 1998.

Chessman, Millan. *Stay Young & Healthy Through Internal Cleansing*, Chessman: San Diego, CA, 1995.

Clement, Brian R. *Living Foods for Optimum Health*, Prima Publishing: Roseville, CA, 1996.

Cobb, Brenda. *The Living Foods Lifestyle*, Living Soul Publishing: Atlanta, GA, 2002.

Cohen, Robert. *Milk the Deadly Poison*, Argus Publishing, Inc.: Oradell, NJ, 1998.

Comby, Bruno, PhD. *Maximize Immunity*, Marcus Books: Queensville, ON, Canada, 1994.

Committee on Diet, Nutrition and Cancer, Assembly of Life Sciences, National Research Council. *Diet, Nutrition and Cancer*, National Academy Press: Washington, DC, 1982.

Cook, Lewis E., Jr., and Yasui, Junko. *Goldot: The Doctrine of Truth: Guidebook of Life — Doctrine of Truth: The Science of Man — A Fundamental Guidebook of Life*, Cook: Oceanside, CA, 1976.

Cordain, Dr. Loren, PhD. *The Paleo Diet: Lose Weight and Get Healthy by Eating the Food You Were Designed to Eat*, J. Wiley: New York, NY, 2002.

Cousens, Dr. Gabriel, MD, with Rainoshek, David. *There Is a Cure for Diabetes: The Tree of Life 21-Day+ Program,* North Atlantic Books: Berkeley, CA, 2008.

Cousens, Dr. Gabriel, MD. *Spiritual Nutrition: Six Foundations for Spiritual Life and the Awakening of Kundalini*, North Atlantic Books: Berkeley, CA, 2005.

Cousens, Dr. Gabriel, MD. *Conscious Eating*, Vision Books International: Santa Rosa, CA, 1992.

Cousens, Dr. Gabriel, MD. *Spiritual Nutrition and the Rainbow Diet*, Cassandra Press: Boulder, CO, 1986.

Da Free John, *Raw Gorilla: The Principles of Regenerative Raw Diet Applied in True Spiritual Practice*, The Dawn Horse Press: Clearlake, CA, 1982.

Devivo, Roman and Spors, Antje. *Genefit Nutrition*, Celestial Arts: Berkeley, CA, 2003.

De Vries, Arnold. *The Fountain of Youth*, Dunlay Publishing Company: New York, NY, 1947.

Diamond, Harvey and Marilyn. *Fit for Life II: Living Health*, Warner Books: New York, NY, 1987.

Diamond, Harvey and Marilyn. *Fit for Life*, Warner Books: New York, NY, 1985.

Diamond, Jared. *Guns, Germs and Steel: The Fates of Human Societies*, Norton: New York, NY, 1999.

Douglass, William C., MD. *Into the Light*, Second Opinion Publishing, Inc.: Atlanta, GA, 1993.

Dries, Jan. *The Dries Cancer Diet: A Practical Guide to the Use of Fresh Fruit and Raw Vegetables in the Treatment of Cancer*, Element Books Inc.: Rockport, MA, 1997.

Dufty, William, *Sugar Blues*, Warner Books: New York, NY, 1975.

Dykeman, Peter A. & Elias, Thomas. *Edible Wild Plants: A North American Field Guide*, Sterling Publishing Co., Inc: New York, NY, 1982.

Ehret, Arnold. *Rational Fasting*, Benedict Lust Publications: New York, NY, 1971.

Ehret, Arnold. *Mucusless Diet Healing System*, Benedict Lust Publications: New York, NY, 1970.

Eisnitz, Gail A. *Slaughterhouse: The Shocking Story of Greed, Neglect and Inhumane Treatment Inside the U.S. Meat Industry*, Prometheus Books: Amherst, NY, 1997.

Feuer, Elaine. *Innocent Casualties: The FDA's War against Humanity*, Dorrance Publishing Co.: Pittsburgh, PA, 1996.

Fredericks, Carlton. *Psycho-Nutrition*, Grosset & Dunlap: New York, NY, 1976.

Fry, T. C. *The Health Formula*, Health Excellence Systems: Manchaca, TX, 1991.

Fry, T. C. and Honiball, Essie. *I Live on Fruit*, Life Science Institute: San Antonio, TX, 1991.

Fry, T. C. and Klein, Dr. David. *Your Natural Diet: Alive Raw Foods*, Living Nutrition Publications: Sebastopol, CA, 2002.

Fuhrman, Dr. Joel, MD. *Fasting and Eating for Health: A Medical Doctor's Program for Conquering Disease*, St. Martin's Press: New York, NY, 1995.

Gallo, Roe, PhD, and Zocchi, Stephen. *Overcoming the Myths of Aging: Lose Weight, Look Great and Live a Happier, Healthier Life*, Roe Gallo Publishing: San Francisco, CA, 2007.

Gallo, Roe, PhD. *Perfect Body: The Raw Truth*, Promotion Publishing: San Diego, CA, 1997.

Gerson, Max, MD. *A Cancer Therapy: Results of Fifty Cases*, Whittier Books: New York, NY, 1958.

Graham, Dr. Douglas, DC. *The 80/10/10 Diet: Balancing Your Health, Your Weight, and Your Life, One Luscious Bite at a Time*, FoodnSport Press: Key Largo, FL, 2006.

Graham, Dr. Douglas, DC. *On Nutrition and Physical Performance: A Handbook for Athletes and Fitness Enthusiasts*, FoodnSport Press: Key Largo, FL, 1999, 2003.

Graham, Dr. Douglas, DC. *Grain Damage*, Dr. Douglas N. Graham: Marathon, FL, 1998.

Gregory, Dick. *Dick Gregory's Natural Diet for Folks Who Eat: Cookin' with Mother Nature!* Harper & Row: New York, NY, 1973.

Griffin, G. Edward. *World without Cancer: The Story of Vitamin B₁₇*, American Media: Westlake Village, CA, 1997.

Haley, Daniel. *Politics in Healing: The Suppression and Manipulation of American Medicine*, Potomac Valley Press: Washington, DC, 2000.

Hawkins, David R. *The Eye of the I*, Veritas: W. Sedona, AZ, 2002.

Hendel, Dr. Barbara and Ferreira, Peter. *Water & Salt: The Essence of Life — The Healing Power of Nature*, Natural Resources, Inc., 2003.

Holick, Dr. Michael F., PhD, MD. *The UV Advantage: The Medical Breakthrough that Shows How to Harness the Power of the Sun for Your Health*, Ibooks, Inc: New York, NY, 2003.

Horowitz, Dr. Leonard G. *Death in the Air: Globalism, Terrorism & Toxic Warfare*, Tetrahedron: Sandpoint, ID, 2001.

Horowitz, Dr. Leonard G. *Emerging Viruses: AIDS and Ebola: Nature, Accident, or Intentional?* Tetrahedron: Rockport, MA, 1997.

Hotema, Hilton. *Man's Higher Consciousness*, Health Research: Pomeroy, WA, 1962.

Hovannessian, Arshavir Ter. *Raw Eating*, Hallelujah Acres Publishing: Shelby, NC, 2000.

Howell, Dr. Edward. *Food Enzymes for Health and Longevity*, Lotus Press: Twin Lakes, WI, 1994.

Howell, Dr. Edward. *Enzyme Nutrition*, Avery Publishing Group, Inc: Wayne, NJ, 1985.

Howenstine, Dr. James A., MD. *A Physician's Guide to Natural Health Products That Work*, Penhurst Books: Miami, FL, 2002.

Hunsberger, Eydie Mae. *How I Conquered Cancer Naturally*, Production House: San Diego, CA, 1975.

Hunt, Dr. Valerie. *Infinite Mind: Science of the Human Vibrations of Counsciousness*, Malibu Publishing Co.: Malibu, CA, 1996.

Iserbyt, Charlotte Thompson. *The Deliberate Dumbing Down of America: A Chronological Paper Trail*, 3d Rsearch Co: Bath, ME, 1999.

Jensen, Dr. Bernard, DC, ND, PhD. *Dr. Jensen's Guide to Diet and Detoxification*, Keat's Publishing: Los Angeles, CA, 2000.

Jubb, Annie Padden and David. *Secrets of an Alkaline Body: The New Science of Colloidal Biology*, North Atlanta Books: Berkeley, CA, 2004.

Jubb, David. *Jubb's Cell Rejuvenation: Colloidal Biology: A Symbiosis*, North Atlanta Books: Berkeley, CA, 2005.

Keck-Borsits, Shelly. *Dying to Get Well: Conventional Medicine FAILED! How Raw Food Reversed My Disease Naturally —Are You Sick & Tired of Being Sick & Tired? — A Medical Cover-Up Exposed! — A Cure to Disease Revealed! — What Your Doctor Isn't Telling You Could Kill You!* Shelly Keck-Borsits: Rensselaer, IN, 2003.

Kelley, Dr. William Donald and Rohe, Fred. *Cancer: Curing the Incurable without Surgery, Chemotherapy or Radiation*, New Century Promotions: Bonita, CA, 2001.

Kennedy, Gordon. *Children of the Sun, A Pictorial Anthology: From Germany to California 1883–1949*, Nivaria Press: Ojai, CA, 1998.

Kenton, Leslie and Susannah. *Raw Energy*, Arrow Books Limited: London, England, 1984.

Kervran, Louis C. *Biological Transmutations, and Their Applications in Chemistry, Physics, Biology, Ecology, Medicine, Nutrition, Agriculture, Geology, Swan House Publishing Co.: Binghamton*, NY, 1972.

Klein, Dr. David. *Self Healing Colitis & Crohn's*, Living Nutrition Publications: Sebastopol, CA, 2005.

Kirby, David. *Evidence of Harm: Mercury in Vaccines and the Autism Epidemic: A Medical Controversy*, St. Martin's Press: New York, NY, 2005.

Krok, Morris. *Fruit: The Food and Medicine for Man*, Essence of Health: Wandsbeck 3631, South Africa, 1984.

Kulvinskas, Viktoras. *Life in the 21$^{st}$ Century*, 21$^{st}$ Century Publications: Fairfield, IA, 1981.

Kulvinskas, Viktoras. *Survival into the 21$^{st}$ Century: Planetary Healers Manual*, 21$^{st}$ Century Publications: Fairfield, IA, 1981.

Lanctôt, Dr. Guylaine, MD. *The Medical Mafia*, Here's the Key, Inc: Morgan, VT, 1995.

Lipton, Bruce, PhD. *The Biology of Belief: Unleashing the Power of Consciousness, Matter and Miracles.* Mountain of Love: Santa Rosa, CA, 2005.

Lyman, Howard F. *Mad Cowboy: Plain Truth from the Cattle Rancher Who Won't Eat Meat*, Scribner: New York, NY, 1998.

Malkmus, George, Rev. *The Hallejuljah Diet: Experience the Ultimate Health You Were Meant to Have,* Destiny Image Publishers: Shippensburg, PA, 2006.

Malkmus, George, Rev., and Dye, Michael. *God's Way to Ultimate Health: A Common Sense Guide for Eliminating Sickness through Nutrition*, Hallelujah Acres Publishing: Eidson, TN, 1995.

Malkmus, George, Rev. *Why Christians Get Sick*, Destiny Image Publishers: Shippensburg, PA, 1995.

Marcus, Erik. *Vegan: The New Ethics of Eating*, McBooks Press: Ithaca, NY, 2001.

McDermott, Stella. *Metaphysics of Raw Foods: Embracing the Natural Food Laws; the Fundamental Principles of Raw Foods; Their Comparative Nutritive Value; the Divine Laws of Dietetics; Methods of Preparing Raw Foods to Serve, Together with Numerous Menus*, Burton Publishing Company: MT, 1919.

Mendelsohn, Dr. Robert, MD. *Confessions of a Medical Heretic*, Contemporary Books: Chicago, IL, 1979.

Mercola, Dr. Joseph, ND, and Levy, Alison Rose. *The No-Grain Diet: Conquer Carbohydrate Addiction and Stay Slim for Life*, Dutton Books: New York, NY, 2003.

Meyerowitz, Steve. *Sprouts, the Miracle Food: The Complete Guide to Sprouting*, Sproutman Publications: Great Barrington, MA, 1999.

Meyerowitz, Steve. *Juice Fasting & Detoxification: Use the Healing Power of Fresh Juice to Feel Young and Look Great: The Fastest Way to Restore Your Health*, Sproutman Publications: Great Barrington, MA, 1999.

Monarch, Matthew J. *Raw Spirit: What the Raw Food Advocates Don't Preach*, Monarch Publishing Company: Granada Hills, CA, 2005.

Moss, Dr. Ralph W., MD. *The Cancer Industry: The Classic Exposé on the Cancer Establishment*, Paragon House: New York, NY, 1989.

Mosseri, Albert. *Mangez Nature Santé Nature*, Les Hygiénistes, 1992.

Murray, Dr. Maynard, MD. *Sea Energy Agriculture*, Acres, USA: Austin, TX, 2003.

Nelson, Dennis. *Food Combining Simplified: How to Get the Most from Your Food*, Nelson's Books: Santa Cruz, CA, 1983.

Nison, Paul. *Raw Knowledge II: Interviews with Health Achievers*, 343 Publishing Company: Brooklyn, NY, 2003.

Nison, Paul. *Raw Knowledge: Enhance the Powers of Your Mind, Body and Soul*, 343 Publishing Company: Brooklyn, NY, 2002.

Nison, Paul. *The Raw Life: Becoming Natural in an Unnatural World*, 343 Publishing Company: New York, NY, 2000.

Nolfi, Dr. Kristine, MD. *Raw Food Treatment of Cancer*, TEACH Services, Inc.: Brushton, NY, 1995.

Oldfield, Harry and Coghill, Roger. *The Dark Side of the Brain: Major Discoveries in the Use of Kirlian Photography and Electrocrystal Therapy*, Element Books, Inc., 1991.

Oski, Frank, MD. *Don't Drink Your Milk! The Frightening New Medical Facts about the World's Most Overrated Nutrient*, TEACH Services, Inc: Brushton, NY, 1983.

Oswald, Jean A. and Shelton, Dr. Herbert M. *Fasting for the Health of It: 100 Case Histories Selected from over 200,000 Clinical Records*, Franklin Books: Bayonet Point, FL, 1983.

Ott, A. True, PhD. *Secret Assassins in Food: The Ninjas of Taste,* Manna Publishing: Ogden, UT, 2005.

Owen, Bob. *Roger's Recovery from Aids: How One Man Defeated the Dread Disease*, Dover: Cannon Beach, OR, 1987.

Patenaude, Frédéric. *The Raw Secrets: The Raw Vegan Diet in the Real World*, Raw Vegan: Montreal, QC, Canada, 2002.

Pearson, R. B. *Fasting and Man's Correct Diet*, Health Research: Pomeroy, WA, 1921.

Pert, Candace. *Molecules of Emotion: Why You Feel the Way You Feel*, Scribner: New York, NY, 1997.

Pfeiffer, Carl C., PhD, MD. *Nutrition and Mental Illness: An Orthomolecular Approach to Balancing Body Chemistry*, Healing Arts Press: Rochester, VT, 1987.

Pottenger, Dr. Francis M., Jr. *Pottenger's Cats: A Study in Nutrition,* The Price-Pottenger Nutrition Foundation: San Diego, CA, 1983.

Price, Dr. Weston A., DDS. *Nutrition and Physical Degeneration: A Comparison of Primitive and Modern Diets and Their Effects*, P.B. Hoeber, Inc: New York, NY, 1939.

Rampton, Sheldon and Stauber, John. *Trust Us, We're Experts! How Industry Manipulates Science and Gambles with Your Future*, Tarcher/Putnam: New York, NY, 2001.

Robbins, John. *Diet for a New America*, H. J. Kramer: Tiburon, CA, 1998.

Rose, Natalia. *Raw Food Life Force Energy: Enter a Totally New Stratosphere of Weight Loss, Beauty, and Health*, Regan Books: New York, NY, 2007.

Rose, Natalia. *The Raw Food Detox Diet: The Five-Step Plan for Vibrant Health and Maximum Weight Loss*, HarperCollins Publishers, Inc: New York, NY, 2005.

Rudell, Wendy. *The Raw Transformation: Energizing Your Life with Living Foods*, North Atlantic Books: Berkley, CA, 2006.

Santillo, Humbart, MH, ND. *Food Enzymes: The Missing Link to Radiant Health*, Hohm Press: Prescott, AZ, 1987.

Schaeffer, Severen L. *Instinctive Nutrition*, Celestial Arts: Berkeley, CA, 1987.

Schauss, Alexander. *Diet, Crime and Delinquency*, Parker House: Berkeley, CA, 1980.

Schmid, Ronald F., MD. *Native Nutrition: Eating According to Ancestral Wisdom*, Healing Arts Press: Rochester, VT, 1994.

Schmid, Ronald F., MD. *Traditional Foods Are Your Best Medicine: Health and Longevity with the Animal, Sea, and Vegetable Foods of our Ancestors*, Ocean View Publications: Stratford, CT, 1987.

Scott, William D. *In the Beginning God Said, Eat Raw Food: Genesis 1:29, a Closer Look*, North Idaho Publishing: Coeur d'Alene, ID, 1999.

Seignalet, Dr. Jean. *L'Alimentation ou la Troisième Médecine* [Nutrition or the Third Medicine], Édition François-Xavier de Guilbert: Paris, France, 2004.

Shelton, Dr. Herbert M., DC. *Food Combining Made Easy*, Willow Publishing, Inc.: San Antonio, TX, 1982.

Shelton, Dr. Herbert M., DC. *The Science and Fine Art of Fasting*, Natural Hygiene Press: Chicago, IL, 1978.

Shelton, Dr. Herbert M., DC. *Health for the Millions*, Natural Hygiene Press: Chicago, IL, 1968.

Shelton, Dr. Herbert M., DC. *Fasting Can Save Your Life*, Natural Hygiene Press: Chicago, IL, 1964.

Shelton, Dr. Herbert M., DC. *The Hygienic System, Vol. III: Fasting and Sunbathing*, Health Research: Pomeroy, WA, 1934.

Shelton, Dr. Herbert M., DC. *The Hygienic System, Vol. I: Orthobionomics*, Dr. Shelton's Health School: San Antonio, TX, 1934.

Shelton, Herbert, M., DC. *The Hygienic Care of Children*, Dr. Shelton's Health School: San Antonio, TX, 1931.

Simontacchi, Carol. *The Crazy Makers: How the Food Industry Is Destroying Our Minds and Harming Our Children*, Tarcher/Putnam: New York, NY, 2000.

Smith, Jeffrey M. *Seeds of Deception: Exposing Industry and Government Lies about the Safety of the Genetically Engineered Foods You're Eating*, Yes! Books: Fairfield, IA, 2003.

Smith, Lendon H. *Dr. Lendon Smith's Low-Stress Diet Book*, McGraw-Hill: Blacklick, OH, 1988.

Somers, Suzanne. *The Sexy Years: Discover the Natural Hormone Connection — the Secret to Fabulous Sex, Great Health, and Vitality for Women and Men*, Random House Large Print: New York, NY, 2004.

Sommers, Craig, ND, CN. *Raw Foods Bible*, Guru Beant Press, San Diego, CA, 2004.

Stitt, Barbara Reed. *Food & Behavior*, Natural Press: Manitowoc, WI, 1997.

Stoycoff, Cheryl. *Raw Kids: Transitioning Children to a Raw Food Diet*, Living Spirit Press: Stockton, CA, 2000.

Szekely, Dr. Edmond Bordeaux, Ed. and Trans. *The Essene Gospel of Peace*, International Biogenic Society: Nelson, BC, Canada, 1981.

Szekely, Dr. Edmond Bordeaux. *The Chemistry of Youth*, Academy Books: San Diego, CA, 1977.

Teitel, Martin, PhD, and Wilson, Kimberly. *Genetically Engineered Food: Changing the Nature of Nature*, Park Street Press: Rochester, VT, 2001.

Tilden, Dr. John H., MD. *Toxemia Explained: The True Interpretation of the Cause of Disease; How to Cure Is an Obvious Sequence*, J. H. Tilden Press, Denver, CO, 1926.

Trudeau, Kevin. *The Weight Loss Cure "They" Don't Want You to Know About*, Alliance Publishing Company: Elk Grove Village, IL, 2007.

Trudeau, Kevin. *More Natural "Cures" Revealed: Previously Censored Brand Name Products That Cure Disease*, Alliance Publishing Group, Inc: Hinsdale, IL, 2006.

Trudeau, Kevin. *Natural Cures "They" Don't Want You to Know About*, Alliance Publishing Group, Inc: Hinsdale, IL, 2004.

Vetrano, Dr. Vivian Virginia, hMD, DC, PhD, DSci. *Errors in Hygiene?!!? T. C. Fry's Devolution, Demise and Why, Interspersed with Salient Facts That Can Save Your Life*, GIH Publishing: Barksdale, TX, 1999.

Vonderplanitz, Aajonus. *We Want to Live*, Carnelian Bay Castle Press: Santa Monica, CA, 1997.

Walford, Dr. Roy L., MD. *Maximum Life Span*, Norton: New York, NY, 1983.

Walker, Dr. Norman, DSc. *Fresh Vegetable and Fruit Juices: What's Missing in Your Body?* Norwalk Press: Prescott, AZ, 1970.

Wigmore, Dr. Ann, DD, ND. *Overcoming AIDS and Other "Incurable Diseases" the Attunitive Way through Nature*, Copen Press: New York, NY, 1987.

Wigmore, Dr. Ann, DD, ND. *The Wheatgrass Book*, Avery Publishing Group, Inc.: Wayne, NJ, 1985.

Wigmore, Dr. Ann, DD, ND. *The Hippocrates Diet and Health Program*, Avery Publishing Group, Inc: Wayne, NJ, 1984.

Wigmore, Dr. Ann, DD, ND. *Be Your Own Doctor: A Positive Guide to Natural Living*, Avery Publishing Group, Inc: Garden City Park, NY, 1982.

Wiley, T. S. *Lights Out: Sleep, Sugar and Survival*, Pocket Books: New York, NY, 2000.

Wolcott, William L. and Fahey, Trish. *The Metabolic Typing Diet: Customize Your Diet to Your Own Unique & Ever Changing Nutritional Needs*, Doubleday: New York, NY, 2000.

Wolfe, David with Good, Nick. *Amazing Grace: The Nine Principles of Living in Natural Magic*, North Atlantic Books: Berkeley, CA, 2008.

Wolfe, David and Holdstock, Shazzie. *Naked Chocolate: The Astonishing Truth about the World's Greatest Food*, Maul Brothers Publishing: San Diego, CA, 2005.

Wolfe, David. *Eating for Beauty: For Women and Men: Introducing a Whole New Concept of Beauty: What It Is, and How You Can Achieve It*, Maul Brothers Publishing: San Diego, CA, 2002.

Wolfe, David. *The Sunfood Diet Success System: 36 Lessons in Health Transformation*, Maul Brothers Publishing: San Diego, CA, 1999.

Yiamouyiannis, John. *Fluoride the Aging Factor: How to Recognize and Avoid the Devastating Effects of Fluoride;* Health Action Press: Delaware, OH, 1993.

Young, Dr. Robert O., PhD, DSc, and Young, Shelley Redford. *The pH Miracle: Balance Your Diet, Reclaim Your Health*, Warner Books: New York, NY, 2002.

Young, Dr. Robert O., PhD, DSc, and Young, Shelley Redford. *Sick and Tired? Reclaim Your Inner Terrain*, Woodland Publishing: Pleasant Grove, UT, 2001.

Zavasta, Tonya. *Quantum Eating: The Ultimate Elixir of Youth*, BR Publishing: Cordova, TN, 2007.

Zavasta, Tonya. *Beautiful on Raw: Uncooked Creations*, BR Publishing: Cordova, TN, 2005.

Zavasta, Tonya. *Your Right to Be Beautiful: How to Halt the Train of Aging & Meet the Most Beautiful You*, BR Publishing: Cordova, TN, 2003.

Zephyr. *Instinctive Eating: The Lost Knowledge of Optimum Nutrition*, Pan Piper Press: Pahoa, HI, 1996.

# Recipe Book Bibliography

Alt, Carol, with Roth, David. *The Raw 50: 10 Amazing Breakfasts, Lunches, Dinners, Snacks, and Drinks for Your Raw Food Lifestyle*, Clarkson Potter, New York, NY. 2007.

Amsden, Matt. *Rawvolution*, HarperCollins Publishers: New York, NY, 2006.

Au, Bryan. *Raw in Ten Minutes*, Trafford Publishing: Victoria, BC, Canada, 2005.

Baird, Lori, Ed. *The Complete Book of Raw Food: Healthy, Delicious Vegetarian Cuisine Made with Living Foods, Includes Over 350 Recipes from the World's Top Raw Food Chefs*, Healthy Living Books: Long Island City, NY, 2004.

Baker, Elizabeth. *The Uncook Book: Raw Food Adventures to a New Health High*, Drelwood Publications: Saguache, CO, 1980.

BidWell, Victoria, and Lundskog, Shirlene. *Brown BagWell & StayWell! (with Love)*, GetWell♥StayWell, America! Concrete, WA, 1991.

BidWell, Victoria. *GetWell Recipes from the Garden of Eden*, GetWell♥Stay Well, America! Concrete, WA, 1987.

Boutenko, Sergei and Boutenko, Valya. *Fresh: The Ultimate Live-Food Cookbook*, North Atlantic Books: Berkeley, CA, 2008.

Boutenko, Sergei and Boutenko, Valya. *Eating without Heating: Favorite Recipes from Teens Who Love Raw Food*, Raw Family Publishing: Ashland, OR, 2002.

Brotman, Juliano. *Raw: The Uncook Book: New Vegetarian Food for Life*, Regan Books: New York, NY, 1999.

Calabro, Rose Lee. *Living in the Raw Desserts*, Book Publishing Co: Summertown, TN, 2007.

Chavez, Gabrielle. *The Raw Food Gourmet: Going Raw for Total Well-Being*, North Atlantic Books, Berkeley, CA, 2005.

Cohen, Alissa. *Living on Live Food*, Cohen Publishing Company, Laguna Beach, CA, 2004.

Cornbleet, Jennifer. *Raw Food Made Easy for 1 or 2 People*, Book Publishing Company, Summertown, TN, 2005.

Cousens, Dr. Gabriel, MD. *Rainbow Green Live-Food Cuisine*, North Atlantic Books: Berkeley, CA, 2003.

Elliott, Angela. *Alive in 5: Raw Gourmet Meals in Five Minutes!* Book Publishing Company: Summertown, TN, 2007.

Ferrara, Suzanne Alex. *The Raw Food Primer*, Council Oak Books: Tulsa, OK, 2003.

Graham, Doug. *The High Energy Diet Recipe Guide*, Nature's First Law: San Diego, CA, 1996.

Hatsis, Marc Anthony. *Ambrosia: Art of Raw Cuisine*, White Crosslet Publishing Company: New York, NY, 2006.

Jubb, Annie Padden and Jubb, David, PhD. *LifeFood Recipe Book: Living on Life Force*, Jubbs Longevity Inc.: New York, NY, 2002.

Kendall, Frances Lillian. *Sweet Temptations Natural Dessert Book: Delicious Desserts That Need No Cooking*, Avery Publishing Group, Inc: Garden City Park, NY, 1988.

Kenney, Matthew. *Everyday Raw*, Gibbs Smith: Layton, UT, 2008.

Kenney, Matthew and Melngailis, Sarma. *Raw Food/Real World: 100 Simple to Sophisticated Recipes,* Regan Books: New York, NY, 2005.

Kulvinskas, Viktoras. *Love Your Body: Live Food Recipes, or How to Be a Live Food Lover*, Hippocrates Health Institute: Boston, MA, 1972.

Levin, James, MD, and Cederquist, Natalie. *Vibrant Living*, GLO, Inc.: La Jolla, CA, 1993.

Maerin, Jordan. *Raw Foods for Busy People: Simple and Machine-Free Recipes for Every Day*, Lulu Press Inc.: Morrisville, NC, 2004.

Malkmus, Rhonda J. *Recipes for Life from God's Garden,* Hallelujah Acres Publishing: Shelby, NC, 1998.

Markowitz, Elysa. *Warming Up to Living Foods*, Book Publishing Company: Summertown, TN, 1998.

Mars, Brigitte. *Rawsome! Maximizing Health, Energy and Culinary Delight with the Raw Foods Diet,* Basic Health Publications, Inc: North Bergen, NJ, 2004.

Patenaude, Frédéric. *Instant Raw Sensations: The Easiest, Simplest, Most Delicious Raw Food Recipes Ever!* Raw Vegan: Montreal, Quebec, Canada, 2005.

Patenaude, Frédéric. *The Sunfood Cuisine: A Gourmet Guide to Raw-Food Vegan Eating*, Genesis 1:29 Publishing: San Diego, CA, 2002.

Phyo, Ani. *Ani's Raw Food Kitchen: Easy, Delectable Living Foods Recipes*, Marlowe & Co: New York, NY, 2007.

Rhio. *Hooked on Raw: Rejuvenate Your Body and Soul with Nature's Living Foods*, Beso Entertainment: New York, NY, 2000.

Rogers, Jeff. *Vice Cream, Over 70 Sinfully Delicious Dairy-Free Delights*, Celestial Arts: Berkeley, CA, 2004.

Rydman, Mary. *Raw and Radiant: Simple Raw Recipes for the Busy Lifestyle*, Outskirts Press: Parker, CO, 2006.

Safron, Jeremy A. *The Raw Truth: The Art of Preparing Live Foods*, Celestial Arts: Berkeley, CA, 2003.

Scott-Aitken, Lynelle. *Raw Food Recipes: No Meat, No Heat,* Green Frog Publishers, 2005.

Shannon, Nomi. *The Raw Gourmet: Simple Recipes for Living Well*, Alive Books: Burnaby, BC, Canada, 1998.

Sheridan, Jameth, ND and Sheridan, Kim, ND. *Uncooking with Jameth & Kim: All Original, Vegan & Raw Recipes & Unique Information about Raw Vegan Foods*, HealthForce Publishing: Escondido, CA, 1991.

Shircliffe, Arnold. *The Edgewater Beach Hotel Salad Book*, The Hotel Monthly Press: Chicago, IL, 1926.

Trotter, Charlie and Klein, Roxanne. *Raw*, Ten Speed Press: Berkeley, CA, 2003.

Underkoffler, Renée Loux. *Living Cuisine: The Art and Spirit of Raw Food*, Avery: New York, NY, 2003.

Vonderplanitz, Aajonus. *The Recipe for Living without Disease,* Carnelian Bay Castle Press: Santa Monica, CA, 2002.

Wandling, Julie. *Thank God for Raw: Recipes for Raw*, Hallelujah Acres Publishing: Shelby, NC, 2002.

Wigmore, Dr. Ann. *Recipes for Longer Life*, Rising Sun Publications: Boston, MA, 1978.

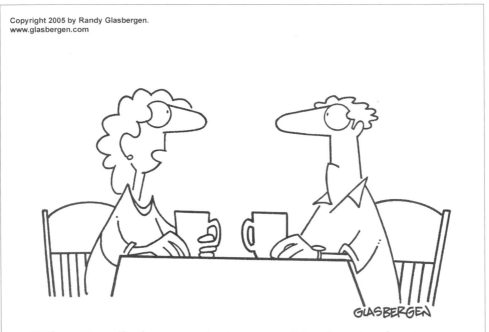

"When I'm dieting, my doctor says it's okay to cheat once in a while. I'm going out with your friend Larry tonight."

# Resource Guide
## Related Web Sites

As those of you who are used to the Internet know, web sites come and go. By the time you read this book, some of these sites may no longer be up. But these are the current ones I have found very useful.

**www.alissacohen.com**

This site sells Alissa's book, *Living on Live Food.* Additionally, there are several "before" and "after" photos of people on the raw diet. There is also a chat room for discussion.

**www.annettelarkins.com**

This web site belongs to Annette Larkins, who gave her testimony in Chapter 2. It has more about her and the products she offers.

**www.buildfreedom.com/rawmain.htm**

This is a very interesting site with links to other major raw food sites. It includes information about the instinctive raw diet and the raw animal food diet (see Appendix C). It has a paragraph about each site and a sort of "who's who" in the raw food world.

**www.cula.edu**

This is the site of City University Los Angeles, P. O. Box 45227, Los Angeles, CA 90045. Phone: 310-671-0783. E-mail: admissions@cula.edu. This educational institution offers graduate degree programs in Nutritional Science, Natural Hygiene, Life Science, Health Care Administration, Public Health, Electromedical Science, Human Studies, Guidance and Counseling, Holistic Care and therapy-oriented majors. Founded in 1974 by Dr. Henry L. N. Anderson, EdD, a natural hygienist and fruitarian student of the late T. C. Fry, DSc, CULA first offered its graduate level degree program in Natural Hygiene in the late 1980s. This degree path remains open to qualified, self-taught and practicing hygienists with college degrees or the equivalent. Although programs and courses have been expanded since, the curriculum CULA first used was created by T. C. Fry, who was bestowed a posthumous honorary Doctor of Science degree in recognition of his many years of service to health seekers.

**www.doctoryourself.com**

This site has a lot of informative articles to help you take responsibility for your health and become your own doctor. It sells an eponymous book.

**www.drday.com**

Anyone who is still skeptical about the power of a raw diet should check out this site. It includes Dr. Day's photos of a very protruding breast tumor while she was busy trying out every sort of alternative health therapy for it. After trying dozens of things, she came upon juice cleansing, wheatgrass and finally Natural Hygiene. She put the principles into action, and her body healed completely. The site sells her numerous videos on the topic from a Seventh Day Adventist Christian perspective.

**www.foodnsport.com**

This site has a lot of interesting articles by notable raw food doctor Doug Graham and word of his upcoming events and lecture appearances, which include a yearly fasting retreat.

**www.fredericpatenaude.com**

This is an informative site with interviews and articles on the subject of raw eating. Site owner Frédéric Patenaude also sells his books, including an excellent and informative recipe book, *Sunfood Cuisine*, and *The Raw Secrets*. His most recent book, *Instant Raw Sensations*, includes fast, delicious recipes that are low in fat. You can also subscribe to his weekly newsletter, which is very informative and has useful tips.

**www.fresh-network.com**

This is a UK-based site. It may not be practical to buy anything here if you live in the US, but it does have some good recipes and articles.

**www.fromsadtoraw.com**

This site offers a lot of information: recipes, answers to frequently asked questions, links, books and magazines, facts and tips.

**www.getwellstaywellamerica.com**

Victoria BidWell's web site offers the largest collection of Natural Hygiene materials ever amassed — 1,000 books and tapes in all — including all of Dr. Shelton's major works, 27 of his live-taped lectures and the complete works of T.C. Fry. The many postings on this web site include case histories, crucial health essays, a gift book of 100 raw recipes and inspirational materials showing the biblical correctness of Natural Hygiene and more. Call her at 360-853-7048.

**www.goneraw.com**

This site was created to help people share and discuss raw vegan food recipes from around the world. It presents some really good and free recipes with color photos and user ratings of the dishes.

**www.greenpeople.org**

This site will link you to your local community supported agriculture (CSA) biodynamic farm, food co-op and health food stores, along with other local resources for obtaining good organic food and ecology-friendly products.

**www.healself.org**

This has numerous articles by Dr. Bernarr Zovluck, DD, DC. You can click on just about any illness or other health topic and read his very informative articles. He has been eating raw foods exclusively for over 50 years and is quite strong and youthful-looking!

**www.health101.org**

This site has a lot of powerful articles on health in addition to sales of books, products and classes. If you click on "articles," I especially recommend the article called "Raw Foods: What Some People Don't Know," which quotes misinformed and ignorant health professionals about the futility of the raw diet, together with Don Bennett's responses clarifying their misconceptions.

**www.livefoodfactor.com**

The web site for this book, it has post-publication updates and additions to the book, as well as articles on the raw food diet. My vision is to expand this site to offer other health books, raw food, a health blog and interviews.

**www.livingnutrition.com**

This site is by noted raw fooder and author Dr. David Klein, PhD. He publishes the raw food magazine *Vibrance*, which you can subscribe to on this site. The site includes a bookstore, health shop and listing of raw food events. He also has another web site: www.colitis-crohns.com.

**www.lovingraw.com**

This site is by a young man who lost 125 pounds on the raw diet! He shares his journey with some videos. The site includes blogs, information and sells some raw foods and appliances.

**www.mercola.com**

This site is run by a doctor who is full of cutting edge knowledge in nutrition and other areas of taking control of your health. You can get on his semi-weekly mailing list, which contains numerous articles. It also has a health information blog.

**www.milksucks.com**

This site is by People for the Ethical Treatment of Animals (PETA) and details how harmful dairy is not only to people, but also to the dairy cows, due to the way they are treated. It includes "Scary Dairy Tales" with testimonials to the perils of a white moustache.

**www.naturalnews.com**

This site is a great place to visit periodically for the latest news regarding health and healthful living, politics and technology. It also has a great compilation of health-related videos, reports, cartoons and news podcasts. (They generously donated cartoons to this book, in fact!)

**www.nelsonsbooks.com**

Dennis Nelson offers a huge variety of alternative health care books to customers who are in business to purchase books wholesale and then sell them retail to health seekers. The web site offers a wide selection of raw food and Natural Hygiene books, including all the classics and the latest publications.

**www.notmilk.com**

Named as a play on the "Got Milk?" dairy ads, this site has dozens of very interesting articles dispelling the milk myth and showing how very hazardous dairy is to our health. The site is by Robert Cohen, who sells his book (also available on audiotape), *Milk the Deadly Poison*, which is loaded with scientific data on the health hazards of dairy consumption.

**www.paulnison.com**

This is the official web site of author and raw food chef Paul Nison, with various resources relating to Paul's health and healing teachings, his lecture schedule, great links and much more.

**www.purehealthandnutrition.com**

This is a great free online newsletter that comes out every Thursday and features tips, tools and advice on the raw-food diet, health and more.

**www.rawandjuicy.com**

This site is by Shelly Keck-Borsits, author of the book *Dying to Get Well*. You can buy the book here or download it for free! The author needs the money from the book sales but is so intent on getting the word out that she freely gives away the book. The site includes a raw chat room, raw recipes and a "raw artist" link.

**www.rawfamily.com**

This is the Boutenkos' site and offers free recipes, frequently asked questions (FAQs), articles, testimonials and links. It also has the Boutenkos' books, DVDs and videos for sale.

**www.rawfood.com**

This is the largest online raw food store, owned by David Wolfe. The items are 100% raw, as he is a 100% raw fooder himself. Imported from all around the world, many of these items are unavailable elsewhere in the USA. He also has the largest selection of raw food books available. In addition, the store sells natural beauty products, tapes, CDs and videos and lists raw food events Wolfe hosts. Also included are links to articles on the raw food diet and related topics, as well as a personals section.

**www.rawfoodinfo.com**

Raw food chef and author Rhio runs this site, at which one could spend hours: it includes a radio podcast from her radio show, articles on the diet, recipes, links, a raw community event calendar, a raw food restaurant directory and "before" and "after" photos of numerous people.

**www.rawfoodlife.com**

This is a very informative site, with links to other raw food sites and related articles published in magazines and professional journals.

**www.rawfoodnews.com**

This site has only some links.

**www.rawfoodplanet.com**

One of the creators of this site is pioneer raw fooder Viktoras Kulvinskas. It is truly a mega-site that is a fantastic resource, especially for travelers since it includes a map of the USA you can click on to find local raw food resources. It even covers quite a few other countries you can click on! Resources on this site include recipes, events calendar, schools, online courses, support and chat groups, books, articles and much, much more.

**www.rawfoods.com** (or **www.living-foods.com**)

This site has plenty of articles, including FAQs about the raw diet, a raw personals for connecting with other raw fooders, a store, free recipes and a chat room.

**www.rawfoodteens.com**

This site is a bulletin board for teenagers going on a raw food diet. There is support for teens, with such issues as eating disorders, weight management, beauty and the struggles of going raw. There will be a chat room later.

**www.rawfoodwiki.org**

This site offers recipes, testimonials, equipment for sale and links.

**www.rawgourmet.com**

This site is by Nomi Shannon, author of the beautiful recipe book *The Raw Gourmet*, which abounds with color photos of her delicious raw food creations. The site has links, recipes, events, kitchen gadgets and books for sale. Sign up for her free seven-part course on eating raw.

**www.rawguru.com**

This site lists raw food leaders and recipes, articles, jokes, games and frequently asked questions. It also sells raw foods, books and equipment. You can also sign up for a newsletter.

**www.rawlife.com**

This is raw food author and lecturer Paul Nison's store. Along with free information, FAQs and recipes, the site sells books, raw food (some hard to find, such as raw cashews), raw chocolates, juicers and other kitchen equipment.

**www.rawreform.com**

This site belongs to Angela Stokes, who presented her testimony in Chapter 2. It includes her E-book for sale, as well as articles.

**www.rawschool.com**

This is raw fooder Nora Lenz's Natural Hygiene web site. Visit here for articles on raw food basics, testimonials, e-mail discussion, T-shirts advertising the raw diet and more.

**www.rawtimes.com**

This site has links to nationwide raw restaurants, raw food stores, raw food machines and supplies, as well as book reviews and other items.

**www.rawvegan.com**

Go to this web site to sign up for a free seven-day e-course (e-mail course) on the raw food diet and learn practical ways to increase your energy and look younger by using the power of raw foods.

**www.rawveganbooks.com**

As the name suggests, this site sells a wide variety of books on the topic of raw veganism. Phone: 800-642-4113.

**www.shazzie.com**

This site has all sorts of information for the raw journey, as well as before and after photos. Shazzie wrote the book *Detox Your World,* which gives information on detoxifying one's environment, as well as on eating raw.

**www.soilandhealth.org**

This online library site contains a wealth of information, including entire books on health that can be downloaded for free.

**www.superbeing.com**

Raw fooder site owner Roger Haeske offers special reports, articles, books, testimonials and a free e-mail newsletter geared to the beginning raw fooder you can sign up to receive.

**www.superchargeme.com**

This site offers the "rawcumentary" DVD *Supercharge Me ... 30 Days Raw*, which won the award for best documentary at the Tofino Film Festival. Jenna Norwood, producer, director and main star of the film, wanted to dress up as a showgirl for Halloween. When she couldn't fit into the costume, she embarked on a raw journey for 30 days, all documented in this entertaining and educational documentary. Watch or download the trailer at this site. The film's contact e-mail address is info@superchargeme.com.

**www.thegardendiet.com**

This site, by long-time raw vegans Storm Talifero, a very muscular bodybuilder, and his family, offers e-books, retreats, photos and DVDs, including their biographical documentary film *Breakthrough*.

**www.thmastery.com**

This is the site of Arnoux Goran, who is mentioned in two testimonials in Chapter 2. It includes articles and recipes and offers courses.

**www.totalhealthsecrets.com**

This site offers information on internal cleansing techniques.

**www.transformationinstitute.org**

This site is a school for Natural Hygiene by Dr. Robert Sniadach. You can purchase his comprehensive correspondence course on this site. It has free FAQs and interviews as well.

**www.welikeitraw.com**

Watch the creative, catchy, hilarious video *Sexy Bitches Like It Raw*, featuring two young female raw eaters singing the praises of the raw diet. BITCHES stands for beautiful, intelligent, talented, compassionate, healthy, empowered, sexy. They offer catering services and plan to post more photos, recipes, and a blog.

**www.wynman.com**

Holistic/preventive dentist Bob Wynman has been a raw eater since 1990. Hr offers dental information from a Natural Hygiene perspective, unconventional political ideas and Nikken wellness products. He also relates the details of his two 40-day water-only fasts.

# Raw Food Chat Groups

The various raw food Internet chat groups are fluid and changeable. They come and go frequently, so this is just a sample of what was available at press time:

http://eat.rawfood.com

http://groups.yahoo.com/group/freshnetgroup/

http://groups.yahoo.com/group/hallelujahdiet/

http://groups.yahoo.com/group/rawfood/

http://groups.yahoo.com/group/rawfoodeaters/

http://groups.yahoo.com/group/rawfoodpower/

http://groups.yahoo.com/group/rawfoodsbeginners/

http://groups.yahoo.com/group/12stepstorawfood/

http://health.groups.yahoo.com/group/100_percent_raw

http://health.groups.yahoo.com/group/rawfoodarticlesarchive/

http://www.rawfoodchat.com

http://www.rawfreedomcommunity.info/forum/

# Resources for Food and Kitchen Supplies

Some raw foods are difficult to find, even at your local health store. It may therefore be necessary to shop online for certain items, such as raw nut butters, sun-dried fruits, unpasteurized oils, raw cashews and others. Kitchen gadgets needed for gourmet dishes (see Chapter 13) are also available at many of these sites. The following lists will also include phone numbers for those who do not have Internet access.

**Acres USA**

P. O. Box 91299, Austin, TX 78709. Phones: 800-355-5313, 512-892-4400, 512-892-4448 (fax). Web site: www.acresusa.com. This is an excellent source of books, tapes and videos for organic farmers and home gardeners. They also publish a monthly magazine. Send for their free catalog.

**Alive Foods**

Web site: www.alivefoods.com. This is an Australian company that sells bee pollen, supplements, hemp oil, books and DVDs about raw food and nutrition.

**Biodynamic Farming and Gardening Association, Inc.**

25844 Butler Rd., Junction City, OR 97448. Phones: 888-516-7797, 541-998-0105, 541-998-0106 (fax). Web site: www.biodynamics.com. E-mail: biodynamic@aol.com. This organization coordinates Community Supported Agriculture (CSA) farms throughout the USA. CSAs supply locally grown organic foods direct from farm to consumer. Call their toll-free number to locate one in your area.

**Blend-Tec USA**

P. O. Box 558, Concrete, WA 98237. Phone: 360-853-7048. E-mail: victoriabidwell@aol.com. Victoria BidWell and I carry every live food preparation machine and gadget on the market at the best prices for *Live Food Factor* friends!

**Country Life Natural Foods**

P. O. Box 489, 52nd St., Pullman, MI 49450. Phones: 800-456-7694, 269-236-5011 and 269-236-8357 (fax). Web site: www.clnf.org. This company sells raw, organic nuts and nut butters, dried organic fruits (some of which are sun-dried and therefore raw) and organic seeds.

**EatRaw**

125 Second St, Brooklyn, NY 11231. Phones: 866-4EATRAW, 866-432-8729, 718-210-0048 and 718-802-0116 (fax). Web site: www.eatraw.com.

This company sells raw food, natural beauty and skin care, kitchen appliances, books, videos and natural cleaning supplies.

## Excalibur Dehydrators

P. O. Box 558, Concrete, WA 98237. Phone: 360-853-7048. E-mail: victoriabidwell@aol.com. Victoria BidWell and I carry every live food preparation machine and gadget on the market at the best prices for *Live Food Factor* friends!

## GetWell♥StayWell, America!

P. O. Box 558, Concrete, WA 98237. Phone: 360-853-7048. Web site: www.getwellstaywellamerica.com. E-mail: victoriabidwell@aol.com. Victoria BidWell offers many healthful snacks, such as premade raw candy bars and crackers. Her own creations found nowhere else include Victory Veggie Vittles, made of 12 kinds of raw and flash freeze-dried vegetables, and four all-raw, no-salt, vegetable seasonings: Veggie Volt! Tomato Bolt! Ginger Jolt! and Instead of Coffee!

## Good Stuff by Mom & Me

13106 Warner Hill Road, South Wales, NY 14139. Phone: 888-797-6865. Web site: www.gimmegoodstuff.com. This company sells a lot of raw, organic, vegan goodies.

## Go Raw

6313 University Ave, San Diego, CA 92115. Phones: 619-286-2446 and 619-286-2446 (fax). Web site: www.goraw.com. This company sells lots of raw crackers, cookies, sprouted and dehydrated seeds, raw granola and more.

## HealthForce Nutritionals

1835A S. Centre City Pkwy, #411; Escondido, CA 92025-6505. Phones: 800-357-2717 and 760-747-8922 (fax also). Web site: www.healthforce.com. This company sells Greener Grasses and Vitamineral Green, both of which are living dehydrated grasses. If you don't have time to make your own wheatgrass, this is the next best thing.

## High Vibe

Phone: 888-554-6645. Web site: www.highvibe.com. They sell raw foods, books and videos concerning the raw lifestyle, natural beauty products and much more.

## Jaffe Brothers Natural Foods

28560 Lilac Road, Valley Center, CA 92082. Phone: 760-749-1133, 760-749-1282 (fax). Web site: www.organicfruitsandnuts.com. In business for over 50 years, this company sells organic nuts, fruits and other dry goods.

## live live & organic

261 East 10th Street, NY, NY, 10009. Phones: 877-505-5504, 212-505-5504. Web site: www.live-live.com. E-mail: info@live-live.com. This organic raw

store sells, among other things, raw food, nontoxic body care products, kitchen appliances, books and DVDs on the raw food diet.

### Live Super Foods

Phone: 800-481-5074. Web site: www.livesuperfoods.com. The sell live super foods such as goji berries, hemp seed, coconut oil.

### Living Nuts

Phone: 207-780-1101. Web site: www.livingnutz.com. For people who are used to eating chips and popcorn with different flavors, these flavored nuts make a great transition food, as well as a great treat for the long-term raw fooder. This company promises to keep providing raw almonds. They will get them from outside the USA, which is now mandating pasteurization.

### Living Tree Community Foods

P. O. Box 10082, Berkeley, CA 94709. Phones: 800-260-5534, 510-526-7106 and 510-526-9516 (fax). Web site: www.livingtreecommunity.com. E-mail: info@livingtreecommunity.com. Not everything is raw. Since things are always changing, you have to e-mail them or call them. They have a large selection of truly raw nuts and truly raw dried fruits. They have a very wide assortment of raw nut and seed butters and olive oil.

### Macaweb

Phone: 888-645-4282. Web site: www.macaweb.com. This company sells various raw, organic foods, including maca, the super food from Peru.

### NatuRAW

851 Irwin Street, Suite 304; San Rafael, CA 94901. Phones: 800-NATURAW (800-628-8729), 415-456-1719 (office), 775-587-8613 (fax). Web site: www.naturaw.com. This company sells raw treats and goodies, supplements, body care and more.

### Orkos

Web site: www.orkos.com/home_EN.php. Within Europe only, these distributors sell instinctive quality, organic produce, nuts, seeds, honey and more.

### Peace Pies

Phone: 619-618-6960. Web site: www.rawpie.com. You certainly don't have to give up pies to be a raw food eater! They sell plenty of raw vegan pies, also sold at the Hillcrest Farmers' Market.

### Raw Life

P. O. Box 16156, West Palm Beach, FL 33416. Phone: 866-RAW-PAUL, 866-729-7285. Web site: www.rawlife.com. Paul Nison sells raw food, books, tapes and videos.

### Seeds of Change

P. O. Box 15700, Santa Fe, NM 87506-5700. Phones: 505-438-8080 and 505-438-7052 (fax). Web site: www.seedsofchange.com. This company sells organic seeds and seeds that have been less hybridized than usual (see Chapter 17).

## Sunfood Nutrition (formerly Nature's First Law)

11655 Riverside Drive, Suite 155, Lakeside, CA 92040. Phone: 800-205-2350, 619-596-7979. Web site: www.rawfood.com. This store carries lots of raw food items you can't find elsewhere, items from all over the world, all organic and 100% raw.

## SunOrganic Farm

411 S. Las Pasas Road, San Marcos, CA 92078. Phone: 888-269-9888, 760-510-8077 and 760-510-9996 (fax). Web site: www.sunorganicfarm.com. This company sells raw nuts, nut and seed butters and dehydrated fruits. Circumstances are always changing, so it is best to call before placing an order to discover which items are truly raw.

## The Raw Bakery

Phone: 800-571-8369. Web site: www.rawbakery.com. This is the only place where I have found truly raw, shredded coconut. It also sells raw cakes and other goodies.

## The Raw Gourmet

P. O. Box 21097, Sedona, AZ 86341. Phone: 888-316-4611. Web site: www.rawgourmet.com. Nomi Shannon sells books, including her highly recommended raw recipe book, as well as useful kitchen gadgets. For more information, see the web site summary at the site listed above.

## The Raw Life

The Raw World, 322 South Padre Juan, Ojai, CA 93023. Phones: 866-RAW-PAUL (866-729-7285) and 818-832-0007 (fax). Web site: www.rawlife.com. Raw food, books, tapes and videos are for sale.

## The Supermarket Coalition

A Project of The Rural Coalition, 1012 14th St., Suite 1100; Washington, DC 20005. Phones: 866-RURAL-80, 202-628-7160, 202-628-7165 (fax). Web site: www.supermarketcoop.com. This web site links to an on-line retail storefront and to various local produce suppliers, such as www.growingpower.org for Milwaukee and Chicago.

## The Watershed Wellness Center

6439 W. Saginaw Hwy., Lansing, MI 48917. Phone: 517-886-0440. Web site: www.watershed.net. This company sells machines that ionize water, making it alkaline for drinking.

## Wayne Gendel

1 Yorkville Ave., Suite 1; Toronto ON M4W 1L1, Canada. Phones: 866-962-4400, 416-962-4400. Web site: www.foreverhealthy.net. E-mail: info@ foreverhealthy.net. Wayne Gendel sells raw/living foods, equipment and supplements. He offers living food recipes, juicers and living water. He also

gives lectures and provides his healthful living manuals, including Forever Healthy Life Extension program, Weight-Loss program and Forever Fit system.

## USDA Farmers National Market Directory

Web site: www.ams.usda.gov/farmersmarkets. Locate a farmers' market in your area.

# Resources for Healing and Fasting Supervision

People who are seriously ill may wish to go to a healing center where they can fast under professional supervision and learn how to eat and prepare live food. Those not seriously ill, but who simply want personal instruction in live food preparation and other healthful living practices, or who simply want to reinforce their own practices, may also choose to attend such a center.

The facilities listed below offer some form of supervised fasting, sometimes on an outpatient basis only, as with Dr. Zovluck. Most of them also offer various educational programs.

Web sites that list doctors who have experience in supervising fasts include www.orthopathy.net/doctors/ and www.naturalhygienesociety.org/doctors.html. Some international contacts may be found at http://sci.pam.szczecin.pl/~fasting/.

## Ann Wigmore Foundation

P. O. Box 399, San Fidel, NM 87049-0399. Phone: 505-552-0595. E-mail: info@wigmore.org. Founded by Ann Wigmore and operated in Boston for 32 years, they are now located in a radiant oasis, high in the desert of enchanting New Mexico.

## Creative Health Institute

112 West Union City Road, Union City, MI 49094. Phones: 866-426-1213, 517-278-6260, 517-278-5837 (fax). E-mail: info@creativehealthinstitute.us. Web site: www.creativehealthinstitute.us. This natural health teaching center, based upon Dr. Ann Wigmore's teachings, provides a natural program of body purification, nutrition and rejuvenation through the use of fresh raw fruits, vegetables, juices, nuts, sprouted seeds, grains, beans, chlorophyll-rich greens and wheatgrass juice.

## Dr. Anthony Penepent, MD, MPH

439 125th Street, 1270 Broadway, #10011; New York, NY 10027. Phone: 212-316-9775. Web site: www.birdflusurvive.com. Dr. Penepent graduated in 1981 from the Grenadan medical school at St. George's University and has a Master of Public Health degree in nutrition from Loma Linda University in California. He studied alternative medicine and Natural Hygiene under Dr. Christopher Gian-Cursio, ND, in New York and began his Natural Hygiene-based practice there in 1986. He was IAHP certified in water fasting and dietary healing in 1989 and is a Member of the International Natural Hygiene Society.

## Dr. Ben Kim

147 Anne St. N, Barrie, ON, Canada L4N2B9. Phone: 705-733-0030. If you are looking for a natural solution to your health condition(s) but cannot visit

the clinic, you can receive personalized guidance from Dr. Kim through his comprehensive consulting service.

### Dr. Bernarr Zovluck, DC, DD

P. O. Box 1523, Santa Monica CA 90406. Phone: 310-396-2914. E-mail: drbernarr@aol.com. Web site: www.healself.org. Dr. Zovluck offers fasting supervision via telephone consultation for those choosing to fast at home, as well as general health consultations.

### Dr. Dimitri Karalis

Hermanus, Cape Province, South Africa. Phones: 27+(0)2854759901, 27+(0)283162978, 27+(0)283161299 (fax). Dr. Karalis has been a naturopathic physician since 1973. He opened the first biologically oriented healing clinic in South Africa and now has a clinic on the coast. He has had great success helping people overcome diseases like arthritis, neuritis, prostate enlargement, migraines, chronic fatigue, insomnia, dyspepsia, diabetes, cancers, depressions, fears, lung disorders, obesity, dermatitis and many other metabolic diseases.

### Dr. Jack M. Ebner, PhD in Biophysiology

P.O. Box 805, Holualoa, Hawaii 96725. Phone: 808-937-1649. E-mail: jack@earthhealthwatch.com. Web site: www.correctivenutrition.com. For the past 15 years, Jack has been offering Natural Hygiene consultations via telephone, e-mail, mail and in his office, as well as fasting supervision in a beautiful, tropical, Hawaiian setting.

### Dr. Joel Fuhrman, MD

4 Walter E. Foran Blvd., Suite 409; Flemington, NJ 08822. Phones: 908-237-0200. 908-237-0210 (fax). E-mail: info@drfuhrman.com. Web site: www.drfuhrman.com. Dr. Fuhrman is a board-certified family physician who specializes in preventing and reversing disease through nutritional and natural methods, has published several books, and publishes an online, monthly newsletter.

### Dr. John Fielder, DO, DC, ND

P. O. Box 901, Cairns, Queensland 4870, Australia. Phones: 07-4093-7989 (617-4093-7989 from outside of Australia). Web site: www.ig.com.au/anl/fielder.html. E-mail: academy.naturalliving@iig.com.au. A practitioner of Natural Hygiene, Dr. Fielder is a graduate of the Naturopathic College of South Australia in osteopathy, chiropractic and naturopathy. He also offers a comprehensive correspondence course in Natural Hygiene.

### Dr. Keki R. Sidhwa, ND, DO

Shalimar 14, The Weavers, Newark-on-Trent, Notts NG2 4RY, England. Phone: 01636-682-941 (011-44-1636-682-941 from the USA). Dr. Sidhwa was founder and director of the former Shalimar Health Home, where he has helped over 25,000 people to overcome their ailments by fasting and following a hygienic lifestyle. Dr. Sidhwa's fasting center is now closed, but he still offers telephone and office consultations.

## Dr. Michel Herskovitz, Health Rehabilitation Specialist

P.O. Box 371053 Las Vegas, NV 89137-1053. Phone: 702-838-9373. E-mail: ephiphanyhouse@hotmail.com. Michel's expertise lies in teaching Natural Hygiene to guests at this home health retreat where she provides the ultimate one-on-one fasting and/or Natural Hygiene intensives. Intensives include daily consultation; a personalized lifestyle program; fitness training; food preparation instruction; raw, organic meals (with cooked transition meals when appropriate or requested), as well as a host of amenities.

Michel is a passionate Christian who believes we are commanded to be good stewards of the body our Lord has given us to perform His good works. All health recommendations are Spirit led and biblically motivated.

## Dr. Stanley S. Bass, ND, DC, PhC, PhD, DO, DSc, DD

3119 Coney Island Ave, Brooklyn, NY 11235. Phone: 718-648-1500. Web site: www.drbass.com. Dr. Bass was certified by the IAHP (International Association of Hygienic Physicians) as a "specialist in fasting supervision and hygienic care" and is a founding board member of the INHS (International Natural Hygiene Society). He has supervised over 30,000 fasts and health recoveries using diet.

## Fasting Center International

Phone: 818-590-2536. E-mail: FastMaster@Fasting.com. Their 20- to 120-day fasts include personal online supervision.

## Hallelujah Acres

P. O. Box 2388, Shelby, NC 28151. Phones: 704-481-1700, 704-481-0345 (fax). E-mail: info@hacres.com. Web site: www.hacres.com. Rev. George Malkmus and his staff publish a free health newsletter and offer classes, including online health education courses, to learn about health and nutrition from a biblical perspective.

## Hawai'i Naturopathic Retreat Center, Inc.

17-502 Ipuaiwaha, Keaau, Hawaii 96749. Phone: 808-982-8202. E-mail: contact@mindyourbody.info. Web site: www.mindyourbody.info. Dr. Maya Nicole Baylac practices privately on the Big Island of Hawaii as a hygienic doctor and psychotherapist. She has practiced Reichian breath work, Gestalt therapy, bioenergetics and meditation in individual and group sessions for 25 years, blending her psychological background and her hygienic practice into a unique mind/body/spirit approach. She supervises detoxification and rebuilding programs with water-only fasting, juice dieting and raw eating during long-term guest visits.

## Hippocrates Health Institute

1443 Palmdale Court, West Palm Beach, FL 33411. Phone: 561-471-8876. E-mail: info@hippocratesinst.org. Web site: www.hippocratesinst.org. Operated by Brian Clement for the past 25 years, this 70-person, in-residence health facility was originally founded by Dr. Ann Wigmore.

## Hummingbird Homestead

22732 NW Gillihan Road, Sauvie Island, OR 97231-3781. Phones: 503-621-3897, 503-621-3781 (fax). E-mail: Jayne@earthworld.com. Hummingbird Homestead, a place of solitude, peace and joy, was founded by Victoria Jayne, LCSW, Reiki Master, NLP Master Programmer, Essene Minister and spiritual seeker. A retreat can include workshops, therapeutic counseling, detoxifying juice diets, raw meals, live foods education, as well as other services and products.

## Linda Sticco's Personal Training Fitness Studio, Inc.

P. O. Box 522, Stroudsburg, PA 18360. Phones: 866-559-2787, 570-688-9998, 570-992-0864 (fax). Web site: www.lsfitness.com. Linda Sticco is a PhD graduate of T. C. Fry's Life Science Health System and Natural Hygiene practitioner. She is also a certified personal trainer and lifestyle fitness coach. A published writer and speaker, she is the author of *The Empowerment Program*. In addition to personal training, Linda conducts telephone consultations designed to help people get the bodies they want, the energy they need and the health they require in order to fulfill their lives' dreams!

## Living Foods Centre

Holmleigh, Gravel Hill, Ludlow SY81QS, UK, Phones: 00944(0)1584 875308, 00944(0)1584 875778 (fax). Director Elaine Bruce, author of *Living Foods for Radiant Health*, is an experienced naturopath teaching residential living foods courses tailored for a UK audience.

## Living Foods Learning Center

P. O. Box 1380, Columbus, NM 88029. Phone: 505-531-2456. Web site: www.livingfoodslearningcenter.com. Using the methods taught to her by Dr. Ann Wigmore, Shu Chan has expanded Dr. Ann's program to create a more effective and accelerated "new" program. A three-week program of hands-on learning, using wheatgrass juice, energy soup, raw foods from their gardens, herbs and rejuvelac to help those who are health challenged build disease-free bodies.

## New-Earth Medicine

Los Angeles, California. Phone: 714-925-1707. E-mail: drzarinazar@yahoo.com. Dr. Zarin Azar, MD, is a medical doctor with a Natural Hygiene approach who takes telephone consultations from clients around the world. Although her specialty is gastroenterology, she welcomes patients with any health issues. Dr. Azar takes a natural holistic approach that focuses on the patient's physical, mental and emotional issues. She offers lifestyle guidance aimed at bringing about the positive changes needed for living in joyful health.

## Optimum Health Institute
There are two Optimum Health Institutes (OHIs):
- OHI San Diego, 6970 Central Ave, Lemon Grove, CA 91945. Phones: 619-464-3346, 619-589-4098 (fax).
- OHI Austin, 265 Cedar Lane, Cedar Creek, TX 78612. Phones: 512-303-4817, 512-303-1239 (fax).

They share the web site www.optimumhealthinstitute.org.

## Our Hygiene Homestead in The Woods
P. O. Box 558, Concrete, WA 98237. Phone: 360-853-7048. E-mail: victoriabidwell@aol.com. Web site: www.getwellstaywellamerica.com. Victoria BidWell has been a Natural Hygiene educator, author and promoter since 1984, having studied under Dr. Vetrano and T. C. Fry. She has just opened a guesthouse/schoolhouse in the Cascade Mountains that accommodates four health seekers who may enjoy these unique features: privacy in a woodsy setting surrounded by national parks and forests; fresh, clean air; blessed quietude; a 2,000 volume book/tape library; fasting; raw juices; raw-only cuisine; hands-on food preparation demonstrations with every meal; personal consultations in overcoming addictions, and finding Hygiene Joy!

See the web site for many pictures of the retreat, its 60 unique features and case histories. I have personally visited Victoria and stayed at Our Hygiene Homestead. It is an amazing wilderness setting! See page 656.

## Sacred Space Healing Center
776 Haight Street (at Scott), San Francisco, CA 94117. Phone: 415-431-0878. E-mail: info@sacredspace-sf.com. The center offers live blood analysis, nutritional counseling and fasting retreats in Puerto Vallarta, Mexico.

## Scott's Natural Health Institute
P. O. Box 361095, Strongsville, OH 44136. Phone: 440-238-3003. Web site: www.fastingbydesign.com. Dr. D. J. Scott, DM, ND, DC, offers therapeutic fasting under professional, scientific supervision, using weekly, precise, scientific, monitoring of disease processes until healing or remission measurably occurs, accomplished by his very advanced, federally licensed, diagnostic laboratory, of which he is the director. He has been in practice for over 50 years and has personally supervised the care of over 40,000 patients. He has fasted, under direct supervision, some 20,000 patients, many of whom were of international origin.

## Tanglewood Wellness Center
Correos Bejuco, Entrega General, Rep. de Panama. Phone: 301-637-4657. E-mail: info@tangelwoodwellnesscenter.com. Web site: www.tanglewoodwellnesscenter.com. Formerly in Bethesda, MD, this fasting center is now located in the Republic of Panama.

## The Arcadia Health Centre
31 Cobah Road, Arcadia, NSW 2159, Australia. Phones: 61-2-9653-1115, 61-2-9653-2678. Web site: www.alecburton.com. Run by Drs. Alec and Ne-

jla Burton, the Arcadia Health Centre is the first and only clinic practicing Natural Hygiene in Australia that is conducted by licensed and certified members of the IAHP (established in 1961). Dr. Burton graduated in chiropractic and osteopathy in England. He is a co-founder of the British Natural Hygiene Society, The Australian Natural Hygiene Society and the International Association of Hygienic Physicians.

### The Gerson Institute

Administrative Office: 316 East Olive, #A; Redlands, CA 92373. Phone: 888-792-0077. E-mail: Mail@wholelifelearningcenter.org. Those at the Gerson Institute have been assisting detoxification and nutritional healing for decades. They also have a new Hawaiian retreat center: 17-502 Ipuaiwaha St., Kea'au, HI 96749. Phone: 808-982-8202 (fax also), 808-280-2537 (cell).

### The Goldberg Clinic

2480 Windy Hill Road, Ste. 203; Marietta, GA 30067. Phone: 770-974-7470. Additional location: 9121 North Military Trail, Ste. 308; Palm Beach Gardens, FL 33410. Phone: 561-722-9637. Dr. Goldberg is a clinical nutritionist, clinical epidemiologist, Diplomate of the American Clinical Board of Nutrition and Certified Natural Hygiene Practitioner.

### Tree of Life Foundation

P. O. Box 778, Patagonia, AZ 85624. Phone: 520-394-2520. Web site: www.treeoflife.nu. The Tree of Life Foundation is headed by Dr. Gabriel Cousens. It also offers seminars, workshops and a master's degree in living foods.

### TrueNorth Health Education and Fasting Center

1551 Pacific Ave, Santa Rosa, CA 95404. Phone: 707-586-5555. Web site: www.healthpromoting.com. Natural Hygiene doctor Alan Goldhamer and his staff have operated the Center for Conservative Therapy, a small in-patient and out-patient residential health education center in Penngrove, California, since 1984. In recent years, they changed the name to TrueNorth. In September 2007, they opened a large facility that takes 50 patients. All have private bedrooms, bathrooms and all the amenities. The kitchen is staffed with live food chefs. Their views are best described in their book *The Pleasure Trap: Mastering the Hidden Force That Undermines Health & Happiness*, by Drs. Douglas J. Lisle and Alan Goldhamer.

# Raw Food Events

Here is a list of raw food events compiled by Victoria Boutenko.

**Vibrant Living Expo**, annual, California, USA. 707-964-2420, www.rawfood chef.com.

**Raw Spirit Retreat**, annual, Oregon, USA. 503-650-4447.

**The Fresh Festival**, annual, United Kingdom, www.fresh-network.com/festival/ index.htm.

**Raw World: International Festival of Raw Food Enthusiasts**, annual, Costa Rica, www.rawworld.org.

**Raw Spirit Festival**, annual, Arizona, USA. 928-708-0784 and 928-776-1497.

# Raw Restaurants

The number of raw restaurants in the USA and Canada has increased so dramatically over the past five years that now there are over 60, I am told. Because there are so many, and they come and go with such fluidity, this listing may not be up-to-date. However, there is a web site that tries to keep up-to-date with the listings of raw food restaurants by state: www.rawfoodinfo.com/directories/dir_rawrests.html.

Another site that contains raw restaurant listings by state (and even by country!) is www.rawfoodplanet.com.

I wish to express my sincere thanks to the owners of both of those sites for giving me permission to reprint their raw restaurant listing at the time of the publication of this book. Please refer to their web site for any updates, as we are sure to see more and more raw food restaurants, just as happened with the vegetarian movement.

I have also added a few restaurants that I knew of which the web site did not have at the time.

Note that some upscale grocery stores, like Whole Foods and Wild Oats, offer seating for eaters, juice and salad/deli bars and of course the produce section, where you can buy fresh fruits to enhance your meal. Check their web sites, or see their telephone numbers listed in the "Raw Franchises" section that follows, to locate one near you.

# United States

## Alaska

### Organic Oasis Restaurant & Juice Bar

2610 Spenard Rd., Ste. B; Anchorage, AK 99503 (next to Inner Dance Yoga). 907-277-7882. Hours: M 11:30AM–7PM, Tu 11:30AM–10:30PM, W-Th 11:30AM–9PM, F-Sat 11:30AM–10PM. It serves organic entrées, soups, salads and raw juices and smoothies with some live entertainment evenings. Includes take out. Nonsmoking.

## Arizona

### Botanica Restaurant

330 E. 7th St., Tucson, AZ 85733 (at Anjoli, ½ block west of Fourth Ave.). 520-623-0913. Raw food restaurant (coming soon), juice bar, yoga studio, bookstore and community center. E-mail: info@anjoli.com. Web site: www.anjali.com.

### Rawsome! Café

234 W. University Drive, Tempe, AZ 85044. 480-496-5959 or 866-RAW-4-LIFE (729-4543). E-mail: info@rawforlife.com.

### Sedona Raw Café

1595 W. Hwy., 89A; Sedona, AZ 86336. Contact Debbie Crick or Candace Peterson: 928-282-2997. Hours: M-F 11AM–8PM, Sun 11AM–6PM. Serves live vegetarian soups, salads, entrées and gourmet desserts. Free Internet access. Web site: www.sedonarawcafe.com.

### Tree of Life Café

771 Harshaw Rd., P. O. Box 1080, Patagonia, AZ 85624. 520-394-2589 and 208-723-5025 (fax). Call for reservations. This is Dr. Gabriel Cousens's raw food restaurant, serving exquisite, very *green*, raw buffet creations fresh from the garden at the healing Tree of Life center. E-mail: cafe@treeoflife. nu. Web site: www.treeoflife.nu.

# California

### Alive Café

1972 Lombard St. (near Webster), San Francisco, CA 94123. 415-923-1052. Vegan, 100% organic, live food cuisine, featuring appetizers, snacks, salads, soups, entrées, desserts, teas and beverages. E-mail: aliveveggie@sbcglobal. net.

### Au Lac Gourmet Vegetarian Restaurant

Mile Square Plaza, 16553 Brookhurst St., Fountain Valley, CA 92708. 714-418-0658. Hours: Tu-Sun 12:00PM–8:45PM. Au Lac is a vegetarian restaurant featuring Vietnamese and Chinese cuisine. Au Lac now offers vegan, raw food dishes. Web site: www.aulac.com.

### Beverly Hills Juice Club

8382 Beverly Blvd., Los Angeles, CA 94122. 323-655-8300. Juices, smoothies and some raw vegan entrées for take out.

### Blissful Cuisine

Carlsbad Village Faire; 300 Carlsbad Village Drive, Ste. 106; Carlsbad, CA 92008. This restaurant serves organic, raw, vegan food.

### Café Gratitude

There are four locations:

- 2400 Harrison St. (at 20th St.), San Francisco, CA 94110.
- 1336 9th Ave. (at Irving), San Francisco, CA 94122.
- 1730 Shattuck Avenue (corner of Virginia), Berkeley, CA 94709.
- 2200 4th St. (near W. Crescent Dr., San Rafael, CA 94901.

415-824-4652. Serving all organic, vegan and mostly live foods! They support local farmers, sustainable agriculture and environmentally friendly products. They also offer food prep classes and catering. Web site: www.withthecurrent.com.

## Café La Vie

429 Front St. (at Cathcart St.), Santa Cruz, CA 95060. 831-429-ORGN (6746). Café La Vie is an all-organic café and bar specializing in raw and mostly-raw vegan cuisine and beverages, including organic beer and wine. Occasional guest chefs and also qualified speakers and workshops on nutritional and wellness topics. Excellent quality raw food staples are available for sale. E-mail: yeyen@lavie.us. Web site: www.lavie.us.

## Café Muse

Located in UC Berkeley Art Museum, 2625 Durant Ave. (near College Ave.), Berkeley (East Bay), CA 94720. 510-548-4366. One-third of the menu is raw food: organic, sustainable and locally grown. Voted most affordable CA cuisine in 2005. Web site: www.rawcafemuse.com.

## Cilantro Live

7820 Broadway, Lemon Grove, CA 91945. They serve raw, organic, vegan food. Web site: www.cilantrolive.com.

## Cru

1521 Griffith Park Blvd. (at Sunset Blvd., Los Feliz area), Los Angeles, CA 90026. 323-667-1551. Hours: 12–10 daily. Organic, raw, gourmet, vegan dishes, including a variety of Oriental and Italian dishes.

## Elixir Tonics & Teas

8612 Melrose Ave, West Hollywood, CA 90069. 310-657-9310. Raw treats, teas and herbal tonics, with an herbal reference library.

## Erewhon Natural Foods Market

7660 Beverly Blvd. #A (east of Fairfax); West Hollywood, CA 90036. 323-937-0777. Organic groceries, produce and salad bar. Raw, kosher and gourmet foods, supplements, macrobiotic, tonic herbs, two nutritionists and herbalists. Good selection of prepared raw foods and raw juice bar. E-mail: erewhonmarket@yahoo.com. Web site: www.erewhonmarket.com.

## Euphoria Loves Rawvolution

2301 Main St. (at the corner of Strand St.), Santa Monica, CA 90405. 310-392-9501. They offer packaged organic raw foods for take out, local delivery or shipping. E-mail: rawvolution@yahoo.com. Web site: www.euphoria company.com.

## Good Mood Food Café

There are two locations:

- 5930 Warner Ave. (crossroad Springdale), Huntington Beach, CA 92649. 714-377-2028. Hours: M-Th 9AM–8PM, F-Sat 9AM–9PM, Sun 10AM–8PM.

- Heritage Plaza; 14310 Culver Dr., Ste. E (between I-5 and Walnut inside Apple a Day Vitamin Shop); Irvine, CA 92604. 949-552-1444. Hours: M-Sat 10AM–3PM. Take out still available after 3PM.

Raw food restaurant with some cooked foods offered. Deli take-out. Also home delivery service and mail order. E-mail: rawgourmet@earthlink.net. Web site: www.goodmoodfood.com/café.htm.

## Green Life Evolution Center

410 Railroad Ave, Blue Lake, CA 95525. 707-668-1781. This is a market that offers prepared raw food items, also juices and smoothies. They will offer a raw food café in the future. Web site: www.greenlifefamily.com.

## Inn of the Seventh Ray

128 Old Topanga Canyon Rd., Topanga, CA 90290. 310-455-1311. Organic cuisine, both raw and cooked, vegan and nonvegan. Features a live foods chef, Angja Aditi. Live food cooking lessons available. Call for details. E-mail: inn@innoftheseventhray.com. Web site: www.innoftheseventhray.com.

## Juliano's Raw Planet

609 Broadway (at 6th), Santa Monica, CA 90401. 310-587-1552. Hours: M-Th 11AM–10PM, F 11AM–11PM, Sat 10AM–11PM, Sun 10AM–10PM. "The world's first organic restaurant certified by QAI (Quality Assurance International), the world leader in organic certification." Also offered are a mail order food catalog and food prep classes. E-mail: email@julianoalive.com. Web site: www.julianoalive.com.

## Leaf Cuisine

There are two locations:

- 11938 W. Washington Blvd., Los Angeles, CA 90066. 310-390-6005.

- 14318 Ventura Blvd. (cross street Beverly Glen), Sherman Oaks, CA 91423. 310-390-6005.

Their food is organic (certified by QAI), vegan, raw and kosher (certified by KCS), with an Italian flair. E-mail: info@leafcuisine.com. Web site: www.leafcuisine.com.

## Living Light Cuisine to Go

Living Light International, 301-B Main St., Fort Bragg, CA 95437. 800-816-2319 or 707-964-2420. Named one of the top 20 vegan restaurants in the country by VegNews! They serve delicious raw, vegan, organic specialties, including salads, entrées, smoothies, juices and sensual desserts. They have a grab-and-go section for food on the run and are open daily 7:00AM–7:00PM. They also sell mail order foods and kitchen supplies and sponsor workshops and retreats. E-mail: info@rawfoodchef.com. Web site: www.rawfoodchef.com.

## Lydia's Lovin' Foods

31 Bolinas Rd., Fairfax, CA 94930. 415-258-9678 and 415-258-9623 (fax). Organic raw and cooked meals. E-mail: info@lydiasorganics.com. Web site: www.lydiasorganics.com.

## Madeleine Bistro

18621 Ventura Blvd., Tarzana, CA 91356. 818-758-6971. Organic, vegan cuisine with some raw options. Web site: http://madeleinebistro.com.

## Millennium Restaurant

580 Geary St. (in Hotel California), San Francisco, CA 94102. 415-345-3900 and 415-345-3941 (fax). This restaurant offers one raw menu item daily, which can be ordered as an appetizer or the main course. If you wish to order other raw items, such as soup, salad, dessert or a different entrée, call three days ahead and speak to the chef. Web site: www.millenniumrestaurant.com.

## Mother's Market

There are presently five locations:

- 2963 Michelson Dr., Irvine, CA 92715. 949-752-MOMS (6667).
- 225 E. 17th St., Costa Mesa, CA 92627. 949-631-4741.
- 19970 Beach Blvd., Huntington Beach, CA 92648. 714-963-MOMS (6667).
- 24165 Paseo de Valencia, Laguna Woods, CA 92637. 949-768-MOMS (6667).
- 10928 Valley Mall, El Monte, CA 91731. 626-443-4314.

800-595-MOMS (6667). These southern California supermarket chain stores, similar to Whole Foods Market, are equipped with juice bars and restaurants that have both vegan and nonvegan cooked entrées along with some raw salad selections to augment your additional produce purchases. All items are also available for take out. Web site: www.mothersmarket.com.

## Naked Apples

784 S. Coast Hwy., Laguna Beach, CA 02651. 949-715-5410. An organic lifestyle boutique and raw foods bar featuring organic raw foods items from soups to desserts, dehydrated nuts, trail mixes, cookies, and other desserts for take-away. They also sell organic clothing.

## Native Foods

There are four locations:

- 2937 Bristol St. (at The Camp), Costa Mesa, CA 92626. 714-751-2151.
- 1110½ Gayley Ave. (at Westwood Village), Los Angeles, CA 90025. 310-209-1055.
- 73890 El Paseo, Palm Desert, CA 92260. 760-836-9396.
- 1775 E. Palm Canyon Dr. (at Smoke Tree Village), Palm Springs, CA 92264. 760-416-0070.

This vegan/vegetarian restaurant offers one raw food option though not on the menu: raw tacos. Web site: www.nativefoods.com.

## 118 Degrees Organic Raw Foods

2981 Bristol St. (at The Camp), Cosa Mesa, CA 92626. 714-754-0718. They serve natural, organic cuisine with a lounge, elixir bar and live music in the SoBeCa district.

## Que SeRAW SeRAW's Retail Store — Fresh Food to Go

1160 Capuchino Ave. (next to Earthbeam Natural Foods on the corner of Broadway and Capuchino, across from the post office), Burlingame, CA 94010. 650-348-7298 (650-FitRaw-8) or 650-400-8590 (cell). Hours: M-F 10–6, Sat 10–4, Sun closed.

## Rancho's Natural Foods

3918 30th St. (North Park), San Diego, CA 92104. 619-298-3339. San Diego's only all-vegan (except honey) grocery. Their raw food deli, vegan deli and juice bar include lots of live vegan foods, and seating is provided.

## Raw Energy Organic Juice Café

2050 Addison St. (between Shattuck and Milvia), Berkeley, CA 94704. 510-665-9464. Offerings include 100% organic juices and smoothies, raw pizza, and one large, raw salad choice. Web site: www.rawenergy.net.

## Taste of the Goddess Café

7373 Beverly Blvd. (inside Priva Hair Salon & One Spa), Los Angeles, CA 90036. 323-933-1400. They offer a full line of raw vegan smoothies, salads, entrées and desserts. They also offer home delivery, catering, classes and nutritional counseling. Web site: www.tasteofthegoddess.com.

## Terra Bella

1408 S. Pacific Coast Hwy. (at Ave. F), Redondo Beach, CA 90277. 310-316-8708. This vegan café features 100% raw gourmet meals. Check out the "green living" reference library in back. Guest speakers and events are on-going. Web site: www.terrabellacafe.com.

## The Greenery

133 Daphne (off Coast Hwy. 101 behind Mozy's Café), Encinitas, CA 92024. 760-479-0996. Hours: M-Sat 11:30–2:00, 6PM–9PM. They serve raw vegan foods. Web site: www.greeneryrawcafe.com.

**Zephyr Vegetarian Café**

340 E. 4<sup>th</sup> St., Long Beach, CA 90802. 562-435-7113. This café offers vegetarian, vegan and raw food.

# Colorado

**Café Prasad**

1904 Pearl St. (located inside the Boulder co-op), Boulder, CO 80302. 303-447-COOP (2667). Some raw food options, juices and salads. Web site: www.bouldercoop.com.

**Turtle Lake Refuge**

848 E. 3<sup>rd</sup> Ave. (at Rocky Mountain Retreat), Durango, CO 81301. 970-247-8395. Raw food lunches are served Tuesdays and Fridays. E-mail: turtlelakerefuge@yahoo.com. Web site: www.turtlelakerefuge.org.

# Connecticut

**Alchemy Juice Bar Café**

203 New Britain Ave., Hartford, CT 06106. 860-246-5700. Lacto, vegan-friendly, organic, take-out, juices, smoothies and salads. Web site: www.alchemyjuicebar.com.

**Blue Green Organic Juice Café**

72 Heights Rd. (located in Equinox Gym), Darien, CT 06820. 203-662-9390. Raw juices, smoothies, nut milks, salads and entrées. Web site: www.bluegreenjuice.com.

# District of Columbia

**Dr. Sunyatta Amen**

Washington, DC 20011. 202-545-8888. Contact person for raw food and vegetarian chefs.

**Source of Life Juice Bar & Deli: Everlasting Life Community Cooperative**

2928 Georgia Ave. NW, Washington, DC 20001. 202-232-1700. Hours: M-Sat 9–9, Sun 11–9. Lectures and cooking classes. Live food and vegan cuisine. Catering available. Web site: www.everlastinglife.net.

# Florida

**Glaser Organic Farms**

3300 Grand Ave. (SW corner of Grand and Margaret), Coconut Grove, Miami, FL. 305-238-7747 and 305-238-1227 (fax). Hours: Sat 10AM until dark. They sell juices, salads and homegrown, organic, prepared raw foods. They also sell by mail order from their online store and offer raw food prep classes locally. E-mail: raw@glaserorganicfarms.com. Web site: www. glaserorganicfarms.com.

### Grass Root Organic Restaurant

2702 N. Florida Ave. (at Columbus Dr.), Tampa, FL 33602. 813-221-ROOT (7668). Hours: Tu-Sat 11AM–9PM. The menu identifies vegan, vegetarian and raw items, including salads and juice bar. E-mail: info@thegrassroot life.com. Web site: www.thegrassrootlife.com.

### Health Station

2500 N. Hwy. A1A, Indialiantic, FL 32903. 321-773-5678. Raw vegan and vegetarian organic and locally grown food.

### Present Moment Café

224 W. King St., St. Augustine, FL 32084. 904-827-4499. Closed Sun-M. Organic, vegan and 100% raw, it features a rotating menu of hummus, parsnip/vegetable sushi, vegetable pasta and pesto, kale salad, pinenut pizza and blueberry parfaits. It also has a juice and smoothie bar, featuring various fruit and nut milks.

### Sunseed Food Co-op

6615 N. Atlantic Ave., Cape Canaveral, FL 32920. 321-784-0930 and 321-799-0212 (fax). Open M-Sat 10AM–6PM. This co-op has raw entrées. Web site: www.sunseedfoodcoop.com.

# Georgia

### Café Life

1453 Roswell Rd. (located in Life Grocery), Marietta, GA 30062. 770-977-9583. Web site: www.lifegrocery.com.

### Lov'n It Live

2796 East Point St., Atlanta, GA 30344. 404-765-9220. Serves only 100% live, organic food. Features occasional live music and poetry, classes and live food support group. Web site: www.lovingitlive.com.

### Mutana Health Café

1388 Ralph D. Abernathy Blvd. (in Mutana Co-Op Warehouse), Atlanta, GA 30310. 404-753-5252. This raw juice and smoothie bar may have relocated by the time you read this. E-mail: mutana@bellsouth.net.

### Totally Rawesome (formerly Everlasting Life Natural Foods Market)

878 Ralph D. Abernathy Blvd., Atlanta, GA 30310. 404-758-1110. Raw food deli.

# Hawaii

**Note:** See the Vegetarian Society of Honolulu Hawaii Vegetarian Dining Guide, featuring over 70 listings (restaurants, health food stores, etc.). E-mail: info@ vsh.org.

### Joy's Place
1993 S. Kihei Rd., Ste. 17 (in Island Surf Building); Kihei, Maui, HI 96753. 808-879-9258. Organic café with free-range meat and raw food options.

### Veg Out
810 Kokomo Rd. (at Haiku Town Center), Haiku, Maui, HI 96708. 808-575-5320. All vegetarian with vegan, raw and wheat-free options. Web site: www.veg-out.com.

# Idaho

### Akasha Organics
160 N. Main St. (inside Chapter One Bookstore), P. O. Box 6454, Ketchum, ID 83340. 208-726-4777 and 208-726-4785 (fax). All meals, juices and smoothies are made with fresh 100% organic ingredients. They also sell supplements and herbs. E-mail: akasha@svidaho.net. Web site: www. akashaorganics.com.

# Illinois

### Charlie Trotter's
816 W. Armitage Ave., Chicago, IL 60614. 773-248-6228, 773-248-6088 (fax). Hours: Tu-Th 6PM-10PM, F-Sat 5:30PM-10PM, occasionally open M. Expensive, mostly cooked, gourmet food, but offers raw dishes upon request. E-mail: info@charlietrotters.com. Web site: www.charlietrotters.com.

### Chicago Diner
3411 N. Halsted St., Chicago, IL 60657. 773-935-6696, 773-935-8349 (fax). This is a cooked food vegetarian restaurant that offers two raw food menu specials every day. Web site: www.veggiediner.com.

### Cousin's Incredible Vitality
3038 W. Irving Park Rd., Chicago, IL 60618. 773-478-6868, 773-478-6888 (fax). Hours: Sun, M, W, Th 4:30PM–10PM, F, Sat 4:30PM–11PM. All vegan, organic, 100% raw restaurant with a Mediterranean flair. Web site: www. cousinsiv.com.

### Karyn's Fresh Corner Café and Karyn's Raw Vegan Gourmet Restaurant
1901 N. Halsted St., Chicago, IL 60614. 312-255-1590. Hours: M-Sun 9AM–9PM. Raw vegan restaurant and grocery. Classes and workshops offered periodically. E-mail: karynraw@aol.com. Web site: www.karynraw. com.

# Maine

### Eden Vegetarian Café

78 West St. (on Mount Desert Island), Bar Harbor, ME 04609. 207-288-4422. Open seasonally April-October. Vegan, mostly organic, locally grown ingredients. Salads and raw food options available. Catering offered. Web site: www.barharborvegetarian.com.

### Little Lad's Bakery

58 Exchange St., Portland, ME 04101. 207-871-1636. See next entry.

### Little Lad's Basket

128 Main St., Bangor, ME 04401. 207-942-5482. "Bangor's only total vegetarian restaurant." They serve "no meat, no fish, no eggs and no dairy." Salads and raw food options available.

# Maryland

### Everlasting Life Health Complex

9185 Central Ave., Ste. A (at exit 15b off the Capitol Beltway); Capitol Heights, MD 20743. 301-324-6900. Lectures and cooking classes. Live food and vegan cuisine. Catering available. Web site: www.everlastinglife.net.

### The Yabba Pot Café and Juice Bar

2433 St. Paul St., Baltimore, MD 21218. 410-662-8638. Locally grown and 100% organic produce, fresh juices and some raw food dishes.

### Zia's Café

13 Allegheny Ave., Towson, MD 21204. 410-296-0799. Serves raw juices, smoothies and some raw food items. Take out and catering available. Web site: www.ziascafe.com.

# Massachusetts

### Chianti Restaurant

285 Cabot St., Beverly, MA 01915. 978-921-2233. This gourmet experience requires calling three days in advance to make reservations with the raw food chef/owner of this traditional Italian restaurant. He is adding more and more raw items to the menu.

### Organic Garden Café and Juice Bar

294 Cabot St., Beverly (45-60 minute drive NE of Boston on the coast), MA 01915. 978-922-0004 (toll free). Hours: Tu 11–8, W-Th 11–9, F-Sat 11–10, Sun 3–7. Features a great selection of raw food items on the menu. Web site: www.organicgardencafe.com.

# Michigan

## Detroit Evolution Laboratory

1434 Gratiot Ave. #1, Detroit, MI 48207. 313-316-1411. Located in the historic Eastern Market, they serve vegan food with some raw dishes and offer raw and macrobiotics food prep classes, yoga lessons and massage. www.detroitevolution.com.

## People's Food Co-op

216 N. Fourth Ave., Ann Arbor, MI 48104. 734-994-9174. Salad bar hours: M-Sat 7AM–9:30M, Sun 9AM–8PM. Organic produce plus soup/salad bar. Web site: www.peoplesfood.coop.

## Seva Restaurant

314 E. Liberty St., Ann Arbor, MI 48107. 734-662-1111. Hours: M-Th 11AM–9PM, F-Sat 11AM–10PM, Sun 10AM–9PM, with brunch served 10AM–3PM. Cooked vegetarian fare with raw salad plates and juices/smoothies.

# Minnesota

## Ecopolitan

2409 Lyndale Ave. S., Ste 2; Minneapolis, MN 55405. 612-87-GREEN (4-7336). Ecopolitan is a completely organic, vegan and raw restaurant and an ecological shop selling natural, nontoxic home and body goods. Reservations recommended. Web site: www.ecopolitan.com.

# Nevada

## Go Raw Café

There are two locations:

- 2910 Lake East Dr., Las Vegas, NV 89117. 702-254-5382.
- 2381 E. Windmill Ln., Las Vegas, NV 89123. 702-450-9007.

Organic, vegan, gourmet live food cuisine. E-mail: owner@GoRawCafe.com. Web site: www.gorawcafe.com.

# New Jersey

## East Coast Vegan

313-A W. Water St. (Garden State Pkwy., Exit 8, at the end of Simply Skin parking lot.), Toms River, NJ 08753. 732-473-9555. Hours: M-Sat 10–7, F 10–8. ECV is NJ's first organic, vegan, 100% raw restaurant. Soups, salads, entrées and desserts. Eat in or take out. Call ahead for faster service. E-mail: info@eastcoastvegan.com. Web site: www.eastcoastvegan.net.

### The Energy Bar Vegetarian Café

307C Orange Rd., Montclair, NJ 07042. 973-746-7003. Fresh juices, smoothies, light vegan food, raw food, desserts, snacks, fresh baby food, school box lunches, some specialty coffee, herbal tea, packaged and pre-pared food, some select nutrition bars and much more. E-mail: info@ kheperfoods.com. Web site: www.kheperfoods.com/energybar.html.

# New Mexico

### Whole Body Café

333 Cordova Rd. (located in the Body Center), Santa Fe, NM 87505. 505-986-0362. Has some raw food selections and juices. E-mail: info@bodyof santafe.com. Web site: www.bodyofsantafe.com/body_cafe.html.

# New York

### Angelica Kitchen

300 E. 12$^{th}$ St. (between 1$^{st}$ and 2$^{nd}$ Ave.), New York, NY 10003. 212-228-2909. Hours: 11:30–10:30 daily. "A minimum of 95% of all food used to prepare our menu has been grown ecologically. In addition, we use no re-fined sugars, no preservatives, no dairy, no eggs, no animal products what-soever." Salads, juices and gourmet raw food entrées on menu. Web site: www.angelicakitchen.com.

### Bonobo's Restaurant

There are two locations:

- 18 E. 23$^{rd}$ St. (at Madison Ave. overlooking Madison Square Park), New York, NY 10010. 212-505-1200.
- Bonobo's Annex, 156 W. 20$^{th}$ St., New York, NY 10011. 212-505-1200.

All food is served with live enzymes intact as Mother Nature intended. We support local farmers. Take out, delivery, catering, skylight, dining room, events. E-mail: eatraw1@aol.com. Web site: www.bonobosrestaurant.com.

### Candle 79

154 E. 79$^{th}$ St., New York, NY 10021. 212-537-7179. Juices, smoothies and a good selection of raw food dishes. Web site: www.candlecafe.com/candle 79.html.

### Caravan of Dreams

405 E. 6$^{th}$ St. (between 1$^{st}$ Ave. and Ave. A), New York, NY 10009. 212-254-1613. Kosher. Good raw food selection. Catering and classes. Web site: www.caravanofdreams.net.

## Counter Vegetarian Bistro

105 1<sup>st</sup> Ave. (between 6<sup>th</sup> and 7<sup>th</sup>), New York, NY 10003. 212-982-5870, 212-982-5870 (fax). Gourmet vegetarian restaurant, some raw. Web site: www.counternyc.com.

## Jandi's Natural Market & Organic Café & Deli

3000 Long Beach Rd., Oceanside, NY 11572. 516-536-5535. Organic vegan, vegetarian and raw food and fresh juices. Web site: www.jandis.com.

## Jubb's Longevity

508 E. 12<sup>th</sup> St. (at Ave. A), New York, NY 10009. 212-353-5000. Live food store, organic juice bar. Web site: www.lifefood.com.

## Organic Soul Café (opening Spring 2007)

Sixth Street Center. 638 E. 6<sup>th</sup> St. (between Aves. B and C), New York, NY 10009. 212-677-1863. Both raw and cooked food. Web site: www.sixth streetcenter.org/cafe_index.html.

## Pure Food and Wine

54 Irving Pl. (at 17<sup>th</sup> and 18<sup>th</sup> St.), New York, NY 10003. 212-477-1010. Vegan, 100% raw food, including take out. Web Site: www.purefoodand wine.com.

## Pure Juice and Takeaway

125½ E. 17<sup>th</sup> St. (between 3<sup>rd</sup> Ave. and Irving Pl.), New York, NY 10003. 212-477-7151. Juices and smoothies. Raw food main dishes and desserts.

## Quintessence

263 E. 10<sup>th</sup> St. (between 1<sup>st</sup> Ave. and Ave. A), New York, NY 10009. 646-654-1823. Quintessence is "a gourmet dining retreat that relaxes and rejuvenates beyond belief. Our food is comprised of some of the most rare and exotic ingredients found on earth. . . . More than just great tasting food, everything served at Quintessence is 100% organic, vegan and raw. . . . Enjoy our spalike environment and experience the essence of food with Quintessence. Web site: www.quintessencerestaurant.com.

## Raw Foods Eatery

118 S. Cayuga St., Ithaca, NY 14850. 607-254-6074. Hours: M-Sat 12:00–5:00PM. Located in picturesque upstate New York in downtown Ithaca. A variety of 100% organic raw food meals, healthful smoothies, and living foods supplies. Includes Everything Wellness Bookstore. E-mail: ewb@earthlink.net.

## Raw Soul Take-Out and Catering

348 W. 145<sup>th</sup> St. (between St. Nicholas and Edgecombe Aves.), Harlem, New York, NY 10031. 212-491-5859. Web site: www.rawsoul.com.

### Soul Restaurant

530 W. 27th St. (in Spirit New York nightclub, New York, NY 10001. 212-268-9477. Nightclub restaurant with raw menu created by raw chef Chad Sarno. Web site: www.spiritnewyork.com.

## Ohio

### Claudia's Natural Food Market

5644 Monroe St., Toledo, OH 43560. 419-534-3343. Hours: M-F 9AM–8PM, Sat 9AM–6PM, Sun 10AM–5PM. Primarily a health food store, it also has a juice and deli bar with some organic, raw, vegetarian entrées and seating. Web site: www.claudiasmarket.com.

### Squeaker's Café & Health Food Store

There are two locations:

- 175 N. Main St., Bowling Green, OH 43402. 419-354-7000.
- 601 N. Main St., Findlay, OH 45840. 419-424-3990.

This health food store also sells prepared vegan and raw deli meals.

## Oregon

### Calendula — A Natural Café

3257 SE Hawthorne Blvd., Portland, OR 97214. 503-235-6800. Vegan/organic, with living foods options.

### Omega Gardens

4036 SE Hawthorne, Portland, OR 97214. 503-235-2551. Super salad bar. Features raw vegan, gourmet dinners. Tu 6–8PM. Call for reservations.

### The Blossoming Lotus

925 NW Davis St. (located in Yoga in the Pearl), Portland, OR 97209. 503-228-0048. Some raw food options. E-mail: info@blpdx.com. Web site: www.blossominglotus.com.

## Pennsylvania

### Arnold's Way

319 W. Main St., Store #4 rear (40 miles N. of Philadelphia); Lansdale, PA 19446. 215-361-0116. The only raw, vegetarian hamburger and steaks! Also: pies, salads, soups, pâtés, wraps, juices and ice creams. Classes and events. Web site: www.arnoldsway.com.

### Kind Café

724 North 3rd St., Philadelphia, PA 19123. 215-922-KIND (5463). 100% vegan, 50% raw and mostly organic. Hours: M-Sat 11–8. Menu features: Live lo mein, happy chicken wrap, raw pizza, chili, living lasagna, raw pies

and vegan smoothies. Books on the shelves, art on the wall and educational classes. E-mail: kc@kindcafe.com. Web site: www.kindcafe.com.

## Loving Life Café

109 Carlisle St., New Oxford, PA 17350. 717-476-LOVE (5683). Hours: Tu-Th 11AM–8PM, F-Sat 11AM–10PM, Sun 11AM–6PM. Living foods restaurant and Natural Zing Store. Menu features: fresh juices, smoothies, shakes, soups, salads, wraps, lasagna, tacos, pizza, ice cream, desserts and much more. All ingredients are nondairy, meat free and as organic as possible. They use no processed or refined sugars and no soy substitutes. They ship raw pies! Sign up to receive their free e-mail newsletter. E-mail: live@lovinglifecafe.com. Web site: www.lovinglifecafe.com.

## Maggie's Mercantile

320 Atwood St., Pittsburgh, PA 15213. 724-593-5056. Hours: M-F 11:30AM–9:00PM. Deli style. Raw, live and organic vegetarian and vegan foods. They say, "Our produce is 90-95% organic. Eat well, live compassionately!" Additional location: 1262 Route 711, Stahlstown, PA 15687. 724-593-5056. Hours: M-F 11:30AM–9:00PM.

## Oasis Living Cuisine

81 Lancaster Ave. (Rt. 30 and Rt. 401, Great Valley Center), Frazer, PA 19355. 610-647-9797, 610-647-2556 (fax). Cooked and raw foods. Not completely vegetarian. Web site: www.oasislivingcuisine.com.

# Texas

## Living Food Bar

801 East Lamar, (at 6th in Whole Foods Market), Austin, TX 76011. 512-476-1206. Hours: 8AM–10PM seven days a week.

## Sunfired Foods

4915 Martin Luther King Blvd., Houston, TX 77021. 713-643-2884.

# Utah

## Living Cuisine Raw Food Bar

There are two locations:

- 2144 S. Highland Dr., Salt Lake City, UT. 801-486-0332.
- 1100 E. Highland Dr. (inside Herbs for Health at the south end of the strip mall complex), Sugarhouse, UT 84106. 801-467-4082.

Fresh, organic, live food.

## Sage's Café

473 East 300 South, Salt Lake City, UT 84111-2606. 801-322-3790. This organic, vegan restaurant serves one raw entrée each night and once a month

a full course raw meal. E-mail: ian@sagescafe.com. Web site: www.sages cafe.com.

### The Food Garden
698 East 300 South, Provo, UT 84606-4908. 801-471-0414. This vegetarian restaurant has a limited selection of raw juices and entrées, but takes special orders upon request. E-mail: agi_habeller@hotmail.com.

## Washington

### Chaco Canyon Café
4761 Brooklyn Ave. NE, Seattle, WA 98105. 206-522-6966. Hours: M-F 8AM–8PM, Sat 9AM–4PM, Sun 10AM–4PM. Their 100% vegan, 95% organic menu includes many raw dishes.

# Canada

## British Columbia

### Gorilla Food
101-422 Richards St. (between Hastings and Pender Sts., downtown), Vancouver, BC, Canada. 604-722-2504. A raw food catering, take out and delivery service. E-mail: info@gorillafood.com and gorillafood@gmail.com. Web site: www.gorillafoods.com.

### Rawdezvous Organic Café
1282 Ellis St., Kelowna, BC, Canada. 250-763-9515 and 250-763-9519 (fax). Hours: Tu-Sat 10AM–7PM, Sun 11AM–5PM. Offers eat in, take out, catering and raw food classes. E-mail: rosemarie@rawdezvouscafe.com. Web site: www.rawdezvouscafe.com.

### Rooted Café
1025 Commercial Dr. (within Eternal Abundance market), East Vancouver, BC, Canada. 604-255-8690. They offer gazpacho soup, living lasagna and pasta, cookies and crackers. The market sells organic produce. E-mail: rooted@shaw.ca.

### Zen Zero Raw Juice Fountain & Raw Food Oasis
407B Fifth St., Courtenay, BC (on Vancouver Island). V9N 1J7. 250-338-0571. They sell fresh raw juices, organic wheatgrass juice and kits to go, real fruit smoothies, salads, sandwiches, gluten/sugar-free goodies and raw food buffet. They also sell dehydrators, juicers and bulk foods. Library and sunny patio.

# Ontario

### Live Organic Food Bar

264 Dupont St. (at Spadina), Toronto, ON M5R 1V7, Canada. 416-515-2002. Closed Mondays. They serve vegan, organic, gourmet raw entrées, desserts, fresh juices and products with catering and delivery upon request. Web site: www.livefoodbar.com.

### Livia Juice Bar and Eatery

55 Mill Street Building 35 (in Lileo clothing store), Distillery District, Toronto, ON M5A 3C4, Canada. 416-413-1410. This juice bar and café is ovo, lacto, vegan-friendly, with juices, salad bar and many raw options. E-mail: info@lileo.ca. Web site: www.lileo.ca.

### Papaya Island

513-A Yonge St. (north of College), Toronto, ON M4Y 1X3, Canada. 416-960-0821. They have fresh, organic juices and smoothies.

### Super Sprouts

720 Bathurst St. W. (at Bloor), Toronto, ON M5S 2R4, Canada. 416-977-7796. They sport a wheatgrass juice bar, sprouts and a bookstore.

### W.O.W. — Wild Organic Way Café & Juice Bar

22 Carden St., Guelph, ON N1H 3A2, Canada. 519-766-1707. This is an all-raw vegan restaurant with a juice bar.

# Québec

### Tout Cru Dans L'Bec

129, 7ᵉ rue Rouyn-Noranda, Québec, QC, Canada J9X 1Z8. 819-764-9843. This restaurant and deli serves organic raw, vegetarian food, including take out. Chef-Owner: Viviane Desbiens. E-mail: toutcrudanslbec@tlb.sympati co.ca. Web site: www.toutcuitdanslebec.com.

# United Kingdom

# England

### The Little Earth Café at TriYoga

6 Erskine Rd., Primrose Hill, London NW3 3AJ, England, UK. 020-7586-0025, 020-7483-3344 and 020-7483-3346 (fax). London's first raw food café. Whole and raw food menu that is meat-free, wheat-free, dairy-free, sugar-free and totally organic. The ingredients used are carefully selected for their healing, revitalizing and energizing properties. E-mail: info@tri yoga.co.uk. Web site: www.triyoga.co.uk/cafe.php.

**Vitaorganic**

74 Wardour St., London V1F 0TE, England, UK. 020-7734-8986. They specialize in 100% vegan, organic, live, enzymatic and gently cooked food with an extensive living/raw menu and juice bar. Web site: www.vita organic.co.uk.

# Raw Chains and Franchises

Some nationwide chains for raw, organic produce include Whole Foods Market and Wild Oats. Jamba Juice is a franchised juice bar. Many of the drinks contain concentrates, but you can request a pure, fresh one. The carrot and orange juices are safe bets.

Check their web sites to find the ones closest to where you live or along the routes you will be traveling. Or you may call their national centers.

For Whole Foods, www.wholefoodsmarket.com, call 512-477-4455.

For Wild Oats, www.wildoats.com, call 800-494-9453.

For Jamba Juice, www.jambajuice.com, call 800-545-9972.

# Glossary

**agglutination** — a reaction in which particles (as red blood cells or bacteria) suspended in a liquid collect into clumps and which occurs esp. as a serologic response to a specific antibody

**ahimsa** — the Hindu/Buddhist philosophy of nonviolence toward any living being

**alliesthethic response** — a change of taste that occurs when one has eaten an initial food to repletion

**allopathic** — pertaining to allopathy, or the use of pharmaceutical drugs to relieve disease symptoms by producing symptoms different from or opposite to those produced by the disease, as practiced by conventional medical practitioners

**amenorrhea** — the absence of menstrual bleeding in women of menstruating age, considered pathological by conventional standards but often found in very healthy, fertile females on a pure uncooked diet

**ankylosing spondylitis** — a disease of the spine that causes the vertebrae to form a solid inflexible column

**antioxidant** — any chemical thought to protect living organisms from the damaging effects of oxidation

**arrhythmia** — a condition in which the heart beats with an irregular or abnormal rhythm

**bioavailability** — the degree to which, or rate at which, a nutrient is absorbed or becomes available at the site of physiological activity after ingestion

**biophotons** — a particle of light (photon) emitted in some fashion from a biological system

*Candida albicans* — a type of parasitic fungus that can form colonies in human tissues when present in excessive amounts

**carcinogen** — a cancer-causing agent

**chakra** — in yoga, one of the centers of spiritual power in the body

**Crohn's disease**  a chronic disease of the intestines, especially the colon and ileum, severely limiting nutritive processes and often characterized by abdominal pains, bleeding, diarrhea and ruptures

**cross-links**  al chemical combinations of sugars and proteins that occur in the presence of heat, either from cooking food or within the body as it ages

**diverticulosis**  an intestinal condition characterized by the presence of numerous *diverticula* (pouches or sacs protruding from the intestinal walls)

*E. coli*  the bacterium *Escherichia coli*, commonly found in the intestines of humans and other animals, at least one strain of which can cause severe food poisoning

**eczema**  a noncontagious inflammation of the skin, characterized chiefly by redness, itching, and the outbreak of lesions that may discharge serous matter and become encrusted and scaly

**edema**  an excessive accumulation of fluid in the body

**enzyme**  a biologically produced catalyst, a protein causing a particular chemical reaction to occur while not being changed itself

**excrete**  to separate and eliminate or discharge (waste) from the blood or tissues or from the active protoplasm

**fibromyalgia**  a syndrome characterized by chronic pain in the muscles and soft tissues surrounding joints, fatigue and also tenderness at specific sites in the body; also called fibromyalgia syndrome, fibromyositis or fibrositis

**free radical**  an atom or molecule missing an electron, a condition that causes it to react with and destroy other molecules it comes into contact with

**frugivore**  an animal that subsists chiefly on fruits

**fruitarian**  a human frugivore

**glycemic index**  a ranking of the rise in blood glucose from various foodstuffs

**goiter**  a noncancerous enlargement of the thyroid gland, visible as a swelling at the front of the neck, often associated with iodine deficiency

**graminivore**  an animal that chiefly consumes grains

**homeostasis**  a relatively stable state of equilibrium among all interdependent components of an organism or system

**hydrogenated**  combined with hydrogen, especially an unsaturated oil combined with hydrogen to produce a solid fat at room temperature

**hygiene**  1: a science of the establishment and maintenance of health
2: conditions or practices (as of cleanliness) conducive to health — *adj* **hygienic**, *n* **hygienist**

**hyperthyroidism**  excessive thyroid function, resulting in increased metabolic rate, enlargement of the thyroid gland, rapid heart rate and high blood pressure

**immunomodulatory**  affecting the functioning of the immune system

**initial food**  a food that is primordially suited to one's biology, usually meaning nonhybridized, not overcultivated and in an unprocessed condition: a whole, raw food that when eaten produces the alliesthetic response in an instinctive eater

**instinctive eater, or instincto**  one who selects which foods to eat chiefly by smell and taste from among initial foods

**jaundice**  a yellowed skin condition resulting from liver pathology

**liquidarian**  one who subsists chiefly on a liquid diet

**liver cleanse**  also called *liver flush* or *gallbladder flush*, may refer to: (1) an equal mixture of vegetable oil and citrus juice, often including various herbs or spices, that causes the liver and gallbladder to spasm, possibly releasing stored stones; or (2) a coffee enema used for the same purpose

**Maillard molecule**  any unnatural chemical produced by cooking food, named after French chemist Louis Maillard

**monomeal**  a meal consisting solely of a single food

| | |
|---|---|
| **mutagen** | an agent or substance that is capable of increasing the frequency of mutation, or change in the DNA sequence of a gene or chromosome |
| **myasthenia gravis** | a disease characterized by progressive fatigue and generalized weakness of the skeletal muscles, especially those of the face, neck, arms and legs, caused by impaired transmission of nerve impulses following an autoimmune attack on acetylcholine receptors |
| **Natural Hygiene** | a natural healing system based on adherence to the biological laws of life, chief of which is that biological organisms are self-healing entities and that disease symptoms are remedial in nature and should therefore be permitted to run their course whenever possible, not suppressed by or ameliorated with drugs or unnecessary surgeries |
| **osteoporosis** | a decrease in bone mass resulting in decreased density and enlargement of bone spaces producing porosity and fragility |
| **Parkinson's disease** | a degenerative disorder of the central nervous system characterized by tremor and impaired muscular coordination |
| **peroxidation** | oversaturation with oxygen resulting in the formation of destructive chemicals known as free radicals |
| **phytochemical** | any chemical found in plants |
| **phytonutrient** | any phytochemical having a beneficial nutritive effect upon health or playing an active role in the prevention or reversal of the disease process |
| **protoplasm** | the organized colloidal complex of substances that comprise the nucleus, cytoplasm, plastids and mitochondria of a cell. |
| **pyrolysis** | the transformation of a substance by the application of heat, as in cooking |
| **SAD** | Standard American Diet — the highly processed, refined and predominantly cooked diet consumed by the typical American |
| **SARS** | Severe Acute Respiratory Syndrome — a serious and highly contagious type of pneumonia |

**trans fatty acid**  a toxic, biologically abnormal saturated or partly saturated fatty acid produced by the hydrogenation of vegetable oils and present in hardened vegetable oils, most margarines, commercially baked foods and many fried foods

**triglyceride**  a naturally occurring fat consisting of three individual fatty acids and one glycerol molecule bound together into a single large molecule; an important energy source forming much of the fat stored by the body, an excess of which in the bloodstream is considered to be a marker for heart disease

**ulcerative colitis**  inflammation of the walls of the bowel accompanied by the formation of ulcers, a condition which can result in permanent bowel damage

**vegan**  one who consumes no animal products, including meat, dairy, eggs and honey, and may even refuse to use anything coming from an animal source, such as leather shoes, fur coats or other such items

**vegetarian**  from the Latin *vegetus*, meaning 'whole, sound, fresh, lively'; one who typically eschews animal flesh consumption, but may consume bee products, eggs (*ovo-vegetarian*), dairy (*lacto-vegetarian*) or both (*ovo-lacto-vegetarian*)

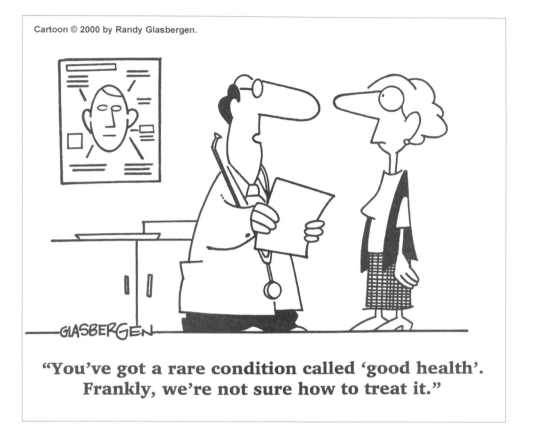

GLASBERGEN

**"You've got a rare condition called 'good health'. Frankly, we're not sure how to treat it."**

Health is a condition of perfect development, a state of wholeness and harmonious development and growth and adaptation of part to part, of organ within the organism, with no part stunted and no part in excess. In this state of organic development lies the perfection and symmetry of beauty. Beauty is but the reflection of wholeness, of health. And is it not easy to demonstrate that the forms and proportions of man and woman, which are in their highest and most perfect state, are also the most beautiful?

—Dr. Herbert M. Shelton (1895-1985)

# Index

**Abel, Dr. Ulrich**, 493, 563
**Abramowski, Dr. O. L. M.**, 149, 563
**acid**, 126, 309, 318, 331, 505
  abscisic, 195
  acetic, 240, 317
  amino, 175, 178, 352, 365, 381, 383, 394,
    523, 524, 527
    creatine, 524
    essential, 178, 352, 479
    lysine, 526
    pool, 178, 271, 381
    taurine, 153
    toxic, 317
    tryptophan, 241
  butyric, 317
  environment, 9, 45, 152, 156, 176, 312,
    314, 331, 332, 368, 381, 401, 471, 473,
    492, 504, 508
  fatty, 376, 481, 621
    essential, 9, 10, 195, 479, 481, 482, 517
    trans, 180, 481, 521, 621
  food, 8, 176, 214, 243, 317, 331, 359, 360,
    361, 400, 482, 507, 520
  formic, 242
  forming, 331, 335, 360, 469, 471, 473, 505
  hydrochloric (HCl), 167, 190, 358, 375,
    504
  lactic, 249, 317, 559
  phytic, 471, 479
  propionic, 317
  stomach, 167, 348, 513
  sulfurous, 242
  uric, 309, 381
**acid/alkaline balance**, 124, 126, 152,
  178, 273, 331, 332, 360, 381, 521, 564
**acne. See symptoms.**
**acrylamide**, 180, 371
**acupuncture**, xxxv, 26, 83, 101, 137,
  138, 197, 291, 373, 392, 494, 496, 497
**addiction**, 88, 89, 97, 107, 108, 247,
  271, 275, 300, 301, 340, 412, 416,
  417, 529, 530, 531, 537, 596
  alcohol, 275, 659
  caffeine. See caffeine.
  drug, 9, 58, 82, 83, 126, 129, 132, 157,
    183, 184, 215, 256, 267, 274, 287, 394,
    400, 401, 488, 516, 530, 659
  enema/colonic, 262
  food, xxxi, xxxiv, xxxviii, xlii, 18, 26, 30, 37,
    42, 44, 67, 70, 89, 99, 110, 116, 173,
    183, 184, 185, 201, 212, 227, 228, 230,
    239, 241, 244, 251, 253, 263, 267, 268,
    274, 279, 299, 300, 302, 303, 369, 376,
    379, 380, 383, 385, 386, 388, 390, 394,

395, 400, 405, 407, 408, 420, 445, 469,
    470, 475, 476, 477, 478, 480, 531, 532,
    533, 534, 535, 536, 538, 563, 565, 570,
    659
  sex, 18, 257
  tobacco, 275
**additives**, xxxvi, 18, 83, 151, 232, 325,
  394, 395, 474, 475, 477, 480, 498
  aspartame, 85, 394, 467, 470, 477, 478,
    479
  baking soda, 482
  BHA, 482
  BHT, 482
  dyes and colorings, 482
  excitotoxins, 85, 250, 394, 477, 480, 564
  MSG, 18, 85, 185, 232, 234, 301, 336, 379,
    394, 401, 403, 420, 467, 477, 478, 480
  natural and artificial flavors, 480, 482
  Olestra, 85, 481, 482
  sucralose (Splenda), 479
  sulfates, 149, 482
  sulfites, 363, 400, 482
**ADHD. See diseases.**
**adrenal glands**, 151, 195, 291, 349,
  361, 391, 392, 402
  secretions. See hormones, adrenal.
**advanced glycation end products.**
  **See AGEs.**
**agave. See sweeteners.**
**AGEs**, 181, 371
**aggression. See symptoms.**
**aging**, 16, 84, 177, 215, 567
  causes, 84, 143, 153, 161, 180, 181, 216,
    323, 327, 334, 342, 363, 372, 381, 402,
    469, 476, 480, 574
  forestalling, 150, 154, 404, 543, 574
  reversal, xli, 316, 513
  symptoms, 168, 181, 189, 192, 542
**AIDS. See diseases.**
**Aimelet, Dr. Catherine**, 509
**air conditioning**, 17, 392
**Airola, Dr. Paavo**, 210, 271, 273, 308,
  563
**albumin. See blood.**
**alcohol**, 9, 83, 87, 106, 109, 129, 157,
  158, 183, 184, 201, 206, 208, 231,
  253, 275, 277, 287, 301, 336, 337,
  348, 400, 411, 422, 465, 471, 476,
  509, 534
  addiction. See addiction.
  symptoms, 275, 391

Alcoholics Anonymous, 184
Alexander, Joe, xxxi, 8, 9, 15, 17, 210, 359, 393, 400, 563
alkaline. *See also acid*, 8, 45, 88, 152, 156, 176, 193, 260, 273, 305, 318, 331, 332, 335, 346, 366, 368, 469, 471, 473, 492, 505, 513, 521, 590
Allen, Woody, 91
allergy. *See symptoms.*
alliesthetic, 507, 617
allopathic, 120, 139, 141, 208, 213, 490, 491, 492, 495, 497, 617
Almond Board of California, 356
ALS. *See diseases.*
Alt, Carol, 11, 36, 231, 370, 388, 563, 575
aluminum. *See minerals.*
Alzheimer's. *See diseases.*
amenorrhea. *See menstruation.*
American Cancer Society, 143, 173, 488
American Heart Association, 168
American Medical Association, 125, 476, 486, 495, 497
American Natural Hygiene Society. *See Natural Hygiene.*
American Red Cross, 207
Americans, xxiii, 19, 29, 81, 104, 116, 117, 121, 135, 169, 180, 183, 206, 207, 208, 209, 250, 256, 263, 264, 275, 312, 322, 323, 338, 371, 372, 381, 387, 388, 467, 469, 471, 473, 476, 480, 481, 485, 490, 495, 499, 529, 537, 542, 553, 564
Amiel, Henri Frédéric, 271
amino acid. *See acid.*
Amsden, Matt, 233, 575
Andrews, Arthur, 289
anemia. *See symptoms.*
Angell, Marcia, 499, 563
angioplasty, 175
Angler, Bradford, 329, 563
anopsology, 20, 140, 183, 318, 323, 370, 389, 394, 406, 466, 470, 474, 497, 506, 507, 508, 509, 510, 511, 513, 514, 515, 519, 522, 565, 572, 574, 579, 589, 619
anthropology, 4, 152, 201, 308, 321, 393, 466, 469
antidepressants. *See drugs.*
antioxidant, 162, 163, 164, 191, 320, 339, 525, 617

anxiety. *See symptoms.*
apathy. *See symptoms.*
apes, 163, 308, 359
Appleton, Nancy, 476, 563
Arlin, Stephen, 219, 563, 582
Army Medical Corps, 487
arteries, 176, 181, 256, 263, 281, 293, 343, 392, 517, 526
arteriosclerosis. *See diseases.*
arthritis. *See diseases.*
aspartame. *See additives.*
asthma. *See symptoms.*
athlete's foot. *See diseases.*
athletics, 7, 11, 72, 150, 156, 215, 231, 289, 345, 360, 372, 375, 381, 404, 478, 567
Atkins, Dr., Robert, 29, 342, 396, 521
attention deficit hyperactivity disorder. *See diseases, ADHD.*
Au, Bryan, 233, 575
Austin, Dr. Harriet, 207
Australia/Australian, 149, 215, 216, 312, 466, 587, 593, 596, 597
autism. *See diseases.*
Azar, Dr. Zarin, 277, 595, 659
Baby, Dr. John, 30
backsliding, 173, 184, 188, 212, 228, 232, 298, 299, 300, 301, 303, 380, 507, 519
bacteria, xxvi, 38, 45, 123, 124, 125, 126, 127, 159, 176, 179, 190, 196, 260, 263, 308, 311, 312, 315, 325, 326, 337, 339, 341, 348, 358, 360, 398, 399, 403, 407, 514, 516, 518, 524, 617
  bubonic plague, 123
  campylobacter, 123
  *E. coli*, 123, 357, 618
  salmonella, 123, 229, 319, 398, 514, 516, 517, 527
Baird, Lori, 233, 575
Baker
  Arthur M., 125, 563
  Elizabeth, 211, 241, 563, 564, 575
baking soda, 482
Baroody, Dr. Theodore, 332, 335, 564
Barton, Clara, 207
Bass, Dr. Stanley S., 160, 313, 314, 517, 529, 594
Batmanghelidj, Dr. Fereydoun, 332, 334
Bealle, Morris, 485, 487, 564
beans. *See legumes.*

**Beard, Dr. John**, 190

**beauty**, 8, 9, 10, 11, 12, 18, 24, 145, 219, 222, 235, 237, 249, 297, 316, 408, 420, 471, 538, 574, 582, 583, 588

**Béchamp, Antoine**, 124, 180

**bee pollen**, 83, 314, 339, 436, 437, 458, 587

**beer**, 83, 275, 601

**behavior modification**, xlii, 240, 244, 245, 268, 274, 299, 301, 529, 531, 532, 535

**Bernays, Edward**, 142, 564

**beta-carbolines**, 182, 183

**Better Business Bureau**, 487

**BHA**, 482

**BHT**, 482

**BidWell, Victoria**, i, ii, xxiii, xxiv, xxv, xxvi, xxvii, xxix, xxxi, xxxii, xxxiii, xxxiv, xxxvii, xxxviii, xliii, 14, 75, 77, 98, 100, 119, 120, 127, 129, 137, 144, 147, 177, 204, 206, 211, 222, 233, 234, 244, 245, 247, 251, 257, 258, 261, 262, 265, 266, 273, 274, 276, 277, 294, 297, 298, 300, 303, 317, 318, 329, 333, 339, 341, 360, 364, 368, 376, 399, 408, 412, 413, 416, 435, 438, 445, 448, 449, 451, 453, 462, 464, 474, 475, 476, 480, 529, 541, 542, 545, 553, 559, 564, 575, 580, 587, 588, 596, 655, 656, 658

**bioacidic**, 151

**bioactive**, 151

**bioelectricity**, 193, 194

**biogenic**, 150, 151, 573

**biophoton**, 145, 192, 194, 310, 326, 328, 329, 337, 374, 617

**biostatic**, 151

**Bircher-Benner**, 203
Dr. Max, 13, 203
Dr. Ralph, 154, 273, 564

**Bland, Dr. Jeffrey**, 103, 564

**Blaylock, Dr. Russell**, 477, 564

**bleeding. See also symptoms**, 76, 206

**blenders**, 236, 384, 396, 429, 436, 444, 457, 482, 504
Blend-Tec, 236, 340, 423, 424, 425, 426, 431, 435, 436, 437, 438, 445, 451, 452, 457, 655
K-Tec, 236
Vita-Mix, 64, 236, 340, 365, 409, 412, 423, 424, 425, 426, 431, 435, 436, 437, 438, 440, 445, 451, 452, 457, 462, 504, 655

**blood**, 6, 8, 42, 76, 105, 114, 124, 130, 155, 176, 180, 183, 253, 258, 260, 265, 273, 277, 278, 293, 294, 309, 331, 339, 359, 402, 406, 479, 544, 545, 552, 618
agglutination, 526, 617
albumin, 349, 351, 381
capillaries, 180, 391, 392, 476
cells, 76, 102, 124, 132, 174, 175, 242, 326, 345, 476, 479, 492, 526, 546, 617
circulation, 11, 12, 47, 118, 196, 367, 391, 392, 393, 415, 526, 549
clots, 526
contaminants, 206, 256, 266, 267, 344, 407, 522
insulin. See insulin.
lipids, 156, 162, 165, 345
location, 392
oxygen, 180, 196, 344, 345, 391
pH, 331, 471, 508
poisoning (toxemia), 105, 107, 109, 111, 114, 115, 120, 131, 137, 149, 163, 183, 208, 248, 266, 303, 378, 381, 392, 397, 405, 422, 507, 530, 543, 544, 547, 548, 559, 573, 621
pressure. See also symptoms, high blood pressure, 26, 30, 42, 92, 155, 156, 158, 170, 171, 256, 265, 272, 547
proteins, 156, 381
C-reactive, 168, 170
hemoglobin, 196
sugar, 63, 169, 170, 214, 328, 344, 345, 402, 469, 618
high. See diseases, diabetes.
low. See hypoglycemia.
tests, 6, 26, 42, 159, 162, 181, 213, 216, 252, 254, 311, 312, 326, 381, 596
transfusion, 76, 102
type, 29, 308, 345, 503
umbilical, 29, 405

**Bloomer, Amelia**, 207

**Bobier, Michael**, 277

**body odor. See symptoms.**

**bodybuilding**, 33, 52, 83, 84, 206, 219, 254, 292, 293, 358, 365, 378, 383, 416, 473, 561, 584

**bone density. See also diseases, osteoporosis**, 52, 169, 212, 505

**bonobos**, 308, 610

**Boutenko**, 29, 62, 196, 211, 212, 329, 385, 504, 565, 582
Igor, 26, 62, 63, 64, 167, 329, 504, 505
Sergei, 9, 62, 63, 212, 233, 329, 384, 385, 473, 482, 575
Valya, 8, 9, 62, 63, 212, 233, 329, 384, 385, 482, 575
Victoria, i, xxix, xxxi, xxxvii, xxxviii, 7, 14,

16, 26, 62, 90, 125, 139, 142, 165, 167, 184, 211, 212, 230, 239, 258, 264, 297, 315, 319, 324, 329, 331, 340, 358, 364, 366, 368, 369, 370, 375, 380, 383, 384, 391, 392, 399, 400, 403, 407, 503, 504, 505, 565, 598, 658, 659

**Bragg, Paul**, 206, 209, 272, 275, 565

**brain. See also mental**, 7, 8, 130, 194, 254, 260, 266, 267, 277, 282, 294, 480, 544, 571
  aging. See aging.
  aneurysm, 89
  cancer. See diseases, cancer.
  chemicals, 14, 182, 294, 368, 383, 470, 481, 535
  composition, 481
  damage, 84, 512
  degeneration, 99, 152, 153, 182, 313, 523, 620
  development, 72, 312, 368, 477
  fog. See symptoms.
  food, 9, 92, 195, 235, 237, 482
  function, xxxvi, 8, 9, 24, 88, 205, 253, 267, 342, 345, 467, 477, 478, 512, 536, 544, 545, 546, 553
  hematoma, 293
  limbic, 267, 302
  pollution, 12, 181, 182, 334, 368, 400, 476, 477, 480
  size, 8, 322
  tumor, 148, 287, 477, 478

**breastfeeding**, 30, 154, 407
**breathing. See lungs.**
**Brekhman, Dr. Israel**, 158
**Britain/British**, 3, 9, 154, 162, 201, 211, 401, 597, 615
**brix**, 338
**Brotman, Juliano**, 18, 232, 394, 575, 602
**Bruce, Elaine**, 565, 595
**Bryant, Dr. Vaughn**, 4
**Bryson, Christopher**, 84, 334, 565
**Buddhism**, 617
**Budwig, Dr. Johanna**, 192
**Bueno, Lee**, 265, 565
**Buhner, Stephen**, 277, 565
**Burger, Guy-Claude**, 20, 183, 389, 395, 398, 400, 506, 507, 508, 509, 510, 514, 515, 519, 565
**Burkitt, Dr. Denis**, 341
**Burton**
  Dr. Alec, 261, 596
  Dr. Nejla, 597
**byproducts**, 109, 110, 125, 134, 145, 173, 175, 180, 183, 248, 251, 260,

278, 317, 326, 334, 379, 387, 396, 471, 525, 528

**cacao. See legumes.**
**caffeine. See also coffee**, 565
  acidity, 400
  addiction, 171, 250, 251, 401, 402
  symptoms, 14, 250, 253, 275, 391, 401, 402

**calories**, 319, 365, 377, 378
  amount of, 11, 18, 24, 85, 89, 159, 165, 169, 176, 187, 310, 338, 344, 379, 396, 459, 479, 481
  counting, 81, 534
  macronutrient composition, 215, 342, 343, 344, 345, 363, 382, 510
  percentage raw, 23, 158, 229, 379
  restriction, 82, 83, 154, 160, 161, 162, 165, 170, 216, 315, 316, 350

**Caloudes, Vern**, 289
**Campbell, Dr. T. Colin**, 102, 115, 140, 188, 373, 381, 382, 467, 488, 565
**Canada**, 83, 129, 176, 215, 221, 356, 393, 495, 566, 571, 573, 575, 576, 577, 590, 592, 599, 614, 615
**Canadian School of Natural Nutrition**, 217

**cancer. See also diseases**, xxxiii, xxxv, xli, xlii, 5, 6, 7, 15, 21, 23, 67, 77, 88, 111, 131, 155, 167, 359, 391, 511, 513
  carcinogens. See carcinogens.
  causes, 117, 159, 161, 168, 174, 180, 181, 182, 184, 193, 196, 212, 219, 263, 308, 316, 320, 321, 322, 326, 331, 335, 344, 371, 374, 381, 397, 401, 467, 469, 472, 476, 481, 488, 489, 492, 506, 508, 516, 519, 522, 524, 525, 526
  history, 466
  incidence, 102, 116, 370, 372, 483, 491
  metastasis, 85, 86
  odors, 474
  prevention, 158, 159, 162, 165, 167, 168, 170, 194, 383, 488, 494
  prostate, 169
  treatment, 129, 137, 140, 160, 486, 492, 493, 494, 495, 499, 570, 593
    calorie restriction, 161
    chemotherapy, 92, 98, 129, 135, 137, 139, 148, 218, 387, 485, 491, 492, 493, 494, 495, 513, 563, 569
    coffee enemas, 156, 238
    cooked food, 119
    enzymatic, 190, 494
    nutrition, 566
    radiation, 135, 139, 387, 492, 494, 495, 569
    raw diet, 148, 156, 160, 161, 171, 184, 187, 194, 195, 203, 204, 212, 218, 230, 373, 379, 387, 390, 505, 506, 511, 512, 513, 567, 568, 571

surgery, 92, 492, 493, 494, 569

*Candida albicans*, 181, 343, 345, 617

capillaries. *See* blood.

carbohydrates, 11, 28, 29, 30, 61, 83, 85, 145, 177, 178, 179, 180, 181, 215, 277, 286, 328, 338, 341, 342, 343, 344, 345, 354, 362, 388, 469, 476, 479, 517, 556, 570
  starch, 20, 175, 178, 179, 180, 183, 189, 190, 205, 207, 259, 260, 263, 268, 318, 327, 338, 365, 377, 396, 470, 525, 526, 528, 555, 556, 557, 558
  adaptation to, 10, 216, 354, 396, 411, 469

carcinogens, 140, 173, 175, 176, 180, 191, 472, 492, 523, 524, 525, 526, 527, 617
  HCAs, 182, 524, 525, 526, 527, 528

carob. *See* legumes.

carotene/carotenoids. *See* vitamins, A (carotene).

Carpenter, Karen, 82

carpets, 266, 367

Carter, Dr. James P., 499, 565

casein
  and cancer, 472, 516
  caseinates, 477, 482
  digestibility, 508, 513, 515, 516

CDC, 371, 487

cell phones, xxxvi, 368

Centers for Disease Control and Prevention, 371, 487

chakra, 14, 276, 617

cheese
  dairy. *See* dairy.
  nut. *See* nuts.
  seed. *See* seeds.

chemistry, 13, 85, 124, 126, 131, 137, 150, 173, 174, 175, 252, 271, 273, 278, 283, 317, 468, 483, 497, 546, 553, 569, 571, 573

chemotherapy. *See* cancer, treatment.

Cherniske, Stephen, 14, 401, 565

Child Protective Services, 30

childhood, 3, 24, 66, 72, 89, 152, 214, 305, 372, 375, 395, 407, 411, 413, 504, 516

children, xxvi, xli, 3, 9, 11, 15, 16, 19, 29, 30, 31, 37, 55, 62, 63, 64, 65, 70, 71, 72, 81, 91, 116, 117, 130, 142, 145, 166, 181, 182, 204, 212, 233, 237, 288, 298, 312, 320, 321, 325, 326, 329, 366, 368, 371, 372, 384, 385, 405, 407, 408, 410, 411, 412,
413, 414, 415, 416, 417, 467, 468, 472, 473, 474, 477, 478, 479, 487, 488, 495, 497, 498, 504, 507, 508, 519, 572, 573

chilliness. *See* symptoms, chills.

chimpanzees, 308, 319, 324, 340, 359, 366, 472, 503, 504, 510, 521

China/Chinese, xxxv, 7, 81, 308, 324, 334, 339, 369, 373, 381, 382, 392, 393, 428, 460, 467, 472, 488, 494, 516, 565, 600

chips, xli, 85, 180, 181, 232, 239, 371, 379, 406, 467, 477, 478, 589
  raw, 457

chiropractic, 26, 75, 106, 205, 215, 220, 221, 291, 440, 486, 593, 597

chlorine, 47, 326, 331, 334, 337, 470, 474, 475

chocolate. *See also* legumes, cacao, 61, 231, 336, 383, 432, 433
  raw, xxxix, 434, 574, 583
  substitute, 432

cholesterol. *See also* symptoms, high cholesterol, 30, 52, 161, 162, 163, 167, 168, 170, 179, 180, 191, 256, 263, 281, 469, 517, 528

chyle, 260, 278

chyme, 260

cigarettes. *See* tobacco.

cilantro. *See* herbs, condiments and spices.

circulation. *See* blood.

Clement, Brian, 9, 189, 193, 204, 213, 331, 339, 565, 595

Cobb, Brenda, 78, 322, 565

Codex Alimentarius Commission, 325, 327, 499, 660

coffee. *See also* caffeine, xxv, 6, 30, 37, 129, 182, 274, 275, 302, 610
  acidity, 331, 400, 401
  addiction, 37, 230, 238, 250, 251, 400, 401, 505, 533
  blood pressure, 401
  decaf, 401
  enema. *See* enema.
  grinder, 237, 430, 431, 435
  maker, 238
  mutagens, 527
  substitute, 464
  ulcer, 400

Coghill, Roger, 194, 571

Cohen
  Alissa, 222, 575, 579
  Robert, 566, 582

cold, common. *See* symptoms.
colema, 261
colic. *See* symptoms, pain.
collagen, 181
colonics, 25, 26, 87, 88, 217, 259, 261, 262, 263, 264
Columbus, Christopher, 98
Comby, Dr. Bruno, 126, 135, 140, 177, 293, 386, 510, 514, 566
condiments. *See* herbs, condiments and spices.
Congress, 181, 323, 325, 338, 476, 496, 500, 501
constipation. *See* symptoms.
Cook, Lewis, 154, 566
cookbooks, 176, 232, 234, 575
cooking, xxxiv, xxxv, xli, 3, 42, 64, 69, 89, 175, 184, 206, 219, 229, 240, 277, 295, 296, 297, 298, 343, 353, 364, 368, 371, 390, 407, 413, 419, 422, 533, 534, 550, 559
  adaptation to, 4, 24, 119, 220, 256, 302, 370, 399
  addiction. *See* addiction, food.
  aromas, 34, 201, 230, 302, 381, 394, 524, 525, 527
  baking, 177, 180, 231, 239, 371, 379, 391, 394, 397, 419, 524, 525, 621
  barbequing, 182, 359, 397, 485, 526
  boiling, 219, 309, 371, 397, 400
  broiling, 175, 181, 182, 526, 527
  dehydrating, 528
  effects of, xxiii, xxxvii, xxxix, xli, xlii, 4, 24, 25, 29, 33, 34, 38, 41, 44, 45, 47, 70, 90, 108, 109, 110, 117, 126, 134, 139, 143, 144, 145, 147, 149, 150, 151, 152, 153, 154, 157, 158, 167, 170, 171, 172, 173, 174, 175, 176, 177, 178, 179, 180, 181, 182, 183, 184, 185, 187, 188, 189, 190, 192, 194, 195, 196, 202, 204, 208, 212, 216, 228, 229, 234, 247, 248, 249, 250, 251, 257, 259, 260, 264, 279, 284, 292, 293, 294, 297, 299, 302, 304, 308, 316, 320, 327, 333, 341, 350, 358, 359, 361, 363, 369, 370, 371, 372, 374, 378, 380, 382, 383, 392, 393, 394, 395, 396, 397, 398, 399, 400, 401, 405, 407, 408, 409, 411, 480, 485, 506, 508, 509, 510, 514, 517, 518, 520, 521, 523, 524, 525, 526, 527, 528, 531, 534, 560, 618, 619, 659
  frying, 41, 61, 85, 181, 182, 229, 371, 379, 397, 419, 524, 525, 526, 527, 528, 621
  grilling, 182, 371, 397, 523, 526, 527
  history of, 3, 4, 6, 148, 201, 218, 393, 404, 521
  microwaving, 177, 238, 371, 397, 419,

    478
    pressure, 397
    reasons to stop, 5, 6, 7, 8, 9, 10, 11, 12, 13, 17, 18, 19, 20, 21, 45, 232, 327
    roasting, 182, 268, 527
    smoking, 182, 478
    steaming, 119, 177, 205, 229, 356, 371, 379, 380, 397
    toasting, 181, 524, 525
Copernicus, Nicolaus, 98
Cordain, Dr. Loren, 469, 566
Cornbleet, Jennifer, 233, 575
Corona, Lou, 189, 213, 308, 339, 375
cortisol. *See* hormones, adrenal.
Cott, Dr. Alan, 277
cough. *See* symptoms.
Cousens, Dr. Gabriel, xxxi, 13, 14, 15, 21, 99, 103, 158, 166, 169, 176, 189, 192, 194, 196, 197, 213, 214, 233, 272, 273, 274, 276, 308, 309, 310, 312, 314, 315, 316, 320, 321, 323, 326, 327, 329, 335, 337, 339, 342, 358, 360, 379, 381, 391, 407, 419, 470, 472, 518, 520, 566, 575, 597, 600
cravings. *See* symptoms.
cream. *See* dairy.
Crohn's. *See* diseases.
cross-linking. *See* proteins.
CSA, 238, 580, 587
cure, 5, 30, 31, 67, 82, 87, 100, 101, 102, 103, 105, 106, 118, 129, 130, 131, 135, 138, 140, 141, 142, 143, 156, 190, 207, 218, 238, 247, 259, 289, 376, 387, 482, 485, 486, 487, 490, 492, 493, 494, 496, 497, 498, 500, 501, 515, 522, 550, 565, 569, 573, 659
Da Free John, 13, 14, 566
dairy, 67, 71, 108, 125, 169, 178, 183, 185, 196, 220, 229, 287, 310, 313, 314, 344, 353, 379, 383, 397, 466, 468, 513, 515, 516, 553, 621
  butter, 175, 180, 241, 512, 558
    raw, 516
  calcium, 242, 473
  casein. *See* casein.
  cattle, 472
  cheese, 38, 82, 99, 175, 297, 350, 353, 355, 398, 508, 515
    cottage, raw, 515
    cream, 380
    goat, 216
    raw, 216, 515
    substitute, 427, 445
  cream, 37, 266, 268, 401, 558

raw, 422, 516
sour, 175
effects of, 11, 26, 29, 41, 154, 165, 166,
  250, 466, 468, 470, 471, 472, 473, 474,
  508, 515, 516, 581, 582
formula, 408
hidden, 394
history of use, 4, 466, 473
hormones added. *See* hormones.
ice cream, 19, 25, 81, 89, 266, 268, 402,
  422
  raw, 237, 238, 422
  substitute, 10, 268, 402, 432, 433, 435, 436,
    448, 577, 612
industry, 381, 466, 468, 471, 472, 473,
  477, 489
kefir, raw, 313, 515
milk, 151, 152, 154, 157, 237, 350, 353,
  401, 408, 409, 411, 422, 466, 471, 472,
  473, 474, 479, 518, 555, 558, 582
  condensed, 152, 153
  evaporated, 152
  goat, 410, 422, 508
  mother's, 30, 154, 382, 395, 407, 408, 409,
    410, 411, 412, 508, 515
  raw, 152, 410, 422, 474, 508
osteoporosis, 473
pasteurized, 152, 154, 157, 229, 355, 408,
  472, 518
raw, 123, 197, 311, 313, 399, 474, 513,
  514, 515, 519, 521, 522
whey, 33, 478, 482
yogurt, 357, 383
  raw, 313, 515

**Darbro, Dr. David**, 389, 490
**Day, Dr. Lorraine**, 97, 171, 190, 494,
  515, 580
**De Vries, Arnold**, 11, 566
**deficiency**, 115, 116
  EFAs, 195, 482
  enzyme, 8, 413
    lipase, 10
  mineral, 335, 336, 338, 360, 361, 396, 471
    calcium, 471, 473
    cobalt, 315
    iodine, 374, 619
    iron, 312
    selenium, 315
    soil, 115, 241, 315, 338, 360, 361, 373
    zinc, 315
  nutrient, 82, 119, 149, 151, 152, 338, 350,
    363, 381
  protein, xxxii, 274, 347, 348, 349, 350,
    351, 361, 362, 382
  protein-calorie, 349
  stomach acid, 358
  vitamin, 154, 326, 338, 482
    $B_1$ (beriberi), 115
    $B_{12}$, 160, 166, 168, 311, 312, 313, 314, 315,
      361, 363, 385, 407, 518
    $B_6$, 312

C (scurvy), 115, 157, 163
D, 160, 313, 314, 367, 385
**degeneration**, 5, 6, 20, 111, 112, 113,
  114, 119, 120, 132, 138, 149, 150,
  151, 152, 154, 155, 157, 174, 177,
  178, 189, 190, 194, 218, 242, 243,
  248, 249, 252, 255, 258, 259, 265,
  285, 286, 290, 316, 340, 349, 372,
  383, 386, 465, 485, 504, 508, 516,
  542, 543, 549, 559, 560, 571
  brain. *See* brain.
  irreversible. *See* disease stages.
  macular. *See* diseases.
**dehydration**, 254, 268, 296, 320, 332,
  333, 377, 383, 394, 402, 421, 428,
  429, 430, 431, 433, 434, 455, 457,
  459, 475, 480, 507, 508, 527, 528
  apple, 242
  apricot, 242, 447
  date, 557
  fig, 242, 447, 557
  food, 333, 464
  fruit, 64, 173, 197, 238, 242, 243, 296, 298,
    299, 344, 355, 359, 360, 361, 362, 365,
    366, 377, 402, 403, 420, 421, 423, 448,
    533, 555, 557, 561, 587, 588, 589, 590
  grape. *See* fruit, raisin.
  greens, 33, 188, 243, 375, 403, 460, 588
  mango, 242, 362
  nuts, 242, 318, 434, 458, 603
  prune. *See also* fruit, plum, 242, 356, 463
  seeds, 242, 318, 403, 455, 588
  tomato, 445, 457
  vegetables, 173, 445, 475, 588
**dehydrators**, 236, 318, 391, 430, 431,
  433, 457, 508, 614, 655
**dental. *See also* teeth**, 120, 144, 259
  college, 266
  deformation, 151
  demineralization, 151, 360, 361
  deterioration, 476
  erosion, 360
  mercury, 375
**deodorant**, 17, 29, 390
**depression**, xxv, 9, 14, 25, 60, 63, 82,
  87, 88, 99, 131, 143, 164, 166, 185,
  203, 241, 303, 311, 313, 331, 351,
  367, 401, 412, 476, 477, 480, 481,
  510, 530, 554, 560, 593
  manic, 9, 474
**detergent**, 17, 266, 335
**detoxification**, 6, 11, 16, 17, 18, 23, 34,
  38, 52, 88, 106, 110, 112, 113, 126,
  131, 132, 155, 185, 188, 191, 197,
  218, 230, 231, 234, 238, 239, 244,

247, 248, 249, 250, 251, 252, 253,
254, 255, 256, 257, 258, 259, 262,
264, 265, 266, 267, 268, 269, 274,
294, 299, 303, 304, 305, 333, 334,
343, 346, 357, 358, 363, 364, 369,
375, 378, 380, 386, 390, 395, 397,
400, 405, 406, 407, 408, 420, 421,
483, 510, 532, 542, 547, 548, 550,
561, 570, 571, 584, 594, 595, 597, 659
environment, 266

**Devivo, Roman**, 144, 334, 507, 519, 566

**DHEA. See hormones.**

**diabetes. See diseases.**

**Diamond**
Harvey, 206, 566
Jared, 314, 566
Marilyn, 206, 566

**diarrhea. See symptoms.**

**Dini, Fouad**, 219, 563

**dioxins**, 515

**disease stages**, 7, 105, 111, 112, 113,
114, 120, 131, 138, 148, 156, 177,
208, 220, 248, 249, 255, 285, 349,
410, 505, 547, 548, 549, 560
enervation. See enervation.
induration (scar tissue), 191, 255, 509, 549
inflammation. See symptoms.
irreversible degeneration. See also
cancer, 549
irritation, 27, 251, 262, 265, 266, 332, 348,
401, 422, 470, 546, 548, 551
toxemia. See blood, poisoning.
ulceration, 5, 72, 254, 348, 349, 400, 401
intestinal, 5, 66, 67, 157, 217, 220, 263, 287, 621
peptic, 76, 77

**diseases. See also symptoms**
ADHD, 84, 182, 320, 321, 334, 478
AIDS, xlii, 5, 86, 116, 138, 140, 148, 171,
196, 204, 387, 402, 487, 494, 510, 568,
573
alcoholism. See also alcohol, 476
ALS, 316, 477
Alzheimer's, 138, 181, 182, 183, 188, 309,
312, 313, 368, 370, 372, 465, 477, 480,
481, 523
ankylosing spondylitis, 166, 289, 617
appendicitis, 287, 341
arteriosclerosis, 149, 175, 188, 334, 343,
381
stenosis, 181
arthritis, 5, 26, 72, 102, 155, 157, 164, 174,
188, 287, 332, 335, 372, 381, 465, 476,
508, 522, 593

osteo, 49, 401
psoriatic, 166
rheumatoid, 63, 159, 162, 466, 469, 509
autism, 138, 477, 487, 509, 511, 569
blue baby syndrome, 69
cancer. See also cancer
bone, 92
brain, 85, 86, 495
breast, 42, 55, 129, 168, 171, 195, 204, 321,
336, 472, 485, 493
cervical, 23
colon, 92, 165, 171, 218, 341
kidney. See also kidneys, 85, 471
leukemia, 326, 387, 472, 512
liver, 87, 92, 286, 472, 525, 526
lung, 85, 159, 374
metastatic, 85, 92, 493
pancreatic, 286, 505
prostate, 336, 472
skin, 160, 161, 367, 397, 493
stomach, 77, 167
throat, 401
thyroid, 55
tongue, 401
cataract, 255, 287, 397, 505
celiac, 469
colon, 67, 159, 217
Crohn's, 166, 217, 220, 397, 569, 618
cystic fibrosis, 102, 103
dementia, 313
dental. See dental.
dermatitis herpetiformis, 469
diabetes, xli, 5, 23, 42, 63, 111, 116, 120,
155, 166, 169, 170, 174, 181, 203, 211,
214, 216, 242, 341, 344, 345, 371, 465,
466, 469, 476, 478, 482, 566, 593
adult onset, 23, 102, 130, 170, 345, 371, 372,
469, 481
juvenile, 169, 170, 345, 472
diverticulosis, 5, 261, 263, 341, 397, 618
emphysema, 111
fibrocystic breast disease, 401
fibromyalgia, 5, 161, 164, 166, 498, 618
gallstones. See gallbladder.
gangrene, 111
glaucoma, 255, 287
gluten intolerance, 469, 470
gout, 5, 72, 308, 522
Grave's, 5
hearing loss, 312, 389
heart, 5, 7, 72, 102, 111, 116, 155, 162,
165, 168, 174, 179, 180, 256, 286, 308,
312, 322, 337, 341, 344, 371, 372, 381,
383, 466, 474, 476, 481, 489, 491, 508,
512, 514, 517, 521, 522, 524, 526, 527,
621
hemophilia, 103, 509
hernia, 341
Hodgkin's, 287
Huntington, 102, 477
infectious. See symptoms.
kidney. See also kidneys, 5, 312, 371, 522

Bright's disease, 203
liver, 312, 400, 479
  Budd-Chiari, 71, 72
  cirrhosis, 87, 102, 471
lupus, 166, 203, 287
macular degeneration, 255
mad cow, 309, 517, 522
multiple sclerosis, 166, 287, 469, 472, 477, 478, 479
muscular dystrophy, 103
myasthenia gravis, 5, 620
osteoporosis. See also bone density, 149, 169, 331, 381, 401, 466, 469, 471, 472, 473, 474, 476, 489, 508, 620
Parkinson's, 138, 182, 205, 288, 321, 477, 478, 620
SARS, 138
schizophrenia, 9, 182, 277, 287, 381, 470
scleroderma, 166
sickle cell, 103
skin. See also symptoms, 5
spasmophilia, 166
thalassemia, 102
thymus, 479
tuberculosis, 203, 209, 222
tumor, 6, 7, 55, 72, 118, 139, 148, 158, 180, 213, 218, 255, 261, 263, 271, 281, 287, 293, 308, 312, 321, 472, 474, 477, 478, 480, 493, 494, 519, 526, 527, 580
DNA, 102, 143, 173, 176, 191, 192, 193, 194, 251, 257, 312, 313, 322, 323, 328, 472, 503, 507, 620
Dohan, T. C., 470
Donaldson, Michael, 165, 314
dopamine, 14
Douglass
  Dr. John, 157, 158, 193
  William C., 368, 566
dressing
  salad, 18, 64, 81, 231, 240, 241, 297, 298, 359, 376, 384, 403, 419, 420, 421, 422, 443, 444, 445, 448, 452, 453, 454, 455, 460, 464, 489, 541
  turkey, 380
Dries, Jan, 7, 187, 194, 359, 374, 391, 567
drug companies, xxxv, xxxvii, xlii, 123, 125, 142, 147, 148, 321, 388, 390, 481, 485, 486, 487, 489, 490, 491, 493, 495, 498, 499, 500, 505, 506
drugs, xxv, xxvi, xxvii, xxxv, xl, 3, 5, 6, 7, 9, 11, 12, 13, 17, 22, 25, 29, 38, 44, 55, 66, 67, 84, 85, 86, 87, 99, 100, 102, 104, 106, 109, 115, 117, 120, 125, 126, 127, 129, 130, 131, 132, 133, 134, 135, 137, 138, 139, 141, 142, 143, 144, 148, 149, 154, 158, 169, 171, 184, 185, 190, 191, 204, 206, 214, 215, 221, 230, 241, 247, 248, 249, 250, 253, 256, 257, 258, 259, 267, 268, 287, 290, 291, 294, 312, 317, 321, 331, 332, 358, 387, 388, 389, 390, 412, 417, 467, 476, 477, 485, 486, 487, 488, 489, 490, 491, 492, 494, 495, 496, 497, 498, 499, 500, 501, 505, 509, 512, 514, 515, 516, 520, 530, 542, 544, 549, 550, 551, 552, 561, 562, 564, 565, 617, 620
  addiction. See addiction.
  alcohol. See alcohol.
  Ambien, 489
  aminophylline, 214
  amphetamines, 17, 24, 82, 659
  analgesic, 139
  antacid, 139
  antibiotics, 38, 104, 133, 141, 309, 399, 472, 473, 474, 513, 520
  antidepressants, 13, 25, 84, 87, 375, 488
  aspirin, 139, 287, 487
  asthma, 82, 83
  Azulfidine, 66, 217
  barbiturates, 130
  caffeine. See caffeine.
  cocaine, 17, 501
  cortisone, 215
  Darvon, 287
  DepoProvera, 498
  depressants, 130
  diabetes, 5
  Ecstasy, 17
  Fosamax, 489
  heroin, 106, 126, 184, 501
  Indocin, 289
  interferon, 85, 86, 87, 88
  laxatives, 139, 304
  Lipitor, 38
  LSD, 17
  marijuana, 17, 501
  methadone, 106
  morphine, 92, 470, 497
  nicotine. See tobacco.
  novocaine, 301
  painkillers, 126, 141, 301, 497
  prednisone, 66, 217
  Prozac, 84, 498, 659
  ribavirin, 87
  Ritalin, 498
  sleeping pills, 87, 551
  tranquilizers, 256
  Valtrex, 5
  Viagra, 489
  withdrawal, 290, 291

**Duerson, Leo**, 291
**Dufty, William**, 476, 567
**dyes and colorings**, 482
**E. coli**, 123, 357, 618
**Ecuador**, 312
**eczema**. *See symptoms.*
**edema**. *See symptoms.*
**EFA**. *See acid, fatty.*
**efficiency**, 9, 262
   digestive, 19, 110, 261, 264, 273, 305,
      317, 382, 547, 548, 553, 561
   farming, 325
   healing, 273, 497
   metabolic, 45, 110, 150, 274, 301, 348,
      392, 400, 546
**Egg Nutrition Board**, 489
**eggs**, 24, 25, 29, 183, 220, 311, 313,
   314, 350, 353, 385, 398, 482, 508,
   512, 514, 516, 517, 518, 522, 558, 621
   acidity, 331
   bacteria, 399, 516, 518
     salmonella, 516, 517
   cholesterol, 517
   lecithin. *See lecithin.*
   raw, xxxviii, 160, 268, 314, 513, 516, 517
   white, 314, 517, 518
   yolk, 160, 314, 510, 516, 517, 518
**Egyptian**, 207, 242, 316
**Ehret, Prof. Arnold**, 8, 16, 115, 203,
   275, 276, 303, 394, 567
**Einstein, Dr. Albert**, 91, 98, 104
**Eisnitz, Gail A.**, 307, 567
**electrolytes**, 262, 474
**electron**, 192, 193, 195, 310, 335, 618
   pi, 193
**Elliott, Angela**, 233, 576
**Enderlein, Dr. Günther**, 124
**enema**, 87, 259, 261, 262, 263, 264
   coffee, 26, 156, 238, 261, 497, 619
   wheatgrass, 261
**energy**, xxiii, xxxiii, xxxix, xli, 3, 7, 12,
   16, 17, 26, 83, 86, 98, 104, 112, 130,
   131, 133, 150, 178, 179, 193, 196,
   250, 276, 278, 294, 335, 340, 367,
   376, 392, 401, 419, 498, 538, 621
   bioelectric, 194
   conservation, 110, 191, 247, 259, 291,
      317, 343, 377, 380, 548, 561
   digestive, 7, 8, 14, 110, 179, 190, 215,
      247, 260, 261, 269, 271, 273, 278, 281,
      283, 285, 363, 365, 381, 382, 468, 476,
      547
   efficiency, 110, 178, 261, 273, 548, 561
   electrical, 15
   enhancers, xxv, xlii, 33, 52, 67, 77, 104,

      105, 106, 107, 109, 111, 112, 113, 114,
      129, 132, 135, 140, 144, 204, 209, 247,
      249, 251, 252, 259, 262, 263, 265, 275,
      279, 285, 289, 302, 304, 305, 317, 365,
      368, 409, 413, 415, 417, 530, 531, 537,
      544, 545, 548, 553, 559, 560, 562, 655,
      659
   kundalini, 276
   life force, 197, 309, 326, 393
   nerve, 114, 251, 252, 272, 277, 278, 281,
      282, 351, 364, 367, 421, 530, 543, 544,
      545, 546, 547, 548, 550, 551, 552, 553,
      554, 555
   nuclear, 326
   reserves. *See reserves.*
   robbers, xxv, 11, 33, 34, 52, 66, 105, 108,
      109, 111, 112, 114, 119, 121, 126, 131,
      132, 250, 251, 284, 317, 332, 402, 489,
      537, 551, 559, 560, 561
   spiritual, 12, 13, 14, 99, 276
   sun, 5, 15, 192, 194, 309, 310, 504, 520
**enervation**, 75, 105, 109, 111, 112,
   120, 133, 138, 181, 249, 251, 257,
   262, 303, 363, 410, 411, 507, 530,
   531, 544, 546, 547, 548, 561
**environment, acid**. *See acid.*
**Environmental Protection Agency**,
   180, 183, 323
**enzyme**, 14, 16, 145, 153, 175, 177,
   178, 188, 189, 190, 191, 240, 242,
   316, 317, 319, 326, 337, 347, 355,
   356, 373, 374, 386, 387, 396, 400,
   404, 421, 480, 517, 568, 572, 618
   deficiency. *See deficiency.*
   destruction, 236, 241
   digestive, 110, 174, 189, 190, 247, 294,
      318, 358, 386, 401, 517
     amylase, 179, 189
     lactase, 508
     lipase, 10, 235, 517
     pepsin, 153
     ptyalin, 153, 179, 411
     rennin, 515
     salivary, 153, 179, 189, 190, 411
     trypsin, 153, 190
     uricase, 309
   fecal, 159, 164
   food, 5, 8, 10, 21, 58, 150, 153, 176, 188,
      189, 190, 395, 396, 397, 398, 402, 610
   inhibitors, 241, 318, 352, 353, 358
     avidin, 517
   liver, 86, 87, 156
   metabolic, 153, 189, 191
   potential, 16, 153, 189, 190, 191, 372, 395
   reserves, 189, 262
   superoxide dismutase, 21
   supplements, xli, 90, 169, 189, 190, 339,
      373, 374, 398

types, 189

**EPA.** *See* **Environmental Protection Agency.**

**epinephrine**, 392

**Eppinger, Dr. Hans**, 150, 193, 194

**Erb, John**, 478

**Eskimo**, 6, 10, 362, 517, 518, 519, 521

**Essene**, 14, 202, 595
bread, 268
Church of Christ, 313
gospel, 202, 573

**essential**
amino acid. *See* acid, amino.
fatty acid. *See* acid, fatty.
oils. *See* oil.

**Esser, Dr. William**, 114

**estrogen.** *See* **hormones.**

**Europe/European**, 123, 148, 159, 171, 190, 194, 203, 207, 274, 320, 323, 368, 381, 393, 470, 474, 499, 508, 519, 522, 589

**excitotoxins.** *See* **additives.**

**exercise**, xlii, 11, 52, 58, 64, 76, 83, 84, 86, 102, 107, 108, 144, 204, 207, 209, 215, 249, 274, 282, 285, 292, 293, 333, 351, 354, 364, 365, 367, 375, 394, 416, 498, 513, 520, 539, 541, 553, 554, 563, 656, 657
aerobic, 196, 254, 365, 378, 416, 561
breathing, 196
heat, 394
jaw, 176, 505
mental, 529, 535, 537
mini-trampoline, 367, 378, 657
needs, 367, 491, 513, 541, 559
slant board, 561, 657
stretching, 76, 281, 365, 367, 378, 416, 534, 561
visualization, 8, 214
weight-bearing. *See* bodybuilding.

**experiments and studies**, xxix, xxxi, xxxv, xxxix, xl, xli, xlii, 4, 7, 8, 10, 19, 97, 100, 102, 103, 115, 147, 148, 149, 150, 151, 152, 153, 154, 155, 156, 157, 158, 159, 160, 161, 162, 163, 164, 165, 166, 167, 168, 170, 171, 172, 173, 174, 181, 182, 183, 188, 190, 195, 201, 202, 203, 212, 213, 238, 239, 243, 271, 286, 300, 308, 309, 311, 313, 314, 315, 319, 320, 321, 322, 324, 326, 334, 337, 338, 360, 363, 367, 373, 376, 378, 381, 382, 387, 397, 398, 401, 403, 405, 407, 466, 467, 472, 478, 479, 480, 481, 487, 488, 489, 490, 491, 493, 497, 503, 508, 509, 510, 512, 515, 516, 517, 518, 519, 521, 523, 524, 525, 526, 527, 565, 571, 660
Roseburg Study, 167, 230, 396, 504

**eyes**, 10, 11, 15, 46, 49, 57, 89, 92, 102, 181, 242, 255, 265, 282, 287, 294, 377, 420, 464, 477, 508, 513
improvement, 65, 255, 287, 404, 504
vision, 275

**Fahey, Trish**, 342, 574

**fasting**, xxvi, 7, 11, 17, 25, 26, 36, 37, 38, 64, 76, 83, 87, 88, 103, 110, 113, 115, 116, 119, 143, 144, 155, 179, 203, 204, 205, 207, 215, 216, 217, 220, 221, 230, 234, 238, 247, 249, 252, 253, 254, 255, 256, 258, 262, 265, 269, 271, 272, 273, 274, 275, 276, 277, 278, 279, 280, 281, 282, 283, 284, 285, 286, 287, 288, 289, 290, 291, 294, 299, 303, 305, 329, 340, 350, 352, 353, 365, 376, 381, 386, 387, 391, 398, 491, 494, 495, 497, 509, 511, 512, 521, 541, 543, 544, 545, 547, 550, 561, 565, 567, 570, 571, 572, 585, 656
clinics, 580, 592, 593, 594, 596, 597
dry, 316
in pregnancy, 286, 406

**fat (cell/tissue)**, 10, 11, 18, 52, 169, 176, 179, 180, 235, 254, 256, 263, 271, 277, 281, 308, 309, 316, 319, 327, 344, 358, 362, 364, 365, 375, 376, 378, 398, 406, 411, 469, 478, 481, 517
overweight. *See* overweight.

**fat (dietary)**, 10, 11, 28, 30, 43, 61, 65, 82, 83, 85, 88, 89, 123, 145, 156, 161, 162, 176, 177, 178, 179, 193, 215, 233, 235, 237, 243, 259, 260, 286, 296, 308, 319, 336, 341, 342, 343, 344, 345, 354, 359, 360, 361, 362, 363, 375, 383, 388, 399, 402, 403, 414, 465, 466, 469, 476, 481, 482, 503, 504, 505, 517, 556, 557, 558, 580
animal, 180, 308, 343, 362, 482, 514, 516, 517, 520, 527
butter. *See* dairy.
heated, 179, 180, 343, 362, 398, 517, 528
lard, 180, 558
lipids, 179, 526, 527
margarine, 180, 482, 558, 621
rancid. *See* rancidity.
saturated, 180, 481, 521, 619, 621

shortening, 482
substitute, 85, 481
trans. *See acid, fatty.*
triglyceride, 168, 179, 256, 376, 621
   LCT, 376
   MCT, 376
unsaturated, 180, 619
**fatigue. See symptoms.**
**fatty acid. See acid.**
**FDA**, 142, 312, 323, 326, 472, 477, 478,
481, 486, 487, 496, 498, 499, 500, 567
**feces**, 152, 159, 261, 264, 515
normal, 260, 265
**Federal Trade Commission**, 487, 496
**fermentation**, 183, 201, 214, 240, 242,
263, 313, 314, 318, 337, 348, 360,
377, 400, 411, 469, 471, 479, 561
**fertility**, 30, 188
infertility. *See symptoms,* 188
plant, 152, 153, 507
**Feuer, Elaine**, 487, 567
**fever. See symptoms.**
**fiber**, 28, 110, 119, 145, 165, 177, 178,
179, 195, 237, 260, 264, 283, 304,
340, 341, 358, 396, 470, 504, 505
psyllium, 341
**fibromyalgia. See diseases.**
**Fieber, Dr. Paul**, 167
**Fielder, Dr. John**, 206, 593
**Finland**, 158, 159, 161, 162, 164
**fish. See meat.**
**flavorings. See additives.**
**flaxseed. See seeds, varieties.**
**Fletcher, Horace**, 245
**flu. See symptoms.**
**fluorine (fluoride)**, 84, 326, 331, 334,
375, 401, 470, 565, 574
**Fontana**, Dr. Luigi, 168, 169
**food**
addiction. *See addiction.*
combining, 107, 109, 232, 233, 242, 248,
249, 287, 290, 297, 298, 304, 317, 318,
348, 353, 362, 365, 369, 373, 402, 415,
421, 422, 503, 541, 544, 555, 556, 561,
572
enzyme. *See enzyme.*
processor, 236, 427, 428, 429, 430, 431,
432, 433, 434, 435, 436, 443, 444, 445,
449, 450, 451, 452, 453, 454, 456, 457,
482
   Cuisinart, 236, 432
**France/French**, 5, 140, 165, 176, 222,
495, 506, 508, 510, 523, 565, 572, 619
**Fredericks, Carlton**, 470, 567
**free radicals**, 21, 176, 180, 181, 193,

618, 620
**freezing**, 41, 202, 238, 241, 366, 402,
431, 432, 433, 434, 561
fruit, 402, 435, 460
   banana, 402, 433, 436
   grape, 433
nuts, 241, 356, 366, 402
seeds, 241, 366, 402
**french fries. See vegetables, potato.**
**fruit**, xxxviii, xxxix, 3, 10, 11, 15, 17, 19,
20, 21, 30, 31, 39, 44, 45, 47, 64, 65,
67, 75, 103, 107, 108, 110, 113, 117,
149, 151, 154, 155, 156, 159, 161,
162, 165, 168, 170, 173, 178, 188,
191, 192, 193, 194, 195, 197, 202,
207, 214, 218, 229, 233, 235, 236,
237, 240, 242, 243, 261, 268, 269,
275, 284, 288, 290, 293, 297, 298,
304, 308, 311, 318, 319, 324, 327,
331, 332, 333, 335, 338, 339, 340,
342, 343, 344, 345, 346, 347, 348,
349, 350, 351, 352, 353, 354, 355,
359, 360, 361, 362, 363, 365, 366,
369, 370, 377, 378, 380, 382, 385,
392, 396, 397, 399, 402, 403, 405,
409, 411, 412, 420, 421, 423, 433,
434, 438, 459, 460, 461, 464, 468,
503, 504, 508, 510, 511, 513, 520,
534, 538, 541, 544, 553, 555, 556,
561, 564, 567, 569, 592, 599, 618, 657
acid, 243, 351, 359, 360, 377, 555, 557
apple, xxxiv, 4, 19, 45, 81, 243, 298, 319,
   324, 411, 414, 434, 438, 442, 448, 452,
   463, 557, 564
apricot, 194, 243, 463, 557
avocado, 10, 65, 89, 178, 194, 195, 230,
   239, 242, 243, 284, 297, 298, 324, 342,
   345, 357, 359, 362, 365, 375, 384, 388,
   397, 403, 411, 424, 425, 426, 427, 432,
   444, 447, 451, 453, 455, 463, 503, 534,
   555, 558
banana, xxvi, 25, 64, 81, 142, 194, 216,
   243, 268, 324, 328, 359, 402, 411, 414,
   422, 432, 435, 436, 437, 441, 442, 443,
   448, 458, 460, 463, 510, 557
berry, 164, 243, 384, 400, 508, 557
   blackberry, 463
   blueberry, 433, 434, 606
   cranberry, 449, 557
   goji, 339, 589
   raspberry, 463
   strawberry, 324, 371, 396, 432, 433, 434, 437,
     439, 463, 557
cherimoya, 243, 557
cherry, 557
citrus, 351, 360

# Index

color, 191
date, xxvi, 216, 237, 243, 324, 327, 355, 370, 378, 383, 384, 420, 424, 431, 433, 434, 436, 441, 445, 457, 463, 482, 507, 557
dehydrated. See dehydration.
durian, 178, 243, 345, 375
fatty, 243
fig, 243, 324, 355, 433, 463, 557
grape, 26, 243, 284, 316, 324, 433, 435, 439, 463, 557, 565
grapefruit, 243, 284, 360, 447, 463, 557
juice. See juice.
kiwi, 194, 243, 434, 463, 557
kumquat, 557
lemon, 29, 216, 237, 242, 243, 272, 331, 355, 360, 400, 441, 447, 451, 557
lime, 243, 360, 447, 557
mango, xxvi, 194, 243, 362, 440, 441, 557
melon, 194, 243, 285, 300, 318, 327, 333, 337, 350, 414, 510, 555, 557
    banana, 557
    canary, 557
    cantaloupe, 243, 557
    casaba, 243, 557
    Christmas, 557
    crenshaw, 243, 557
    honeyball, 557
    honeydew, 243, 350, 557
    muskmelon, 243, 557
    nutmeg, 557
    persian, 557
    pie, 557
nectarine, 324, 463, 557
nonsweet, 45, 344
olive, 10, 89, 232, 241, 243, 298, 342, 345, 359, 362, 366, 375, 384, 388, 403, 431, 451, 453, 455, 459
orange, 194, 237, 243, 264, 284, 360, 384, 403, 441, 443, 449, 463, 557
papaya, 194, 243, 448, 557
passion, 510
peach, 243, 324, 434, 463, 557
pear, 243, 298, 422, 442, 449, 463, 557
persimmon, 194, 222, 243, 435, 463, 557
pineapple, 194, 437, 463, 507, 534, 557
plum, 243, 557
pomegranate, 463, 557
pomello, 557
raisin, 242, 324, 414, 420, 433, 442, 447, 448, 449, 452, 458, 482, 557
ripe, 361
sapote, 557
subacid, 243, 555, 557
sulfured, 242
sweet, 243, 327, 344, 361, 363, 377, 476, 555, 557
tangelo, 463, 557
tangerine, 463, 557
tree, 471

tropical, 194, 345
unsulfured, 242
watermelon, 76, 243, 278, 284, 285, 327, 350, 414, 557
wild. See wild.
fruitarian, 149, 155, 160, 202, 203, 215, 308, 312, 313, 338, 346, 347, 359, 385, 506, 563, 579, 618
Fry, T. C., xxxiii, xxxiv, 67, 68, 77, 107, 114, 117, 205, 206, 209, 215, 217, 222, 244, 251, 261, 278, 346, 361, 376, 377, 382, 445, 453, 489, 542, 553, 567, 573, 579, 580, 595, 596, 658
FTC, 487, 496
Fuhrman, Dr. Joel, 142, 567, 593
fungi, 88, 124, 125, 190, 469, 476, 518, 617
    aflatoxin, 472
    fungicide, 176, 219, 320, 321, 322, 325, 507
    mushroom, 329, 400, 558
        wild, 329
Galant, Dr. Laurence, 67
Galileo, 98
gallbladder, 88
    detoxification, 254, 619
    stones, 88, 341, 619
Gallo, Roe, 78, 211, 214, 215, 567
Gandhi, Mahatma, 203, 276
Garden of Eden, 3, 4, 14, 202, 219, 233, 265, 312, 422, 509, 575, 658
garlic. See herbs, condiments and spices.
Gendel, Wayne, 590, 659
genetic, xxv, xxvi, xxxviii, 4, 21, 42, 92, 100, 101, 102, 103, 114, 116, 118, 126, 139, 151, 173, 174, 180, 183, 191, 221, 258, 262, 263, 272, 308, 311, 312, 313, 315, 316, 321, 323, 326, 342, 345, 357, 359, 396, 469, 474, 506, 516, 519, 526, 564, 620
    modification (GMO), 36, 139, 191, 321, 322, 323, 324, 470, 480, 507, 508, 572, 573
germ, 69, 115, 143, 174, 305, 314, 326, 357, 398, 509, 518, 544, 566
    theory, 101, 103, 104, 121, 123, 124, 125, 138, 208, 542
German/Germany, 6, 7, 27, 73, 124, 125, 149, 150, 163, 182, 188, 192, 203, 204, 272, 275, 326, 328, 331, 334, 382, 493, 563
Gerson
    Dr. Max, 156, 203, 482, 497, 567

Institute, 26, 203, 238, 479, 597

**GI. See glycemic, index.**

**Gian-Cursio, Dr. Christopher**, 160, 314, 592

**gluten**, 466, 468, 470, 482, 524
intolerance. See diseases.

**glycemic**, 327, 482
high, 327, 344, 361, 363, 469
hypoglycemia. See hypoglycemia.
index (GI), 327, 328, 345, 618
low, 169, 214, 242, 344

**Goldhamer, Dr. Alan**, 597

**Gonzalez, Dr. Nicholas**, 190

**Goran, Arnoux**, 55, 58, 584

**gorillas**, 13, 14, 219, 313, 333, 344, 359, 566

**Graham**
Dr. Douglas, 7, 19, 30, 107, 114, 116, 215, 217, 233, 251, 296, 327, 328, 343, 344, 345, 360, 361, 363, 382, 470, 471, 559, 567, 568, 576, 580
Dr. Sylvester, 206, 207, 208

**grains**, 19, 20, 29, 64, 108, 156, 157, 179, 193, 206, 215, 229, 268, 326, 327, 350, 366, 396, 399, 465, 466, 468, 469, 470, 471, 476, 508, 524, 553, 557, 558, 568, 592, 619
acidic, 8, 473
amaranth, 268, 469
barley, 469, 478
buckwheat, 268, 431, 469
cereal, 408, 466, 468, 469, 471, 557
corn, 91, 179, 207, 212, 216, 304, 322, 323, 324, 327, 365, 379, 397, 411, 425, 442, 455, 463, 482, 557, 558
chips, 232
cornbread, 41
flour, 482
popcorn, 82, 89, 379, 390, 403, 478, 589
flour, 250, 331, 341, 343, 524
history of use, 4
kamut, 469
millet, 268, 469
oat, 275, 356, 469
quinoa, 268, 468, 469
rice, 154, 216, 396
wild, 357, 469
rye, 469
spelt, 469
triticale, 469
wheat, 11, 38, 84, 165, 185, 216, 229, 268, 324, 326, 380, 383, 394, 397, 431, 466, 467, 468, 469, 470, 471, 480, 482, 508, 524, 607
biscuit, 180
bread, 47, 154, 180, 181, 185, 231, 240, 295, 328, 379, 466, 468, 471, 525
Essene, 268

Ezekiel, 231
cake, 185, 363, 379, 394, 408, 471, 482
cookie, 81, 82, 239, 471
cracker, 81, 206, 239, 240, 363, 420
doughnut, 89, 471
flour, 29, 41, 47, 229, 482
grass, 10, 150, 160, 195, 196, 213, 243, 375, 376, 403, 494, 574, 580, 588
pancake, 214
pasta, 47, 85, 231, 366, 390, 471

**graminivore**, 344, 466, 619

**Grandison, Ronnie**, 215

**Greece/Greek**, 5, 202, 207
Aristotle, 276
Herodotus, 21, 202
Hippocrates, 5, 144, 145, 369, 503
Pelasgians, 21, 202
Plato, 202, 276
Pythagoras, 202, 203, 276
Socrates, 202, 276, 417

**Gregory, Dick**, 7, 16, 210, 276, 568

**Griffin, G. Edward**, 493, 568

**Guinness**, 171

**Guyton, Dr. Arthur**, 381

**Haag**
Dr. Gregory, xxiii, xxvii, 77, 114, 256
Dr. Tosca, xxiii, xxvi, xxvii, 114, 120, 256, 406, 408, 409, 415, 416

**Haeske, Roger**, 222, 584

**Hahnemann, Dr. Samuel**, 249

**hair**, 3, 10, 138, 155, 195, 349, 382, 508
color, 12, 64, 75, 87, 204, 266, 503, 513
growth, 6, 10, 509
loss. See symptoms.

**Haley, Daniel**, 499, 568

**Hallelujah**
Acres, 164, 165, 218, 314, 372, 494, 568, 570, 576, 577, 594
Diet, 29, 165, 369, 399, 586

**Harrelson, Woody**, 10, 91

**Hartman, Thom**, 471

**Hawkins, David**, 141, 568

**headache. See symptoms.**

**heart**, xl, 70, 120, 176, 195, 212, 287, 292, 293, 294, 363, 517, 547, 617
angioplasty, 175
arrhythmia, 63, 211, 286, 389, 401, 546, 617
attack, 7, 42, 131, 214, 219, 291, 292, 293, 402, 474
blood pressure. See blood.
bypass, 291
congestive failure, 181, 474
disease. See diseases.
racing, 301, 401
rate, 272
stimulants. See stimulation.

stroke, 42, 85, 86, 219, 474, 526
symptoms. *See* symptoms.
**Hebrews**, 14
**heirloom**, 216, 323, 327, 329
**Hendel, Dr. Barbara**, 240, 568
**herbicides**, 143, 219, 309, 320, 321, 322, 324, 325
**herbs, condiments and spices**, 38, 45, 65, 83, 84, 87, 129, 138, 139, 175, 194, 297, 329, 341, 369, 373, 376, 393, 420, 421, 477, 478, 479, 491, 504, 561, 601
  agave, 436, 437, 454
  basil, 377, 420, 444, 445, 450, 455, 464
  burdock, 216
  cacao. *See* legumes.
  carob. *See* legumes.
  cilantro, 242, 376, 420, 423, 425, 430, 431, 441, 443, 444, 445, 449, 450, 451, 453, 457, 459, 460, 461, 503
  cinnamon, 293, 431, 433, 434, 442, 443, 455
  cloves, 293, 433
  cumin, 456
  curry powder, 429, 444
  dandelion, 216, 473
  dill, 377, 423, 454, 456, 464
  ephedra, 487, 516
  garlic, 88, 167, 242, 336, 363, 421, 423, 424, 425, 426, 429, 443, 445, 449, 450, 451, 452, 454, 456, 457, 459, 460, 558, 561
  ginger, 88, 242, 433, 440, 441, 442, 443, 450, 454, 464, 475, 487, 588
  horsetail grass, 474
  hot. *See also* pepper, 250, 268, 421, 561
  liquid smoke, 429
  milk thistle, 87
  mint, 434, 442, 450, 453
  miso. *See* soy.
  mustard, 336, 359, 419, 429, 444, 452, 454
  nama shoyu. *See* soy.
  nutmeg, 433, 434, 443
  oregano, 420, 455
  paprika, 456
  parsley, 242, 420, 424, 441, 442, 445, 454, 464, 503
  pepper. *See also* vegetables
    black, 336, 429, 534
    cayenne, 336, 430, 437, 438, 444, 449, 454, 457, 460
    chili, 336, 426, 429
    hot, 558, 561
  peppermint, 433, 434, 437
  salt, xxxix, 11, 45, 154, 229, 230, 232, 240, 241, 250, 268, 283, 304, 333, 336, 337, 341, 369, 374, 383, 396, 397, 403, 409, 421, 465, 466, 467, 474, 475, 476, 480, 482, 534, 542, 561, 568
    Celtic sea, 240, 336, 337, 420, 451, 455, 457, 475
    Himalayan, 240, 337, 420, 455, 475
    sea, 476
    substitute, 449, 475
    toxicity, 18, 29, 240, 253, 255, 333, 337, 468, 470, 474, 475, 476, 564
  sea vegetables. *See* vegetables.
  soy sauce. *See* soy.
  stevia. *See* sweeteners.
  thyme, 420, 450
  toxicity, 422
  turmeric, 426
  vanilla, 432, 435, 437, 443, 482
  vinegar, 240, 336, 453
    apple cider, 88, 240, 420, 421, 423, 426, 443, 444, 452, 454, 456
    toxicity, 240
  watercress, 428
  yerba maté, 401
**Hertel, Dr. Hans**, 397
**Hesse, Hermann**, 203
**Hilton, Conrad**, 209
**Hinduism**, 14, 617
**Hippocrates**, 5, 144, 145, 369, 503
  Diet, 150, 574
  Health Institute, 9, 10, 176, 187, 189, 204, 213, 220, 243, 576, 594
**Hodge, Dr. J. W.**, 497
**Holick, Dr. Michael**, 367, 568
**Hollywood**, xlii, 10, 232, 263, 275
**Holmes, Dr. Oliver Wendell, Sr.**, 500
**homeopathy**, 26, 208, 222, 291, 486
**homocysteine. *See* proteins.**
**honey. *See* sweeteners.**
**Honiball, Essie**, 385, 567
**hormones**, 5, 6, 14, 25, 177, 182, 195, 271, 272, 294, 362, 392, 404, 482, 546
  abscisic acid. *See* acid.
  added, 9, 166, 472
  adrenal
    adrenaline, 257, 310, 335, 522, 560
    cortical, 179, 195
    cortisol, 291, 402
    epinephrine, 392
    norepinephrine, 392
  balance, 9, 182, 351
  DHEA, 402
  estrogen, 321, 336, 479
  growth, 168, 169, 170, 469, 546
  insulin. *See* insulin.
  leptin, 169, 376
  replacement, 55, 375, 488
  serotonin, 84, 272
  steroid, 179, 219, 291, 309, 392, 474, 513, 520

Horowitz, Dr. Leonard, 487, 568
hospital, 22, 24, 25, 38, 66, 71, 76, 82,
    86, 92, 101, 102, 103, 104, 118, 138,
    141, 142, 149, 165, 214, 261, 291,
    372, 389, 467, 490, 491, 492, 498,
    501, 512
Hotema, Hilton, 13, 370, 568
Hovannessian, A. T., 29, 204, 392, 568
Howell, Dr. Edward, 8, 10, 16, 150,
    153, 173, 174, 189, 190, 197, 517, 568
Howenstine, Dr. James, 191, 568
Hull, Dr. Janet Starr, 478
Human Genome Project, 103
hunger, 64, 154, 227, 232, 280, 283,
    296, 298, 323, 329, 352, 388, 402,
    403, 410, 469, 492, 507, 533, 546
    excess, 11, 176, 183, 185, 348, 361, 388
    false, 255, 333, 388, 541
    genuine, xxvii, 110, 244, 253, 255, 264,
        265, 271, 284, 297, 333, 340, 365, 387,
        391, 409, 411, 462, 531, 532, 541
    protein, 348, 351
Hunsberger, Eydie Mae, 171, 195,
    204, 568
Hunt, Dr. Valerie, 197, 568
Hunzakuts, 150, 308, 316
Hurt, William, xxxii
hybridization. See also genetic,
    modification, 216, 323, 327, 328,
    329, 346, 360, 470, 590
hydrochloric acid. See acid,
    hydrochloric (HCl).
hydrogen peroxide, 196, 237, 241
hydrogenation, 29, 180, 467, 481, 482,
    619, 621
hydrotherapy, 208, 262, 318
hygeotherapeutics, 207, 208
hygiene. See Natural Hygiene.
hypertension. See symptoms, high
    blood pressure.
hypnosis, 141, 218, 417, 418
hypoglycemia, 82, 88, 216, 218, 242,
    293, 361, 363, 374, 402, 420, 467,
    476, 479, 482, 520
hysterectomy, 25
ice cream. See dairy
    maker, 237, 435
India, 14, 19, 20, 157, 197, 202, 233,
    276, 326, 359, 369, 472
indigestion. See symptoms.
induration. See disease stages.
infection. See symptoms.
infertility. See symptoms.

inflammation. See symptoms.
inorganic, 176, 374, 386, 474, 489
insecticide, 320, 323
insects, 308, 311, 313, 321, 323, 326,
    375, 503, 508
    eggs, 311
insomnia. See symptoms.
instinct, 8, 140, 183, 243, 257, 267,
    288, 290, 324, 346, 352, 394, 395,
    400, 406, 470, 506, 507, 508, 511,
    514, 549, 551, 554
instinctive eating/instinctotherapy.
    See anopsology.
insulin, 63, 85, 120, 130, 169, 170, 195,
    203, 216, 286, 294, 327, 328, 342,
    345, 361, 363, 420, 469, 476, 478, 479
    blood, 170, 469
    overdose, 63
    resistance, 344, 345
International Association of Hygienic
    Physicians (IAHP). See Natural
    Hygiene.
intestines, 175, 190, 196, 255, 278,
    311, 340, 348, 514, 515, 521, 618
    fermentation, 348, 471
    large, 259, 260, 261, 263, 264, 471
    small, 115, 178, 179, 190, 259, 260, 264,
        311, 312, 317, 318, 339
IQ, 165, 321
irradiation, 192, 216, 325, 326, 327,
    371, 380, 499, 660
    grains, 326
    meat, 326, 387
    spices, 380
irritation. See disease stages.
Iserbyt, Charlotte Thompson, 495, 568
Italy/Italian, 369, 392, 471, 601, 602,
    608
Jackson, Dr. James, 207
JAMA, 486, 489, 490, 491
Jennings, Dr. Isaac, 206, 207, 208
Jensen, Dr. Bernard, 210, 247, 256,
    568
Jesus, 14, 202, 275
Jones, Dr. Hardin B., 492
Jubb
    Annie, 180, 193, 216, 569, 576
    David, 180, 193, 216, 217, 319, 328, 339,
        345, 569, 576
juice, xli, 7, 10, 37, 77, 171, 197, 209,
    236, 237, 271, 272, 273, 278, 279,
    282, 283, 284, 285, 290, 299, 333,
    338, 340, 341, 346, 357, 365, 377,
    403, 410, 411, 422, 448, 480, 504,

# Index

534, 555, 561, 573, 592, 599, 600, 601, 602, 603, 604, 605, 606, 607, 608, 609, 610, 611, 612, 613, 614, 615, 616, 619
additives, 357, 383, 478
apple, 88, 438, 439, 440, 442, 446, 447, 448
beet, 430, 446
cabbage, 440
carrot, 422, 424, 438, 440, 446, 616
celery, 438, 439, 440, 446
citrus, 441
cucumber, 446, 447
dehydrated, 460
diet, xxvi, 7, 26, 67, 83, 87, 113, 230, 256, 271, 272, 273, 274, 276, 283, 284, 290, 299, 343, 377, 388, 516, 570, 580, 594, 595
digestive, 153, 190, 318, 334, 348, 561
    gastric, 19, 167, 259, 348
    pancreatic, 260, 505
fruit, 7, 67, 237, 274, 410, 411, 437, 438, 447, 448, 494
grape, 191, 439, 440
grapefruit, 10, 420, 421, 446
green, 45, 240, 473
lemon, 237, 357, 420, 421, 423, 424, 426, 429, 434, 441, 443, 444, 446, 447, 448, 449, 450, 451, 452, 454, 455, 456, 522, 533
lime, 420, 421, 426, 441, 448, 450, 454
mango, 440
noni, 339
orange, 237, 298, 410, 422, 429, 433, 436, 437, 440, 443, 446, 457, 616
pasteurized, 357
pear, 439
pineapple, 446, 447
rejuvelac, 595
tangelo, 446
tomato, 439, 441, 442, 446, 447
vegetable, 67, 273, 274, 358, 396, 410, 448, 494, 513
watermelon, 410
wheatgrass, 10, 196, 243, 339, 386, 592, 595, 614, 615
juicer, 45, 236, 237, 243, 409, 439, 450, 504, 583, 590, 614, 655
    centrifugal, 433
    Champion, 438, 442, 448, 450
    citrus, 237
    masticating, 236
    Norwalk, 209
    Omega, 236, 450
    SoyaJoy, 237, 436
Juliano. See Brotman.
Jurek, Tawana, 387
Just, Adolph, 203

karma, 310, 312, 520
Keck-Borsits, Shelly, 143, 498, 569, 582
Kelley, Dr. William Donald, 21, 494, 569
Kellogg, Dr. John Harvey, 114, 207, 263
Kennedy, Gordon, 203, 569
Kenney, Matthew, 233, 576
Kenton, Leslie and Susannah, 9, 11, 13, 569
Kervran, Louis, 474, 569
ketosis, 254
kidneys. See also diseases, kidney, 38, 132, 187, 248, 254, 407, 480
    cancer. See diseases, cancer.
    degeneration, 242
    dialysis, 120
    enlarged, 479
    healing, 203
    impairment, 181, 286, 381, 476, 546
    inactive, 474
    infection, 38
    stones, 254, 287
Kirby, David, 487, 569
Kirlian imaging, 194, 216, 571
Klaper, Dr. Michael, 521
Klein
    Dr. David, xxxi, 66, 114, 217, 397, 466, 567, 569, 581, 659
    Roxanne, 232, 577
Kollath, Prof. Werner, 149, 188, 373
Kouchakoff, Dr. Paul, 175
Krok, Morris, 359, 392, 569
K-Tec. See blenders.
Kuhne, Louis, 203
Kulvinskas, Viktoras, 8, 41, 204, 213, 569, 576, 583
kundalini, 13, 276, 332, 566
Kuratsune, Dr. Masanore, 154
lactation, 312, 349, 354, 407, 409, 412
lactose intolerance, 472, 474, 508
Lai, Dr. Chiu-Nan, 193
Laibow, Dr. Rima, 325
LaLanne, Jack, 206, 209, 481
Lanctôt, Dr. Guylaine, 495, 569
laws, biological, 15, 155, 190, 218, 219, 389, 489, 549, 570, 620
lead. See minerals.
Leakey
    Richard, 359
    Robert, 308
Leape, Dr. Lucian, 491
learning disabilities, 334, 470, 477,

478, 481, 487
**lecithin**, 482
  egg, 517
  soy, 482
**legumes**, 8, 183, 344, 350, 366, 396
  cacao. *See also* chocolate, 339
    raw, 336, 339, 434, 435
  carob, 383, 431, 432, 433, 434, 435, 437,
    461
  coffee bean. *See also* coffee, 527
  garbanzo, 365
  green bean, 82
  lima bean, 557
  mung bean, 558
  pea, 324, 365, 463, 557, 558
    snow, 428, 463
    sugar snap, 463, 558
  peanut, 268
    butter, 268, 403, 432
  soy. *See* soy.
  sprouts. *See* sprouting.
  string bean, 558
**leptin**, 169, 376
**leukocytes**, 174
  leukocytosis, 174, 175
**Levine, Dr. V. E.**, 10
**Life Science Health System**, 206, 209,
  251, 542, 595
**lifespan**, 5, 20, 21, 22, 84, 139, 150,
  189, 215, 218, 257, 315, 321, 370,
  387, 469, 573
  extension, 161, 181
  longevity, 20, 21, 150, 308, 316, 339, 370,
    568, 572
**Lindlahr**
  College, 262
  Dr. Henry, 501
**Linus Pauling Institute**, 160, 373
**Lipton, Dr. Bruce**, 102, 368, 498, 569
**liver**, 38, 71, 72, 87, 102, 132, 156, 168,
  178, 180, 221, 248, 278, 311, 314,
  346, 392, 407, 471, 514, 546, 619
  bile, 88, 254, 260
  cleansing, 26, 38, 88, 238, 254, 619
  disease. *See* diseases.
  enzymes, 86, 87, 156
  pulse, 392
  supplements, 87
**longevity. *See* lifespan.**
**Loomis, Dr. Howard**, 175
**lotions**, 3, 367
**Lundskog, Shirlene**, 298, 575
**lungs**, 119, 248, 287, 301, 305, 407,
  415, 516, 546, 593
  bad breath. *See* symptoms.
  breathing, 19, 52, 85, 86, 92, 123, 138,

145, 183, 196, 197, 215, 253, 254, 265,
  286, 292, 293, 332, 415, 416, 516, 536,
  560, 594
**Lyman, Howard**, 19, 321, 477, 569
**lymph**, 10, 248, 260, 266, 267, 278,
  367, 378, 479, 548, 561, 656
**lysine. *See* acid, amino.**
**MacDonald, John**, 156
**Macfadden, Bernarr**, 75, 77, 206
**macrobiotics**, xxxv, 392, 494, 601, 609
**Maerin, Jordan**, 233, 576
**Maillard**
  Louis Camille, 175, 523, 619
  molecules, 175, 523, 526, 527, 619
**make-up**, 11, 12, 46, 49, 367
**Malkmus, Rev. George**, 13, 15, 114,
  164, 171, 211, 218, 329, 369, 379,
  389, 399, 408, 493, 494, 569, 570,
  576, 594
**Malngailis, Sarma**, 17, 233, 576
**malnutrition. *See also* deficiency**, 9,
  31, 102, 115, 124, 185, 192, 491, 492
**Manek, Hira Ratan**, 31
**Marcus, Erik**, 29, 570
**Mars, Brigitte**, 233, 393, 576
**Maslow, Abraham**, 107
**Mattson, Dr. Mark**, 271
**Mayo Clinic**, 321
**McCandless, Chris**, 329
**McCarrison, Sir Robert**, 157
**McDougall, Dr. John**, 343
**Mead, Margaret**, 227
**meat**, 8, 17, 23, 24, 29, 31, 37, 38, 41,
  42, 66, 67, 86, 108, 142, 143, 151,
  152, 177, 178, 181, 182, 183, 185,
  195, 201, 206, 219, 229, 231, 260,
  287, 290, 297, 307, 308, 310, 312,
  326, 331, 344, 350, 353, 371, 376,
  379, 383, 385, 387, 390, 396, 397,
  399, 413, 420, 466, 468, 473, 475,
  478, 505, 508, 515, 516, 518, 520,
  521, 522, 525, 553, 558, 569, 621
  adaptation to, 354, 506, 508, 512, 513,
    518, 519, 520, 521
  additives, 9, 166, 308
  contamination, 309, 325, 514, 515, 518,
    522
  dehydrated, 508
  effects of, 25, 26, 70, 182, 196, 204, 218,
    220, 250, 251, 308, 309, 310, 313, 358,
    382, 383, 473, 506, 508, 512, 513, 519,
    520, 521, 523, 524, 526, 527, 528
  environmental costs, 19, 20, 310, 521,
    522

ethics of eating, 307, 310, 312, 511, 520
fish, 29, 82, 170, 182, 183, 195, 309, 316,
    375, 383, 397, 500, 515, 520, 521, 524,
    527
history of, 308
industry, 19, 381, 466, 477
kosher, 310, 522
parasites, 201, 308, 514, 515, 522
raw, 10, 123, 151, 160, 308, 311, 314, 386,
    387, 399, 508, 512, 513, 514, 518, 519,
    520, 521, 522
sources, 522
substitute, 232, 233, 384, 430, 464, 612
**medication. See drugs.**
**meditation,** 8, 13, 14, 16, 47, 204, 218,
    219, 247, 257, 276, 281, 294, 313,
    511, 545, 594
**memory,** 81, 137, 138, 187, 239, 266,
    267, 268, 302, 413, 486, 538
cellular, 274
genetic, 506
improvement, 8, 26, 33, 41, 265, 277
loss, 134, 311, 401, 546
**Mendelsohn, Dr. Robert S.,** 489, 501,
    570
**menopause,** 6, 41, 195, 215
**menstruation,** 5, 24, 349
amenorrhea, 163, 617
bleeding, 4, 30, 46, 163, 617
PMS. See symptoms.
**mental,** 346, 554
adjustment, 98, 144, 538
fog. See symptoms, brain fog.
function, xli, xlii, 3, 7, 8, 9, 12, 13, 16, 22,
    23, 24, 27, 33, 34, 37, 39, 41, 43, 46, 65,
    66, 77, 88, 109, 121, 126, 129, 130, 132,
    217, 250, 251, 253, 254, 257, 265, 267,
    269, 271, 276, 277, 278, 279, 280, 281,
    282, 294, 303, 305, 320, 321, 342, 343,
    345, 360, 380, 406, 407, 419, 477, 529,
    530, 533, 535, 536, 538, 542, 545, 551,
    565, 659
habit, 177, 378, 383
healing, 148, 277, 288, 498, 531, 595
health, xxv, xxxix, xl, 7, 9, 47, 68, 83, 84,
    91, 100, 142, 157, 203, 363, 389, 404,
    468, 470, 474, 481, 571, 659
institution, 467, 470
programming, 9, 72, 77, 173, 208, 300,
    343, 406, 416, 417, 488, 535, 536, 537
resolve, 227
rest, 544, 545
retardation, 487, 511
**Mercola, Dr. Joseph,** 335, 469, 490,
    517, 570
**mercury. See minerals.**
**metabolic type,** 26, 342

**metastasis. See cancer.**
**Mexico/Mexican,** 26, 83, 150, 203,
    210, 215, 265, 320, 321, 369, 441,
    481, 494, 497, 596
**Meyer, Prof. B. J.,** 155, 156
**Meyerowitz, Steve,** 276, 570
**microwaving. See cooking.**
**microzyma,** 124, 180
**migraine. See symptoms.**
**milk. See dairy.**
**mind. See mental.**
**minerals,** 70, 145, 177, 187, 214, 243,
    274, 325, 338, 344, 346, 347, 360,
    412, 480
absorption, 176, 188, 316, 335, 338, 375
aluminum, 183, 320, 470, 474, 480
arsenic, 325, 499
balance, 187, 273, 360, 476
bioactivity, 176, 187
bone, 152, 168, 176, 331, 473, 474
bromine, 331
cadmium, 515
calcium, 84, 151, 152, 176, 237, 242, 319,
    320, 331, 403, 436, 471, 473, 477, 479,
    482, 496
    sources, 473, 474
cobalt, 313, 315
copper, 331, 479
deficiency. See deficiency.
depletion. See also deficiency, 149,
    152, 188, 241, 331, 335, 338, 360, 361,
    373
food, 45, 47, 83, 149, 150, 339, 360, 361,
    373
importance, 338
inorganic, 187, 188, 335, 336, 475
iodine, 55, 156, 240, 331, 374, 475, 619
iron, 115, 183, 312, 320, 331, 479, 482
lead, 320, 334
magnesium, 319, 320, 331, 339, 471, 473,
    479
manganese, 320
mercury, 266, 315, 316, 375, 470, 477,
    487, 515, 569
    removal. See teeth.
phosphorus, 8, 331, 473
potassium, 149, 319, 331
reserves, 272
selenium, 241, 315, 320, 374
silicon, 331, 474
sodium, 45, 161, 188, 319, 331, 333, 337,
    406, 474, 475, 476, 477, 482, 534
    sources, 406, 475
soil, 19, 39, 241, 324, 338, 339, 360, 361,
    373
sulfur, 242, 331
supplements, 169, 188, 373, 386, 499

taste, 361
trace, 320, 337, 474
zinc, 149, 241, 315, 479
sources, 241
**mini-trampoline. See exercise.**
**moderation,** 161, 163, 178, 206, 248,
274, 292, 302, 344, 397, 468, 519, 544
**mold,** 124, 181, 229, 237, 241, 266,
319, 356, 469
**Monarch, Matthew,** 12, 16, 570
**monkeys,** 16, 139, 157, 308, 359, 526
**monomeal,** 47, 299, 336, 397, 541,
619
**monosodium glutamate. See
additives.**
**Monsanto,** 321, 322, 472
**Moore**
Demi, 10, 232
Dr. Barbara, 392
Michael, 495
**Mormons,** 14, 203
**morning sickness. See pregnancy,
nausea.**
**Moscow Psychiatric Institute,** 277
**Moss, Dr. Ralph W.,** 117, 493, 499, 570
**Mosseri, Albert,** 115, 570
**mouse,** 102, 156, 157, 158, 160, 161,
188, 271, 313, 373, 398, 472, 478, 526
**mouthwash,** 17, 390
**MS. See diseases, multiple sclerosis.**
**MSG. See additives.**
**mucus. See also phlegm,** 30, 67, 115,
203, 263, 348, 516
forming, 401, 518
lining, 348, 391, 422
**multiple sclerosis. See diseases.**
**Murray, Dr. Maynard,** 39, 338, 570
**mushroom. See fungi.**
**mutagens,** 173, 175, 176, 181, 182,
308, 394, 472, 523, 524, 525, 526,
527, 620
HAAs, 525
**mycotoxins,** 180, 360, 469, 518
**National Cattlemen's Beef
Association,** 489
**National Health Association. See
Natural Hygiene.**
**National Institute on Aging,** 271
**National Institutes of Health,** 117
**Native American,** 6, 214, 511, 512
**Natural Hygiene,** xxiii, xxiv, xxv, xxvi,
xxvii, xxix, xxxiii, xxxiv, xxxvii, xxxviii, xl,
xliii, 6, 67, 75, 77, 100, 104, 105, 106,
113, 115, 117, 145, 171, 184, 197,
201, 204, 205, 206, 207, 208, 209,
215, 217, 220, 221, 222, 233, 234,
240, 241, 242, 252, 254, 262, 263,
272, 273, 276, 277, 279, 280, 281,
282, 283, 284, 285, 286, 289, 291,
293, 303, 317, 333, 341, 364, 381,
382, 406, 408, 409, 411, 413, 417,
419, 421, 438, 445, 462, 494, 498,
504, 530, 533, 538, 541, 542, 543,
544, 559, 579, 580, 582, 584, 585,
592, 593, 594, 595, 596, 597, 620,
655, 657, 658, 659
American Natural Hygiene Society, 75,
205, 221, 261
Canadian Natural Hygiene Society, 221
International Association of Hygienic
Physicians (IAHP), 221, 592, 594, 597
International Natural Hygiene Society,
592, 594
National Health Association, 205, 221
school, 585, 593
**Nature's First Law,** 38, 157, 219, 489,
506, 563, 576, 590
**naturopathy,** 38, 55, 209, 286, 290,
291, 378, 471, 593, 595
**nausea. See symptoms. See also
pregnancy.**
**Navratilova, Martina,** 215
**Navy Bureau of Medicine,** 487
**Nazariah, Brother,** 313
**Nelson, Dennis,** 317, 318, 570, 582
**nerve energy. See energy.**
**neurotransmitter. See brain,
chemicals.**
**Newsome, Dr. William,** 176
**nicotine. See tobacco.**
**Nightingale, Florence,** 115, 207
**Nikolayev, Dr. Yuri,** 277
**Nison, Paul,** 23, 78, 220, 235, 363, 397,
570, 582, 583, 589
**nitrogen balance,** 347, 351
**Nobel Prize,** 189, 192, 331, 487, 492
**Nolfi, Dr. Kristine,** 171, 230, 390, 571
**norepinephrine,** 392
**Norway,** 215
**Null, Dr. Gary,** 490, 491
**nutrition, nonfood sources,** 47
**nuts,** xxiii, xxxix, 30, 45, 64, 65, 72, 103,
107, 110, 113, 170, 178, 193, 197,
202, 229, 232, 233, 236, 237, 238,
240, 242, 261, 269, 284, 290, 296,
297, 298, 299, 308, 311, 319, 324,

333, 339, 340, 342, 344, 345, 346,
347, 349, 350, 351, 352, 356, 360,
361, 362, 363, 375, 377, 378, 384,
388, 397, 402, 403, 409, 411, 412,
421, 431, 434, 436, 438, 439, 440,
450, 464, 475, 503, 504, 507, 508,
519, 534, 538, 544, 553, 555, 558,
561, 592
acidity, 8, 331
benefits, 10, 21, 150, 155, 164, 195
   cholesterol, 162, 165, 168
butter, 236, 242, 297, 298, 363, 366, 403,
   411, 423, 424, 426, 429, 431, 436, 443,
   444, 445, 448, 450, 451, 452, 453, 454,
   455, 587, 589
   almond, 423, 424, 432, 443, 444, 446, 458,
      459, 482
   brazil, 447
   cashew, 446
   coconut, 10, 241, 376, 388, 403, 432, 437,
      482
   pecan, 446
   walnut, 446
calcium, 242, 473
   almond, 242
cheese, 420, 450
   macadamia, 430, 450, 459
cream, 238
   coconut, 238, 359
dehyrated. See dehydration.
digestibility, 235, 241, 318, 319, 352, 353,
   354, 358, 359, 397, 402, 403, 513, 521
environmental impact, 19
milk, 37, 236, 237, 365, 401, 409, 412, 414,
   422, 432, 436, 437, 441, 449, 541, 605,
   606
   almond, 426, 437
   coconut, 30, 238, 400, 435, 441
oil. See oil.
peanut. See legumes.
protein, 183, 343, 358, 362, 365, 382
sources, 587, 588, 589, 590
storage, 237, 242
   freezing, 241, 356, 366, 402
varieties
   almond, 168, 319, 356, 424, 425, 428, 429,
      431, 432, 433, 434, 443, 446, 458, 463, 589
   brazil, 241, 323, 434, 447, 463
   cashew, 356, 424, 428, 435, 440, 446, 456,
      463, 482, 583, 587
   chestnut, 557
   coconut, 30, 397, 431, 434, 441, 458, 482,
      557, 590
   filbert (hazelnut), 463
   macadamia, 168, 319, 447, 450, 456, 459
      cheese, 431
   pecan, 353, 434, 442, 450, 453, 455, 463
   pine, 456, 606
   pistachio, 168
   walnut, 168, 239, 433, 434, 438, 439, 441,
      452, 460, 463

   weight gain, 375
   weight loss, 10, 89
**O'Donnell, Rosie**, 219
**obesity. See also overweight**, xli, 5, 8,
   10, 23, 28, 60, 61, 63, 102, 116, 158,
   219, 268, 286, 316, 466, 593
   cats, 386
   causes, 10, 155, 176, 185, 216, 334, 341,
      396, 469, 474, 476, 478, 546
   statistics, 371, 372
**odor**, 263, 415, 511, 514
   body. See symptoms
   stool, 258
**oil. See also fat**, 142, 187, 263, 287,
   336, 340, 343, 375, 403, 561
   canola, 482
   coconut, 241, 376, 432, 437, 453, 589
   cod liver, 151
   corn, 376
   cottonseed, 482
   fish, 527
   flaxseed, 193, 237
   heated, 29, 180, 297, 343, 356, 363, 467,
      481, 526, 527, 619, 621
   hemp, 587
   linseed, 129
   mineral, 470
   olive, 88, 231, 240, 242, 329, 345, 356,
      423, 424, 429, 431, 443, 444, 445, 450,
      451, 452, 453, 454, 455, 456, 589
   palm, 481
   petroleum, 310, 322, 337, 471, 486
   raw, 197, 356, 380
   snake, 499
   soybean, 376, 482
   vegetable, 39, 156, 175, 340, 376, 453,
      503, 526, 558, 587, 619
**Oldfield, Harry**, 194, 571
**Olestra. See fat (dietary), substitute**
**omnivorous**, 41, 42, 161, 164, 307,
   343, 344, 346, 465
**open-mindedness**, xxvii, xxxvii, 9, 15,
   296
**organic**, 107, 266, 297, 320, 475, 588,
   594
   beer, 601
   chemistry, 174
      minerals, 187, 475
   clothing, 603
   food, 9, 36, 192, 197, 208, 214, 216, 230,
      237, 238, 239, 241, 300, 310, 319, 324,
      337, 338, 339, 340, 366, 387, 511, 522,
      588, 605, 614
      apple, 145, 319
      banana, 324
      benefits, 319, 320, 321, 322, 324, 328
      berries, 320

cheese, 216
cost, 319, 388, 399
dehydrated, 242
eggs, 516
grains, 469
grape, 26, 316
greens, 315, 403
herbs, 420
industry, 388
meat, 512, 513, 518, 520, 522
melons, 320, 383
milk, 508
nuts, 238
olive, 241
restaurants, 600, 601, 602, 603, 604, 605, 606, 607, 608, 609, 611, 612, 613, 614, 615, 616
seeds, 242, 323
sources, 325, 326, 327, 522, 580, 587, 588, 589, 590
spices, 421
spinach, 319
standards, 325, 326, 339
tea, 401
vanilla, 432
wax, 322
wine, 36, 316, 400, 601
gardening, 17, 44, 150, 587
oxygen, 196
seeds, 660
**Organic Gardening**, 44
**Orkos**, 508, 522, 589
**osteopathy**, 517, 593, 597
**osteoporosis. See diseases.**
**Oswald, Jean**, 256, 287
**Ott, True**, 335
**Overeaters Anonymous**, 299
**overeating**, 6, 61, 64, 110, 116, 176, 241, 244, 275, 304, 337, 343, 344, 346, 349, 353, 359, 360, 361, 362, 363, 365, 377, 388, 412, 422, 507, 510, 519, 529, 531, 532, 533, 534, 535, 536, 537, 538
**overweight. See also obesity**, 6, 10, 11, 18, 23, 38, 45, 52, 57, 58, 61, 62, 81, 85, 154, 158, 161, 163, 176, 179, 258, 297, 304, 316, 371, 386, 406, 469, 478, 479, 481, 532
**oxygen**, 70, 176, 194, 196, 310, 331, 391, 620
blood. See blood.
depletion, 196, 241, 345
**PAHs**, 182
**pain. See symptoms.**
**paint, nontoxic**, 367
**Pakistan**, 276
**pancreas**, 174, 189, 190, 286, 312, 328, 342, 345, 346, 361, 363, 420, 478, 479, 505

cancer. See diseases.
enlargement, 153, 190
secretions. See insulin. See also enzyme, digestive.
**Pangaia**, 511
**paradigms**, xl, 97, 98, 99, 105, 112, 114, 118, 120, 126, 134, 140, 141, 144, 145, 148, 187, 253, 272, 278, 283, 376, 490, 494, 495, 550, 551, 658
**parasites**, 125, 126, 514, 617
tapeworm, 126, 514
**Parkinson's. See diseases.**
**Pasteur, Dr. Louis**, 124, 125, 542
**pasteurization**, 81, 124, 125, 175, 195, 219, 231, 266, 297, 356, 357, 371, 380, 401, 589
almond, 356
dairy. See dairy.
juice. See juice.
**Pasztai, Dr. Arpad**, 322
**Patenaude, Frédéric**, 222, 233, 241, 296, 302, 313, 334, 400, 571, 576, 580
**Paul, Dr. Ron**, 501
**Pauling, Dr. Linus**, 161
**peanuts. See legumes.**
**peas. See legumes.**
**Pelasgians**, 21, 202
**Penney, J. C.**, 209
**Pert, Candace**, 368, 571
**Pester, Bill**, 203
**pesticides**, 9, 143, 151, 176, 219, 308, 309, 315, 319, 320, 321, 322, 323, 324, 325, 337, 405, 498, 507, 515, 520, 660
DDT, 258, 320
**pets**, xlii, 20, 143, 156, 309, 386, 387, 413, 522
birds, 183
cats, 103, 143, 386, 387
dogs, 23, 143, 387
**pH**, 335
balance, 124, 331, 332, 574
blood. See blood.
saliva. See saliva.
urine. See urine.
**phlegm**, 41, 87, 88, 115, 203, 254, 305, 314, 508, 516
**phytochemicals**, 21, 191, 374, 620
lycopene, 191, 396
phytoestrogens, 479, 480
quercetin, 191
resveratrol, 21, 191, 316
**pineal gland**, 15, 16
**pituitary**, 349

**pizza**, 25, 212, 408, 464, 471
  raw, 232, 236, 268, 363, 385, 407, 430,
    431, 459, 604, 612
**placebo effect**, 148, 207, 486, 498,
  499
**plaque**, 188, 255
  arterial, 256
  brain, 523
  dental. *See* teeth.
  intestinal, 263, 268, 516
**PMS. See symptoms.**
**Poland/Polish**, 168
**Popp, Dr. Fritz**, 192, 328
**Pottenger, Dr. Francis M., Jr.**, 103, 151,
  152, 153, 190, 195, 571
**prana**, 15, 197, 276
**prayer**, 13, 16, 57, 89, 213, 218, 219,
  281, 313, 511, 545
**pregnancy**, 12, 24, 25, 41, 288, 312,
  334, 354, 405, 406, 409, 477, 478, 488
  cravings, 25, 406
  delivery, 25, 29
  labor, 3, 6, 24, 509
  miscarriage, 23, 326, 406, 479
  nausea, 24, 406
  weight gain, 24, 25, 29
**preservatives. See additives.**
**Price, Dr. Weston A., DDS**, 152, 504,
  518, 519, 571
**prisoners**, 9, 154, 204, 205, 332, 334,
  398, 407, 467
**prostate**, 169, 255, 288, 336, 472, 593
**proteins**, 30, 85, 145, 160, 161, 167,
  177, 178, 179, 188, 189, 193, 263,
  271, 286, 308, 309, 318, 339, 342,
  343, 346, 347, 348, 349, 350, 351,
  352, 353, 354, 365, 382, 411, 412,
  477, 478, 553, 555, 556, 557, 558
  acidity, 520
  animal, 30, 156, 160, 308, 309, 314, 382,
    466, 472, 473, 478, 506, 513, 516, 519,
    520
  complete, 518
  C-reactive. *See* blood, proteins.
  cross-linking, 181, 182, 523, 524, 618
  deficiency. *See* deficiency, protein.
  digestion, 190
  foods, 183, 331, 344, 350, 352, 358, 382,
    383, 478, 482, 504
  heating, 175, 176, 181, 182, 183, 316,
    382, 479, 518, 525, 526, 527
  homocysteine, 168, 312, 314
  muscles, 383
  requirements, xlii, 33, 87, 160, 170, 274,
    309, 338, 342, 343, 344, 345, 347, 348,

    350, 352, 362, 381, 382, 385, 517, 519
  reserves. *See* reserves.
  supplements, 33, 85, 153, 343, 383, 478
**psyllium**, 341
**PubMed**, 147, 148, 156, 158, 159, 161,
  162, 163, 164, 165, 167, 168, 170,
  314, 315, 321, 360, 528
**Pulitzer Prize**, 314, 487
**pulse**, 30, 256, 265, 392, 547
**putrefaction**, 196, 214, 260, 263, 307,
  352, 381, 474
**Quality Low Input Food Project**, 320
**radiation. See cancer, treatment.**
**radura**, 326
**Rampton, Sheldon**, 141, 571
**rancidity**, 237, 263, 356, 362, 399, 517
**rash. See symptoms.**
**Reagan, Nancy**, 135, 500
**Recommended Daily Allowance
  (RDA)**, 347, 352
**refractometer**, 338
**rendering**, 309, 522
**reserves**, 112, 252, 391, 550, 551
  alkaline, 331
  conservation, 406
  digestive, 361
  energy, xxiv, xxxiv, xxxvii, 13, 14, 17, 18,
    25, 26, 34, 37, 42, 44, 49, 52, 58, 63, 65,
    72, 75, 85, 86, 87, 88, 104, 105, 109,
    111, 112, 114, 118, 119, 120, 131, 132,
    133, 134, 137, 139, 142, 145, 154, 158,
    171, 184, 188, 189, 203, 204, 211, 216,
    218, 227, 229, 247, 248, 249, 250, 251,
    255, 256, 257, 258, 259, 262, 263, 272,
    278, 280, 281, 283, 285, 286, 293, 301,
    303, 304, 305, 308, 317, 349, 350, 352,
    359, 361, 365, 372, 377, 378, 379, 384,
    386, 388, 393, 398, 404, 406, 410, 415,
    427, 530, 536, 543, 547, 548, 551, 553,
    559, 584, 595
  enzyme, 189, 262
  nutrient, 252, 272, 273, 278, 279, 280, 406
  protein, 272, 349, 350, 351, 352
  robbers, 301
**retracing**, 255, 267, 268, 334, 494
**Rhio**, 355, 385, 577, 582
**Richardson, Dr. William**, 196
**Richter**
  John, 204
  Vera, 204
**rickets. See symptoms.**
**Robbins, John**, 19, 310, 571
**Robinson, Dr. Arthur**, 160, 161
**Rockefeller**
  Foundation, 486

John D., 485, 486, 487, 564
**Rose**
Ken, 346
Natalia, 11, 13, 18, 118, 185, 197, 231, 317, 378, 397, 408, 571
**Roseburg Study. See experiments and studies.**
**Rosedale, Dr. Ron**, 521
**Rush, Dr. Benjamin**, 496
**Russia/Russian**, 62, 63, 308, 364
**SAD**, 19, 28, 31, 37, 55, 69, 89, 108, 109, 110, 116, 117, 143, 154, 155, 212, 215, 220, 227, 238, 248, 250, 251, 253, 259, 261, 264, 274, 278, 284, 298, 327, 340, 341, 343, 376, 388, 389, 411, 413, 414, 415, 417, 421, 438, 440, 445, 447, 448, 464, 475, 533, 534, 541, 544, 547, 552, 558, 620, 659
**salad dressings. See dressing, salad.**
**saliva**, 26, 153, 179, 189, 259, 265, 302, 351, 381, 387, 411
enzymes. See enzyme.
pH, 331
**salivary glands**, 157, 351
**salmonella. See bacteria.**
**salt. See herbs, condiments and spices.**
**Sarelli, Joseph**, 275
**scar. See disease stages, induration.**
**Schaeffer, Severen**, 4, 326, 466, 470, 474, 507, 509, 510, 519, 572
**Schauder, Dr. Peter**, 188
**Schauss, Alexander**, 474, 572
**Schenck, Susan**, i, ii, xxiii, xxiv, xxv, xxvi, xxvii, xxix, xxxviii, xxxix, xl, 81, 104, 113, 120, 405, 421, 655, 657, 658, 659, 660
**Schweitzer, Dr. Albert**, 203
**Scott, Dr. David J.**, xl, 114, 119, 220, 221, 252, 253, 276, 278, 280, 284, 287, 440, 555, 596
**Scott's Natural Health Institute**, 220, 252, 440, 596
**Sears, Dr. Barry**, 85, 342
**seasonality**, 242, 337, 362, 380, 391, 394, 521
**seaweed. See vegetables, sea.**
**seeds**, xxxix, 15, 18, 30, 47, 64, 65, 103, 107, 110, 113, 178, 193, 197, 202, 229, 233, 236, 237, 240, 242, 243, 261, 269, 284, 290, 308, 311, 319, 323, 328, 333, 339, 340, 342, 344, 345, 346, 347, 349, 350, 352, 354, 356, 360, 361, 362, 363, 375, 377, 378, 384, 388, 409, 411, 412, 421, 436, 438, 443, 475, 503, 504, 508, 519, 538, 544, 553, 555, 558, 561, 660
acidity, 8, 331
benefits, 10, 21, 164, 195
butter, 242, 366, 411, 423, 448, 451, 589, 590
sesame, 446
calcium, 242, 473
sesame, 242
celery, 464
cheese, 420, 450
flax, 204
pumpkin, 450
chips
flax, 457
crackers, 588
flax, 204, 241, 242, 403, 449, 450, 457, 459, 460
cream, 238
sesame, 237
dehyrated. See dehydration.
digestibility, 241, 318, 319, 352, 353, 354, 358, 359, 397, 513, 521
environmental impact, 19
heirloom, 329
milk, 236, 237, 432, 436, 437, 449
sesame, 237, 424, 426, 473
oil. See oil.
protein, 183, 343, 362, 365, 382
sources, 587, 588, 589, 590
sprouting. See sprouting.
storage, 237, 242
freezing, 241, 366, 402
tahini, sesame, 356, 380, 423, 426, 427, 428, 443, 449
varieties
alfalfa, 430
flax, 9, 193, 195, 237, 298, 299, 304, 341, 426, 430, 445, 455, 457, 517
grains. See grains.
hemp, 266, 458, 519, 589
mustard, 444, 452
pumpkin, 241, 450, 451, 452
sesame, 304, 403, 428, 431, 436, 449, 453, 454, 455, 473, 474
sunflower, 157, 241, 297, 329, 353, 403, 427, 430, 446, 451, 454, 455, 458, 463
**Seignalet, Dr. Jean**, 165, 166, 572
**seizures. See symptoms.**
**Selye, Dr. Hans**, 294
**sensitivity**, 24, 157, 185, 214, 266, 301, 302, 303, 305, 380, 420, 478, 516
**serotonin. See hormones.**
**Seventh Day Adventists**, 171, 207, 494, 580
**Sexauer, Hermann**, 204

**shampoo**, 266, 367, 390
**Shannon, Nomi**, 233, 430, 577, 583, 590
**Shelton, Dr. Herbert M.**, xxiv, xxv, xxvi, xxxviii, 6, 11, 25, 75, 76, 77, 91, 107, 114, 115, 135, 138, 145, 171, 204, 205, 206, 208, 209, 221, 227, 250, 256, 262, 265, 276, 277, 280, 284, 286, 287, 288, 289, 290, 302, 318, 332, 377, 408, 541, 553, 562, 571, 572, 580, 658
**Shircliffe, Arnold**, 422, 577
**Sidhwa, Dr. Keki**, 593, 594
**Sikinger, Maximilian**, 204
**Silverstone, Alicia**, 10
**skin**, 179, 188, 195, 248, 265, 287, 294, 301, 407, 430, 431, 544, 547
  cancer. See diseases.
  care, 334, 367, 588
  eczema. See symptoms.
  itch. See symptoms.
  moles, 504
  pimples. See symptoms, acne.
  pustule, 118, 254, 386
  texture, 3, 6, 10, 11, 12, 26, 27, 36, 46, 49, 57, 58, 88, 138, 155, 181, 235, 254, 265, 275, 297, 349, 351, 362, 382, 469, 471, 477, 504, 618, 619
  wart. See symptoms.
**sleep**, xxxii, 88, 92, 131, 171, 207, 253, 278, 282, 353, 406, 408, 409, 410, 416, 547, 559, 560, 561
  after eating, 8, 64, 85, 185, 303, 304, 467
  deprivation. See also symptoms, insomnia, 86, 171, 259, 363, 489, 546
  function, 554
  needs, xliii, 6, 11, 20, 21, 49, 52, 65, 71, 88, 107, 108, 109, 204, 205, 247, 248, 249, 253, 257, 281, 285, 299, 304, 357, 363, 364, 365, 367, 376, 404, 491, 504, 541, 545, 546, 547
  purpose, 545, 546, 547, 551, 553
  quality, 23, 26, 41, 47, 87, 161, 164, 167, 196, 241, 301, 363, 392, 400, 401, 402, 477, 486, 492, 512, 516, 593
  walking, xli, 28, 30, 370, 489
**Smart Recovery**, 300
**Smith**
  Dr. Dorothy, 490
  Dr. Lendon H., 474, 573
  Jeffrey M., 323, 572
  Joseph, 14, 203
**smoking**
  food. See cooking.
  tobacco. See tobacco.
**smoothie**, 25, 240, 299, 314, 357, 365,

369, 384, 385, 397, 402, 403, 414, 436, 437, 440, 441, 442, 448, 459, 460, 599, 600, 602, 604, 605, 606, 607, 608, 609, 610, 611, 613, 614, 615
  green, 65, 90, 167, 230, 231, 237, 243, 264, 366, 375, 403, 503, 504, 505, 658
**Sniadach, Dr. Robert**, 184, 206, 381, 585
**soap**, 17, 266, 367, 415
**social pressure**, 202, 364, 370, 498
**Somers, Suzanne**, 375, 573
**Soria, Cherie**, 222
**South Africa**, 155, 156, 563, 569, 593
**South Korea**, 222
**soy**, 183, 322, 473, 481
  bean, 420
  extracts, 478
  GMO, 323
  lecithin. See lecithin.
  milk, 311
  miso, 240, 242, 336, 337, 420, 423, 426, 430, 433, 444, 454
  nama shoyu, 336, 420, 423, 424, 426, 430, 443, 454, 457
  oil. See oil.
  protein, 478, 482
  sauce, 336, 420, 478
  tempeh, 240, 337, 428
  tofu, 37, 371, 480
**spaghetti**, 237
  raw, 232, 237, 427, 445, 461, 464
**Spatuzzi, Gabriel**, ii, xxxi
**spices. See herbs, condiments and spices.**
**spirituality**, xli, 3, 13, 14, 15, 16, 27, 33, 45, 47, 60, 68, 83, 84, 90, 99, 100, 191, 202, 203, 213, 214, 218, 253, 254, 271, 275, 276, 280, 309, 312, 313, 340, 343, 360, 404, 520, 530, 531, 535, 562, 565, 566, 595
**spirulina**, 193, 240, 311, 339, 436
**Spors, Antje**, 144, 334, 507, 519, 566
**sprouting**, xxxix, 65, 107, 110, 113, 164, 240, 261, 268, 290, 296, 332, 339, 399, 403, 411, 423, 438, 463, 464, 475, 508, 521, 538, 561, 570, 615, 660
  benefits, 150
  garbanzo, 365
  grains, 20, 150, 193, 197, 231, 240, 357, 362, 375, 382, 431, 468, 470, 519, 557, 558
  legumes, 20, 150, 240, 362, 375, 382, 519, 592
  lentil, 365, 463
  methods, 237, 318

mung bean, 428, 463, 558
nuts, 240, 353
seeds, 145, 150, 188, 240, 241, 242, 318,
  353, 366, 402, 427, 430, 458, 588, 592
  alfalfa, 463, 558
**Spurlock, Morgan**, 185
**stamina**, 7, 8, 11, 150, 155, 158
**Standard Oil**, 486
**starch. See carbohydrates. See also**
  **vegetables.**
**starvation**, 11, 81, 161, 203, 276, 279,
  280, 310, 348, 388, 395, 398, 405,
  406, 470, 471, 492, 512, 543, 550
**Stauber, John**, 141, 571
**Steiner, Rudolph**, 15, 191
**stent**, 139, 175
**Stern, Howard**, 219
**steroids. See hormones.**
**stevia. See sweeteners.**
**Sticco, Linda**, 595, 659
**stimulation**, 6, 14, 82, 83, 110, 130,
  133, 166, 175, 247, 250, 251, 252,
  253, 257, 261, 262, 267, 273, 275,
  282, 302, 335, 336, 340, 341, 367,
  374, 378, 388, 392, 395, 410, 421,
  469, 477, 478, 516, 529, 530, 531,
  534, 545, 546, 548, 550, 551, 619
  natural, 15, 194, 196
**Stitt, Barbara Reed**, 468, 573
**stomach**, 8, 49, 64, 76, 77, 179, 190,
  255, 260, 276, 278, 318, 331, 334,
  340, 348, 352, 358, 362, 377, 388,
  391, 403, 422, 513, 533
  ache. See symptoms, pain.
  acid. See acid.
  cancer. See diseases, cancer.
  tumor, 180
**Stoycoff, Cheryl**, 408, 573
**Streep, Meryl**, 145
**stress**, 12, 13, 21, 33, 71, 75, 76, 77, 83,
  89, 102, 109, 142, 175, 178, 179, 182,
  205, 254, 257, 272, 282, 294, 303,
  304, 312, 331, 347, 352, 354, 365,
  368, 377, 380, 382, 403, 420, 437,
  466, 474, 481, 488, 491, 522, 547, 554
**strikes, medical**, 491
**stroke. See heart.**
**studies. See experiments and**
  **studies.**
**sucralose (Splenda). See additives.**
**sugar. See sweeteners.**
  blood. See blood.
**sulfates, sulfites. See additives.**

**Sumner, Dr. James B.**, 189
**sungazing**, 31, 47
**sunscreen**, 367
**sunshine**, xlii, 11, 45, 47, 57, 76, 99,
  106, 107, 108, 169, 177, 192, 204,
  206, 248, 314, 332, 367, 385, 416,
  541, 542, 544, 554, 559, 561, 657
**super foods**, 303, 338, 339, 340, 360,
  373, 589
**supplements**, xli, 17, 33, 45, 70, 84, 86,
  129, 144, 169, 173, 188, 204, 228,
  303, 313, 315, 327, 338, 339, 340,
  373, 374, 375, 393, 474, 475, 480,
  494, 499, 520, 590, 601, 607
  charcoal, 304
  enzyme. See enzyme.
  herbal, 373, 499
  liver, 87
  mineral. See minerals.
  probiotic, 264, 314, 315
  sources, 589
  vitamin, 90. See vitamins.
**surgery**, xxvi, xl, 99, 100, 102, 115, 120,
  139, 141, 142, 144, 206, 388, 389,
  493, 542, 549
  appendix, 139
  avoiding, xli, 57, 58, 67, 138, 139, 213,
    491, 494, 509, 513, 569, 620
  brain, 293
  bypass, 175
  cancer. See cancer, treatment.
  colostomy, 139
  ear, 473
  gallbladder, 88, 139
  heart, 139, 343
  hysterectomy, 139
  laser, 23
  nasal, 258
  oral, 151
  reconstructive, 25, 102
  replacement, 102
  thyroid, 55
  tonsillectomy, 139
  tumor, 139
**Swedish/Sweden**, 149, 180
**sweeteners**
  agave, 37, 197, 237, 240, 242, 420, 421,
    424, 429, 430, 432, 434, 435, 444, 454,
    456, 457, 479, 482
  aspartame. See additives.
  corn syrup, 467, 481, 482
  cornstarch, 482
  date. See fruit.
  dextrose, 482
  honey, 36, 170, 197, 237, 240, 242, 268,
    272, 287, 324, 327, 356, 357, 374, 384,

398, 401, 403, 420, 421, 424, 430, 431,
432, 433, 434, 436, 437, 443, 444, 452,
454, 455, 457, 460, 508, 510, 511, 512,
513, 558, 589, 604, 621
maltose, 482
maple syrup, 356
molasses, 482
stevia, 242, 401, 420, 421, 437, 479
sucralose (Splenda). See additives.
sugar, 29, 31, 36, 37, 38, 41, 81, 175, 178,
179, 181, 183, 220, 229, 230, 232, 242,
250, 251, 263, 289, 327, 331, 336, 341,
343, 344, 345, 346, 357, 360, 361, 379,
383, 394, 396, 399, 409, 411, 414, 420,
465, 466, 468, 469, 473, 476, 479, 480,
482, 498, 523, 524, 526, 534, 556, 558,
563, 574, 618
disguised, 481
fruit, 216, 344, 347
industry, 389
syrup, 556, 558
**Switzerland**, 154, 157, 174, 203, 392,
397, 506, 564
**Swope, Dr. Mary Ruth**, 466
**symptoms.** *See also* **diseases**
acne, 3, 6, 37, 118, 166, 213, 218, 254,
304, 370, 481
aggression, 152, 182
allergies, 3, 6, 23, 27, 38, 53, 63, 72, 82,
84, 134, 152, 158, 166, 214, 218, 296,
323, 370, 469, 474
amenorrhea. See menstruation.
anemia, 5, 76, 115, 157, 287, 401
pernicious, 115
angina, 287, 474
anorexia, 57, 82
anxiety, 13, 36, 84, 138, 313, 339, 401,
412, 477, 481
apathy, 182, 349, 382
arrhythmia. See heart.
asthma, xli, 5, 23, 63, 82, 83, 166, 211,
214, 469, 476, 477, 516
athlete's foot, 3, 6, 88, 304
bad breath, 6, 44, 304, 508
bleeding
gums, 45, 151, 176, 313, 361
intestinal, 66, 67, 220, 618
menstrual. See menstruation.
bloat, 46, 49, 235, 317, 318, 358, 396, 481
body odor, 6, 44, 47, 218, 255, 265, 304,
317, 474
brain fog, 7, 24, 26, 88, 303, 305, 342,
345, 477, 478
bulimia, 82, 83
bursitis, 287
cellulite, 10, 12, 88
chicken pox, 395
chills, 126, 254, 258, 359, 391, 392, 394,
509

cold sores, 6, 254
colitis, 5, 66, 67, 68, 111, 119, 157, 217,
220, 263, 287, 341, 397, 569, 621
coma, 86, 370, 512
common cold, xxxv, 6, 24, 25, 46, 70,
111, 126, 131, 133, 138, 155, 214, 218,
254, 305, 357, 395, 407, 411
conjunctivitis, 166
constipation, 3, 25, 26, 89, 139, 213, 262,
263, 303, 304, 317, 340, 341, 357, 358,
370, 380, 471, 521
cough, 86, 131, 254, 301
cramp, 24, 41, 66, 255
cravings. See also addiction, 18, 25, 29,
30, 36, 65, 157, 167, 183, 184, 185, 229,
230, 231, 239, 264, 266, 267, 268, 271,
274, 299, 333, 334, 361, 371, 372, 380,
388, 403, 406, 407, 459, 469, 473, 476,
504, 505, 508, 510, 519
Crohn's, 68
cyst, 118, 287
dandruff, 6, 218
dental. See dental.
depression. See depression.
dermatitis, 593
diarrhea, 25, 26, 66, 67, 111, 126, 235,
263, 340, 357, 358, 395, 401, 469, 477,
479, 508, 618
dry mouth, 351
dyslexia, 33, 511
dyspepsia, 593
earache, 24, 395, 407
eczema, 23, 166, 287, 505, 618
edema, 63, 154, 164, 166, 255, 304, 337,
349, 351, 382, 474, 475, 561, 618
encephalitis, 138
fatigue, 42, 85, 102, 109, 111, 153, 189,
190, 203, 216, 218, 240, 250, 251, 262,
311, 317, 327, 342, 345, 349, 361, 363,
388, 395, 401, 402, 480, 503, 541, 554,
618, 620
chronic, 38, 102, 164, 228, 344, 351, 361,
402, 512, 560, 593
fever, 24, 254, 256, 357, 395, 407, 412
flu, 6, 104, 111, 126, 133, 138, 155, 183,
218, 254, 305, 357, 411
gas, 46, 49, 66, 235, 263, 317, 318, 395,
471
gastritis, 317
goiter, 157, 619
hair loss, 87, 351
hallucination, 126, 470, 546
headache, 84, 85, 111, 134, 139, 237,
253, 256, 287, 293, 294, 301, 304, 357,
370, 388, 397, 401, 476, 477
heart attack. See heart.
hemorrhoid, 31, 37, 218, 287, 341
herpes, 5, 6
high blood pressure, 5, 42, 156, 157, 158,

171, 218, 337, 401, 469, 474, 475, 476, 619
hypoglycemia. See hypoglycemia.
indigestion, 111, 139, 235, 317, 318, 370, 386, 422, 469
infection, 6, 84, 158, 174, 323, 398, 469, 473, 491, 492, 497, 508, 509, 514
  bladder, 23
  candida, 181, 343, 344, 345, 617
  chronic, 25
  E. coli, 357
  ear, 38, 473
  fungus, 312
  hepatitis C, 86, 87, 512, 513
  kidney. See also kidneys, 38
  parasite, 514
  salmonella, 514, 516
  sinus, 38, 218, 254, 288, 305, 473
  strep, 473
  tonsillitis, 23
  yeast, 26, 181, 196, 345
infertility, xli, 23, 29, 152, 188, 372
inflammation, 6, 21, 68, 138, 158, 168, 169, 181, 220, 349, 509, 546, 548, 549, 618, 621
insomnia, 23, 41, 82, 87, 241, 253, 275, 339, 363, 401, 477, 546, 593
irritable bowel syndrome, 166, 397, 469
itch, 63, 134, 254, 301, 477, 548, 618
jaundice, 5, 203, 619
jet lag, 6, 88
lactose intolerance, 472, 474, 508
libido loss, 257, 498
liver
  abscess, 271
measles, 395
meningitis, 89, 218, 287
migraine, 23, 25, 203, 478, 498, 593
mumps, 395
nausea. See also pregnancy, 76, 126, 255, 275, 301, 477
neuritis, 593
obesity. See obesity.
overeating. See overeating.
overweight. See overweight.
pain, xxxix, 42, 46, 72, 76, 83, 84, 85, 89, 92, 105, 111, 120, 130, 134, 139, 141, 145, 206, 215, 230, 255, 262, 263, 267, 287, 289, 292, 293, 301, 303, 304, 325, 370, 376, 389, 412, 497, 500, 509, 516, 542, 548, 549, 553, 561
  abdominal, 25, 408, 472, 618
  acupuncture, 497
  arthritis, 164
  asthma, 516
  $B_{12}$ deficiency, 311, 313
  back, 89
  ear, 38
  enemas, 497
  fibromyalgia, 161, 164, 498, 618
  indigestion, 234
  labor, 3, 4, 6, 24

  menstrual, 4, 24, 41
  psychological, 13, 57, 505
  stomachache, 77, 245, 388, 395
panic attack, 313, 401, 477, 533
paranoia, 9, 311
PMS, 3, 5, 6, 85, 88, 370, 401, 474
pneumonia, 214, 620
polyps, 118, 261, 263
proctitis, 138
prostate enlargement, 255, 593
pyorrhea, 381
rash, 63, 254, 259, 395, 408, 469, 477
reflux, 318
rhinitis, 166
rickets, 152
seizures, 152, 477, 478, 512
sigmoiditis, 138
snoring, 287
sore throat, 481
stress. See stress.
tinnitus, 401
ulcer, 548. See disease stages, ulceration.
urticaria, 166
varicose veins, 63, 287, 341, 476, 561
vomiting, 76, 126, 254, 275, 386, 406, 477, 492
wart, 64, 118, 504
whooping cough, 289, 290
Szekely, Dr. Edmond Bordeaux, 114, 150, 151, 210, 382, 573
tapeworm, 126, 514
tastebuds, 18, 53, 179, 229, 232, 267, 279, 284, 336, 376, 394, 395, 401, 421, 464
taurine. See acid, amino.
tea, 30, 129, 275, 400, 401, 600, 601, 610
  addiction, 400, 401, 533
  kombucha, 337, 400
  symptoms, 275
teeth. See also dental, 47, 176, 410, 411, 412
  anesthesia, 301
  brushing, 359, 360, 560
    electric, 560
  canine, 308
  chewing, 176, 505
  crooked, 151, 176
  demineralization, 176, 359, 360, 471
  deterioration, 149, 157, 176, 338, 349, 351, 361, 469, 560
  enamel, 351, 360
  extraction, 504
  flossing, 45, 403, 560
  grinding, 401
  loose, 44, 313
  loss, 346, 361

mercury removal, 266
perfection, 519, 560
plaque, 176, 403, 560
regrowth, 212
sensitivity, 64, 503, 504
**Teflon**, 183
**testimonials**, xxv, xxix, xxxi, xli, xlii, 23, 78, 215, 235, 499, 505, 581, 582, 583, 584, 660
  Boutenko, Victoria. *See also* Boutenko, xxxvii, 62
  Christy, Samara, 57
  Jessica, 24
  Klein, Dr. David. *See also* Klein, xxxi, 66
  Lambart, Ric, 69
  Larkins, Annette, 41, 579
  McCright, Mike, 44
  Nash, Jackie, ii, xxxi, 52
  P., Al, xxxi, 33, 458, 461
  Pettaway, Dana, xxxi, 36
  Raquel, 23
  Schenck, Susan, 81
  Schrift
    Amy, 46
    Sandra, 49, 434
  Smith, Jenny, 28
  Stokes, Angela, 60, 583
  Tadič, Marie, 25, 370
  Tye, Tim, 37
  Vetrano, Dr. Vivian V. *See also* Vetrano, xxxvii, 75
  Wood, Paula, 55
**Thai**, 232, 369
**Thoreau, Henry David**, 207
**thymus**, 479
**thyroid**, xli, 55, 84, 152, 240, 374, 480, 619
  hyper, 63, 211, 287, 619
  hypo, 61, 240, 334, 351, 401, 469, 479
**Tilden, Dr. John**, 114, 160, 206, 208, 253, 377, 501, 559, 573, 658
**tobacco**, 184, 371
  addiction. *See* addiction.
  nicotine, 109, 129, 140, 157, 253, 275, 301, 331
  smoking, xxv, 9, 36, 83, 158, 159, 182, 185, 275, 300, 301, 312, 374, 400, 488, 509
**toothpaste**, 29, 47, 375, 390
**toxemia. *See* blood, poisoning (toxemia).**
**toxicosis. *See also* blood, poisoning (toxemia)**, 105, 543
**toxins**, ii, 8, 11, 12, 13, 38, 44, 103, 105, 106, 112, 113, 114, 116, 117, 118, 126, 132, 139, 145, 155, 174, 176,

182, 193, 194, 195, 196, 203, 232, 248, 249, 251, 253, 254, 255, 256, 257, 258, 261, 263, 264, 266, 267, 271, 272, 274, 277, 279, 286, 299, 301, 302, 303, 304, 305, 308, 312, 314, 319, 321, 323, 325, 326, 332, 333, 334, 340, 367, 372, 374, 375, 378, 380, 386, 391, 396, 405, 407, 470, 471, 476, 497, 505, 515, 516, 520, 544, 546, 548, 552
  endogenous, 109, 110, 117, 118, 119, 126, 133, 174, 248, 249, 251, 259, 317, 331, 348, 371, 383, 410, 421, 530, 544, 548, 549, 551, 559, 560, 562
  exogenous, 109, 110, 117, 118, 126, 129, 132, 133, 174, 182, 248, 249, 250, 251, 253, 259, 266, 333, 334, 348, 371, 410, 421, 530, 544, 547, 548, 549, 551, 559
**trail mix**, 241, 242, 296, 298, 369, 402, 458, 459, 461, 507, 603
**Trall, Dr. Russell**, 206, 500
**trans fat. *See* acid, fatty.**
**transfusion. *See* blood.**
**transit time, digestion**, 7, 304
**transitioning**, xxvii, xlii, 20, 44, 52, 145, 210, 227, 228, 229, 230, 231, 232, 235, 236, 237, 256, 258, 299, 333, 336, 343, 358, 359, 361, 362, 386, 391, 394, 402, 408, 421, 438, 462, 464, 468, 505, 557, 561, 573, 589, 594
**Tree of Life Foundation**, 166, 597
**Trotter, Charlie**, 232, 577, 607
**Trudeau, Kevin**, 129, 321, 376, 479, 481, 488, 496, 522, 573
**tryptophan. *See* acid, amino.**
**tumor. *See* diseases.**
**Twain, Mark**, xxxvi, 300
**ulcer. *See* disease stages, ulceration.**
**Underkoffler, Renée Loux**, 233, 577
**United Nations**, 310, 327, 499
**University of Kuopio**, 158, 159, 161, 162, 163, 164
**unpasteurized**, 242, 268, 336, 380, 420, 423, 424, 426, 430, 431, 433, 443, 444, 445, 450, 451, 452, 453, 454, 587
**urine**, 152, 159, 161, 181, 254, 265, 415, 525
  pH, 156, 331, 504
**US Public Health Service**, 487
**USDA**, 242, 356, 477
**vaccination**, 11, 29, 30, 72, 104, 123, 125, 138, 204, 375, 395, 477, 487,

488, 497, 511, 569

**varicose veins. See symptoms.**

**vegan**, xxix, xxxv, 20, 25, 29, 30, 31, 36, 37, 38, 55, 60, 67, 71, 72, 159, 160, 161, 162, 163, 164, 165, 166, 168, 169, 213, 214, 215, 216, 218, 237, 239, 241, 310, 311, 312, 313, 314, 315, 334, 337, 339, 343, 346, 375, 381, 382, 385, 405, 407, 420, 505, 506, 508, 513, 514, 515, 516, 517, 518, 519, 520, 521, 570, 571, 576, 577, 584, 588, 589, 600, 601, 602, 603, 604, 605, 606, 607, 608, 609, 610, 611, 612, 613, 614, 615, 616, 621

**vegetab les**
mushroom, 558

**vegetables**, xxxix, 10, 11, 17, 19, 21, 30, 47, 49, 64, 65, 67, 75, 103, 107, 108, 110, 113, 119, 149, 151, 154, 156, 159, 161, 162, 164, 165, 167, 168, 170, 173, 177, 178, 179, 188, 191, 192, 193, 194, 197, 205, 206, 207, 214, 218, 229, 233, 235, 240, 243, 269, 284, 288, 290, 293, 297, 298, 304, 308, 311, 324, 331, 332, 333, 335, 339, 340, 343, 344, 345, 346, 347, 349, 350, 351, 352, 353, 358, 359, 360, 365, 371, 378, 379, 380, 382, 383, 396, 397, 400, 403, 405, 409, 411, 412, 421, 422, 423, 425, 427, 438, 443, 445, 449, 451, 452, 454, 455, 459, 460, 464, 468, 478, 503, 508, 513, 521, 534, 538, 541, 544, 553, 555, 561, 564, 567, 572, 592, 606, 657
artichoke, 558
asparagus, 452, 557
beans. See legumes.
beet, 216, 237, 243, 304, 327, 328, 365, 414, 427, 430, 454, 464, 557
bok choy, 216, 426, 453, 463, 558
broccoli, 25, 167, 168, 178, 229, 336, 396, 426, 427, 428, 449, 450, 463, 473, 558
brussels sprouts, 168, 558
cabbage, 167, 168, 242, 396, 428, 452, 453, 454, 463, 558
sauerkraut, 168, 240, 337
carrot, xxxiv, 77, 81, 119, 167, 216, 237, 243, 298, 324, 327, 328, 329, 336, 365, 380, 384, 394, 396, 403, 411, 424, 425, 427, 428, 429, 430, 433, 449, 450, 452, 453, 454, 457, 461, 464, 503, 557
cauliflower, 324, 336, 426, 453, 456, 461, 463, 558
celery, 240, 284, 298, 324, 336, 369, 377, 378, 406, 411, 420, 421, 423, 424, 425, 428, 430, 438, 441, 447, 448, 453, 455, 457, 461, 463, 464, 475, 555, 558, 561
cream, 236
salt, 449, 475
chard, 240, 473, 475, 558
collard, 41, 503, 558
colors, 191
cucumber, 45, 232, 243, 284, 298, 324, 377, 403, 423, 425, 451, 461, 463, 507, 511, 558
dehydrated \t See dehydration., i
digestibility, 358, 396
dip, 449, 450
eggplant, 243, 430, 431, 558
greens, 8, 45, 47, 64, 65, 162, 178, 188, 196, 197, 237, 243, 273, 298, 308, 311, 313, 315, 318, 319, 331, 332, 339, 342, 344, 349, 354, 358, 359, 366, 377, 383, 403, 409, 421, 442, 473, 503, 504, 505, 519, 558, 592
beet, 503
jerusalem atrichoke, 557
jicama, 414, 455
juice. See juice.
kale, 25, 64, 168, 216, 315, 336, 426, 437, 438, 453, 473, 503, 504, 558, 606
kohlrabi, 463, 558
leek, 558
legumes. See legumes.
lettuce, 82, 278, 284, 296, 345, 371, 377, 412, 414, 430, 442, 448, 452, 463, 473, 503, 507, 555, 558, 561
maca, 339, 589
mushroom, 329, 400
wild, 329
mustard greens, 558
nonstarchy, 297, 344, 365, 377, 411, 525, 555, 556, 558
oil. See oil.
okra, 41, 243
onion, 242, 336, 363, 421, 426, 427, 428, 429, 430, 431, 441, 445, 449, 450, 451, 452, 453, 454, 455, 464, 558, 561
parsley, 242, 420, 424, 441, 442, 445, 454, 464, 503
parsnip, 557, 606
pea. See legumes.
pepper
bell, 45, 243, 284, 424, 425, 426, 427, 428, 430, 431, 447, 448, 449, 450, 451, 452, 453, 454, 455, 463, 558
black. See herbs, condiments, and spices.
cayenne. See herbs, condiments, and spices.
chili. See herbs, condiments, and spices.
jalapeño, 336, 426, 451
potato, 10, 19, 89, 99, 119, 144, 175, 180,

181, 216, 290, 322, 323, 324, 327, 328, 365, 379, 390, 391, 406, 419, 525, 557
  chips, 180, 371, 379, 478, 481
  french fries, 37, 99, 180, 181, 185, 371, 396
  substitutes, 232, 456, 461
pumpkin, 557
radish, 427, 428, 558
root, 216, 243, 327
rutabaga, 557
scallion, 558
sea, 240, 311, 331, 339, 406, 420, 421, 424, 426, 429, 430, 443, 444, 445, 449, 450, 451, 452, 454, 456, 457, 475
  algae, 240, 269, 311, 339
  arame, 240, 454
  chlorella, 376
  dulse, 240, 339, 421, 425, 426, 430, 443, 444, 449, 475
  hijiki, 240
  kelp, 240, 421, 475
  nori, 240, 311, 339, 427, 430, 443, 449, 460
  wakame, 240
spinach, 240, 319, 324, 406, 425, 436, 437, 442, 444, 449, 452, 453, 459, 461, 463, 464, 473, 475, 503, 558
sprouts. See sprouting.
squash, 45, 179, 216, 243, 427, 450, 557, 558
  acorn, 557
  banana, 557
  buttercup, 557
  crookneck, 558
  gold nugget, 557
  hubbard, 557
  patty pan, 558
  spaghetti, 237, 557
starchy, 180, 410, 556, 558
sugar
  beet, 467
  cane, 467
sweet potato, 365, 557
tomatillo, 447, 448
tomato, 41, 45, 176, 216, 243, 284, 371, 384, 396, 403, 411, 424, 426, 427, 428, 429, 430, 431, 439, 441, 445, 446, 447, 448, 451, 453, 455, 457, 461, 463, 464, 475, 507, 555, 557, 588
turnip, 243, 365, 557
wild. See wild.
yam, 237, 365, 557
zucchini, 119, 237, 243, 425, 427, 428, 449, 450, 453, 463, 558, 564
**vegetarian**, 15, 19, 23, 29, 41, 42, 70, 71, 85, 149, 160, 164, 165, 168, 182, 204, 208, 220, 307, 308, 309, 310, 311, 313, 314, 343, 346, 350, 358, 375, 381, 405, 413, 505, 506, 511, 513, 518, 519, 520, 521, 522, 575, 599, 600, 604, 605, 606, 607, 608, 609, 611, 612, 613, 614, 615, 621

  lacto-ovo, 313
**Vegetarian Times**, 313
**veterinarian**, 143, 386, 387
**Vetrano, Dr. Vivian V.**, i, ii, xxvii, xxix, xxxi, xxxiii, xxxvii, xxxviii, 75, 100, 103, 104, 106, 114, 115, 120, 129, 133, 137, 140, 177, 187, 205, 208, 209, 221, 222, 247, 249, 256, 261, 264, 272, 273, 277, 280, 284, 285, 286, 291, 300, 303, 317, 318, 319, 327, 332, 339, 346, 361, 364, 376, 382, 408, 409, 413, 416, 438, 464, 504, 541, 542, 545, 573, 596, 658
**Vietnamese**, 600
**villi**, 260
**Vinci, Leonardo da**, 137
**Virchow, Dr. Rudolph**, 125
**viruses**, xxvi, 5, 86, 87, 123, 125, 126, 131, 138, 190, 196, 324, 386, 387, 487, 542, 544, 568
  HIV. See also diseases, AIDS, 126, 139
  SIV, 139
**vision. See eyes.**
**visualization**, 8, 214, 218, 274, 422, 534, 536
**vitamins**, xli, 25, 70, 145, 149, 150, 154, 176, 177, 187, 242, 313, 316, 326, 338, 347, 373, 402, 412, 480, 481
  A (carotene), 163, 374, 396
  absorption, 188, 312, 375
  B, 83, 187, 479
  $B_1$ (thiamine), 149, 482
  $B_{12}$ (cobalamin), 71, 115, 116, 166, 168, 311, 312, 313, 314, 315, 339, 346, 363, 385, 407, 479, 505, 518, 520
  $B_{17}$ (laetril), 493, 568
  $B_2$ (riboflavin), 150, 482
  $B_6$ (pyridoxine), 150, 312
  biotin, 517, 518
  C, 160, 161, 163, 187, 344, 359, 373, 374, 396, 525
  D, 168, 169, 314, 367, 385, 473
  deficiency. See deficiency.
  depletion, 396
  E, 160, 163, 525
  flavonoids, 191
  folic acid, 150, 482
  niacin, 482
  pyrroloquinoline quinone, 188
  reserves, 272
  supplements, 149, 188, 312, 313, 373, 374
**Vita-Mix. See blenders.**
**Voltaire, François**, 5
**vomiting. See symptoms.**

**Vonderplanitz, Aajonus**, 123, 139, 233, 241, 258, 259, 268, 329, 374, 399, 476, 511, 512, 513, 515, 517, 518, 520, 521, 573, 577

**Walford, Dr. Roy L.**, 315, 370, 573

**Walker, Dr. Norman**, 209, 573

**Warburg, Dr. Otto**, 331

**wart. See symptoms.**

**water**, xlii, 11, 19, 26, 30, 86, 87, 99, 106, 107, 108, 113, 117, 119, 125, 144, 145, 155, 174, 177, 180, 195, 202, 206, 207, 214, 215, 231, 237, 241, 247, 248, 260, 261, 262, 272, 273, 274, 275, 277, 278, 282, 283, 284, 285, 287, 289, 290, 299, 304, 310, 316, 318, 319, 326, 332, 333, 334, 335, 336, 337, 351, 356, 362, 367, 375, 377, 378, 381, 386, 392, 397, 398, 400, 401, 402, 415, 416, 423, 424, 425, 426, 429, 430, 431, 436, 437, 438, 439, 441, 442, 443, 444, 447, 448, 450, 451, 452, 453, 454, 455, 456, 457, 464, 475, 482, 504, 509, 515, 522, 533, 542, 544, 555, 559, 560, 590, 594
   alkaline, 335
   childbirthing, 509
   chlorinated. See chlorine.
   distilled, 29, 241, 280, 334, 335, 336, 438, 534, 553, 655
   fluoridated. See fluorine (fluoride).
   ionized, 335, 590
   mineral, 444
   reverse osmosis, 334, 335, 336
   sea, 338, 339
   spring, 241, 334, 335, 336

**weight**
   gain. See also pregnancy, 10, 24, 33, 41, 57, 61, 62, 63, 64, 82, 84, 216, 240, 254, 257, 342, 343, 352, 358, 361, 363, 364, 365, 370, 375, 383, 479, 480
   ideal, 3, 9, 10, 86, 358, 375
   loss, xli, 5, 6, 9, 10, 11, 18, 23, 24, 25, 29, 33, 38, 41, 44, 52, 57, 58, 60, 61, 63, 65, 81, 86, 89, 92, 118, 155, 158, 159, 161, 163, 164, 171, 179, 215, 244, 254, 257, 258, 271, 283, 313, 343, 349, 358, 363, 364, 375, 376, 377, 383, 386, 404, 469, 479, 481, 509, 526, 529, 533, 543, 550, 563, 564, 565, 566, 567, 571, 573, 581

**weightlifting. See bodybuilding.**

**Weiss, Harvey**, 99

**wheatgrass. See grains, wheat. See** also juice, wheatgrass.

**Whitaker, Dr. Julian**, 488

**White, Ellen**, 207

**Wigmore, Dr. Ann**, 10, 20, 41, 150, 156, 160, 187, 204, 213, 216, 243, 573, 574, 577, 592, 595

**wild**, 511
   animals, 15, 16, 20, 70, 76, 139, 163, 174, 190, 308, 329, 333, 340, 359, 366, 372, 386, 392, 393, 398, 503, 509, 514, 515, 518
   foods, 192, 216, 328, 362, 400
   fruits, 469, 507
   grains, 469
   meats, 469, 520
   plants, 216, 328, 329, 399, 563, 567
   rice. See grains, rice.
   vegetables, 45, 47, 329, 469, 503, 660
     carrot, 329

**Wilde, Stuart**, xxxv

**Wiley**
   Dr. Harvey, 242
   T. S., 182, 363, 476, 481, 493, 574

**wine**, 36, 191, 240, 275, 316, 363, 400, 601

**Wolcott, William L.**, 342, 574

**Wolfe, David**, xxxi, 8, 15, 18, 22, 219, 231, 302, 308, 316, 336, 338, 339, 342, 374, 471, 474, 563, 574, 582

**World Health Organization**, 23, 180, 338, 499

**World Trade Organization**, 499

**Wright, Tony**, 171

**Yasui, Junko**, 154, 566

**yeast**, 124, 469
   infection. See symptoms.
   nutritional, 83, 311, 312, 314, 315, 477

**yerba maté**, 401

**Yiamouyiannis, John**, 84, 334, 574

**yoga**, 14, 47, 68, 84, 197, 202, 312, 313, 332, 367, 375, 609
   kundalini, 332

**Young, Dr. Robert O.**, 7, 124, 125, 308, 331, 332, 574

**Zavasta, Tonya**, 11, 16, 222, 316, 385, 420, 574

**Zephyr**, 370, 507, 510, 511, 519, 574

**Zocchi, Stephen**, 215, 567

**Zone Diet**, 85

**Zovluck, Dr. Bernarr**, 176, 205, 209, 291, 292, 293, 581, 592, 593

# The Hygiene HighJoy Hotline: 360-855-7232

## From Victoria BidWell at the HighJoy Homestead

Dear Health Seekers! We love you! How can we be of use to you beyond our book? Christian husband and wife team Ken and Sandra Chin have been GetWell friends since 1984. In 2002, they purchased a ½-acre property where my *Captain HighJoy America!* horse and I could live and carry on our calling to help health seekers. This blessed property is located in the wilderness of the Cascade Mountains of Washington State. My workers and I have cleared the land, built anew and recycled buildings for use as the GetWell♥StayWell, America! Headquarters. From our recycled shipping building, we will be answering the Hygiene HighJoy Hotline and sending out educational materials in our Homes across America Campaign! Susan and I want to share our many services offered through the Hygiene HighJoy Hotline in this — one of my last lists!

• I will answer your personal situation questions that fall within my scope as a health educator of the ten energy enhancers. I do not play doctor.

• I will refer you to a list of qualified doctors and health education counselors who can help with your personal situation issues that fall beyond my scope as a health educator of the ten energy enhancers.

• I will discuss your need for special educational materials to speed your personal situation progress, while referring to my offerings of 1,000 Natural Hygiene books, courses, audio tapes, compact discs, videos, charts, wheels and more.

• I will advise you concerning your special needs to set up your victory kitchen. And I will do a cost comparison to give you our best price quotes for major healthy home products: juicers, the Blend-Tec and Vita-Mix machines, food dehydrators, water distillers, the BodySlant, the Needak mini-trampoline and virtually all other major purchases. We offer special prices and wonderfully useful GetWell gifts with these major purchases you make directly through us.

• I will offer you a special savings for your personal copy of *The Health Seekers' YearBook with The Best of Common Health Sense.*

• I will be thrilled to share with you how to get more copies of *The Live Food Factor* into your circle of friends and help you make the arrangements for ordering these additional copies. Susan and I have special prices so that no one is left out and all can benefit from the teachings in our lifesaving book!

# Victoria BidWell's Vita-Mix Code: 06-000271

I have used the Vita-Mix since 1990. I use it every day. When you order your Vita-Mix directly through the company at phone 800-848-2649 and give my name and Vita-Mix Code above, you get two treats: free shipping and a gift from Susan and me. Or you can call me directly, and I will place your Vita-Mix order for you and get your gift out to you right away!

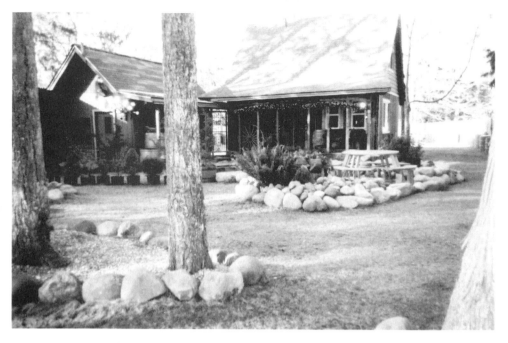

# Our Hygiene Homestead in The Woods

## Call "The Wilderness Woman," Victoria BidWell, at 360-853-7048.

## See Fun Photos at www.getwellstaywellamerica.com.

Some of the many unique features of Our Hygiene Homestead in The Woods:

- A double-gated, 6-7 foot high and solid board cedar fence for privacy
- A rustic elegance and woodsy theme throughout the buildings and ½ acre
- Private scheduling for "one-person-only" use of Our Hygiene Homestead
- Group scheduling for "3 to 4 persons use" of Our Hygiene Homestead
- Year around assisted hygienic living available
- The perfect setting to take yourself on a fast with Victoria's assistance
- A kitchen completely empty of food while you are fasting
- Two private bedrooms overlooking the woods, 1 with a wood-burning stove
- A large "takes 2 bedroom" upstairs
- All rooms throughout completely renewed from ceiling to walls to floors
- An old-fashioned, metal and enameled, deep bathtub for relaxation
- Beds that elevate the feet and/or provide gentle massage
- Private, feel-good, by donation massage available
- Tape and CD players with headphones at every bedside for Hygiene lectures
- Sleeping in without being awakened for an untimely consultation
- A heavenly massage lounge recliner for lymphatic exercise and relaxation
- A victory kitchen with all the machines and gadgets for — Fun! Fun! Fun!

- Your hands-on experience in gourmet creations, supervised by Victoria
- One set of dishes with a fruits and veggie theme, 1 with a wilderness theme
- Cloth napkins for dining elegance experiences
- Dining joys enhanced with a variety of dishes and glasses and cups
- Open invitation food preparation demonstrations by Victoria
- An awesome, huge butcher's block, now recycled for live foods
- Our Homestead book/video/tape/CD library of 2,000 individual titles
- Friendly fires in wood-burning stoves in library and living room
- A free, long-distance phone located in the library for your personal use
- Televisions for VCR videos and DVDs on Natural Hygiene
- No junk TV going day and night to divert your healing focus
- The GetWell♥StayWell, America! Bookstore at The HighJoy Homestead
- A private place solarium on the ½ acre for total-body sunbathing
- A grassy, mossy, user-friendly ½-acre lawn for bare-footing
- Comfy outdoor lounges for sitting and lying around
- A wilderness-themed, covered and carpeted back deck for outdooring
- A potbellied wood stove on the back deck for roughing it enjoyment
- Two life-sized, howling wolf statues on the back deck to keep you company
- An on-deck dining spot for communing with nature while eating
- A custom-made picnic table pit in the open yard to seat 8
- A big hammock between 2 tall trees to sway you in the breezes
- A *Dances with Wolves*-sized, open campfire pit to seat several or just one
- Peace and quiet from morning through night with rural life sounds only
- A bird apartment complex and houses along the fence for bird watching
- Mild Western Washington Cascade Mountain temperatures
- No wet and sticky humidity and never too hot and never too cold
- No flesh-eating insects and no poisonous snakes
- Fresh and pure air — nonstop oxygenated by thickets and woods
- Both large and standard-sized BodySlants for antigravity relaxation
- Exercise mats for stretching and other ground uses
- The Needak rebounder mini-trampoline for more antigravity exercise
- A long driveway on the premises for mild walking exercise
- Charming community back roads and trails for walking adventures
- Endless exercise adventures in nearby national and state parks and forests
- Wilderness hiking and fresh lake swimming just minutes away by car
- The cutoff Bronco Buckboard for open-air travel on wilderness outings
- A bald eagle sanctuary and festivals attracting tourists every year
- A herd of protected elk often greeting you as you enter Concrete
- Starry, starry skies on the cloudless, clear nights
- Individual needs and rates as discussed with Victoria
- Endless high joy exercises if you want an extreme attitude adjustment
- Our author Susan Schenck has visited us and endorses our programs!

We enjoy much more. But you get the idea. We're in Concrete heaven up here! With just a little more than a covering contribution — you are invited to share the blessings offered at Our Hygiene Homestead in The Woods.

# Final Encouragements from Victoria BidWell

Dear Health Seekers and Live Food Enthusiasts: GOOD WORK! You have made it all the way through to the end of our book! And we hope you will never see or be quite the same — all for the best in your bodies, minds and spirits, of course. We dearly hope you have given up the medical mentality at its very worst as your primary health care system of choice and that you have made the paradigm shift to — *Health by Healthful Living!*

I call *The Live Food Factor* "our book" in the very widest sense of the term: Susan is "our author" with 6 years of going raw, researching and writing. I am "our final Natural Hygiene editor and contributor and assistant editor" with 2,400 hours of wildly intense work over 24 months and with countless hours of work put into my teachings created since 1983 and used throughout our book. Bob Avery is "our editor in chief" with all his editing, formatting, computering and exhaustive indexing. Dr. Vetrano is "our editor and contributor" of the priceless Natural Hygiene teachings throughout our book as she brings 60 years of doing right and living raw with her. Victoria Boutenko is "our contributor" with her 15 years of Raw Family experiences, *12 Steps to Raw Foods* and green smoothie teachings. Dr. Shelton, Dr. Tilden, T. C. Fry and many Natural Hygiene and raw food teachers past and present are "our giants" on whose shoulders we — "The Four Horsewomen of the Live Food Revolution" — all stand and to whom we all owe so much. The 300 GetWell♥StayWell, America! Friends are "our heroes" for sending their money for 600 copies a year ahead of this new edition's creation, which monies freed me up to work on our book. And you all are "our new friends in health!" So while this book is copyrighted in her name, and "Susan Schenck" stands on the cover as the author "with" me, in the widest sense, *The Live Food Factor* is "our book," a product of persons throughout history and the new millennium masterpiece of truth and proof, of inspiration and love, all of which is now owned by all of us!

Personally, I was called by God, in no uncertain voice, to take on this enormous project and do all in my power to lift the book up so that our teachings within would be true to Nature, human health and Natural Hygiene. I knew I could help with my English teacher talents and gifts. I look at *The Live Food Factor: The Comprehensive Guide to the Ultimate Diet for Body, Mind, Spirit & Planet*, now in its final, fabulous form, as "a Great Gift from God" — to serve as a blessing for all of us who choose life and do right by going back to the Garden of Eden plan for our health and happiness. I encourage you all, on behalf of us "Four Horsewomen of the Live Food Revolution." Love yourselves: Choose life. We hope you will follow through with every good and loving impulse you get to share the truth and proof in this God-given book. It is a totally natural human inclination to want to share a good thing. And now, at our book's end, please ask yourselves: "Do we ever have a good thing to share — or what?" Please don't hold back the reins. Run free to greener pastures with the truth! Have fun!

## Choose Life! Do Right! Eat Live! And Get High!

# It's Detox Time!

Wanting to experience higher states of consciousness and the joys they bring is part of the natural human condition. But taking toxic, mind-altering substances as shortcut tactics to get high brings addiction with dreadful downsides too horrible for words. Only health by healthful living will get us a natural high!

*Addiction* means 'bondage to a self-destructive thought or habit'. It has been part of the human condition after the Beginning and has been practiced throughout the millennia. In America, taking the geographical cure and spending time in a rehabilitation facility is a highly accepted and now popular practice for alcoholics, illegal and prescription drug addicts and persons with eating disorders. Being addicted used to bear a social stigma. But lately, going to a detox center is a glamorous status symbol among movie celebrities and politicians alike coming off their favored drugs, from amphetamines and alcohol to Prozac and eating disorders. Nowadays nobody questions the need for going into detox or the benefits to be derived for one's body, mind and spirit.

Today — it's detox time for us health seekers, too! It's time to see the need, the benefits and even the glamour and especially the fun of detoxing for superlative health and high joy! *The Live Food Factor* has proven, without a scientific doubt, that the cooked SAD food supply is toxic, contaminated with protoplasmic poisons and addictive. In glorious opposition, the raw food diet — best practiced as Natural Hygiene teaches — is health enhancing, poison free and nonaddicting. Hopefully, our book has inspired you to go to 50% raw today and work up towards 100% raw tomorrow. In so doing, all detoxification and healing events and wondrous side effects are your blessings to claim!

# Susan and I Answer, "Where Do We Go from Here?"

• Attend a raw foods/Natural Hygiene retreat and get firsthand education and hands-on experience.

• Go into consultation with Dr. Zarin Azar, MD; Dr. Dave Klein, PhD; Linda Sticco, PhD; Wayne Gendel; myself, or another of the many well-versed counselors to receive the education, support and inspiration via phone and/or e-mail detox help.

• Use Victoria Boutenko's revised *12 Steps to Raw Foods*. I edited it and endorse it. Her teachings will further help you break SAD food addiction and detox.

• And the very most important of all single things to do next: get *The Health Seekers' YearBook with The Best of Common Health Sense*. In studying and applying the teachings therein, you become your own detox doctor! You will need this book's further teachings not in *The Live Food Factor*. You will want the breakfast, lunch and dinner menus for every day of the year, without repetition, and its hundreds of recipes and endless recipe formulas for health seekers. This book will lay out for you the year in detox while you eat the raw food diet and practice all ten of Natural Hygiene's energy enhancers. Fun!

# Author Contact Information

I love nothing more than teaching people how to go raw! I am available for speeches, workshops, seminars and radio shows. I will go anywhere to lecture and do workshops if you or your group can make provisions for my travel expenses! I am also available for raw coaching! It is my mission to spread the truth about how easy it is to get healthy. In fact a further project might be a documentary based on this book, especially if I can find investors.

Please contact me if you are interested in any of the above.

## info@livefoodfactor.com

## sschenck@alumni.Indiana.edu

Also, please take time to visit www.healthfreedomusa.org and sign the petitions to stop Codex Alimentarius from irradiating our food supply and poisoning it with more pesticides. Learn to become independent from the "food grid" by making your own sprouts from organic seeds, foraging for wild greens and growing your own food.

Stay tuned to my website www.livefoodfactor.com for any updates to what is happening in the raw food movement and any new studies that come out.

Your victories and testimonials relating to your own raw journey are welcomed, as are any comments about the book or diet. Maybe you would like to contribute to my next book.

While I welcome all reader feedback, please be advised that personal replies are not guaranteed.

Best wishes on your raw journey! Stay raw, live long, *be free*!